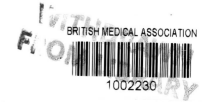

Operative
Thoracic Surgery

Operative
Thoracic Surgery

SIXTH EDITION

Edited by

Larry R. Kaiser, MD, FACS
The Lewis Katz Dean
The Lewis Katz School of Medicine at Temple University
Philadelphia, Pennsylvania, United States

Sarah K. Thompson, MD, PhD, FRCSC, FRACS
Discipline of Surgery
University of Adelaide
and
Royal Adelaide Hospital
Adelaide, Australia

Glyn G. Jamieson, MS, MD, FRACS, FRCS, FACS
Discipline of Surgery
University of Adelaide
Royal Adelaide Hospital
Adelaide, Australia

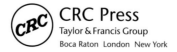 CRC Press
Taylor & Francis Group
Boca Raton London New York

CRC Press is an imprint of the
Taylor & Francis Group, an **informa** business

First published in 1956 by Butterworths Heinemann
Second edition 1968
Third edition 1976
Fourth edition 1982

Fifth edition published in 2006 by Hodder Arnold, an imprint of Hodder Education

CRC Press
Taylor & Francis Group
6000 Broken Sound Parkway NW, Suite 300
Boca Raton, FL 33487-2742

© 2018 by Taylor & Francis Group, LLC
CRC Press is an imprint of Taylor & Francis Group, an Informa business

No claim to original U.S. Government works
Printed and bound in India by Replika Press Pvt. Ltd.

Printed on acid-free paper

International Standard Book Number-13: 978-1-4822-9957-1 (Pack – Book and Ebook)

Library of Congress Cataloging-in-Publication Data

Names: Kaiser, Larry R., editor. | Jamieson, Glyn G., editor. | Thompson, Sarah K., editor.
Title: Operative thoracic surgery / [edited by] Larry R. Kaiser, Glyn Jamieson, Sarah K. Thompson.
Other titles: Separated from (work): Rob & Smith's operative surgery. | Rob & Smith's operative surgery series.
Description: Sixth edition. | Boca Raton : CRC Press, [2016] | Series: Rob & Smith's operative surgery series | Separated from Rob & Smith's operative surgery.
5th ed. 1993-[2006] | Includes bibliographical references.
Identifiers: LCCN 2016042751| ISBN 9781482299571 (hardcover bundle : alk. paper) | ISBN 9781482299595 (eBook VitalSource) | ISBN 9781482299588 (ebook pdf).
Subjects: | MESH: Thoracic Surgical Procedures.
Classification: LCC RD536 | NLM WO 500 | DDC 617.5/4059--dc23
LC record available at https://lccn.loc.gov/2016042751

Visit the Taylor & Francis Web site at
http://www.taylorandfrancis.com

and the CRC Press Web site at
http://www.crcpress.com

"For Lindy: who after all these years still is trying to figure out how I do these books"
LK

"For Amelia: my most enthusiastic supporter"
ST

"For Elizabeth (1942-2010)"
GJ

Contents

SECTION II ESOPHAGEAL SURGERY

Contributors

Abbas E. Abbas, MD, FACS
Division of Thoracic Surgery
Department of Thoracic Medicine and Surgery
Temple University School of Medicine
Philadelphia, Pennsylvania, United States

Derek Alderson, MD, FRCS
Emeritus Professor of Surgery
University of Birmingham
and
Honorary Consultant Surgeon
University Hospitals NHS Trust
Queen Elizabeth Hospital
Birmingham, United Kingdom

Erdoğan Atasoy, MD
Department of Surgery
University of Louisville School of Medicine
and
Affiliated Surgeon
Kleinert Kutz and Associates Hand Care Center
Christine M. Kleinert Institute
Louisville, Kentucky, United States

Andrew Barbour, PhD, FRACS
Surgical Oncology Group
University of Queensland
and
Upper Gastro-Intestinal and Soft Tissue Unit
Princess Alexandra Hospital
Brisbane, Australia

Julianne S. Barlow, BSc
Division of Thoracic Surgery
Brigham and Women's Hospital
Boston, Massachusetts, United States

Alessandro Brunelli, MD
Department of Thoracic Surgery
St. James's University Hospital
Leeds, United Kingdom

Raphael Bueno, MD
Division of Thoracic Surgery
Brigham and Women's Hospital
Harvard Medical School
Boston, Massachusetts, United States

Adrienne Camp, BSc
International Mesothelioma Program
Division of Thoracic Surgery
Brigham and Women's Hospital
Boston, Massachusetts, United States

Claudio Caviezel, MD
Department of Thoracic Surgery
University Hospital Zurich
Zurich, Switzerland

Robert James Cerfolio, MD, FACS, FCCP
Division of Cardiothoracic Surgery
University of Alabama at Birmingham
Birmingham, Alabama, United States

Aaron M. Cheng, MD, FACS
Division of Cardiothoracic Surgery
Department of Surgery
University of Washington
Seattle, Washington, United States

Geoffrey S. Chow, MD
Department of Surgery
Northwestern Medicine
Chicago, Illinois, United States

Anna Maria Ciccone, MD, PhD
Department of Thoracic Surgery
"Sapienza" University of Rome
Sant'Andrea Hospital
Rome, Italy

Antonio D'Andrilli, MD
Department of Thoracic Surgery
"Sapienza" University of Rome
Sant'Andrea Hospital
Rome, Italy

Jean Deslauriers, MD, FRCS(C)
Department of Thoracic Surgery
Centre Hospitalier Laval
Québec City, Canada

Peter G. Devitt, MBBS, MS, FRCS, FRACS
Discipline of Surgery
University of Adelaide
Royal Adelaide Hospital
Adelaide, Australia

André Duranceau, MD
Department of Surgery
Université de Montreal
and
Department of Surgery
Division of Thoracic Surgery
Centre Hospitalier
Universitaire de Montreal
Montreal, Québec, Canada

Wentao Fang, MD
Department of Thoracic Surgery
Shanghai Chest Hospital
Jiaotong University Medical School
Shanghai, People's Republic of China

Juan J. Fibla, MD, PhD
Thoracic Surgery Department
University of Barcelona Hospital Idc Salud Sagrat Cor
Barcelona, Spain

Hugh A. Gelabert, MD
Division of Vascular and Endovascular Surgery
David Geffen UCLA School of Medicine
Los Angeles, California, United States

Marco Ghionzoli, MD, PhD
Pediatric Surgery Department
Meyer Childrens' Hospital and University of Florence
Florence, Italy

Peter Goldstraw, FRCS
Department of Thoracic Surgery
Royal Brompton Hospital
and
Thoracic Surgery
Imperial College, London, United Kingdom

Abel Gómez-Caro, MD, PhD
Department of General Thoracic Surgery
University Hospital Clínic de Barcelona
Barcelona, Spain

S. Michael Griffin, MD, FRCS
Northern Oesophago Gastric Cancer Unit
Royal Victoria Infirmary
Newcastle upon Tyne, United Kingdom

Ewen A. Griffiths, MD, FRCS
Department of Upper Gastrointestinal Surgery
University Hospitals Birmingham NHS Foundation Trust
and
Department of Surgery
Queen Elizabeth Hospital
Birmingham, United Kingdom

Brechtje A. Grotenhuis, MD, PhD
Department of Surgery
Erasmus University Medical Center
Rotterdam, Netherlands

Jorge Hernández, MD
Thoracic Surgery Department
University of Barcelona Hospital Idc Salud Sagrat Cor
Barcelona, Spain

Konrad Hoetzenecker, MD, PhD
Department of Thoracic Surgery
Medical University of Vienna
Vienna, Austria

Arnulf H. Hölscher, MD, FACS, FRCS
Department of Visceral and Vascular Surgery
University of Cologne Medical School
Cologne, Germany

Young K. Hong, MD
Department of Surgery
Division of Surgical Oncology
University of Louisville Hospital
Louisville, Kentucky, United States

John G. Hunter, MD, FACS
Division of General and Gastrointestinal Surgery
Department of Surgery
Oregon Health and Science University
and
Digestive Health Center
Oregon Health and Science University
Portland, Oregon, United States

Maxim Itkin, MD, FSIR
Radiology Department
Hospital of the University of Pennsylvania
Philadelphia, Pennsylvania, United States

Glyn G. Jamieson, MS, MD, FRACS, FRCS, FACS
Discipline of Surgery
University of Adelaide
Royal Adelaide Hospital
Adelaide, Australia

Gregory J. Jurkovich, MD, FACS
Department of Surgery
UC Davis Health System University of California
Sacramento, California, United States

Larry R. Kaiser, MD, FACS
The Lewis Katz Dean
The Lewis Katz School of Medicine at Temple University
Philadelphia, Pennsylvania, United States

Walter Klepetko, MD
Department of Thoracic Surgery
Medical University of Vienna
Vienna, Austria

Benjamin Knight, MbChB, FRCS
Oesophago-gastric and Bariatric Surgery
Queen Alexandra Hospital
Portsmouth, United Kingdom

John C. Kucharczuk, MD
Division of Thoracic Surgery
Department of Surgery
Hospital of the University of Pennsylvania
Philadelphia, Pennsylvania, United States

Zhigang Li, MD
Department of Thoracic Surgery
Shanghai Chest Hospital
Jiaotong University Medical School
Shanghai, People's Republic of China

Jun-Feng Liu, PhD
Department of Thoracic Surgery
Fourth Hospital of Hebei Medical University
Shijiazhuang, People's Republic of China

Sheraz Markar, PhD, MRCS, MSc, MA
Department of Academic Surgery
St. Mary's Hospital
Imperial College
London, United Kingdom

M. Blair Marshall, MD
Division of Thoracic Surgery
MedStar Georgetown University Hospital
and
Georgetown University School of Medicine
Washington DC, United States

Reza Mehran, MD, FRCS(C), FACS
Department of Thoracic and Cardiovascular Surgery
University of Texas M. D. Anderson Cancer Center
Houston, Texas, United States

Antonio Messineo, MD
Pediatric Surgery Department
Meyer Childrens' Hospital and University of Florence
Florence, Italy

Fernando Mier, MD
Division of General and Gastrointestinal Surgery
Department of Surgery
Oregon Health and Science University
and
Digestive Health Center
Oregon Health and Science University
Portland, Oregon, United States

Laureano Molins, MD, PhD
Thoracic Surgery Department
University of Barcelona Hospital Idc Salud Sagrat Cor
and
Thoracic Surgery Department
University Hospital Clínic de Barcelona
Barcelona, Spain

Scott M. Moore, MD
Trauma and Acute Care Surgery
Denver Health Medical Center
and
University of Colorado Denver School of Medicine
Denver, Colorado, United States

Paula Moreno, MD, FETCS
Thoracic Surgery and Lung Transplantation Unit
University Hospital Reina Sofia
Cordoba, Spain

Alex Nagle, MD, FACS
Division of Gastrointestinal & Oncologic Surgery
Northwestern University Feinberg School of Medicine
Chicago, Illinois, United States

Carlos A. Pellegrini, MD, FACS, FRCSI (Hon.)
Department of Surgery
University of Washington
Seattle, Washington, United States

Christian G. Peyre, MD
Division of Thoracic and Foregut Surgery
Department of Surgery
University of Rochester School of Medicine and Dentistry
Rochester, New York, United States

Frederic M. Pieracci, MD, MPH, FACS
Trauma Center
Denver Health Medical Center
and
University of Colorado Denver School of Medicine
Denver, Colorado, United States

Erino Angelo Rendina, MD
Department of Thoracic Surgery
"Sapienza" University of Rome
Sant'Andrea Hospital
Rome, Italy

William G. Richards, PhD
Division of Thoracic Surgery
Brigham and Women's Hospital
Boston, Massachusetts, United States

Nabil P. Rizk, MD, MPH, MS
Division of Thoracic Surgery
Hackensack University Medical Center
Hackensack, New Jersey, United States

Gaetano Rocco, MD, FRCSEd, FEBTS, FCCP
Department of Thoracic Surgical and Medical Oncology
Division of Thoracic Surgery
Istituto Nazionale Tumori
Fondazione Pascale
Istituto di Ricerca e Cura a Carattere Scientifico
Naples, Italy

Valerie W. Rusch, MD
Thoracic Surgery Service
Department of Surgery
Memorial Sloan Kettering Cancer Center
New York, New York, United States

Amber L. Shada, MD
General Surgery/MIS Division
University of Wisconsin School of Medicine and Public Health
Madison, Wisconsin, United States

Jon Shenfine, PhD, FRCS, FRACS
Discipline of Surgery
University of Adelaide
Royal Adelaide Hospital
Adelaide, Australia

Joseph B. Shrager, MD
Department of Cardiothoracic Surgery
Division of Thoracic Surgery
Stanford University School of Medicine
Stanford, California, United States

J. Rüdiger Siewert, MD
Department of Surgery
Technical University of Munich
Munich, Germany

B. Mark Smithers, FRACS, FRCSEng, FRCSEd
University of Queensland
and
Upper Gastro-Intestinal and Soft Tissue Unit
Princess Alexandra Hospital
Brisbane, Australia

Nathaniel J. Soper, MD
Department of Surgery
Northwestern Medicine
Chicago, Illinois, United States

Aravind Suppiah, MD, FRCS
Discipline of Surgery
Royal Adelaide Hospital
Adelaide, Australia

Lee L. Swanström, MD, FACS, FASGE, FRCSEng (Hon.)
GI/MIS Division
The Oregon Clinic
Portland, Oregon, United States
and
Institute of Image Guided Surgery
IHU-Strasbourg
Strasbourg, France

Sarah K. Thompson, MD, PhD, FRCSC, FRACS
Discipline of Surgery
University of Adelaide
and
Royal Adelaide Hospital
Adelaide, Australia

Iain Thomson, FRACS
University of Queensland
and
Upper Gastro-Intestinal and Soft Tissue Unit
Princess Alexandra Hospital
Brisbane, Australia

Eric Vallières, MD, FRCSC
Division of Thoracic Surgery
Swedish Cancer Institute
Seattle, Washington, United States

J. Jan B. van Lanschot, MD, PhD
Department of Surgery
Erasmus University Medical Center
Rotterdam, Netherlands

Camilla Vanni, MD
Department of Thoracic Surgery
"Sapienza" University of Rome
Sant'Andrea Hospital
Rome, Italy

Federico Venuta, MD
Division of Thoracic Surgery
"Sapienza" University of Rome
Policlinico Umberto I
Rome, Italy

Shajahan Wahed, MD, FRCS
Northern Oesophago-Gastric Cancer Unit
Royal Victoria Infirmary
Newcastle upon Tyne, United Kingdom

David Ian Watson, MBBS, MD, PhD, FRACS, FAHMS
Department of Surgery
Flinders University
and
Oesophago-Gastric Surgery Unit
Flinders Medical Centre
Adelaide, Australia

Thomas J. Watson, MD, FACS
Division of Thoracic and Esophageal Surgery
Department of Surgery
Medstar Washington
Georgetown University School of Medicine
Washington DC, United States

Walter Weder, MD
Department of Thoracic Surgery
University Hospital Zurich
Zurich, Switzerland

Benjamin Wei, MD
Division of Cardiothoracic Surgery
University of Alabama at Birmingham
Birmingham, Alabama, United States

Bas P. L. Wijnhoven, MD, PhD
Department of Surgery
Erasmus University Medical Center
Rotterdam, Netherlands

Jennifer L. Wilson, MD
Department of Thoracic Surgery
Beth Israel Deaconess Medical Center
Harvard Medical School
Boston, Massachusetts, United States

Douglas E. Wood, MD
Division of Cardiothoracic Surgery
Department of Surgery
University of Washington
Seattle, Washington, United States

Giovanni Zaninotto, MD, FACS
Department of Academic Surgery
St. Mary's Hospital
Imperial College
London, United Kingdom

Yifan Zheng, MD
Division of Thoracic Surgery
Brigham and Women's Hospital
Boston, Massachusetts, United States

Chenxi Zhong, MD
Department of Thoracic Surgery
Shanghai Chest Hospital
Jiaotong University Medical School
Shanghai, People's Republic of China

Illustrators

Kelly Casssidy, BA (Hon.), MMAA

Angela V. Christie, FMAA

Francesca Corra, MMAA

Peter Cox, NDD, MMAA

Gillian Lee, FMAA, Hon. FIMI

Gillian Oliver, FMAA

Amanda Williams, BA (Hon.), FMAA

Preface

It would not be unreasonable to ask why another book, when so much information may be accessed online. Indeed, videos of almost any operative procedure are now easily available. So, the question is begged, why a Sixth Edition of this venerable text, *Operative Thoracic Surgery*? The difference lies in the expertise embedded in each chapter of this book, provided by internationally known, widely geographically dispersed surgeons who literally reveal at least some of their tricks and, in some cases, their secrets. Once you read a chapter you may very well wish to access online videos of a particular procedure, but you will do so armed with the insights provided by the world experts who have contributed to this book. This Sixth Edition is much more than a text since each expert author provides specific technical details of an operative procedure, accompanied by accurate and beautifully drawn illustrations. Much has changed in our field since publication of the Fifth Edition in 2006, evidenced by the addition of new chapters. Minimally invasive approaches have matured and, in many cases, surpassed traditional open approaches. Take, for example, the first chapter formerly entitled, *Thoracic incisions*, which now carries the title, *Modern thoracic approaches: minimally invasive thoracic surgery*. New chapters on robotic approaches to lobectomy and uniportal video-assisted thoracoscopic surgery have been added, in addition to a chapter on outpatient thoracic surgery. The section on esophageal surgery has been entirely revised with many new authors and a new editor, Sarah Thompson, working with us. New chapters on laparoscopic antireflux surgery and laparoscopic large hiatus hernia repair join other chapters detailing new and improved minimally invasive techniques. We are especially pleased to include a chapter on per oral endoscopic myotomy (POEM) for achalasia, a procedure that has the potential to render obsolete the open or laparoscopic Heller myotomy. This new edition is timely, accurate and up-to-date and should be a welcome addition to the library of both trainees and senior surgeons. Once again our publisher, and in particular Miranda Bromage, has been more than just helpful (indispensable, is the word which comes readily to mind!), and the drawings of Gillian Lee and her team continue to add immeasurably to the written content.

Larry R. Kaiser, MD, FACS
Sarah K. Thompson, MD, PhD, FRCSC, FRACS
Glyn G. Jamieson, MS, MD, FRACS, FRCS, FACS

Thoracic surgery

Modern thoracic approaches: minimally invasive thoracic surgery

M. BLAIR MARSHALL

INTRODUCTION

Chapters written on thoracic incisions have historically dealt with the traditional approaches used in the practice of thoracic surgery. These are standard incisions that provide exposure to the common thoracic pathologies. These have changed relatively little in the previous decades and have been written about in previous versions of this text and others; I will not review these approaches here but refer you to the previous versions of this text.

Modern approaches, strategies for less invasive means of managing thoracic pathology have continued to grow over the past two decades, and these ongoing developments will be addressed by this chapter. These will be broken down by anatomic location: pulmonary resections; wedge excision and hilar dissections; and mediastinal approaches, anterior and posterior, including the intraoperative strategies to facilitate working through these smaller incisions. The reasoning for this is that given the limited access through small incisions, operative planning for these less invasive approaches must take into account the location of the pathology; hindrances to access; hindrances for instrumentation; strategies for resection; and reconstruction, when needed. When compared with an open approach, a minimally invasive approach itself may be considered a hindrance; however, the magnified view, ability to use angled cameras to change perspective, as well as the markedly decreased pain and recovery time commonly associated with these approaches more than justify their use.

THORACOSCOPY VERSUS LAPAROSCOPY

Although those who pioneered the field of minimally invasive thoracic surgery did not have general surgical experience in minimally invasive surgery, that is not true of today's trainees. In transitioning from minimally invasive

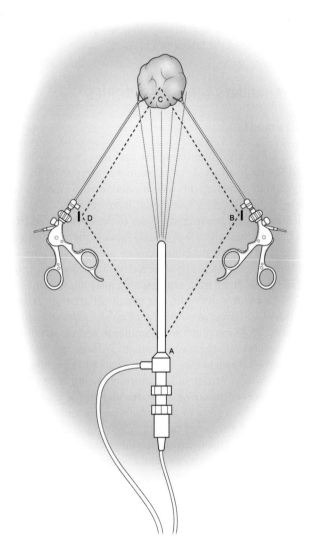

1.1 Baseball diamond concept for orientation of minimally invasive ports and camera location in relation to pathology.

intra-abdominal surgery to thoracic surgery, there are some important differences.

Minimally invasive approaches are typically taught with the baseball diamond concept in mind (see **Figure 1.1**). This is where the camera typically resides at the base of the diamond and the surgeon operates with two instruments on either side, through ports placed at points B and D. The pathology is typically located at point C. This approach is kept in mind when planning thoracoscopic and laparoscopic procedures; however, important adjustments are made due to location within the chest, limitations of the bony fixed chest wall, and span of operative pathology. For example, complete intrathoracic dissection of the esophagus requires much more movement than a laparoscopic cholecystectomy where the operative field is fairly small. Also, unlike most abdominal approaches, as the complexity of the intrathoracic procedures performed increases, we add extra ports and frequently move the camera from one area to another to maximize visualization. Lastly, as many thoracic procedures are performed with the patient in the lateral decubitus position, visuospatial challenges are created when working under camera guidance, in particular when surgeons are on opposite sides of the table.

INSTRUMENTS AND ACCESSORIES

Instruments

Given the limits of the size of the incisions currently being used for video-assisted thoracoscopic surgery (VATS), traditional open instruments have limited functionality within these small incisions. Traditional instruments need to be oriented along the intercostal space to function. Those who use them in these situations quickly learn of their limitations as the sizes of their incisions become progressively smaller. Additional instruments have been developed specifically for VATS. These differ from laparoscopic instruments, as early VATS procedures often did not use insufflation of carbon dioxide (CO_2), thus maintenance of an airtight seal was not required. VATS instruments are similar to open instruments with alterations to the hinge points to facilitate use between the intercostal spaces (see **Figure 1.2**). In addition, they are available with a variety of curvatures allowing access to all of the spaces of the chest, in particular to the chest wall. Access to certain areas of the parietal pleura and chest wall is limited with the use of straight laparoscopic instruments. VATS-specific instruments are provided through a variety of vendors and some are more cumbersome than others—one should try out these instruments prior to committing to purchasing.

After many years of performing minimally invasive thoracic surgery, we have incorporated standard laparoscopic instruments into all of our procedures, having found they provide a number of advantages. Specifically, their hinge point is always at the end closest to the operator's hand when the instrument is within the thoracic cavity; they

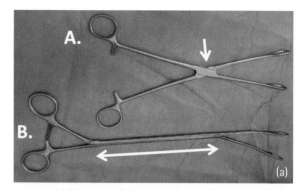

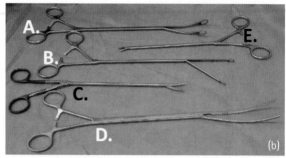

1.2a–b (a) Photograph of standard ring forceps (A) and minimally invasive ring forceps (B). Note the long, narrow shaft that can work easily within the intercostal spaces. (b) Additional VATS instruments with similar mechanisms including the ring (A), 5 mm ring forceps (B), scissors (C), vascular clamp (D), and thorascopic needle driver (E).

work through the 5 mm ports; and they come in a variety of lengths, from 20 to 45 cm. Additionally, most hospitals already have several sets of these instruments, so they do not require an additional capital purchase. When working with both hands from the posterior and anterior aspect of the chest, or for hilar work when the patient is in the lateral decubitus position, we have found the standard laparoscopic length does not work particularly well. However, we have found pediatric laparoscopic instruments to be of use when working at the hilum, as that length is ideally suited for most adult patients (see **Figure 1.3a and b**).

When working in the anterior or posterior mediastinum, the length of the standard laparoscopic instruments works well. In particular, for video-assisted thymectomy or minimally invasive esophagectomy, the length of these instruments tends to be advantageous allowing one to work superiorly to dissect the cervical horns of the thymus gland or, for an esophageal resection, to dissect the entire length of the intrathoracic esophagus, from diaphragm to thoracic outlet.

Ports

For port access, we use a metal trocar with a collar we have modified so that it does not interfere with the trocar angularity (see mediastinal resections below). When using CO_2

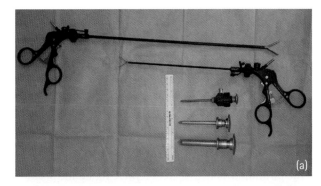

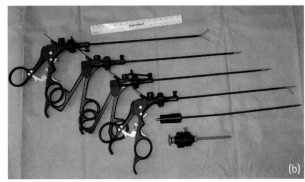

1.3a–b (a) Standard laparoscopic instruments above and the smaller pediatric length below with the 3 mm, 5 mm, and 10 mm ports. (b) Variety of shorter 3 mm laparoscopic instruments, including a hook cautery at the bottom.

insufflation, one must use either metal ports with an adapter for insufflation, as with the 3 mm ports (see **Figure 1.3a and b**), or disposable laparoscopic trocars. Although the latter add to the expense of the procedure, they can be particularly useful in the obese patient where metal trocars are often too short to completely traverse the chest wall. For the utility incision, which is larger than a typical port, we use a soft-tissue retractor such as the Alexis wound protector (Applied Medical Resources Corporation, Rancho Santa Margarita, California, United States). Although purists argue that this is not "true" VATS, and may not be necessary in the thin older individual, it is particularly useful in larger patients.

Camera

We use a 30-degree 5 mm endoscope with a high-definition camera, as the current optics are so good we have found little use for the 10 mm camera. The 30-degree angle allows for improved visualization through rotation of the lens. Today, additional endoscopes are available that strategically address challenges associated with the camera view, such as the EndoEYE (Olympus New Zealand Ltd., Auckland, New Zealand) and three-dimensional viewing VITOM 3D Karl Storz GmbH and Co. KG, Tuttlingen, Germany). In our experience, although conceptually attractive, the location of the articulation joint for the EndoEYE endoscope can

interfere with the operative procedure, so we have not yet found this technology useful. This is particularly true for the smaller patient. As well, operation of this initial prototype is not intuitive. Future improvements will probably address these limitations.

CO_2 insufflation

The use of CO_2 insufflation in chest surgery has become progressively more popular. We use it frequently and find that it facilitates a number of maneuvers when working within the confines of the chest. In contrast to an intra-abdominal procedure, where the insufflated pressure limit is set at 15 mmHg, for intrathoracic procedures, we go no higher than 10 mmHg, as any higher pressure often results in hypotension due to restriction of venous return to the right atrium.

When performing thoracic surgery without single lung ventilation, CO_2 insufflation creates a large enough pneumothorax to provide a working space. This is particularly useful for bilateral VATS sympathectomy, where the patient is positioned supine.

When performing thymectomy, the addition of insufflation remarkably improves visualization of the anterior mediastinum. When working on the left side, the intrathoracic pressure obtained with insufflation is enough to push the heart toward the right to create sufficient working space. As well, it allows visibility of the inferior aspect of the neck beneath the heads of the clavicles (see **Figure 1.4**). With the use of CO_2 insufflation, we perform VATS thymectomy without lung isolation but feel that, for those without experience, using CO_2 in the chest it is more safely performed with lung isolation.

Insufflation of CO_2 during VATS diaphragmatic plication allows for increased intrathoracic space, as the CO_2 displaces the diaphragm inferiorly allowing for better visualization.

For other mediastinal procedures, we also use a continuous flow of CO_2 to assist in the evacuation of smoke from the chest during cautery dissection. Lastly, when lung isolation proves to be difficult and the anesthesiologist is working on

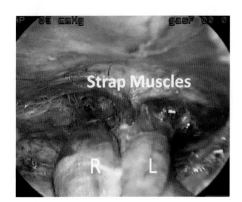

1.4 View into cervical region during thymectomy; (r) right superior and (l) left superior horns of the thymus.

addressing endobronchial tube placement, CO_2 insufflation provides enough space to allow intrathoracic work to continue.

POSITIONING

Surgeon and assistant

For the majority of chest procedures, the surgeon and assistant traditionally have worked on opposite sides of the table. However, when using a thoracoscopic approach, with the camera providing the view from the surgeon's side of the table, the assistant is often working at a disadvantage, as their view is reversed. This is mitigated by having the surgeon and assistant stand on the same side, while the scrub nurse is on the opposite side of the table. Depending on the size of the patient, this may be a challenge for hilar work but can work well in the teaching setting. One can readily demonstrate a particular maneuver or other teaching point during the operation, such as methods of maneuvering the articulated stapler. For resection of posterior and anterior mediastinal masses, we routinely keep the surgeon and assistant on the same side.

Patient positioning

Positioning for VATS approaches has also evolved over the past decade. A discussion of positioning should incorporate two critical aspects: (1) the position of the patient's chest/body, and (2) the position of the arm/scapula. Traditional incisions were typically performed either with the patient in the supine position for a transsternal approach or lateral decubitus position for the majority of the remaining procedures. With the latter position, the arm was brought across the patient to pull the scapula to the most cephalad position. Today, with less invasive approaches, positioning has become much more nuanced and is used to optimize muscle sparing and the minimally invasive approach.

One can view the approach to traditional and modern positioning of the chest/body by thinking of the patient as a frontal plane. Supine positioning would represent 1 degree of the frontal plane. Rotation of the chest would correspond to the angle created between the frontal plane supine and in the position, where 0 degrees represents supine positioning, lateral decubitus positioning represents 90 degrees, and prone positioning represents 180 degrees (see **Figure 1.5**).

SUPINE (0 DEGREES)

Supine positioning for VATS is most commonly used for bilateral sympathectomy. Once the drapes are placed, the back is elevated to a semi-Fowler's position to allow the lungs to fall away from the apex of the chest. In addition to sympathectomy, the supine position may also be used for simple procedures such as pleuroscopy with biopsy, bullectomy, or mechanical pleurodesis. We use this typically when we are doing a bilateral procedure, as the single position eliminates the time needed to change positions and re-prep and drape the patient. Other traditional procedures such as sternotomy or mediastinoscopy are also best performed with the patient supine. The latter has been extended to include transcervical approaches to lymph node dissection, excision of mediastinal masses, and thymectomy, but even pulmonary resections have been performed through a transcervical approach.

SEMISUPINE (30–45 DEGREES)

The use of a vacuum-secured beanbag facilitates these more challenging positions. We most often employ this position for anterior approaches to the mediastinum, including

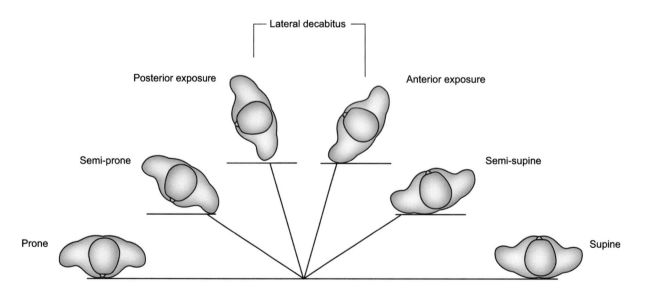

1.5 Range of positioning for strategies used in minimally invasive thoracic surgery.

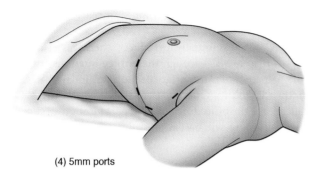

(4) 5mm ports

1.6 Positioning for left VATS thymectomy. Notice the arm by the patient's side and the exposed neck.

thymectomy and the resection of anterior mediastinal masses. We typically place the patient on top of the vacuum-secured beanbag and roll the support under the chest (see **Figure 1.6**). The arm typically is placed along the chest on the bed when there is the potential for access to the neck or anterior chest, such as for those patients with thymoma or other anatomic complexities when adding a cervical incision may be needed. The semisupine position allows for the instruments to move in an unobstructed fashion when working toward the diaphragm. When access to the neck is not needed, the arm can be brought across the patient's chest, facilitating unhindered movement of the instruments.

LATERAL DECUBITUS (ANTERIOR 80 DEGREES; POSTERIOR 100 DEGREES)

We consider the lateral decubitus position to be two different positions: anterior exposure and posterior exposure. The anterior version can be adapted from the classic posterolateral position. This is done by lifting the arm of the patient once in lateral decubitus then rotating the patient so that the anterior axillary line is at the most superior position. This provides three advantages: (1) the intercostal spaces are relatively wider anteriorly than posteriorly, thus more anteriorly placed incisions may minimize trauma to the intercostal nerves; (2) the ipsilateral axilla is opened up and the latissimus moved to a more posterior position, so that it can be entirely spared; and (3) an axillary utility port is more cosmetically acceptable than a posterior utility port (see **Figure 1.7a**).

The traditional lateral decubitus (posterior exposure) approach for a posterolateral thoracotomy is probably the most common position used by thoracic surgeons. However, we reserve it for minimally invasive approaches to the posterior mediastinum—specifically, the resection of posterior mediastinal masses, exposure of the esophagus, or other pathology in this location (see **Figure 1.7b**).

In particular, when using this position, rotating the bed to a steeper angle enlists the force of gravity to assist in keeping the lung away from the operative field.

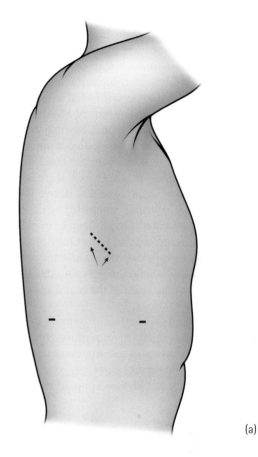

(a)

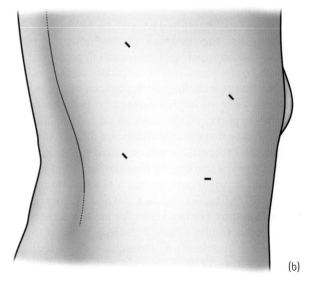

(b)

1.7a–b (a) Healed incision after a right VATS basilar segmentectomy. The utility port is anterior, just below the axilla, marked by the arrows. (b) Healed incision following a posterior mediastinal approach.

PRONE (180 DEGREES)

Prone positioning is advocated by some, in particular for the thoracic dissection during a minimally invasive esophagectomy. It has the advantage of allowing gravity to facilitate certain aspects of the dissection. The lung will be out of the way, and the trachea will also essentially fall away from the esophagus. We have found this useful for esophageal dissection during minimally invasive esophagectomy when a cervical anastomosis is planned. However, placing an intrathoracic anastomosis with the patient in the prone position adds additional complexity to an already difficult operation. One should be well versed in minimally invasive procedures, as the management of bleeding, should it be encountered during these approaches, may create additional challenges. In our experience, we do not think that the small advantage offered on occasion by the purely prone position outweighs the disadvantage. As well, there is also the possibility of using the semiprone, 120-degree position, where the patient is again securely supported by a vacuum bag and the bed can be rotated several degrees in either direction to have the patient reach an almost fully prone position or rotated in the opposite direction to have the patient reach the decubitus position. This combines the advantages of prone positioning with the safety of the lateral approach, allowing for conversion.

Thoughtful consideration of optimal positioning and its impact on the operative procedure, combined with the anticipated hindrances of each approach with the appropriate instrumentation must be carefully considered in advance to successfully use less invasive approaches.

PORT PLACEMENT

When planning port placement, several factors must be taken into consideration. In planning a minimally invasive procedure, the chest wall, ribs, sternum, and scapula must be treated as potential hindrances to access and must be thoughtfully considered. In addition, certain intrathoracic structures, including the diaphragm, heart, and lungs themselves, may be injured during port placement. When introducing ports into the chest, we ask to hold all ventilation to ensure that the trocar does not inadvertently enter the lung parenchyma. As well, one must take into account the challenges of working on the chest wall from inside the chest. This is particularly true for VATS first rib resection, other VATS chest wall resections, and VATS following previous thoracotomy. The latter is similar to VATS decortication, which shares similar technical challenges related to lysing adhesions to the chest wall throughout the pleural space. The broadest area of the chest can be particularly challenging without curved or articulating instruments.

LOCATION OF INCISIONS

Specific incision location will be covered by the individual chapters corresponding to the operative procedures. However, an overview of approaches to incision placement will be discussed.

When VATS was initially introduced, there was a standard for port placement. Through these three incisions, a finger could palpate the entire surface of the lung. Today, this is less strictly adhered to. One must consider the objectives and challenges of the procedure and how port location, in concert with positioning, will best address these issues.

Parenchymal resections (wedge and lobectomy)

Ports for parenchymal wedge resection are most commonly placed in a standardized location, no matter the location of the pathology. Essentially, all of the lung may be palpated through one of the three port incisions. This approach holds true for the majority of parenchymal wedge resections performed today.

Placement of ports for wedge resection must take into account whether the procedure is being done strictly for diagnostic purposes or as a prelude for a VATS lobectomy. If so, one should place the superior port along the line where a potential utility incision will be located. Are there multiple nodules to be removed? What are the ergonomic challenges related to the stapler, chest wall, and intercostal spaces; what additional instrumentation will be needed; and where are the nodule(s) located (see **Figure 1.8**)? Strategies to aid in the resection of challenging locations include placement of a diaphragm traction suture, placement of a suture through the nodule to provide better access and counter traction, division of the inferior pulmonary ligament, and partial division of the fissure. Also, one must consider whether digital palpation of the lesion will be necessary to identify the nodule. If so, port placement should reflect this planning if the nodule is in a particularly challenging location.

When performing VATS lobectomy, we place the utility port directly over the hilum—at the level of the pulmonary

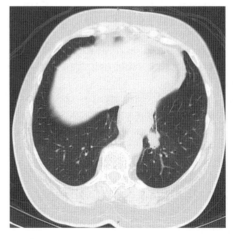

1.8   Challenging location for a VATS wedge resection. Here, the stapler is fired from the superior anterior port site.

vein for an upper lobectomy and just below the level of the fissure for a lower lobectomy. This allows for direct access to the most critical part of the dissection, the hilar vascular structures. Also, if needed, this location facilitates conversion to a thoracotomy. We use an anterior approach to VATS lobectomy and segmentectomy, routinely using the anterior inferior port for placement of the stapler, as the intercostal spaces are larger and the stapler may produce less trauma to the intercostal nerve than when placing the stapler through the considerably narrower posterior aspect of the intercostal space. Lastly, the utility port should be inferior to the point of the dissection at the hilum to facilitate working under camera guidance.

Although the camera is placed through the anterior inferior port for the majority of the dissection, we may move it to other ports to more easily accomplish more complex resections.

Mediastinal resections

ANTERIOR

For the anterior mediastinum, the patient is positioned semisupine but may be rotated to lateral decubitus, in particular if there is additional pathology to address. The left is our preferred side to approach thymectomy because of the commonly encountered large amount of thymic tissue that extends into the aortopulmonary window. This is most easily resected through a left-sided approach. However, if there is a mass such as a thymoma that is more prominent on the right, we will proceed from the right side. We also do not hesitate to place an additional port on the opposite side when necessary. Typically, we use three or four ports depending on the challenges presented by each case. In females, when possible, care is taken to conceal incisions in the axilla or inframammary crease (see **Figure 1.9**).

Unlike traditional port placement, when working at the hilum for thymectomy and other anterior pathology, the trajectory of the ports can play a significant role in decreasing torque on the intercostal nerves. The inframammary ports are placed in a more tangential position to avoid the heart and facilitate dissection that extends up to and above the level of the clavicular heads in order to completely remove the cervical horns of the thymus gland. Depending on the needs of the dissection, it is not uncommon to remove and replace a port through several different intercostal spaces while working through the same skin incision. This avoids unnecessary torque on the ribs or intercostal nerves. In addition, we frequently move the camera to optimize the view of the right side of the chest, the cervical region, or the left chest.

POSTERIOR

Approaches to the posterior mediastinum most commonly are used for sympathectomy, esophagectomy, or masses in the paravertebral location.

We use a fairly standard four-port approach that uses two 5 mm ports, or one 10 mm port if needed, and typically a 3 mm port. This allows for management of esophageal diverticula and myotomies, posterior mediastinal masses, and other pathologies. (see **Figure 1.10**).

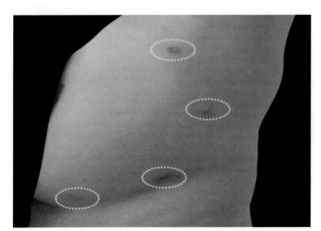

1.9 Healed incision following VATS thymectomy for myasthenia gravis. As there is no thymoma, the thymus is morcellated prior to extracting.

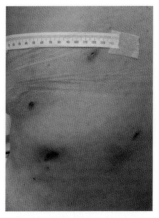

1.10 Postoperative incisions for a posterior mediastinal approach. Note the use of a variety of port sizes to minimize trauma to the intercostal nerves.

LAPAROSCOPIC APPROACHES

We use laparoscopy for mobilization of the gastric conduit during esophagectomy. However, with experience, we have progressively performed more of the intrathoracic esophageal dissection through the hiatus. Distal esophageal diverticula and and the accompanying myotomy can be managed entirely through the hiatus as well as Morgagni hernia and other paraesophageal hernia (see **Figure 1.11a through d**). The visibility achieved through the hiatus is excellent. We typically add a hand port (GelPort, Applied Medical

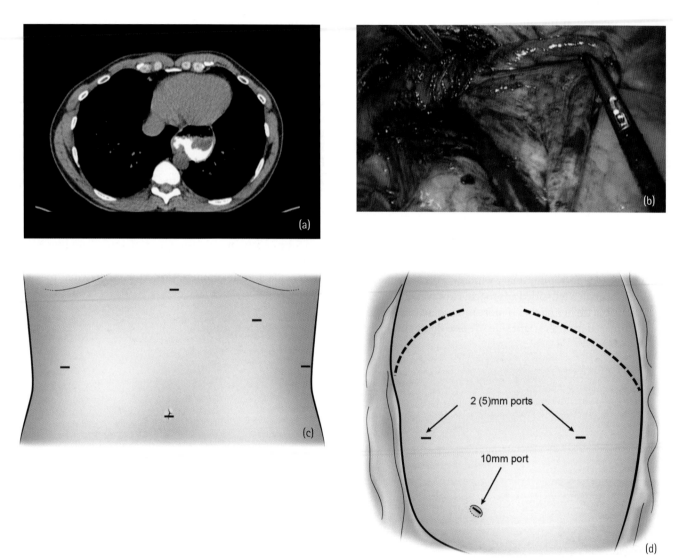

1.11   Laparoscopic transhiatal approach to the mediastinum. (a) Computed tomography scan demonstrating a large diverticulum. (b) Diverticulum delivered through the hiatus into the abdomen prior to resection. (c) Postoperative incisions in the same patient. Here, multiple ports are placed along the left costal margin to allow for maximal intrathoracic dissection. (d) Immediate postoperative image demonstrating port placement for laparoscopic Morgagni hernia repair. We perform these most often as outpatient procedures.

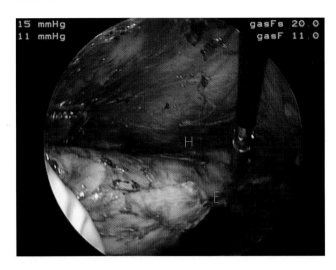

1.12 Intraoperative laparoscopic view into mediastinum for transhiatal esophagectomy in a patient with end-stage achalasia; (h) heart, (e) esophagus.

Resources Corporation). to allow for tactile feedback—so critical for reduction and repair of giant paraesophageal hernias and other more complicated procedures—that enhances what we already achieve thanks to the excellent magnified view and the ability to see well into the mediastinum (see **Figure 1.12**). For all of these approaches, we have found split-leg positioning, with the operator between the legs, offers a distinct advantage over the standard supine position (see **Figure 1.13**).

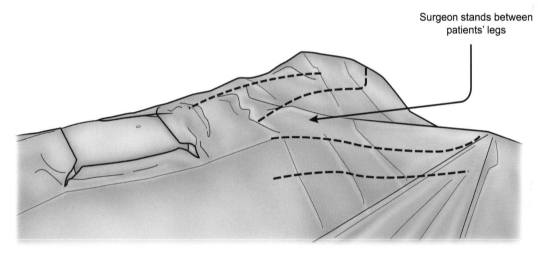

Surgeon stands between patients' legs

1.13 View of a patient in the split-leg position.

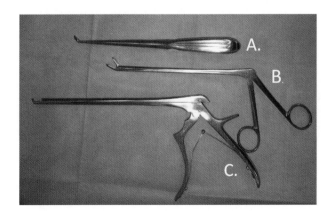

1.14 Instruments that facilitate minimally invasive chest wall resection: (a) angled elevator, (b) pituitary rongeur, (c) Kerrison rongeur.

Minimally invasive chest wall resections

For minimally invasive chest wall resections in particular, operative planning and recognition of hindrances are critical to ensure success. We often borrow orthopedic and neurosurgery instruments, as they are specifically designed to work through these smaller incisions—in particular, the Kerrison rongeur and pituitary rongeur (see **Figure 1.14**). These rongeurs both have long narrow shafts and a hinge mechanism that is not blocked by the chest wall. As well, the burr saw, often used for burr holes, can be an effective tool for sawing though ribs.

CONCLUSIONS

Given that minimally invasive surgery involves procedures performed through ports, incisions, per se, are not the critical aspect of these less invasive approaches. Positioning and strategies to minimize hindrances must be carefully considered when planning the operative procedure. Today, thoracic surgeons have a myriad of approaches to use in the management of thoracic pathology. The ideal approach is selected based on consideration of a number of factors related to the patient and the surgeon. As a surgeon becomes progressively more comfortable working under camera guidance, the complexity of pathology that can be safely managed through minimally invasive approaches increases. As one sees the benefits to patients afforded by these minimally invasive approaches, the desire to continue to push the envelope continues to increase.

2

Pectus deformities

ANTONIO MESSINEO AND MARCO GHIONZOLI

Pectus excavatum and pectus carinatum, which represent the two main anterior chest wall deformities, are often associated with systemic weakness of the connective tissues and poor muscular development of the human trunk, including chest, abdomen, and spine. Both forms have, therefore, a markedly increased association with scoliosis and connective tissue disorders such as Marfan and Ehlers–Danlos syndromes.

Pectus excavatum, as its name suggests, presents with an excavated, sunken, or funnel chest and accounts for around 84% of all deformities (see **Figure 2.1**). Classifications allow us to differentiate asymmetric/symmetric, localized/diffuse, and long/short defect.

Pectus carinatum, a chest wall protuberance, which constitutes approximately 13% of chest wall deformities, presents in two forms: (1) the more frequent chondrogladiolar defect (which can be symmetric or asymmetric) (see **Figure 2.2**), and (2) the rarer, upper defect, the chondromanubrial one (see **Figure 2.3**).

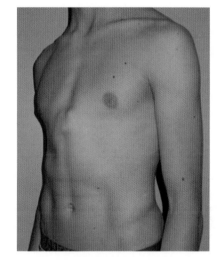

2.2

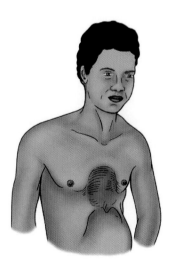

2.1

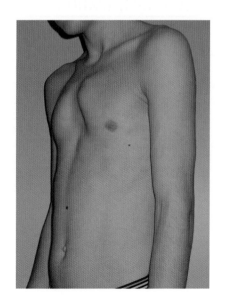

2.3

PECTUS EXCAVATUM REPAIR

In the 1920s, Ferdinand Sauerbrucha, pioneer in thoracic surgery, performed the first pectus repair using the bilateral costal cartilage resection and sternal osteotomy technique. He advocated the use of external traction for 5–6 weeks to hold the sternum in its corrected position and prevent recurrence. This technique was soon used by other surgeons in Europe and rapidly gained popularity in the United States as well.

Two decades later, Ravitch published his experience with eight patients in which he had used a radically extended modification of Sauerbruch's technique. Since the sternum was cut loose from all its attachments, he hypothesized that the sternum would no longer sink back into the chest and considered the use of external traction unnecessary. Such a modified procedure, however, was accompanied by an increased recurrence rate. To overcome this problem, in the 1950s, Wallgren and Sulamaa proposed the use of a slightly curved stainless-steel bar as an internal support. In the same period, J. Alex Haller drew attention to the risk of acquired asphyxiating chondrodystrophy in very young patients who had undergone the Ravitch procedure. This report prompted many surgeons to refrain from performing open pectus repair in young children, preferring to wait until the pubertal period. Moreover, many surgeons reverted to a procedure that entailed a decreased amount of cartilage resection and a more limited skin incision, the so-called modified Ravitch procedure.

In 1998, Nuss published his revolutionary experience with a minimally invasive technique that did not require any cartilage resection or sternal osteotomy: this procedure relied on internal bracing, with a curved stainless-steel bar inserted, under thoracoscopic view, through two lateral chest incisions.

PRINCIPLES AND JUSTIFICATION

The majority of children with pectus excavatum are asymptomatic; they are referred because they experience psychological distress and have a negative body image. A small subset complains of nonspecific chest pain and shortness of breath. These patients present with a very characteristic pattern: rounded shoulders, sloped ribs, potbelly and sunken chest. The excavatum defect is often associated with scoliosis and heart displacement toward the left hemithorax.

PREOPERATIVE ASSESSMENT AND PREPARATION

Chest computed tomography scanning or thoracic magnetic resonance imaging provides an accurate assessment of anatomical situation. The ratio of the distance between the sternum and vertebral bodies and the transverse diameter of the chest through the deepest portion of the defect may be used to calculate (Haller index). In normal children, this index is less than 2.5, whereas the index may range from 3 to 7 in those with severe deformities. The asymmetry index should also be calculated to determine the severity of defect.

Simultaneous pulmonary and cardiac evaluation has shown that a severe deformity can cause compression of the right side of the heart, resulting in right-ventricular outflow distortion. The vast majority of children show normal pulmonary function at rest, while a few individuals with severe deformities may have mild restrictive patterns.

In patients with pectus excavatum, the appropriate selection of children who will benefit from defect correction still remains the main issue. Surgical indications include chest pain and/or dyspnea on exertion, cosmetic concerns, and psychological disturbance. We believe that repair should be performed in early adolescence, after pubertal growth spurt, when patients are mostly aware of their body image and can exhibit strong motivation to undergo the operation.

ANESTHESIA

Chest wall reconstruction is performed under general anesthesia with or without thoracic epidural analgesia.

RAVITCH PROCEDURE

The modified Ravitch operation involves the resection of all abnormal costal cartilages, a concept that is applicable equally to excavatum and carinatum deformities. The sternum is displaced by longitudinal cartilage overgrowth, and, therefore, once it has been freed from such deformed cartilage, a fracture of its anterior table is required to restore a normal position.

Ravitch procedure technique

INCISION

1. A transverse, rather than vertical, incision through the deepest or prominent portion of the defect is used.

SKIN AND MUSCLE FLAPS

2. Following adequate subcutaneous dissection, which starts in the midline and moves laterally, pectoralis muscle flaps are created, exposing the costochondral junction. The defect may involve many ribs, but usually only cartilages from the 5th to the 8th bilaterally are altered. A minimum of four cartilages for each side should be excised (see **Figure 2.4**).

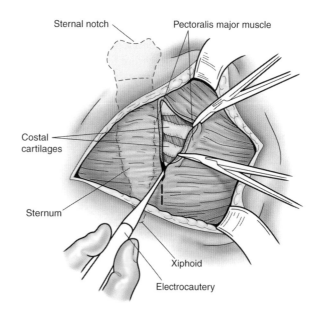

2.4

SUBPERICHONDRIAL RESECTION OF THE DEFORMED CARTILAGES

3. At each involved cartilage, perichondrium is longitudinally incised, exposing the deformed cartilage (see **Figure 2.5a**). Caution is taken to avoid entering the pleural space. Each altered cartilage is resected from the ossified part to the sternal attachment. The perichondrium should be preserved as a template for the new cartilage growth (see **Figure 2.5b**).

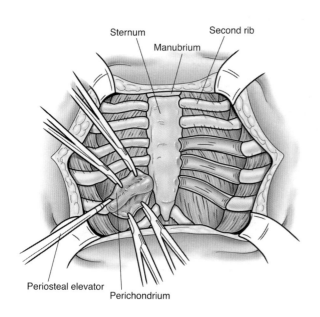

2.5a

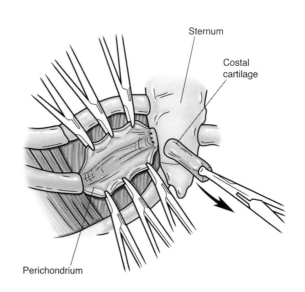

2.5b

MOBILIZATION OF THE STERNUM

4. The xiphoid is exposed and elevated, and the retrosternal plane is bluntly developed, reflecting the pleura and pericardium away from the sternum (see **Figure 2.6a**). The intercostal muscles and perichondrial bundles are detached from the sternum from xiphoid to the highest involved ribs (see **Figure 2.6b**).

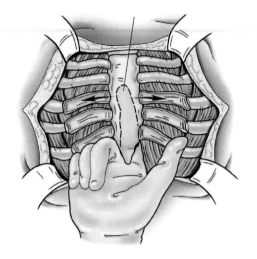

2.6a

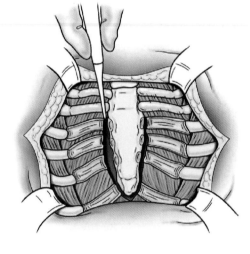

2.6b

5. A single oblique or transverse wedge osteotomy of the anterior table of the twisted sternum allows sternal rotation up to neutral position. Occasionally, a second anterior table osteotomy is required. The sternal periosteum is then sutured to further secure the sternum in its new flat position (see **Figure 2.7**).

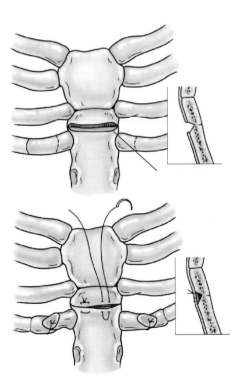

2.7

6. In adolescents, especially when they are affected by connective tissue abnormalities, it is recommended that a substernal stainless-steel bar be placed beneath the distal sternum and secured to the ribs (**Figure 2.8**). The defect between sternum and resected bundles should be closed, approximating such tissues (see **Figure 2.9**).

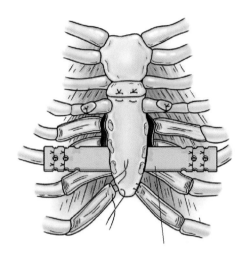

2.8

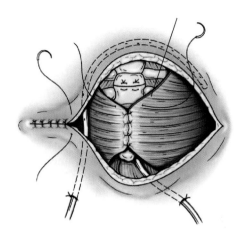

2.9

Postoperative care

Costal cartilages may regenerate within 2 months; therefore, contact sports should be avoided during this period. In patients with steel-bar strut placement, the device is usually removed after 6–8 months.

Outcome

At the present time, the Ravitch procedure should be reserved for adult patients who have a very rigid chest wall and severe defect for whom the Nuss procedure is considered inappropriate or too risky. Indications may include patients who have had a failed Ravitch procedure or those who have undergone a sternotomy. However, variants of the Nuss technique, such the one reported by Hans Pilegaard suggesting a more anterior approach in adults with severe pectus excavatum, allow the minimally invasive approach to be performed in nearly every patient.

RAVITCH PROCEDURE FOR PECTUS CARINATUM

In the case of chondrogladiolar defect of pectus carinatum, the general concept of the modified Ravitch operation also applies. Once a subperichondrial resection of all deformed cartilages is obtained and the sternum has been detached from the perichondrial and intercostal muscles attachments, an anterior sternal osteotomy is performed, allowing the sternum to be fractured and displaced posteriorly.

In the case of a chondromanubrial deformity, a technique described by Shamberger and Welch should be used. Cartilages are resected, starting from the second cartilage and going inferiorly, then a large osteotomy is performed in the region of maximal sternal protrusion.

MINI-INVASIVE REPAIR OF PECTUS EXCAVATUM (MIRPE)

This technique was described by Nuss in 1998 and since then it has rapidly become the gold standard operation for patients with severe pectus excavatum. In the three centers most experienced with this technique (Children's Hospital of The King's Daughters, Norfolk, VA, United States; Seoul St. Mary's Hospital, The Catholic Universtiy of Korea, Seoul, South Korea; and Institut for Klinisk Medicin- Hjerte-, Lunge- og Karkirurgi, Aarhus, Denmark), more than 4000 procedures with different variations have been performed in the last 15 years.

The term "mini-invasive" was used by Nuss to indicate that cartilages were not removed and that the surgical approach, using lateral incision, avoided any anterior scar.

MIRPE technique

1. The patient is positioned on the operating table, and the most depressed area of the sternal plate and the preferred entrance and exit points at the chest ridge are identified (see **Figure 2.10**).

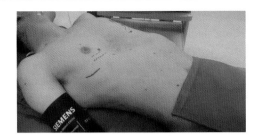

2.10

2. On both sides, in the posterior axillary line, a 5 mm trocar is inserted and carbon dioxide (CO_2) is inflated at pressure running from 4 to 6 mmHg. Through such accesses, a 30-degree thoracoscope is shifted from one side to the other to verify the deepest point of sternal depression in order to be able to choose the preferred entrance and exit points and to visually guide the procedure

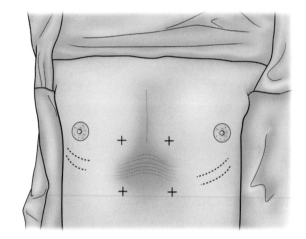

2.11a

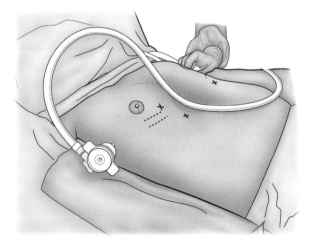

2.11b

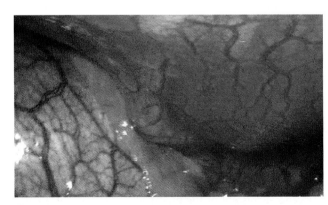

2.11c

3. Once the placement locations are defined and the bar is bent to the desired shape, 3 to 4 cm curved skin incisions are made bilaterally at the midaxillary line (in the female, an inframammary incision is preferred), and a subcutaneous tunnel is created up to the entrance points on the chest ridges (see **Figure 2.12a**). If the incision is at the level of pectoralis muscles, a submuscular tunnel is created up to a convenient intercostal space (see **Figure 2.12b**).

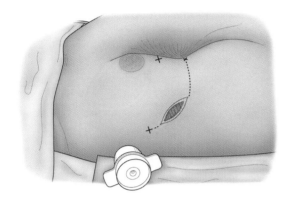

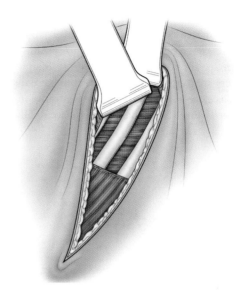

2.12a

2.12b

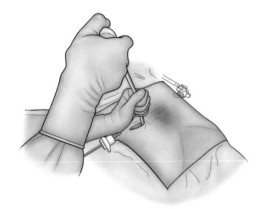

2.13a

4. A metal introducer is pushed through the entrance intercostal point on the right chest ridge to dissect intrapleurally a plane separating the sternum from the pericardium, thus creating a tunnel through the anterior mediastinum (see **Figure 2.13a and b**). The introducer tip is then pushed out at the chosen left intercostal space (see **Figure 2.13c**).

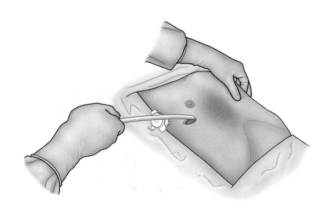

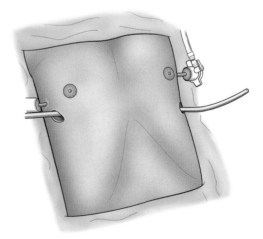

2.13b

2.13c

5. A plastic tube is tightly attached from one side to the introducer tip and from the other to the customized bar and the introducer is pulled backward, allowing the bar passage through the mediastinal tunnel from left to right (see **Figure 2.14a**). The bar is inserted with the concave side up (see **Figure 2.14b**), then it is rotated 180 degrees around its axis, thus pushing the sternum up (see **Figure 2.14c through e**). Stainless-steel stabilizers are routinely inserted on both bar ends and pushed as close as possible to the bar entrance in the chest (see **Figure 2.14f**). Stabilizers are eventually fixed

to intercostal muscles by interrupted polyglactin sutures. An additional bar is introduced at surgeon's judgment, taking into account the length of the defect and the rigidity of the chest wall. In cases in which a second bar is required, a single stabilizer for each bar is placed, one for each side.

Pilegaard reports it may be necessary to use three bars in adult patients. In case of asymmetrical pectus excavatum, HyungJoo Park suggests bending the bar asymmetrically to obtain a complete and satisfactory result.

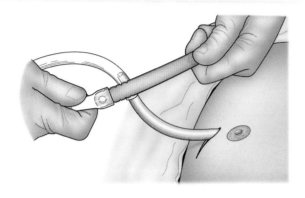

2.14a

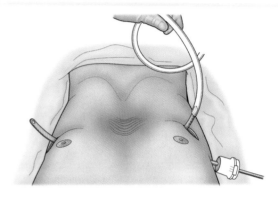

2.14b

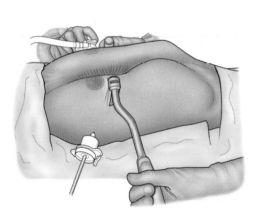

2.14c

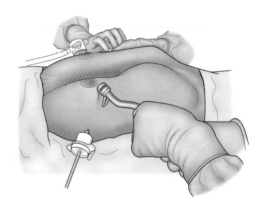

2.14d

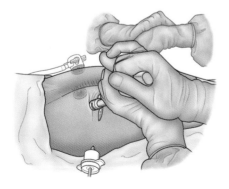

2.14e

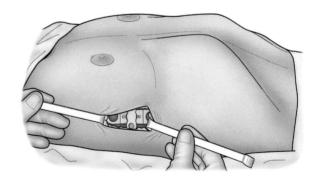

2.14f

Postoperative care

Postoperative pain is managed with epidural analgesia and nonsteroidal anti-inflammatory drugs. The follow-up plan requires outpatient visits at 1, 6, 12 and 24 months. Light physical activity is reintroduced 1 month after surgery and contact sports are allowed after 6 months. Chest X-rays are taken postoperatively in all patients to document the result of the procedure and to allow assessment of the position of the bar during the follow-up period.

Outcome

This operation is considered minimally invasive; however, no one must think that recovery from this procedure is always simple. Postoperative pain control can be quite challenging, at times requiring multimodal pain management such as epidural and patient-controlled analgesia.

A recent meta-analysis estimates complications occur in approximately one-third of patients who undergo MIRPE, most of which are minor; specifically, residual pneumothorax, pleural effusion, pneumonia, pericarditis, wound infection, bar shift, or transient Horner's syndrome. Conversely, there are a few reports detailing major complications, such as liver lacerations or perforations, bilateral empyema, bacterial pericarditis, or thoracic outlet-like syndrome and cardiac perforations.

Postoperative evaluation demonstrates a significant improvement in pulmonary function tests. Many patients note a significant improvement in self-confidence and self-esteem within a few weeks after surgery.

Bar removal

The bar is removed by reopening both lateral incisions at, or at about, 3 years after the insertion.

After bar removal, the majority of patients report great satisfaction with the result.

NONSURGICAL TREATMENT OF PECTUS CARINATUM

Alongside the evolution of the surgical techniques for the correction of pectus carinatum, the concept of noninvasive treatment via external bracing of the deformity has been developed. The idea of a nonsurgical corrective treatment was based on the fact that in pectus excavatum, forces acting within the chest wall early in puberty are markedly reduced in comparison with those present in adults, thus allowing a potential reshaping of the sternum and costal cartilage by external compression applied over the deformity. Several devices have been developed to facilitate this nonsurgical approach.

Abramson procedure

As noted earlier, the traditional surgical correction of pectus carinatum involves removing portions of the cartilage and creating a sternal osteotomy to reconfigure the chest wall.

A minimally invasive technique, which was first proposed in 2005 by Horatio Abramson, is based on the Nuss procedure. A special bar, similar to the Nuss bar with different stabilizer, was designed for this purpose.

The correction of the chest contour and simultaneous lateral expansion of the depressed costochondral arches are achieved using a submuscular metal bar that compresses the protruding chest wall and remodels the chest shape. The bar is laterally fixed using two special stabilizers with three holes, which are matched with the holes in the bar, so that the bar may be fixed on each side with stainless-steel screws under different pressure.

The most appropriate time to apply this technique is during the rapid growth of puberty. This technique is difficult to use in patients having a pectus carinatum with a stiff chest wall.

3

Thoracic trauma

SCOTT M. MOORE, FREDERIC M. PIERACCI, AND GREGORY J. JURKOVICH

HISTORY

Almost all historical accounts of chest trauma are within the context of war and conflict. The oldest surgical treatise on record is the *Edwin Smith Surgical Papyrus* from around 3000 BC, which predates Hippocrates by approximately 1000 years and is believed to have been a handbook for the treatment of injuries sustained during military campaigns. However, few if any of these ancient writings effectively address intrathoracic injuries, as they mainly deal with extremity and soft-tissue wounds. Hemothorax and pneumothorax were first described about 200 years ago, and evacuation by either incisional drainage or tube placement was standard practice by the 1870s, with the development of underwater-seal drainage devices coming not long after. Ludwig Rehn described the first cardiorrhaphy for a penetrating injury in 1896. However, most of the major operations that will be described in this chapter have been innovations of the twentieth century, with guidelines for the management of penetrating thoracic trauma not established until World War II.

PRINCIPLES AND JUSTIFICATION

Trauma is the leading cause of death in individuals aged 1 to 44 years old, making it the number-one cause for productive life-years lost. Thoracic trauma is second only to head injury as a cause of death in the injured patient, with an overall mortality of 8.4% among those who present to the hospital. However, the burden of disease is likely to be much higher if one takes into account prehospital deaths and inhospital deaths in patients with multiple injuries, in which case thoracic trauma contributes to an estimated 50% of trauma-related deaths. Reflecting the importance of promptly addressing thoracic wounds, the systematic approach to the thoracic trauma patient is well described in all nine editions of *Advanced Trauma Life Support*.[1] While less than 10% of blunt and only 10%–15% of penetrating chest injuries will require an operation, the lifesaving maneuvers of tube decompression, flail chest and open pneumothorax management, and airway control are essential skills for any surgeon. This chapter will describe procedures that are essential to the management of the thoracic trauma patient.

PREOPERATIVE ASSESSMENT AND PREPARATION

As with all trauma patients, the initial approach to the patient with a suspected chest injury involves a primary survey in which immediately life-threatening problems are identified and corrected as they are found. Assessment of the patient proceeds in the systematic "ABC" fashion—beginning with *airway*, followed by *breathing*, and ultimately *circulation*. British military surgeons faced with the devastating problem of improvised explosive devices and exsanguinating extremity injuries have advocated revising the ABC of trauma care to the "CABC" with the first emphasis being on *catastrophic hemorrhage control*, often with an extremity tourniquet.[2] Injuries that must be addressed at this stage include upper airway injuries, open and tension pneumothorax, massive hemothorax, flail chest, and cardiac tamponade. Diagnosing these conditions may only require physical exam (e.g., tension pneumothorax), but many will require more detailed evaluations such as bedside ultrasound or even thoracotomy (e.g., cardiac tamponade) to diagnose and adequately treat.

Following completion of the primary survey, and with the use of adjuncts to the physical exam such as radiography and ultrasound, a more detailed secondary evaluation is done to search for potentially life-threatening problems such as simple pneumothorax, hemothorax, pulmonary contusion, tracheobronchial injuries, aerodigestive injury, blunt cardiac injury, aortic injury, and diaphragmatic injury.

One of the more challenging aspects at this stage involves choosing only the essential examination maneuvers, radiologic studies, and laboratory measurements that will direct the necessary actions to stabilize the patient, while omitting time-consuming tests that are both unlikely to change management acutely and may place patients at risk by subjecting them to long periods remote from resources. To this end, an understanding of the value of the various exam maneuvers, imaging modalities, and laboratory studies will help in expediting the initial work-up of the thoracic trauma patient, and minimize delay should an operation be necessary.

We briefly mention the tertiary survey at this point, to emphasize the need to review the physical exam, laboratory and radiographic findings, and adequacy of therapeutic plans for all documented injuries at an early stage in the hospital course, preferably within 24 hours of admission, to ensure no injuries were missed during the initial evaluation and recovery is proceeding as expected.

Key examination findings

Evaluations for airway patency and presence of breath sounds are essential components of the primary survey. In a hypotensive patient with unilateral absence of breath sounds, especially if accompanied by hyperresonance, a tension pneumothorax should be strongly suspected and a tube thoracostomy immediately performed. Alternatively, decreased unilateral breath sounds but without hyperresonance may represent hemothorax. The appearance of distended neck veins can signify one of four potentially life-threatening conditions: (1) tension pneumothorax, (2) pericardial tamponade, (3) coronary air embolism, or (4) cardiac contusion with pump failure. Beck's triad describes the classic exam findings of cardiac tamponade: muffled heart sounds, hypotension, and distended neck veins. Unfortunately, only 50% of patients with cardiac tamponade will demonstrate just one of these findings, and muffled heart sounds are often difficult to discern in the noisy trauma bay. Kussmaul's sign (increased venous pressure with inspiration) and pulsus paradoxus (>10 mmHg decrease in systolic pressure with inspiration) are also characteristic of cardiac tamponade, but neither exam finding is sensitive. Exam findings of flail chest include paradoxical movement of the involved chest wall segment during the respiratory cycle. The detection of crepitance by simple palpation may help determine if a patient has rib fractures with underlying parenchymal lung injury. Lateral and anteroposterior compression of the chest wall is a useful maneuver for evaluating chest wall injuries, and the absence of pain in this setting essentially rules out clinically significant rib fractures. Distinguishing tension pneumothorax from cardiac tamponade in a trauma patient with hypotension is an essential skill of the trauma surgeon, since most inexperienced evaluators will jump to the conclusion that the hypotension is caused by blood loss.

Imaging studies

The application of ultrasound in the initial trauma evaluation (i.e., focused assessment sonography in trauma—FAST) can circumvent many of the difficulties associated with diagnosing cardiac tamponade by physical exam alone, having 97% sensitivity and 100% specificity for the presence of hemopericardium.[3] Currently, the supine portable chest X-ray is a vital portion of the secondary survey, allowing a rapid assessment for pneumothorax, hemothorax, rib fractures, great vessel injuries (widened mediastinum), and diaphragmatic rupture (presence of nasogastric tube in the chest). For penetrating injuries, using radiopaque labels to mark the wounds can greatly facilitate determining the missile tract, and plain X-rays are very useful for identifying retained bullets and bullet fragments. The extended focused assessment sonography in trauma, or eFAST, includes a sonographic evaluation for pneumothorax and has reported sensitivities of 98%, compared with 75% for the traditional supine chest X-ray, and has the potential to further increase the efficiency of the initial trauma evaluation.[3] As with all ultrasound studies, FAST and eFAST are significantly operator dependent, and there is an inadequate literature honestly addressing the false-negative rate of ultrasound in the emergency trauma setting. Formal echocardiography may be required in cases of questionable cardiac function (e.g., cardiac contusion, acute coronary syndrome); however, these evaluations are time-consuming and often unnecessary in the initial surgical decision-making.

The initial work-up for blunt thoracic aortic injuries begins with the chest radiograph, which has a reported sensitivity of 81%–100% and specificity of 60% for blunt aortic injury.[4] The characteristic findings of blunt-traumatic aortic injury include widening of the mediastinum to greater than 8 cm at the level of the aortic knob, obscuring of the aortic knob, depression of the left mainstem bronchus, displacement of the trachea at the T4 level, and presence of an apical pleural cap. Aortography was the preferred method for detecting aortic injuries until advances in computed tomographic angiography (CTA) technology and training caused a relative shift in this practice. Modern computed tomography (CT) equipment can obtain thin-slice (3–5 mm) cross-sectional imaging from the base of the skull to the pubic symphysis in less than 1 minute with a sensitivity and specificity that rivals aortography, making CTA the initial screening modality of choice at most centers for patients at high risk for aortic injuries. Furthermore, the images obtained by CTA can be reconstructed and used to plan endovascular interventions should an aortic injury be identified. While the location for blunt aortic injury is at the level of the ligamentum arteriosum in the vast majority of cases, injuries can occur at any site where the aorta is relatively fixed, and can also occur in regions adjacent to severe spinal column injuries.[5]

Penetrating wounds that traverse the mediastinum or are in the vicinity of the heart or great vessels require a methodologic work-up. These injuries should be suspected on any patient with a penetrating wound within the area bounded by the sternal notch superiorly, nipples laterally, and costal margin inferiorly (known traditionally as "the box"). FAST exam should be performed in the trauma bay to detect hemopericardium, with the caveat that false negatives can result when there is communication between the pericardial and pleural spaces.[6] Assuming patient stability, CTA provides excellent evaluations of the thoracic vasculature and also anatomic detail regarding the path of the offending object. Bullet fragments can occasionally cause significant signal artifact, and, in these circumstances, it is sometimes necessary to perform traditional aortography. If injury to the aerodigestive tract is suspected based on the CT results, then laryngo-tracheo-bronchoscopy and esophagography should be performed. Combining endoscopy with contrast studies of the esophagus has a near 100% sensitivity for detecting esophageal injuries.

ANESTHESIA

The patient that presents with hemodynamic collapse in the trauma bay does not require any anesthetic agents, though placement of an endotracheal tube should occur concurrently with resuscitative maneuvers, if not already done by prehospital personnel. For urgent operations done for major hemorrhage, the patient should be completely prepped and draped and the surgical team ready to make an incision prior to administration of anesthetic agents, due to the relatively high chance of cardiovascular collapse on anesthetic induction.

OPERATION

Bedside procedures for pneumothorax and hemothorax

Pneumothorax occurs when air enters the pleural space, usually as a result of parenchymal lung injury in the setting of rib fractures or penetrating trauma. In this setting, simple pneumothorax seen on plain chest X-ray should be treated by tube thoracostomy. Pneumothorax not seen on chest X-ray but seen on subsequent chest CT (known as "occult" pneumothorax) does not require thoracostomy in a hemodynamically normal patient without respiratory embarrassment. Rather, it can be safely followed on serial chest X-ray. Importantly, a simple pneumothorax can quickly convert to a life-threatening tension pneumothorax, especially in the setting of general anesthesia and positive-pressure ventilation. Hemothorax is characterized as either simple (<1500 mL) or massive (>1500 mL), and if evident on plain chest X-ray should be treated by tube thoracostomy. The utility of draining smaller volumes of uncomplicated hemothorax that are only visible on chest CT remains controversial. The risk of introducing infection and pain must be weighed against the benefit of lung expansion and retained

fluid evacuation. In our practice, we generally recommend evacuation of those hemothoraces estimated to be greater than 500 mL.

NEEDLE THORACOSTOMY

Decompression of a tension pneumothorax can be accomplished rapidly by placement of a large bore angiocatheter in the second intercostal space at the midclavicular line. However, in some patients with particularly thick chest walls, the length of commonly available angiocatheters (5 cm) may not be adequate to reach the pleural space.[7] Furthermore, the midclavicular line may not be the ideal location in such individuals; instead, the midaxillary line may provide a shorter distance for intrapleural insertion.[8] Tube thoracostomy is always required following successful needle thoracostomy, which invariably results in a simple pneumothorax regardless of whether one existed prior to its placement. Percutaneous approaches using the Seldinger technique (i.e., needle, wire, tube) and pigtail catheters have been advocated by some for pneumothorax without blood; however, such tubes are prone to kinking and can become clogged with even small quantities of blood within the pleural space. Due to these limitations, most busy trauma centers favor formal tube thoracostomy as the primary treatment modality for pneumo- and hemothorax.

TUBE THORACOSTOMY

Preparation for tube thoracostomy should include skin disinfection with an alcohol-based 2% chlorhexidine solution, and the field should be widely draped, with the surgeon wearing sterile gloves, cap, gown, and face mask. The patient in extremis (e.g., tension pneumothorax) may require abbreviated skin preparation and draping. The value of antibiotics prior to chest tube insertion for preventing pneumonia or empyema is debated. This is exemplified by guidelines from the Eastern Association for the Surgery of Trauma, which initially recommended presumptive antibiotics when first released in 2002, while the updated guidelines in 2012 retracted this recommendation based on poor quality and conflicting data.[9]

The optimal site is typically at the fifth intercostal space (nipple level in males) just anterior to the midaxillary line. Local anesthetic should be liberally infiltrated into the skin, subcutaneous tissues, intercostal muscles, and pleura. A 2–3 cm horizontal incision is made and a Kelly clamp is used to dissect through the tissues in the direction of the intended interspace, taking care to dissect just over the top of the lower rib. Once the pleura is reached, it should be bluntly punctured forcefully, ideally with a finger, but in a controlled fashion so as to avoid injury to underlying lung. Generous spreading of the tract with the Kelly clamp at this point will greatly facilitate tube placement. A gloved finger should then be inserted into the pleural space. This maneuver may provide several pieces of useful information including confirmation of intrapleural placement, diagnosis of cardiac tamponade (left side), diagnosis of diaphragmatic rupture, and sweeping away of any adhesions. The chest tube is then clamped at its tip and directed through the tract and into the pleural space. As trauma patients often have a combination of both fluid and air in the pleural space (i.e., hemopneumothorax), the tube should be directed along the posterior chest wall toward the apex. Spinning the tube during advancement helps prevent lodgment into the fissure, and fogging of the tube confirms intrapleural placement. The tube is then secured with heavy suture, attached to a water-seal drainage device, and covered with an occlusive and sterile dressing. Authorities have historically recommended large bore chest tubes (36–40 Fr) for treatment of hemothorax, though no studies have supported this assertion, and studies have shown no difference between small (20–32 Fr) and large (36–40 Fr) tubes for successful evacuation of hemothorax.[10] The need for emergent operative exploration is based on both initial output (>1000 mL for penetrating and >1500 mL for blunt) and subsequent output (>300 mL per hour for 2 consecutive hours for both blunt and penetrating). Finally, emergent operative exploration is indicated for lower outputs in the setting of hemodynamic instability.

Temporizing measures for cardiac tamponade

Adjunctive procedures such as pericardiocentesis and subxiphoid pericardiotomy (see "Subxiphoid pericardiotomy" subsection) were historically used mostly for the diagnosis of hemopericardium, although these procedures have been supplanted in this role by pericardial ultrasound due to the latter's high sensitivity and noninvasiveness. Effective treatment for cardiac tamponade mandates immediate decompression and repair of the underlying cardiac injury, which requires either a sternotomy or thoracotomy incision. Though transfer to the operating room is preferred, some patients will require immediate intervention in the trauma bay (i.e., emergency department thoracotomy [EDT]—see "ED thoracotomy" subsection). The role of pericardiocentesis as a therapeutic procedure is less clear, but most centers have abandoned therapeutic pericardiocentesis due to concerns over delays in definitive operative intervention. Occasionally, experienced surgical personnel are not immediately available or ultrasound results are equivocal, and decompression of cardiac tamponade by pericardiocentesis is necessary. Furthermore, a single-center experience recently reported that performance of pericardiocentesis in the emergency department (ED) does not delay definitive therapy and that early relief of cardiac tamponade leads to improvements in patient hemodynamics.[11]

PERICARDIOCENTESIS

This procedure is performed using sterile technique and a long (at least 15 cm) 16- to 18-gauge angiocatheter, with continuous electrocardiographic monitoring throughout the procedure. The skin is entered at a 45-degree angle and 1–2 cm inferior and to the left side of the xiphocondral junction. The needle is advanced slowly in the direction of the left shoulder until blood is withdrawn, signifying entry into the pericardial sac. As much blood should be removed as possible, and then a catheter attached to a three-way stopcock left in place. The Seldinger technique may be used for placement of the pericardial catheter, or it may be inserted directly over the needle. Inadvertent injury to the myocardium during needle advancement or during aspiration will be detected by ST-T wave changes on the electrocardiogram monitor, which should prompt immediate withdrawal of the needle. The utility of pericardiocentesis for both diagnostic and therapeutic purposes can be limited by the difficulty in aspirating clotted blood within the pericardial sac. Furthermore, although temporary relief of symptoms may occur, all trauma patients with acute cardiac tamponade ultimately require complete examination of the heart and cardiorrhaphy of any injuries.

OPERATION

Major procedures for thoracic trauma

POSITIONING

The choice of incision influences positioning; however, unstable patients should remain in the supine position, as lateral positioning limits access to the superior mediastinum and opposite hemithorax, compromises ventilation of the dependent lung, results in pooling of blood within the contralateral bronchial tree, and limits exploration of other body cavities. For stable patients undergoing planned thoracotomy, lateral positioning facilitates posterolateral exposure, but flexion of the bed should only be performed if spinal injury has been excluded. All patients undergoing exploratory surgery following trauma should be prepped from the neck to the knees to permit full access to incidentally discovered injuries and, if needed, exposure for saphenous vein harvesting.

INCISIONS

Injury mechanism, patient stability, anticipated intrathoracic pathology, and associated nonthoracic injuries will dictate the most appropriate incision:

- *Left anterolateral thoracotomy* provides the most options for immediate resuscitative maneuvers in the pulseless trauma patient, regardless of the underlying pathology, and is especially useful for penetrating cardiac wounds leading to cardiovascular collapse. With the exception of a diagnosis of cardiac tamponade, this is the "workhouse" incision for the unstable trauma patient with suspected intrathoracic trauma. This incision is easily extended to a transsternal bilateral anterolateral (aka "clamshell") thoracotomy if needed, as described next.
- *Transsternal bilateral anterolateral thoracotomy* (i.e., "clamshell thoracotomy") is useful in the salvaged patient undergoing EDT, as it allows the surgeon to address right thoracic injuries and improves overall exposure to the left chest and mediastinum. The sternum is transected with a Lebsche knife followed by suture ligation of the internal

mammary arteries and veins, and the incision is carried through the fifth intercostal space on the right side. The main limitation of the clamshell thoracotomy is the limited exposure of the aortic arch vessels. This exposure can be improved by a superior sternotomy extension.

- *Median sternotomy* is versatile for addressing thoracic trauma due to its excellent exposure of the right heart, ascending aorta and arch, and arch vessels, and the relative ease of opening and closing. It may also be extended into the neck or supraclavicular fossa for exposure of the innominate artery, and proximal subclavian and common carotid arteries. However, exposure of posterior mediastinal structures is very limited, and cross-clamping of the descending thoracic aorta is not possible.

- *Right posterolateral thoracotomy* provides the best exposure of the right lung, trachea, carina, right and proximal left mainstem bronchi, and proximal and middle esophagus. The right heart is also easily accessible, though the left lung, distal left airways, descending thoracic aorta, aortic arch, arch vessels, and left heart are not accessible through this incision.

- *Left posterolateral thoracotomy* provides ideal exposure of the left lung and hilum, descending thoracic aorta, distal esophagus, and distal left mainstem bronchus. As mentioned, left thoracotomy does not afford access to the right chest, and the posterolateral incision further limits exposure to the right heart, though the left heart chambers are accessible.

- *Left trapdoor thoracotomy* combines a left anterolateral thoracotomy incision and partial sternotomy with left supraclavicular extension. Though controversial due to its associated morbidity, this incision can prove useful in the specific circumstance where a resuscitative thoracotomy has been performed and an injury is encountered in the proximal left subclavian artery. The sternocleidomastoid and strap muscles are transected during the supraclavicular extension to provide full exposure, and care must be taken to avoid injury to the left phrenic nerve that runs along the surface of the anterior scalene muscle.

ED (RESUSCITATIVE) THORACOTOMY

The development of well-organized prehospital trauma systems has led to increased survival among individuals sustaining major penetrating and blunt injuries. This has increased the proportion of trauma patients suffering a witnessed cardiac arrest during their ED evaluation or minutes prior to their arrival. EDT is a resuscitative maneuver with the goal of stabilizing the patient for transport to the operating room, where either definitive repair or damage control of thoracic injuries can be accomplished. The goals of EDT vary based on the mechanism of injury and can include a combination of the following: release of cardiac tamponade; control of hemorrhage from cardiac wounds; internal cardiac compression; cross-clamping of the pulmonary hilum in the setting of major lung hemorrhage, air embolism, or massive bronchopleural fistula; and cross-clamping of the descending thoracic aorta to maximize coronary and cerebral perfusion and limit hemorrhage from the lower torso and extremities. The best outcomes occur in those sustaining penetrating stab wounds to the heart where cardiac tamponade is the principle cause of cardiovascular collapse, whereas the most dismal outcomes occur in blunt-trauma patients whose pulses were lost prior to arrival to the ED. Though indications for EDT vary between trauma centers, most would agree that EDT should not be performed if prehospital personnel were required to perform cardiopulmonary resuscitation for more than 10 minutes for blunt trauma, and for more than 15 minutes for penetrating mechanisms. The essential instruments for EDT include a No. 10-blade scalpel, Finochietto retractor, toothed forceps, Mayo scissors, Satinsky (or DeBakey) vascular clamps (at least two), long needle holder and 2-0 polypropylene sutures, and a Lebsche knife and mallet. Other materials that may be needed include silk ties, Teflon pledgets, and a skin stapler.

1. EDT is performed through a left anterolateral thoracotomy through the fifth intercostal space, which is just below the nipple in males and in the inframammary crease in females. The incision should start just to the right side of the sternum and be carried horizontally across the left chest until just beyond the nipple, at which point the incision is angled gently toward the left axilla. (See **Figure 3.1**.)

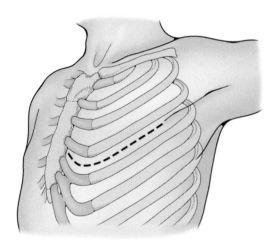

3.1

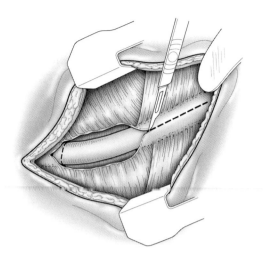

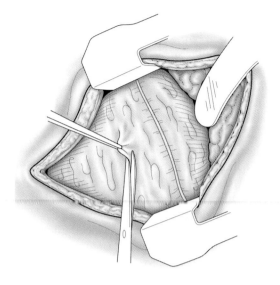

3.2

2. Once the intercostal muscles are reached, either the scalpel or scissors can be used to complete the incision (see **Figure 3.2**).

3.3

3. If a penetrating cardiac wound is suspected, attention should be immediately directed toward release of cardiac tamponade and repair of cardiac wounds. A low threshold for extension to a bilateral anterior thoracotomy should be maintained if a cardiac wound is suspected. This will allow for maximal exposure of the injured area. The pericardium can be quite tense and may require a scalpel to incise. The pericardiotomy is then extended vertically in a direction parallel and anterior to the phrenic nerve. (See **Figure 3.3**.)

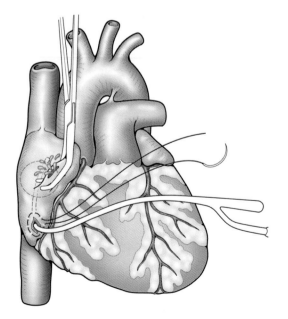

4. Complete delivery of the heart from the pericardial sac not only allows for more thorough examination and control of cardiac injuries but also facilitates open cardiac massage in the setting of cardiac arrest. Intracardiac injection of epinephrine (1 mg) may also be employed, as well as cardiac defibrillation (20–50 J) using internal paddles positioned on the anterior and posterior aspects of the heart. Finally, intra-atrial infusion of blood products may be achieved via cannulation of either atrial appendage around a purse-string stitch and using a Foley catheter. (See **Figure 3.4**.)

If hemorrhage from a great vessel is determined as the cause for the arrest, the initial priority should be hemorrhage control by direct pressure.

3.4

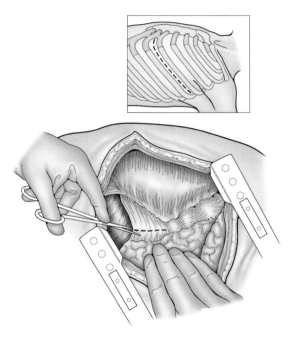

3.5

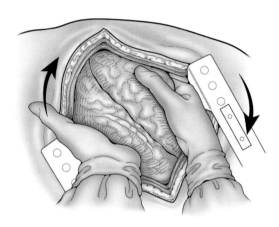

3.6

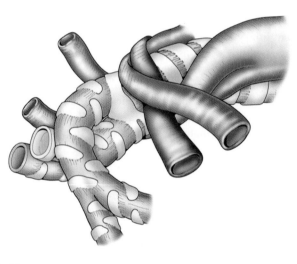

3.7

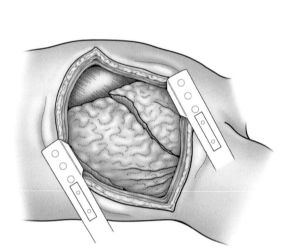

3.8

5. In the case of air embolism, major pulmonary hemorrhage, or bronchopleural fistula, the pulmonary hilum can be controlled by applying a vascular clamp, by performing a pulmonary hilar twist, or by direct digital compression. (See **Figures 3.5 through 3.8.**) These maneuvers may be facilitated by division of the inferior pulmonary ligament.

Clamping of the descending thoracic aorta is usually accomplished below the pulmonary hilum, and is facilitated by creating a defect within the overlying parietal pleura using scissors or the narrow end of a vascular clamp. Creating such a defect ensures the vascular clamp is completely across the aorta and helps prevent dislodgement of the clamp during transport. The flaccid aorta is the first structure anterior to the thoracic spine. Though some advocate division of the inferior pulmonary ligament prior to cross-clamping, we have not found this to be necessary. If return of spontaneous circulation is obtained (perfusing rhythm with systolic blood pressure >70 mmHg), then the patient is transported to the operating room for more definitive repair of injuries.

SUBXIPHOID PERICARDIOTOMY

Subxiphoid pericardiotomy, also referred to as "pericardial window," should be performed in the operating room under sterile conditions and adequate lighting. A 10 cm midline incision through skin and subcutaneous tissue is made overlying the xiphoid process, and the latter is dissected free so that it may be grasped with a Kocher clamp and retracted in a cephalad direction. Fatty tissue in the subxiphoid space can then be bluntly dissected along with the use of frequent digital palpation to direct the dissection toward the cardiac impulse. Once the pericardium is visualized, which is facilitated by placing the patient in reverse Trendelenburg position at this stage, it should be grasped firmly with two Allis clamps. A 1 cm longitudinal incision is then made between the clamps, with care taken to avoid inadvertent injury to the underlying epicardium. Immediate return of straw-colored pericardial fluid indicates the absence of blood and a negative window, whereas bloody effluent is a positive result and mandates extension to a sternotomy for full exploration and cardiorrhaphy. Absence of any fluid from the pericardiotomy should raise suspicion of clotted blood within the pericardial sac, and should be investigated by insertion of a suction catheter. If a negative result is obtained and sternotomy is not required, the pericardiotomy is closed with several simple interrupted polyglactin sutures, followed by closure of the incision.

CARDIORRHAPHY

Repair of cardiac injuries is typically performed through either median sternotomy or left anterolateral thoracotomy. Atrial injuries can be temporarily controlled by digital occlusion of the defect or by placement of a vascular clamp, and definitive repair is usually possible by simple running or purse-string sutures. Due to their relatively anterior location, the ventricles are the most commonly injured cardiac chambers in patients sustaining precordial penetrating wounds.

6. Temporary control of hemorrhage from the ventricles is best accomplished by finger occlusion. For left ventricular wounds encountered in the trauma bay during EDT, skin staples can sometimes prove useful for temporary control if the laceration is linear and the edges approximate during diastole. Foley-balloon occlusion has also been described, though care must be taken not to extend the wound. In the right ventricle, a running or horizontal mattress repair with 3-0 polypropylene suture is recommended, and use of pledgets is often not necessary if sutures are placed accurately. In contrast, repairs of the thicker-walled left ventricle typically do require pledgets, and use either vertical mattress sutures or deeply placed horizontal mattress sutures followed by a continuous epicardial stitch. Hemostatic glues may serve as a useful adjunct to suture repairs. (See **Figure 3.9**.)

Injuries that are adjacent to coronary arteries must be repaired without occluding the vessel, which can be accomplished by using horizontal mattress sutures lateral and deep to the vessel in a manner that avoids encircling the vessel.

OPEN REPAIR OF AORTIC INJURIES

Ascending aortic disruptions are usually due to a penetrating mechanism and as a whole are rare due to the high on-scene lethality of the injury. They are best approached through a median sternotomy with neck extension for adequate distal control. Small anterior injuries may be repairable by primary closure with 4-0 polypropylene suture, whereas more extensive injuries will require cardiopulmonary bypass and an interposition graft. Blunt injuries to the descending thoracic aorta most commonly occur just distal to the origin of the left subclavian artery. Open repair is performed using a left posterolateral thoracotomy through the fourth interspace, and can be done without the use of left heart bypass ("clamp and sew" technique), though rates of paraplegia are significantly reduced if distal perfusion is maintained throughout the repair. In either case, proximal control of the injury is obtained by dissection of the proximal aorta and left subclavian artery, followed by isolation of the descending thoracic aorta. Division of the ligamentum arteriosum and dissection between the lesser curve of the aortic arch and the proximal right pulmonary artery can facilitate exposure for proximal clamp placement. Care should be taken to avoid injury to the vagus, recurrent laryngeal, and phrenic nerves, whose locations may be obscured in the midst of a large hematoma. A DeBakey aorta clamp is applied between the left subclavian and common carotid arteries followed by occlusion of the left subclavian with an umbilical tape and clamping of the descending thoracic aorta for distal control. The hematoma is then entered and the aortic injury assessed

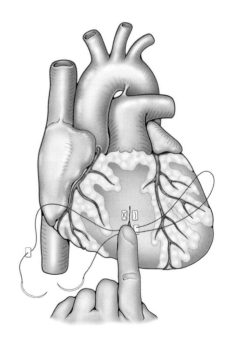

3.9

for either primary aortorrhaphy or repair by interposition graft (85% of cases).

ENDOVASCULAR REPAIR OF AORTIC INJURIES

Endovascular repair is increasingly used for patients with traumatic aortic injury, now surpassing the use of open repair. Endovascular repair offers the potential benefit of a durable repair while avoiding the morbidity of thoracotomy, aortic cross-clamping, and cardiopulmonary bypass, all of which are suboptimal in the trauma patient with limited physiologic reserve and other life-threatening injuries. Even with advancements in open technique and increased use of distal aortic perfusion, at least two meta-analyses have reported lower mortality (8%–9% vs 19%) and decreased paraplegia rates (0.5%–3.0% vs 3%–9%) with endovascular repair.[12,13] Furthermore, though the first 15 years of endovascular treatment for aortic injuries was limited by device availability and required the off-label use of devices originally designed for abdominal aneurysms, the recent development of devices specific for thoracic aortic pathology is expected to further advance this novel treatment for aortic injuries.

REPAIR OF GREAT VESSEL INJURIES

Injuries to the innominate, proximal common carotid, and proximal subclavian arteries can occur secondary to both blunt and penetrating mechanisms, though these patients rarely survive long enough to reach the ED. Median sternotomy with various forms of cervical extension typically provide adequate access for proximal and distal control. The innominate and right subclavian arteries are accessed through a right supraclavicular extension, which involves division of the sternocleidomastoid and strap muscles from the sternum and clavicle. The thymus is divided in the midline and the left brachiocephalic vein either dissected free and retracted or ligated to provide the needed exposure. The right phrenic and vagus nerves—which lie on the surface of the anterior scalene muscle and anterior aspect of the subclavian artery, respectively—are vulnerable during this dissection. The origin of the right common carotid can be exposed by lateral retraction of the right internal jugular vein; however, more complete exposure is accomplished by a vertical extension along the anterior border of the right-sided sternocleidomastoid. Left common carotid exposure can be more challenging along its proximal extent due to the overlying left brachiocephalic vein, which can either be retracted medially while the left internal jugular vein is retracted laterally, or ligated. Exposure of the left subclavian can be suboptimal through a median sternotomy due to its posterior take-off from the aortic arch, although a left supraclavicular extension with division of the sternocleidomastoid and strap muscles can facilitate this exposure. As on the right, the phrenic and vagus nerves are vulnerable and should be identified and protected. For more distal exposure, it is sometimes necessary to resect the medial third of the clavicle.

7. Innominate artery injuries tend to be proximal in blunt trauma and distal in penetrating wounds; regardless, repair can be completed without cardiopulmonary bypass or heparinization, as innominate cross-clamping is tolerated well. If lateral or patch repair cannot be done, then bypass exclusion is performed from the ascending aorta to the distal end of the innominate, with oversewing of the innominate at its origin. (See **Figures 3.10a through c**.)

Injuries to the subclavian arteries almost always require an interposition graft due to the friability of these vessels and inability to adequately mobilize for primary repair. In contrast, common carotid injuries often can be mobilized and repaired primarily, though interposition grafting may be required for destructive injuries. While common carotid clamping is generally tolerated well, heparinization is recommended to avoid cerebral embolization.

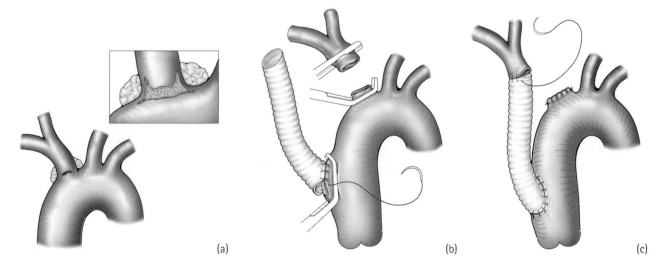

(a)   (b)   (c)

3.10a–c

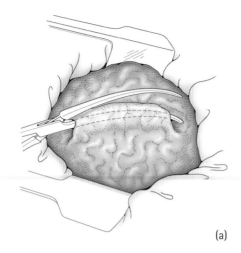

(a)

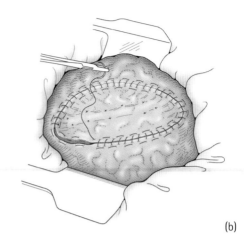

(b)

3.11a–b

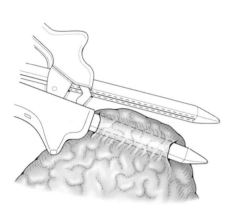

3.12

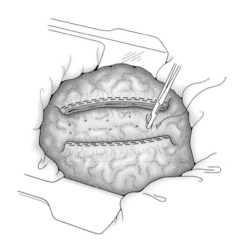

3.13

REPAIR OF PARENCHYMAL LUNG INJURY

Lacerations to the lung parenchyma can occur from blunt or penetrating mechanisms. Chest tube placement with reexpansion of the lung often leads to adequate hemostasis without the need for operative intervention. Massive or ongoing losses, especially if accompanied by hemodynamic instability, require operative control. Anatomic resection (e.g., lobectomy, pneumonectomy) is usually unnecessary and bleeding can almost always be controlled by more limited interventions. Small superficial lacerations can often be oversewn with a continuous monofilament suture (e.g., pneumorrhaphy), whereas deeper parenchymal injuries may require wedge resection or tractotomy.

8. Tractotomy is particularly useful in the treatment of gunshot wounds, where the injury tract is opened using a linear stapling device or between two vascular clamps, and any bleeding vessels or disrupted airways along the opened tract are selectively ligated with 4-0 polypropylene suture. If clamps are used, then the tissue within the clamp is oversewn with 0 polypropylene suture. (See **Figures 3.11b and b, 3.12 and 3.13.**)

Tractotomy should not be used in missile tracts that involve the lung hilum, which are usually best treated by formal lobectomy. Full exploration and control of hilar injuries often requires opening of the pericardium for control of the pulmonary artery and vein. Every effort should be made to perform as limited a resection as possible, as mortality increases with the extent of resection and approaches 100% for pneumonectomy in the setting of traumatic shock.

REPAIR OF TRACHEOBRONCHIAL INJURIES

While rare, tracheobronchial injuries carry a high mortality and can be very challenging to manage. Penetrating injuries have a higher likelihood of injury to the cervical trachea, whereas blunt trauma most commonly injures the distal trachea and carina (within 2.5 cm of the carina 80% of the time). Subcutaneous emphysema may be present on exam and tube thoracostomy classically results in a large continuous air leak without complete resolution of pneumothorax on chest X-ray. Airway management must be undertaken with caution, as careless attempts at blind intubation can worsen the injury. Emergent flexible bronchoscopy should be undertaken, without the use of sedatives or paralytics in awake patients with functional airways, and the trachea and mainstem bronchi must be examined circumferentially to precisely localize the injury. If the airway must be secured, an endotracheal tube can be guided over the bronchoscope and beyond the injured segment under direct vision. Urgent tracheostomy may also be performed depending on the extent and level of injury; alternatively, tube placement directly through the injury itself may be the simplest and most efficient strategy to secure the airway. In general, tracheobronchial injuries that involve more than one-third of the airway circumference should be repaired surgically; in contrast, small injuries that involve less than one-third of the circumference may be successfully managed nonoperatively, especially in unstable patients or those unlikely to tolerate thoracotomy.

Injuries to the proximal half of the trachea are exposed through a cervical collar incision, whereas the more distal trachea, carina, right mainstem bronchus, and proximal left mainstem bronchus are approached through a right posterolateral thoracotomy through the fourth or fifth interspace. Distal left mainstem bronchial injuries (>3 cm from carina) should be repaired through a left posterolateral incision at the fifth interspace.

Devitalized tissue should be debrided and a primary end-to-end anastomosis performed using interrupted absorbable suture (e.g., 3-0 polyglactin) with knots tied on outside of the airway. Mobilization of the trachea may be necessary to ensure a tension-free and airtight anastomosis, and can be done by blunt dissection anterior and posterior to the trachea while preserving the blood supply laterally. Up to one-half of the trachea, and the entirety of either mainstem bronchi, can be resected if necessary to achieve a tension-free repair. For intrathoracic repairs, the suture line should be buttressed with a flap of pericardial fat, intercostal muscle, or pleura, especially if a concomitant esophageal repair is performed.

REPAIR OF ESOPHAGEAL INJURIES

Esophageal injuries in the setting of trauma are usually secondary to penetrating wounds, though they can occur with blunt mechanisms. While iatrogenic esophageal perforations may be successfully managed nonoperatively and some centers have advocated stent placement in carefully selected patients, the rarity of traumatic esophageal injury and the high frequency of associated injuries (88%) make operative management the standard approach for these injuries.

The cervical esophagus is best approached through a left neck incision, whereas the proximal intrathoracic esophagus is most easily accessed by right posterolateral thoracotomy.

The distal third is best approached through a left posterolateral thoracotomy. For cervical repairs, the esophagus is exposed by lateral retraction of the sternocleidomastoid and dissection in the prevertebral plane, with care to avoid injury to the recurrent laryngeal nerve that is located in the tracheoesophageal groove.

9. Once the defect is found, it is essential to visualize the full extent of mucosal injury, which is usually larger than the defect in the muscular layer. Any nonviable tissue should be debrided and the mucosal and muscular defects then repaired, primarily in two layers. For intrathoracic esophageal injuries, the lung is retracted and the mediastinal pleura is opened widely to facilitate exposure, with division of the azygos vein necessary for access to more proximal injuries. Repair is then performed in a similar fashion to that of the cervical esophagus, except that intrathoracic repairs should be buttressed with a pleural or muscular flap (e.g., intercostal, latissimus dorsi). Placement of drains is recommended for all esophageal repairs. Rarely, a definitive esophageal repair is not possible due to extensive devitalization, longstanding contamination, or patient instability; in these cases, temporizing measures, including wide drainage and placement of a T-tube into the esophagus, with its distal end exteriorized to create a controlled esophageal fistula, can be life-saving. (See **Figure 3.14a through b**.)

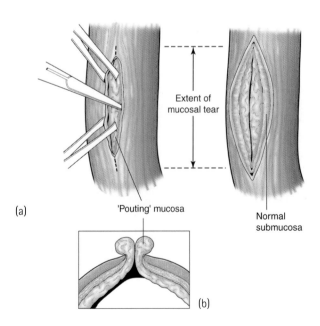

(a)   'Pouting' mucosa   Extent of mucosal tear   Normal submucosa   (b)

3.14a–b

REPAIR OF CHEST WALL INJURIES

Operative repair for chest wall injuries has primarily focused on surgical stabilization of rib fractures (SSRF) in the setting of flail chest, which is defined as three or more consecutive ribs with fractures in two or more places. Several studies, albeit small in size, have found favorable outcomes following SSRF, including reduced pneumonia rates, decreased duration of mechanical ventilation, decreased length of intensive care unit (ICU) stay, decreased need for tracheostomy, and lower medical costs.[14–16] Though these studies mostly focused on critically ill trauma patients with flail chest, evidence suggests that even isolated rib fractures can progress to long-term disability and chronic pain, and that SSRF may have the potential to abrogate this progression.[17,18] Furthermore, simple rib fractures in the elderly can be especially high risk, which increases proportionately with the number of ribs fractured.[19,20] To better define which patient population is at risk for complications from rib fractures and provide an objective tool that may help inform the decision to proceed with SSRF, we devised a scoring system known as "RibScore".[21] The RibScore assigns one point for each of the following anatomic characteristics: six or more ribs fractured, flail chest, bilateral fractures, first rib fracture, three or more displaced fractures, and fracture in each anatomic area (i.e., anterior, lateral, and posterior). This system has the advantage that a score can be assigned immediately following CT imaging of the chest, and does not depend on demographic or other clinical variables, which may not be readily available for all trauma patients on presentation. This timeliness allows immediate risk stratification of patients and facilitates early operative intervention in patients without competing clinical concerns. Ongoing studies are defining the RibScore that predicts which patients will benefit the most from SSRF.

Surgical planning for SSRF depends on a detailed assessment of the fracture pattern on CT imaging. The optimal timing for SSRF is somewhat controversial, and several studies have performed fixation within 1 week of injury while others have waited until clinical variables (e.g., failed ventilator wean) become apparent. As inflammation around the fractures peaks between 3 and 5 days postinjury, and pain from rib movement during respiration can cause progressive splinting, atelectasis, and potential respiratory failure, we strive to perform SSRF within 72 hours of patient presentation. Ideally, patients without hemodynamic instability or other competing operative priorities should be transported directly from the trauma bay to the operating room for SSRF. For anterior fractures, patients are placed supine and an anterolateral thoracotomy incision is used. For isolated lateral fractures of three to five contiguous ribs, an 8–10 cm longitudinal incision centered over the middle fracture provides adequate exposure, whereas a combination of lateral and posterior fractures involving five or more contiguous fractures is best exposed through a standard posterolateral thoracotomy incision. We routinely perform SSRF on all fractures within the operative field, though some other groups have advocated fixing only one side of a flail segment or repairing every other rib in the setting of multiple contiguous fractures. Muscle division should be minimized in all cases. For anterior fractures, the subpectoral plane can be developed to provide exposure; alternatively, posterior and lateral fractures can be accessed by bluntly dissecting and reflecting the latissimus dorsi posteriorly and splitting the fibers of the serratus anterior to gain exposure to the fractured segments. Rib fragments should only be exposed for about 3–5 cm on both sides of the fracture, as excessive dissection of muscle and periosteum can disturb blood supply and inhibit healing. Following exposure of the fractured segments, right-angle clamps are then placed deep between the ribs on both sides of the fracture, and gentle traction is applied until the fractured ends are aligned ("double right-angle" technique). Fixation is then performed using one of several commercially available plating systems. For systems that use screws, depth gauges should be used to select the proper screw length, and a specialized drill and drill guide assist in ensuring holes are perpendicular and at proper depth to achieve bicortical penetration. Locking screws should be used to prevent screws from being displaced. For difficult to reach areas, use of a drill guide is often not possible and a right-angle drill and screwdriver may be required. In all cases, holes must be drilled at a right angle to the rib. A minimum of six screws should be used for each plate, with at least three screws positioned on both sides of the fracture. In addition, plates should sit flush with the rib. Most commercially available plating systems have precontoured plates for each rib; however, these are typically designed for anterolateral fractures and plate bending is often necessary for posterior fractures. For all cases of SSRF, we routinely evacuate any hemothorax that is visible on CT and place a 24 Fr straight chest tube in a position remote from the fracture repair. We also use paravertebral analgesic catheters to assist with postoperative pain control.[22]

Sternal fractures were once considered a major risk factor for occult thoracic injuries such as cardiac contusion or great vessel injury. Prior to widespread implementation of three-point restraints in cars, the most common cause for sternal fractures was rapid deceleration and steering-wheel impaction; however, most sternal fractures commonly seen are a result of seat-belt impingement. Consequently, sternal fractures in contemporary practice are less often associated with severe injuries, and can often be managed on an outpatient basis with oral analgesics. Operative repair of sternal fractures is sometimes indicated for significant displacement and overlap, or when associated with rib fractures deemed appropriate for SSRF, and can be accomplished using principles of exposure and plating systems similar to those used in SSRF.

POSTOPERATIVE CARE

Patients who have undergone operative intervention for thoracic trauma generally require admission to an ICU. Attention should be directed toward resuscitation while avoiding volume overload, which may be facilitated by various invasive and noninvasive monitoring devices and serial evaluation of the base deficit and serum lactate levels. Major hemorrhage is common in patients sustaining thoracic trauma, and trauma-induced coagulopathy can be a significant challenge in these patients. The appropriate use of blood components such as fresh frozen plasma and platelets is essential to achieving favorable outcomes in such severely injured patients. Frequent laboratory evaluation of coagulation, preferably with thromboelastography, allows precise correction of coagulopathy while avoiding the harmful effects of excess blood-product administration. As heat loss can be substantial throughout a patient's initial evaluation and in the operating room, establishing and maintaining normothermia is also critical in the postoperative ICU setting. Many patients will require continued mechanical ventilation for respiratory support. Decision-making regarding the optimal timing for ventilator weaning should take into account the increased risk associated with prolonged ventilator support (e.g., increased mechanical stress on pulmonary repairs, ventilator-associated pneumonia, deconditioning) while recognizing that the multiple-injured patient often has competing issues (e.g., head injury) that may preclude early extubation.

OUTCOME

The outcome for patients undergoing operative intervention for thoracic trauma generally depends on the severity of the initial physiologic insult, the specific thoracic injuries requiring surgical repair, and the severity of associated injuries. Emerging techniques such as the endovascular treatment of aortic injuries lack long-term results, and will need to be closely scrutinized as these repairs become more common. Similarly, the outcomes for repairs for chest wall injuries are unclear due to a lack of high-quality studies comparing operative management to nonoperative treatment strategies.

REFERENCES

1. *ACS. ATLS Student Course Manual.* 9th edn. Chicago: American College of Surgeons; 2012.
2. Ministry of Defence. *Clinical Guidelines for Operations.* Joint Service Publication 999. London: Ministry of Defence; 2012.
3. Blaivas M, Lyon M, Duggal S. A prospective comparison of supine chest radiography and bedside ultrasound for the diagnosis of traumatic pneumothorax. *Acad Emerg Med.* 2005; 12: 844–9.
4. Woodring JH. The normal mediastinum in blunt traumatic rupture of the thoracic aorta and brachiocephalic arteries. *J Emerg Med.* 8: 467–76.
5. Bashir M, McWilliams RG, Desmond M, Kuduvalli M, Oo A, Field M. Blunt aortic injury secondary to fragmented tenth thoracic vertebral body. *Ann Thorac Surg.* 2013; 95: 2161–4.
6. Baker L, Almadani A, Ball CG. False negative pericardial Focused Assessment with Sonography for Trauma examination following cardiac rupture from blunt thoracic trauma: a case report. *J Med Case Rep.* 2015; 9: 155.
7. Harcke HT, Pearse LA, Levy AD, Getz JM, Robinson SR. Chest wall thickness in military personnel: implications for needle thoracentesis in tension pneumothorax. *Mil Med.* 2007; 172: 1260–3.
8. Inaba K, Branco BC, Eckstein M, Shatz DV, Martin MJ, Green DJ, Noguchi TT, Demetriades D. Optimal positioning for emergent needle thoracostomy: a cadaver-based study. *J Trauma.* 2011; 71: 1099–103; discussion 1103.
9. Moore FO, Duane TM, Hu CK, Fox AD, McQuay N Jr, Lieber ML, Como JJ et al. Presumptive antibiotic use in tube thoracostomy for traumatic hemopneumothorax: an Eastern Association for the Surgery of Trauma practice management guideline. *J Trauma Acute Care Surg.* 2012; 73: S341–4.
10. Inaba K, Lustenberger T, Recinos G, Georgiou C, Velmahos GC, Brown C, Salim A, Demetriades D, Rhee P. Does size matter? A prospective analysis of 28-32 versus 36-40 French chest tube size in trauma. *J Trauma Acute Care Surg.* 2012; 72: 422–7.
11. Jones TS, Burlew CC, Stovall RT, Pieracci FM, Johnson JL, Jurkovich GJ, Moore EE. Emergency department pericardial drainage for penetrating cardiac wounds is a viable option for stabilization. *Am J Surg.* 2014; 207: 931–4.
12. Lee WA, Matsumura JS, Mitchell RS, Farber MA, Greenberg RK, Azizzadeh A, Murad MH, Fairman RM. Endovascular repair of traumatic thoracic aortic injury: clinical practice guidelines of the Society for Vascular Surgery. *J Vasc Surg.* 2011; 53: 187–92.
13. Fox N, Schwartz D, Salazar JH, Haut ER, Dahm P, Black JH, Brakenridge SC et al. Evaluation and management of blunt traumatic aortic injury: a practice management guideline from the Eastern Association for the Surgery of Trauma. *J Trauma Acute Care Surg.* 2015; 78: 136–46.
14. Marasco SF, Davies AR, Cooper J, Varma D, Bennett V, Nevill R, Lee G, Bailey M, Fitzgerald M. Prospective randomized controlled trial of operative rib fixation in traumatic flail chest. *J Am Coll Surg.* 2013; 216: 924–32.
15. Tanaka H, Yukioka T, Yamaguti Y, Shimizu S, Goto H, Matsuda H, Shimazaki S. Surgical stabilization of internal pneumatic stabilization? A prospective randomized study of management of severe flail chest patients. *J Trauma.* 2002; 52: 727–32; discussion 732.
16. Granetzny A, Abd El-Aal M, Emam E, Shalaby A, Boseila A. Surgical versus conservative treatment of flail chest. Evaluation of the pulmonary status. *Interact Cardiovasc Thorac Surg.* 2005; 4: 583–587.
17. Mayberry JC, Kroeker AD, Ham LB, Mullins RJ, Trunkey DD. Long-term morbidity, pain, and disability after repair of severe chest wall injuries. *Am Surg.* 2009; 75: 389–94.
18. Fabricant L, Ham B, Mullins R, Mayberry J. Prolonged pain and disability are common after rib fractures. *Am J Surg.* 2013; 205: 511–15; discussion 515–16.
19. Bulger EM, Arneson MA, Mock CN, Jurkovich GJ. Rib fractures in the elderly. *J Trauma.* 2000; 48: 1040–6; discussion 1046–7.
20. Flagel BT, Luchette FA, Reed RL, Esposito TJ, Davis KA, Santaniello JM, Gamelli RL. Half-a-dozen ribs: the breakpoint for mortality. *Surgery.* 2005; 138: 717–23; discussion 723–5.
21. Chapman BC, Herbert B, Rodil M, Salotto J, Stovall RT, Biffl W,

Johnson J et al. RibScore: A novel radiographic score based on fracture pattern that predicts pneumonia, respiratory failure, and tracheostomy. *J Trauma Acute Care Surg.* 2016; 80: 95–101.

22. Pieracci FM, Rodil M, Stovall RT, Johnson JL, Biffl WL, Mauffrey C, Moore EE, Jurkovich GJ. Surgical stabilization of severe rib fractures. *J Trauma Acute Care Surg.* 2015; 78: 883–7.

4

Chest wall masses and chest wall resection

ANNA MARIA CICCONE, CAMILLA VANNI, FEDERICO VENUTA,
AND ERINO ANGELO RENDINA

HISTORY

The first known chest wall resection to remove a thoracic tumor is believed to have been performed by Osias Aimar in 1778. Rehn at the beginning of this century reported a very high incidence of complications and quoted a 20% mortality rate, similar to that reported by Quenue and Longuet in 1989. The first report of chest wall resection in the United States was by Parham in 1889. From the early to the middle years of the twentieth century, limited numbers of resections of chest wall tumors were reported. In 1921, Hedgeblom described his experience of 313 cases, of which 73% were malignant. Twenty years later, O'Neal and Ackerman reported 96 cases of tumors of the ribs and of the sternum. Another large experience was reported by Hockemberg in 1953, who observed and treated 205 cases of chest wall tumors. Respiratory complications and sepsis were the most common and serious problems at that time.

The modern era of chest wall resection began late in the 1960s, thanks to the improvement in surgical techniques and anesthesia, the introduction of antibiotics and intensive care units, and the development of new methods of reconstruction. Extensive resection of the chest wall became possible with more acceptable morbidity and mortality. Furthermore, better understanding of the natural history, biological variability of the cell types, and the use of radiation and chemotherapy allowed for better treatments and improved results.

PRINCIPLES AND JUSTIFICATION

Primary chest wall tumors have been estimated to represent less than 1% of all tumors. The majority of them originate from the cartilage or bone, but they can develop in any of the histological elements of the thorax, including muscle, nerve, and soft tissue. Moreover, neoplasms of the external thorax could be a metastatic lesion from a previously treated or occult primary tumor. Approximately 60% of primary chest wall tumors prove to be malignant. The principal requirement for adequate local control of chest wall tumors remains wide local excision. With the available skeletal and soft tissue reconstructive techniques, even large lesions can be successfully resected with adequate margins. Although the primary purpose of these operations is a curative resection, a significant number of symptomatic patients can benefit from palliative resection. A key element is a multidisciplinary approach by the thoracic surgeon, reconstructive surgeon, medical oncologist, and radiotherapist.

Epidemiology and classification

Although chest wall tumors are uncommon, they consist of a variety of both benign and malignant lesions. They may be primary or metastatic or may involve the chest wall by contiguous spread from adjacent disease, most often lung[1] or breast cancer.

MALIGNANT PRIMARY TUMORS

In adults, the most common primary malignant lesions are chondrosarcoma, plasmacytoma, and fibrosarcoma. *Chondrosarcoma* frequently appears as a large lobulated excrescent mass arising from a rib, with scattered calcification seen on imaging studies. As with other cartilaginous tumors, chondrosarcomas commonly develop from the costochondral junction, and radiographically they may be indistinguishable from an osteochondroma or chondroma. *Plasmacytoma* is less frequent than chondrosarcoma, but the systemic disease, multiple myeloma, is frequently seen to involve several ribs as well as the sternum. The lesions of plasmacytoma or multiple myeloma typically appear as well-defined lytic lesions associated with extrapleural soft masses, similar to most metastatic lesions. In advanced plasmacytoma, marked erosion, expansion, and destruction of the bony cortex is often present, sometimes with a thick ridging around the periphery, creating a soap bubble appearance. *Fibrosarcoma* is the most common malignant tumor of the chest wall arising from the soft tissue in adults. However, in most earlier series, cases identified as fibrosarcoma probably included many that would now be classified as malignant fibrous histiocytoma, as well as spindle cell tumors such as malignant schwannoma or synovial sarcoma. Fibrosarcoma often presents as a mass of soft tissue density associated with necrotic low density areas; foci of calcification may be present. Approximately 15% of malignant schwannomas develop in the trunk, and about one-third occur on the anterior chest wall. Like their benign counterparts, they appear as rounded or elliptical masses adjacent to the rib. Any radiographic evidence of bony destruction is indicative of a malignant process.

Less common primary chest wall tumors seen in the adult population are *osteosarcoma, liposarcoma,* and *angiosarcoma*. In children and adolescents, the most common primary tumor of the chest wall is *Ewing's sarcoma*, which generally presents as a lytic and sometimes expansile lesion of a rib or clavicle with associated new bone formation and a soft tissue mass. Frequently, pleural effusion, fever, and general symptoms are present. Ewing's sarcoma is also seen as the most common metastatic tumor of the bony thorax. Other less common primary malignant tumors in the pediatric age group are osteosarcoma, rhabdomyosarcoma, and mesenchymoma.

BENIGN TUMORS

Approximately half of all chest wall tumors are benign, and the majority of them are of cartilaginous origin, namely *chondromas, enchondromas,* and *osteochondromas*. These lesions are often incidentally found on chest X-ray done for unrelated purposes. Malignant degeneration is rare in solitary lesions, but it may occur in as many as 5%–20% of cases in inherited syndromes such as multiple osteochondromatosis or enchondromatosis. *Fibrous dysplasia* is the most common bone tumor or tumor-like condition of the ribs, accounting for 20%–30% of all benign bone tumors of the chest wall. Fibrous dysplasia probably originates from the bone-forming mesenchyme. The disease usually presents as a painless lytic lesion, often with a localized area of bone expansion, located in the posterior aspect of the rib. Less common benign bone tumors of the chest wall include *eosinophilic granuloma; osteoblastoma; hemangioma,* usually located in a vertebral body; and *chondroblastoma*. The most common benign soft tissue tumor of the chest wall is the *lipoma,* which generally occurs deep in the soft tissue, just outside the parietal pleura, and often with an intrathoracic and extrathoracic component connected by an isthmus of tissue between the ribs. *Neurofibromas* and *schwannomas* most commonly occur in the posterior mediastinum, but they can originate from the intercostal or other nerves of the chest wall. These tumors usually appear as well-circumscribed spherical or elongated masses, causing sometimes widening of the neural foramina, as well as pressure, erosion, and spreading of adjacent ribs. Evident bone destruction indicates a malignant differentiation.

METASTATIC DISEASE

Metastatic lesions are the most common tumors occurring in the chest wall and are seen more frequently than either primary malignant or benign tumors. In the adult population, the most common metastatic chest wall lesions are those arising from lung, breast, kidney, or prostate cancers. With the exceptions of prostate and breast cancers, the majority of metastatic chest wall tumors are lytic. In children, neuroblastoma, leukemia, and Ewing's sarcoma are the most common metastatic lesions presenting as chest wall masses.

PREOPERATIVE ASSESSMENT AND PREPARATION

Symptoms and physical findings

Approximately 20% of patients with chest wall tumors are asymptomatic and their tumors are incidental findings. The most common referred symptom is pain, present in 50%–60% of patients with enlarging masses. General symptoms (e.g., weight loss, asthenia, fever) are inconstant. Physical examination should be aimed at evaluating the tumor location and size and the possible involvement of contiguous organs. Malignant tumors are usually fixed to the bony thorax. The location of the lesion may suggest the histological type of the tumor. Usually, cartilaginous tumors arise along the costochondral junctions in the anterior aspect of the chest. Masses away from the osteocartilaginous structures are usually of soft tissue origin.

Diagnosis

Radiographic evaluation of a chest wall tumor is critical to determine the origin of the mass (i.e., cartilage, bone, soft tissue), as well as an aid to planning for surgical or non surgical therapy. A standard *chest radiograph* can be used to localize the lesion and obtain some information about the status of the lung fields and the pleural cavity (pleural effusion). *Computed tomography* (CT) is the most valuable tool for the evaluation of chest wall neoplasms because of the excellent resolution and the appearance of images in the axial plane. CT defines, albeit incompletely, the relationship between the tumor and the contiguous structures, though distinguishing invasion from simple abutment remains problematic. Examination of the lung windows will help to determine the presence of synchronous metastatic disease. Mediastinal or bone windows provide the best information on the dimensions and density of the tumor and allow for an assessment of bone destruction. CT is also valuable to assess the relation of the tumor to the chest wall musculature, helping in chest wall reconstruction planning. *Magnetic resonance imaging* can add significant information because of a greater contrast resolution for soft tissues and the ability to gain images in multiple planes: it is the gold standard for the study of neurogenic tumors of the posterior mediastinum and pulmonary superior sulcus tumors (Pancoast tumor). Useful data can also be recorded on the nature of the tumor. Technetium-99m whole-body bone scintigraphy should be performed in all cases of chest wall tumor to detect bone metastases or primary osteogenic neoplasms. Positron emission tomography may, in fact, be more useful in determining the presence of metastatic disease. Combined with CT, the Positron Emission Tomography (PET) co-registered scan provides additional valuable information in those malignancies with high metabolic activity.

Current opinion suggests that all chest wall tumors should be considered malignant until proven otherwise, and when possible, wide excision should be carried out. Usually, small lesions can be resected totally without preliminary biopsy. For larger lesions, preoperative histological diagnosis should be obtained. Fine needle aspiration biopsy or core-cutting biopsy is used. The latter has higher accuracy (96%) than fine needle aspiration. If these techniques do not yield a definitive diagnosis, an incisional biopsy is justified and performed through a transverse incision, which can easily be excised at the time of the definitive resection.

Preoperative evaluation

Chest wall resection and reconstruction constitute a major procedure with a risk of life-threatening complications. Accurate preoperative assessment is therefore crucial, because it allows detection and treatment of correctable problems and permits the surgeon to individualize the postoperative management. Risk factors may be cardiovascular, pulmonary, or nutritional.

CARDIAC EVALUATION

In general, the cardiac risk for a chest wall operation is similar to that of any major surgical procedure. A history of recent myocardial infarction or poorly controlled congestive heart failure is a contraindication to elective chest wall resection.

PULMONARY EVALUATION

A good history is essential and should include questioning on smoking, chronic conditions, infections, dyspnea on exertion, and any other symptoms suggesting respiratory impairment. All patients undergoing chest wall resection will have some degree of postoperative ventilatory dysfunction because of the disruption in chest wall mechanics. Routine preoperative evaluation should include chest X-ray, arterial blood gas analysis, and spirometry before and after bronchodilation.

NUTRITIONAL ASSESSMENT

Malnourished patients have a higher incidence of postoperative complications. In general, it is advisable to delay the operation as long as is required to correct malnutrition. Body weight, serum albumin levels, serum transferrin, and total lymphocyte count can be useful.

CHEST WALL RESECTION AND RECONSTRUCTION

Planning the operation is dependent on the assessment of several factors:

- Exact histological diagnosis
- Extent of chest wall involvement
- Previous history of chemotherapy, radiation, or surgical operation at the site of the disease
- Patient medical conditions, performance status, and comorbidities
- Aim of the treatment: cure or palliation

A combined preoperative evaluation by both the thoracic surgeon and the plastic surgeon is advisable to discuss the need, availability, and feasibility of soft tissue coverage in cases of extensive chest wall resection, taking into account the need to draw on alternative reconstructive solutions for repeat resections.[2] The most recent oncological data encourage an aggressive surgical approach even after several local recurrences.

Regarding patients for whom palliative resection is planned and who have an incurable tumor, two main points should be considered: first, although long-term survival is not expected, local excision and tumor control can improve the quality of life; second, patients whose symptoms are correlated to compression of the lung or other organs clearly show improvement in symptoms and quality of life after palliative resection. These findings justify surgical treatment, especially when nonsurgical options are of little or no benefit.

Patient's position

Positioning of the patient for a chest wall resection depends on the location of the chest wall tumor. The patient is positioned and draped on the operating table so that both resection and reconstruction are facilitated. For anterior lesions, the patient may be kept in the supine position, with slight lateral elevation to assist in thoracotomy. The majority of chest wall lesions are most easily resected with the patient positioned as for posterolateral thoracotomy.

ANESTHESIA

Standard inhalation and narcotic techniques can be used for chest wall operations. Selective ventilation using a double lumen tracheal tube is extremely useful, especially to define any adhesions between the chest wall tumor and the underlying lung and to aid the exploration of the chest cavity as well as the resection. Epidural analgesia is usually very useful in the management of postoperative pain.

OPERATION

Tumor resection

Traditionally, the *skin incision* was placed to avoid the tumor, but it is well known nowadays that the incision can safely be made over the tumor to improve the exposure and reduce the vascular damage to the cutaneous area if the skin is spared. In fact, resection of skin and subcutaneous tissues is necessary only if the tumor is adherent to or has penetrated these structures or to excise previous scars, including biopsy sites. The skin overlying previously irradiated tumors should be resected. During the dissection, it is preferable to include one normal musculofascial plane between the skin and the lesion. However, muscle not adherent to the chest wall (i.e., latissimus dorsi, pectoralis major, scapular muscles) should be spared if not involved.

The pleural cavity is usually entered anteriorly one intercostal space below or above the first uninvolved rib, and the intrathoracic extension of the tumor is evaluated by finger palpation. The presence or absence of adhesions to the lung and pleural effusion can also be assessed by this initial thoracotomy, as well as the relation of the tumor to the ribs that will serve as the superior, medial, and lateral margins. Adhesions between the lung and the chest wall should not be violated; they can be easily divided after complete or almost complete mobilization of the chest wall mass.

1. After the chest has been assessed, and the rib above where the intercostal incision was made is judged to be clear of tumor, the incision is extended anteriorly and posteriorly. It is most advantageous to establish the anterior margin as the initial part of the resection. The cephalad and caudad margins of the resection are one normal rib superiorly and inferiorly. The extent of lateral margins is controversial. Usually, 3–4 cm of grossly normal tissue with microscopic evaluation of the margins by frozen section is considered sufficient. The dissection is facilitated by taking segments anteriorly of each rib to be resected, as this permits assessment of the margin and provides additional space to carry out the resection. The ribs are most easily divided using a costotome or a guillotine bone cutter; the intercostal bundle is encircled and divided between ties of non absorbable suture. The intercostal muscle may be divided between ribs using electrocautery. When a rib is clearly involved by the tumor, it should be completely excised with its cartilaginous articulation, because it is not possible to predict the marrow extension of the tumor. Excision of skin and muscle is necessary only if the tumor is adherent to or has penetrated these structures or to excise previous scars, including biopsy

sites. The skin overlying previous irradiated tumors should be resected. During the dissection, it is preferable to include one normal musculofascial plane between the skin and the lesion. However, muscle not adherent to the chest wall (i.e., latissimus dorsi, pectoralis major, scapular muscles) should be spared if not involved. (See **Figure 4.1.**)

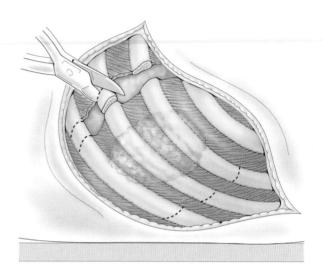

4.1

After all of the rib segments are resected and all intercostal bundles are secured, the portion of the chest wall should be completely free except for any attachments to the lung or diaphragm. If the tumor extends posteriorly toward the spine, it may be necessary to disarticulate the head and neck of the rib from the vertebral body and transverse process and ligate the intercostal bundle at the level of the vertebral foramen. Disarticulating the head and neck of the rib requires incising the cartilaginous junction between the rib and transverse process, placing an osteotome in that space and using the vertebral body as a fulcrum to separate the rib. Segments of pleura and pericardium are included in the resection if involved. Utilizing standard surgical stapling devices, the lung can be divided so the resection will include any adhesions. The diaphragm can be widely excised and reapproximated using mattress sutures. Involvement of the subscapular muscle or the scapula itself can be approached by removing the scapula partially or totally, with resuturing of the uninvolved muscles to the residual chest wall. *En bloc* removal of the tumor is an important criterion for a complete resection.

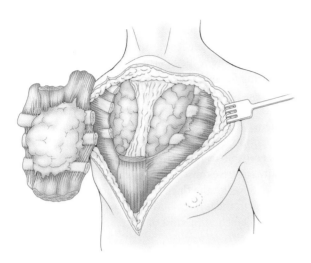

4.2

2. Tumors of the sternum are evaluated preoperatively for involvement of underlying structures. The skeletal resection of sternal tumors encompasses 2–4 cm of rib in addition to the affected portion of the sternum. It is preferable to keep part of the sternum intact if the margin of resection is safe, and it is advisable to save one or both superior epigastric vessels to retain the option of using the rectus abdominis muscle flap for the reconstruction. (See **Figure 4.2.**)

Reconstruction

After completion of the resection, skeletal stabilization is carried out, followed by soft tissue coverage if needed. Basic surgical principles include adequate hemostasis and drainage of the pleural cavity, protection of the pedicle flap from extrinsic compression, approximation of tissues without tension, and measures that prevent air leak.

In planning the reconstruction of chest wall defects based on the criterion of biomimesis, several factors should be considered:

- The structure of the underlying defect
- The location and size of the defect
- The aim of the operation (palliation or cure)
- The general condition of the patient
- Previous surgical procedure that may interfere with the choice of the flap for reconstruction
- Prior radiation therapy that may change the quality of the skin and may require full-thickness resection of the irradiated field
- Prior chemotherapy that could reduce the patient's immune response, making it more susceptible to infection of the prosthesis to be implanted.

SKELETAL RECONSTRUCTION

For limited resections of 5 cm or less, especially when located on the posterior chest wall, no rigid replacement is necessary because usually no physiological effects will occur after the resection. Larger defects can require some rigid support to obtain structural chest wall stability sufficient to preserve the cardiorespiratory function, reduce the paradoxical respiration, and maintain physiological chest capacity in patients with a long life-expectancy. Anterior, lateral, or posteroinferior defects of more than three ribs usually need skeletal reconstruction. Posterior defects under the scapula and the large muscles of the back do not usually require bony stabilization. Sternal and sternoclavicular resection causes significant paradox, and reconstruction should be carried out also to protect the underlying mediastinal structures.

Many different types of autogenous or synthetic materials have been used over the years for skeletal reconstruction.[3] The ideal characteristics of the material for skeletal reconstruction should be durability, availability, adaptability to any size and shape, nonreactivity, resistance to infections, translucency to X-rays, incorporation by body tissue, and ease of use. *Bone grafts* have proved to be very durable. The ribs offer the best bone grafts for chest wall reconstruction, as they are rigid and not rejected by the body. The disadvantages of using autogenous bone grafts are pain and possible instability in the area of harvesting. As a result of the widespread use of cryopreserved bony homografts in orthopedic surgery, interest in homologous biomaterials for reconstructive thoracic procedures has been recently renewed. Their use is still limited by the lack of availability of bone banks and high cost.

Over the years, various *alloplastic materials* have been used, such as metal, stainless steel, tantalum, Lucite, and fiberglass. Titanium implants (e.g., plates, bars) are widely used for their malleability and resistance to stabilize and restore the continuity of the thoracic cage. Although all these prostheses are able to prevent flail chest, they are extremely rigid, in contrast to the chest wall, and this issue creates special problems (e.g., erosion, destruction of the contiguous structure) and even extrusion through the overlying skin or interiorly. Therefore, when using these materials, it is important to interpose biological or synthetic patches to cover the underlying visceral compartment, especially with anterior defects or with partial or total sternal resection. Often, for their ease of use, *synthetic materials* have been preferred, in the form of flexible meshes (e.g., Prolene, Marlex, Gore-Tex, PTFE, polyglactin). These prostheses differ in caliber and construction. Marlex mesh is a single knit fabric, rigid in only one direction and stretchable in the opposite direction. Prolene mesh is a double stitch knit and is rigid in all directions. These meshes can be sutured to the defect margins, tightly enough to be semirigid. The mesh is incorporated into the chest wall by infiltration of its interstices with fibrous tissue. Gore-Tex is a soft tissue patch, impervious to air and water, ideal for a large defect associated with pneumonectomy. PTFE is an inert plastic material with watertight/airtight properties that supplies structural stability and visceral protection. Polyglactin is a woven absorbable mesh that provides temporary support. In recent years, research on implantable *biocompatible prosthetic materials* led to the development of porcine and human acellular collagen matrices. These patches are characterized by natural organic fibrous architecture that allows a physiological incorporation into the host. In addition, their increased resistance to infection makes them indicated in reconstructive surgery of immunocompromised patients and in the replacement of infected prostheses.

3. When a rigid chest wall reconstruction is necessary, a *Marlex/methylmethacrylate sandwich* can be used. Two pieces of Marlex mesh are prepared slightly larger than the defect. Methyl methacrylate is then prepared until it begins to thicken and is spread over one layer of the Marlex to a size smaller than the defect. To complete the composite, the second layer of Marlex mesh is placed

over the methyl methacrylate. It will take 5–10 minutes to harden; during this time, the mesh can be molded to the shape of the defect and sutured to the edges. Muscle and skin closure is then performed.

Seroma formation requiring long-term drainage has been associated with the Marlex sandwich technique. Infection, if it occurs with alloplastic materials, dictates immediate removal of the prosthesis. With either mesh alone or the composite, infections first can be treated conservatively using drainage and irrigation, which is usually effective most of the time. If removal is required after 6–8 weeks, the thick fibrous reaction formed in response to the foreign body can be rigid enough to prevent flail chest in most of cases. (See **Figure 4.3**.)

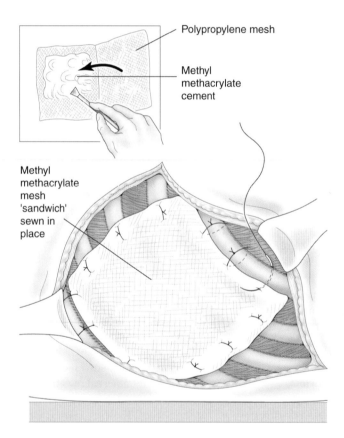

Polypropylene mesh

Methyl methacrylate cement

Methyl methacrylate mesh 'sandwich' sewn in place

4.3

SOFT TISSUE RECONSTRUCTION

After completion of skeletal stabilization, if primary closure cannot be performed, muscle transposition is the optimal method to accomplish soft tissue reconstruction. The most commonly used muscle flaps are the pectoralis major, latissimus dorsi, and transverse rectus abdominis muscle. The size and location of the chest wall defect and preservation of the blood supply to the flap dictate the appropriate reconstruction. Schematically, the thorax can be divided into three areas: sternal, anterolateral, and posterior.

4. In the *sternal region*, the defects are usually full thickness and require skeletal and soft tissue reconstruction because of the proximity of the skin to the underlying bone. The *pectoralis major muscle* is the most frequent flap used in such defects. The pectoralis can be taken simply as a muscle flap or as a myocutaneous flap because of the multiple perforators entering the skin through the muscle. The pectoral branch of the thoracoacromial artery contributes the major blood supply. Release of the humeral tendon of the muscle provides a wider mobilization and rotation. For larger defects located over the mid sternum, bilateral pectoral muscle flaps may be used. When the pectoralis major is not available and one of the superior epigastric vessels is preserved, a transverse or vertical rectus abdominis flap is a good alternative. (See **Figure 4.4a through c**.)

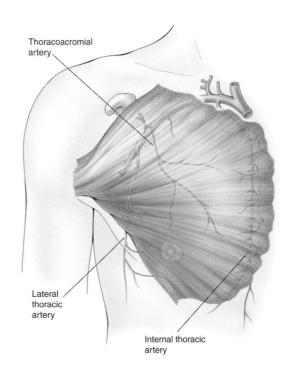

4.4a

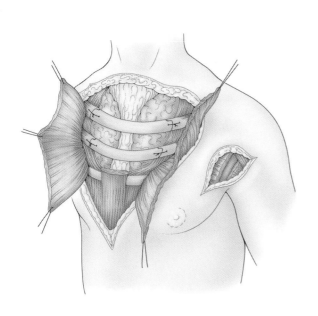

4.4b

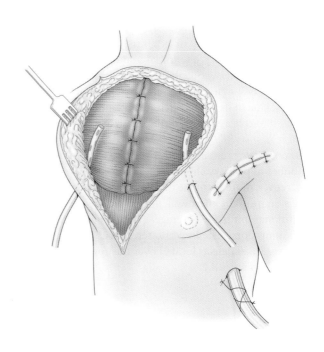

4.4c

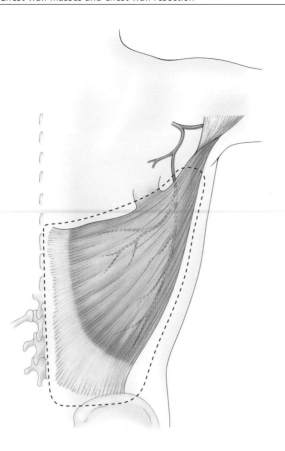

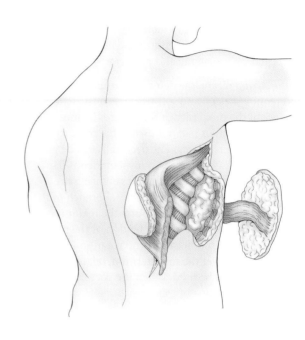

4.5a

4.5b

5. *Anterior* and *lateral* are the most common defects
   after chest wall tumor resection. The muscle flap
   of choice is the *latissimus dorsi*, which can be used
   as a myocutaneous flap or as a muscular flap. The
   thoracodorsal artery, a terminal branch of the
   subscapular artery, contributes the major blood supply,
   but it can be carried on the serratus collateral vascular
   plexus. Due to its long pedicle, a latissimus dorsi flap can
   be used to cover any area of the chest. (See **Figure 4.5a
   and b.**)

6. *Posterior defects* are infrequent because of the small
   number of primary chest wall lesions in this area.
   Moreover, more than one musculofascial layer separates
   the skin from the chest wall, decreasing the need for
   additional soft tissue coverage. The flap of choice is the
   latissimus dorsi. The *trapezius* remains an alternative
   to cover small defects located over the upper half of the
   back. (See **Figure 4.6.**)

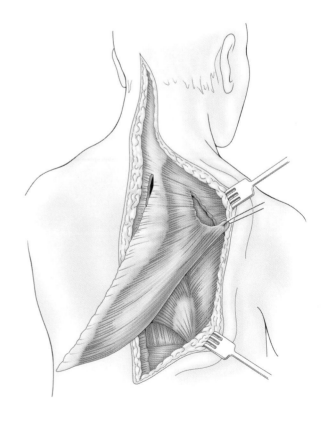

4.6

A. Right gastroepiploic
artery pedicle

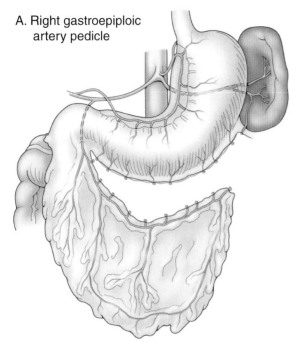

4.7a

B. Left gastroepiploic
artery pedicle

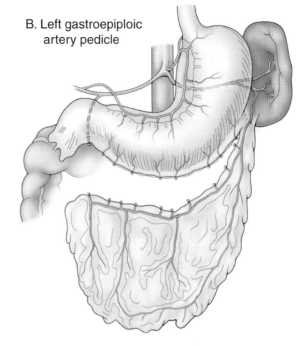

4.7b

C. Bipedicle

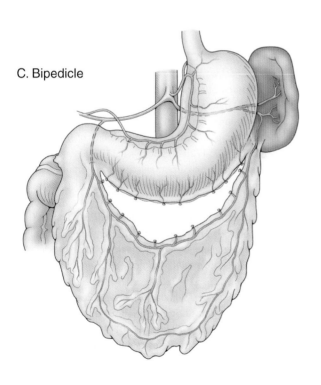

4.7c

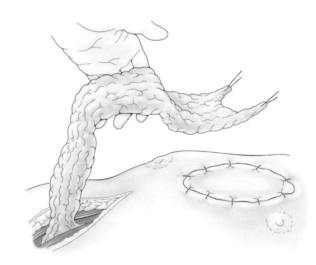

4.7d

7. When muscle flaps are not available or large enough, the *omentum* based on the right or left epiploic vessels can be placed over bone grafts or mesh.[4] This tissue is very vascular, and when adequately mobilized, it can reach any area of the thorax. The main disadvantage is the need to open the abdomen to prepare it. Omentum will not provide chest wall stability. The recently described technique of omental flap transposition, performed through a thoracotomy approach by a radial incision in the diaphragm, avoids the additional laparotomy. (See **Figure 4.7a through d.**)

POSTOPERATIVE CARE

Although chest wall resection and reconstruction constitute a major operation, the postoperative morbidity and mortality rates are low. Complications are usually due to infection and partial graft failure, if soft tissue coverage with a flap has been used. Total graft failure is uncommon. Three areas require special attention in the postoperative management: cardiovascular, respiratory, and nutritional. Common cardiovascular problems are blood pressure irregularities, arrhythmias, heart failure, and myocardial infarction. Hypotension should be avoided and can result in irreversible ischemia of the flaps used in reconstruction. Arrhythmias are common, especially in older patients, and are usually correlated with electrolyte imbalances, hypoxia, and fluid overload. Congestive heart failure is usually the result of fluid overload. Pulmonary management is directed to secretion management and maintaining adequate respiratory function and to recognizing and treating eventual complications. Early extubation, aggressive pulmonary toilet and physiotherapy, pain control and prophylaxis for deep venous thrombosis represent the goals of postoperative care. The patient must be provided with excellent nutritional support; if necessary, supplemental parenteral or enteral nutrition can be employed.

OUTCOME

Once the histological type of tumor has been determined, the appropriate therapeutic plans must be prepared. Most primary and metastatic chest wall tumors can be treated by surgical resection as a first line of treatment.[5] In selected cases, preoperative or adjuvant chemotherapy, radiation, or a combination of both can play an important role.

Chondrosarcoma is the most common malignant tumor, representing 20% of all chest wall tumors. Chondrosarcomas are usually solitary and localized at the level of the costochondral or sternochondral junction. The natural history of this tumor usually consists of slow growth and a risk of local recurrence after resection. The 10-year overall survival rate reported in a series from Memorial Sloan Kettering Cancer Center was 64%; 96% for patients undergoing wide excision, 65% after local excision, and only 14% after palliative resection.[6] This tumor is extremely radio- and chemo-resistant.

Osteogenic sarcoma occurs mainly during childhood and adolescence and is characterized on imaging by typical cortical destruction, periosteal elevation, and extraosseous extension. This tumor is highly vascularized and often accompanied by pulmonary metastases. For these reasons, protocols of neoadjuvant chemotherapy and adjuvant chemotherapy plus radiation therapy have been proposed.[7] Although survival advantages have not been documented, a decrease in local recurrence rate has been observed with a multimodal therapy regimen.

Plasmacytoma represents 15%–30% of all chest wall tumors, presenting most frequently in middle-aged to older patients. This tumor is very responsive to chemotherapy and radiation, and obtaining a tissue diagnosis is the only role for surgery. The majority of patients with plasmacytomas unfortunately either have, or will develop, multiple myeloma. The overall 5-year survival rate currently reported by the Surveillance, Epidemiology and End Results Program of National Cancer Institute (SEER) is 48.5%.

Soft tissue sarcomas of various types represent 20% of malignant lesions of the chest wall. Surgery alone is associated with a high rate of local recurrence (20%). Recent investigations have evaluated the impact of adjuvant therapies (radiation with or without chemotherapy). In a National Cancer Institute study,[8] the disease specific survival after combined surgery and radiation therapy approach was 64% at 5-years. A wide surgical resection margin is mandatory in order to achieve the best disease-free survival rate, as reported by Gross et al.[9]

Desmoid tumors are well-differentiated fibrosarcomas and have a high incidence of local recurrence if not widely resected. In the Mayo Clinic experience[10] recurrence developed in 89% patients with positive surgical margins compared to 18% with negative margins. After radical resection, long term survival rates are excellent.

Ewing's sarcoma is markedly vascular with large areas of necrosis and is considered quite radiosensitive. Despite radiosensitivity, the prognosis before the advent of chemotherapy was poor (5%–15% 5-year survival). Currently, surgical resection is considered the first-line therapy followed by local radiation and chemotherapy. Local control of the disease is usually excellent, and the overall 5-year survival rate is close to 60%.[11]

REFERENCES

1. Allen MS. Chest wall resection and reconstruction for lung cancer. *Thoracic Surgery Clinics*. 2004; 14: 211–16.
2. Mansour KA, Thourani VH, Losken A, Reeves JG, Miller JI Jr, Carlson GW, Jones GE. Chest wall resections and reconstruction: a 25-year experience. *Annals of Thoracic Surgery*. 2002; 73: 1720–5; discussion 1725–6.
3. Rocco G. Overview on current and future materials for chest wall reconstruction. *Thoracic Surgery Clinics*. 2010; 20: 559–62.
4. Shrager JB, Wain JC, Wright CD, Donahue DM, Vlahakes GJ, Moncure AC, Grillo HC, Mathisen DJ. Omentum is highly effective in the management of complex cardiothoracic surgical problems. *Journal of Thoracic and Cardiovascular Surgery*. 2003; 125: 526–32.
5. Warzelhan J, Stoelben E, Imdahl A, Hasse J. Results in surgery for primary and metastatic chest wall tumors. *European Journal of Cardiothoracic Surgery*. 2001; 19: 584–8.
6. McAfee MK, Pairolero PC, Bergstralh EJ, Piehler JM, Unni KK, McLeod RA, Bernatz PE, Payne WS. Chondrosarcoma of the chest wall: factors affecting survival. *Annals of Thoracic Surgery*. 1985 Dec; 40(6): 535–41.
7. Bielack SS, CaRRIE d, Hardes J, Schuck A, Paulussen M. Bone

tumors in adolescents and young adults. *Current Treatment Options in Oncology.* 2008 Feb; 9(1): 67–80.

8. Bagaria SP, Ashman JB, Daugherty LC, Gray RJ, Wasif N. Compliance with National Comprehensive Cancer Network guidelines in the use of radiation therapy for extremely and superficial trunk soft tissue sarcoma in the United States. *Journal of Surgical Oncology.* 2014 Jun; 109(7): 633–8.

9. Gross JL, Younes RN, Haddad FJ, Deheinzelin D, Pinto CA, Costa ML. Soft-tissue sarcomas of the chest wall: prognostic factors. *Chest.* 2005; 127: 902–8.

10. Abbas AE, Deschamps C, Cassivi SD, Nichols FC 3rd, Allen MS, Schleck CD, Pairolero PC. Chest-wall desmoid tumors: results of surgical intervention. *Annals of Thoracic Surgery.* 2004; 78: 1219–23; discussion 1219–23.

11. Smith SE, Keshavjee S. Primary chest wall tumors. *Thoracic Surgery Clinics.* 2010; 20: 495–507.

5

Thoracic outlet syndromes

HUGH A. GELABERT AND ERDOĞAN ATASOY

A VASCULAR APPROACH

Introduction

A renewed interest in thoracic outlet syndrome (TOS) has been evident with an increased number of publications in the recent literature. Advances in standardization of diagnostic criteria and evaluation, advances in surgical technique, as well as formulation of treatment algorithms have resulted in improved results of treatment.

History

Initial reports of aberrant cervicobrachial findings date to the Greek physician Galen (Aelius Galenus, ca. 129–ca. 200) and the Renaissance anatomist Andreas Vesalius (1514–1564), who described the presence of cervical ribs. There was more modern recognition by the anatomist François-Joseph Hunauld (1701–1742), who reported the association of cervical ribs with upper extremity symptoms.

Sir Astley Cooper (1768–1841) is credited with describing symptoms resulting from arterial vascular compression due to a cervical rib.[1]

Spontaneous venous thrombosis of the axillary and subclavian veins was described independently by the English surgeon Sir James Paget (1814–1899) and the Austrian internist Leopold von Schrötter (1837–1908). The term "Paget–Schroetter syndrome" was coined by the English surgeon Edward Stuart Hughes in 1948 in an effort to aggregate disparate reports of spontaneous upper extremity venous thrombosis.

The term "thoracic outlet syndrome" was coined by Peet in 1956.[2] This recognized the common denominator of anatomical compression at the thoracic outlet as the mechanism resulting in the variety of presentations that had previously been separately enumerated: scalenus anticus syndrome, costoclavicular syndrome, backpack palsy, and neurovascular compression syndromes. The first rib was recognized as the fulcrum against which the brachial plexus, subclavian artery, and subclavian vein were compressed.

The surgical approaches to first rib resection then followed. O. T. Clagett in 1962 described the use of posterior high thoracoplasty for first rib resection.[3] David. B. Roos published the initial description of transaxillary first rib resection in 1966,[4] and Robert. J. Sanders described the supraclavicular resection of a first rib in 1985.[5]

Principles and justification

PREOPERATIVE ASSESSMENT

Clinical diagnosis

The clinical diagnosis of neurogenic TOS is based on the presence of core symptoms of pain or paresthesias extending from the base of the neck to the hand. These symptoms are frequently exacerbated by overhead or forward use of arms in tasks such as driving or typing. Physical examination is characterized by sensitivity to palpation or percussion over the brachial plexus at Erb's point. Additional examination findings may include loss of the radial pulse with arm abduction, fatigue or symptom reproduction with overhead stress testing, or upper extremity limb tensioning.

Vascular presentations most commonly include thrombotic events. In the venous system, this includes thrombosis of the subclavian vein with secondary pain, swelling, and cyanosis of the limb. On the arterial side, the presentation ranges from digital ischemia from repeated microembolization to major artery thrombotic occlusion and limb threat.

Testing

The diagnosis of TOS has diverged along vascular and neurological lines. Neurological diagnosis has relied principally on physical examination and clinical judgment along with nerve conduction studies and response to anterior scalene muscle blocks.

Nerve conduction testing has evolved from the initial measurement of conduction velocities to the more recent use of somatosensory evoked potentials across the thoracic outlet and median antebrachial cutaneous sensory nerve amplitudes. These remain limited in their sensitivity and specificity. Image or electrophysiologically guided anterior scalene muscle block with local anesthetic remains the most sensitive and specific test with which to diagnose neurogenic TOS.

Imaging for the diagnosis of thrombotic vascular presentations of TOS has relied on catheter-based arteriography and venography to identify areas of compression and occlusion of arteries and veins. The concomitant use of thrombolysis allows rapid, nonsurgical dissolution of thrombus. At the same time, this allows identification of the site of compression or other pathology within either the venous or arterial system.

More recent use of magnetic resonance imaging (MRI) and computed tomography angiogram (CTA) allow for diagnosis of compression in non-occluded vessels. MRI has been used extensively in the diagnosis of both occluded vessel and neurogenic TOS, identifying features such as edema of the brachial plexus cords and displacement of the brachial plexus by various compressive elements.

Initial management and indications for surgical intervention

Initial management of neurogenic TOS relies on physical therapy and risk-factor modification (most commonly workplace ergonomic assessment and correction). This is often supplemented with medication to manage pain. If this fails to relieve symptoms, scalene muscle block testing is used to provide relief of symptoms and to confirm the diagnosis. Surgical decompression is then the best alternative to achieve symptomatic relief when the conservative management has failed.

Vascular presentations are managed with anticoagulation and thrombolysis. Arterial thrombosis may be effectively relieved by surgical thrombectomy. This is followed by diagnostic angiography and surgical decompression. Surgical decompression of the thoracic outlet is necessary for all vascular presentations where TOS compression of the subclavian vessels is confirmed.

Choice of surgical approach

Transaxillary first rib resection is very effective in decompressing the thoracic outlet for the neurogenic, arterial, and venous presentations of TOS. In vascular cases that require reconstruction of the subclavian vessels, separate supraclavicular and infraclavicular incisions are needed. This is usually not necessary for those who present with venous occlusion but is more commonly required in arterial presentations, which often include the finding of aneurismal dilatation of the artery. Venous occlusion may most often be managed with balloon angioplasty following rib resection.

The supraclavicular rib resection allows for effective decompression of neurogenic TOS. It is limited in that the anterior portion of the first rib is not reliably removed via this approach. For this reason, the *paraclavicular* (supra- and infraclavicular incisions) approach has been adopted for vascular presentations.[6] In this operation, a secondary incision is made beneath the clavicle to allow removal of the most anterior portion of the first rib.

The posterior high thoracoplasty approach has proven most useful for the resection of a residual posterior rib segment in patients who present with recurrent or persistent neurogenic symptoms.[7]

Operations

FIRST RIB RESECTION: TRANSAXILLARY APPROACH
Conceptual approach

The transaxillary approach allows for resection of the entire first rib ("cartilage to cartilage") with minimal need for distraction of the brachial plexus and minimal risk to the phrenic and long thoracic nerves.

In essence, the operation requires identification and division of three muscles: the subclavius, the anterior scalene, and the middle scalene. The rib is divided in its midportion to allow distraction of the anterior and posterior segments to facilitate dissection.

Execution

The patient is placed in lateral decubitus with the intended surgical side up. An axillary roll, bean bag, and pillows are used for padding and support. The index limb (hand, arm, shoulder, axilla, and chest wall) is prepped and draped into the field. The limb is abducted away from the chest by a surgical assistant or a mechanical arm holder.

The incision is placed inferiorly in the axilla, purposely trying to avoid axillary contents, extending from the lateral border of the pectoralis major to the lateral border of the latissimus dorsi. (See **Figure 5.1a**.)

The incision is carried down onto the chest wall. Once in the areolar plane of the chest wall, the dissection is carried up to the apex of the axilla with the use of a Kitner dissector. In the course of this dissection, the intercostal brachial cutaneous nerve is often encountered. We attempt to preserve this by gently retracting or mobilizing by partially dividing entrapping intercostal muscles in the second interspace.

On reaching the apex of the axilla, the subclavian vein is identified. In front of this lies the subclavius muscle ligament attaching onto the first rib. Behind the vein lies the anterior scalene muscle. These are dissected free of surrounding tissue using a Kitner dissector. The anterior scalene muscle is divided over a right angle. The subclavius muscle tendon is elevated over a tonsil clamp and divided.

A Haight–Alexander periosteal elevator is used to remove intercostal muscle from the lateral margin of the rib. The goal of this dissection is to remove the rib along with its periosteum to prevent regrowth of bone.

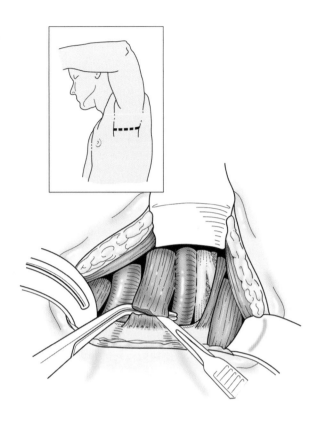

5.1a

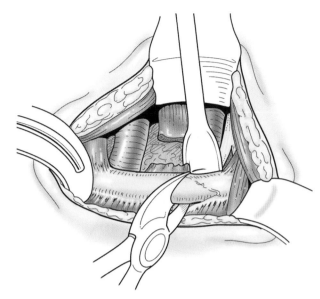

5.1b

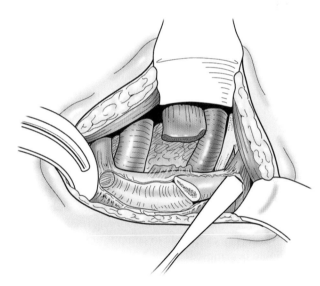

5.1c

This dissection is carried out anteriorly toward the sternum and posteriorly toward the transverse process at the base of the first rib. The same elevator is used to dissect the pleura away from the inferior aspect of the first rib. Finally, the elevator may be used to remove the lateral aspect of the middle scalene muscle from the dorsal surface of the rib. It is not used to remove the more medial portion of the middle scalene muscle, as this would potentially jeopardize the lower trunks of the brachial plexus.

The medial portion of the middle scalene muscle is dissected away from the brachial plexus with a right-angle clamp. It can then be elevated with the right-angle clamp and divided with scissors.

At this point, the brachial plexus, subclavian artery, and vein should be clearly evident as well as the first rib. A right-angle clamp is passed beneath the rib and rotated so that the tip of the clamp is on the medial aspect of the rib and can be used to sweep away any remnant attachments.

A Roos nerve root protector is placed between the inner aspect of the rib and the neurovascular structures to protect these, while Bethune rib shears are used to transect the rib in its midportion.

The Bethune rib shears may again be used to transect the rib anteriorly near the costochondral junction. (See **Figure 5.1b**.)

Using the periosteal elevator, the posterior remnant of the first rib is cleared of remaining middle scalene muscle. The rib may then be grasped with a rongeur and excised back to the articulation with the transverse process. To avoid injury, it is important to clearly visualize the T1 nerve root as it lies inferior to the rib. (See **Figure 5.1c**.)

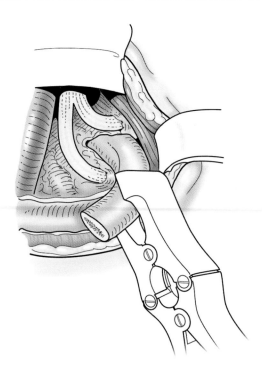

5.1d

An alternative method of removing the posterior rib segment is to use the small box rongeur to grasp the rib and twist the rib to disarticulate it. This separates the rib from the transverse process and allows removal. Typically, a small residual portion remains and may be removed with a narrow Dale rongeur. (See **Figure 5.1d.**)

Following removal of the rib, the last portion of the case requires examination of the brachial plexus, subclavian artery, and subclavian vein to assess for any residual fibrous bands, which may contribute to compression. If identified, these should be removed.

A catheter is placed for intra-incision infusion of local anesthetic. The incision is normally closed over a 10 Fr round fluted drain.

FIRST RIB RESECTION: SUPRACLAVICULAR APPROACH
Conceptual approach

The supraclavicular approach has the advantage of being familiar to most vascular surgeons. The position of the patient is similar to that which is considered a neutral body position with a direct anterior to posterior approach.

The operation essentially requires resection of two muscles (anterior and middle scalene) and removal of the posterior aspect of the first rib. The phrenic and long thoracic nerves are prominently displayed and must be protected. The operation requires gently retracting the brachial plexus in order to expose the middle scalene. For these reasons, nerve injuries are of concern and occur with a significantly greater incidence following the conceptual approach than following the transaxillary approach.

The supraclavicular exposure does not allow for resection of the anterior aspect of the first rib. Accordingly, in instances of venous TOS, an additional infraclavicular incision is also required.

Execution

The patient is positioned supine with a folded sheet beneath the shoulder to reduce traction of the brachial plexus (see **Figure 5.2a**).

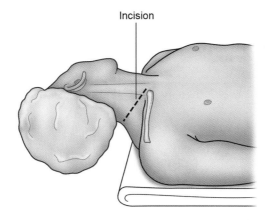

Incision

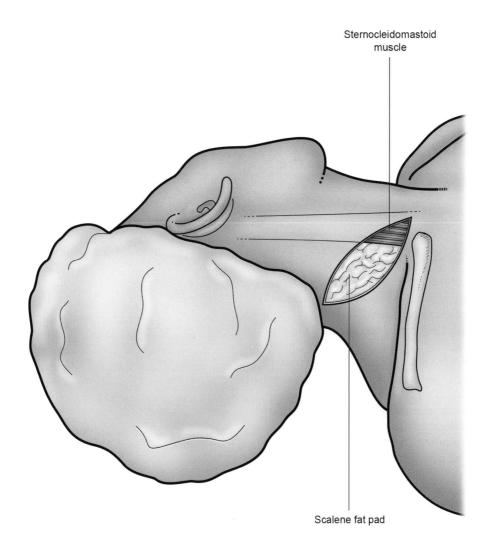

Sternocleidomastoid
muscle

Scalene fat pad

5.2a

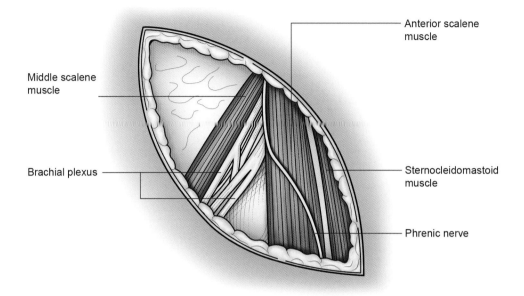

Anterior scalene
muscle

Middle scalene
muscle

Brachial plexus

Sternocleidomastoid
muscle

Phrenic nerve

5.2b

The incision begins at the lateral margin of the sterno-cleidomastoid muscle about 2 cm above the clavicle and extends transversely, directed posteriorly.

A subplatysmal flap is elevated and beneath this the scalene fat pad is encountered.

The fat pad is mobilized away from the lateral margin of the internal jugular vein. Care is taken to identify and seal any leak of lymph fluid that may occur.

As the scalene fat pad is reflected laterally, the anterior surface of the anterior scalene muscle is revealed. It is normally covered by layers of connective tissue. Within these layers is the phrenic nerve. The phrenic nerve will course from the superior lateral margin of the scalene muscle toward the inferior medial aspect of the muscle. A nerve stimulator helps confirm the identity of the nerve. Attention should be paid to identifying and preserving an accessory branch of the phrenic nerve, which occasionally arises from the C5 nerve root. (See **Figure 5.2b.**)

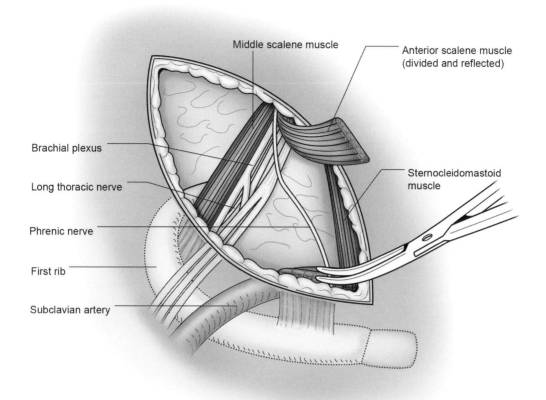

Middle scalene muscle

Anterior scalene muscle
(divided and reflected)

Brachial plexus

Sternocleidomastoid
muscle

Long thoracic nerve

Phrenic nerve

First rib

Subclavian artery

5.2c

The margins of the anterior scalene muscle are dissected with a Kitner dissector and the insertion of the muscle onto the first rib is identified. The muscle should be transected as close to its insertion as possible. It is then mobilized by grasping the cut edge and gently retracting cephalad. Care is taken to protect the phrenic nerve from distraction. Once retracted, the anterior scalene muscle is divided at its upper attachment and removed. (See **Figure 5.2c.**)

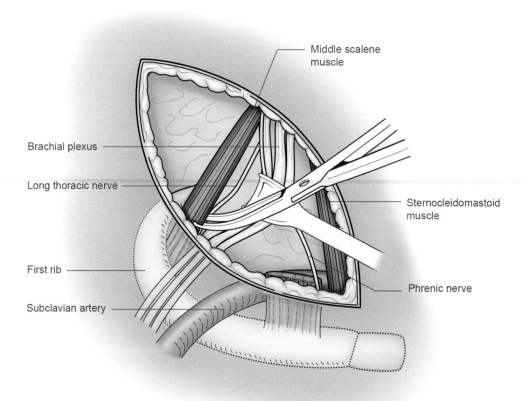

Middle scalene muscle

Brachial plexus

Long thoracic nerve

Sternocleidomastoid muscle

First rib

Phrenic nerve

Subclavian artery

5.2d

Next, the middle scalene muscle is identified posterior to the C5 nerve root and upper border of the brachial plexus. It is dissected away from the brachial plexus with blunt dissection. Attention is paid to identifying the long thoracic nerve as it arises from the brachial plexus (C5, C6) and dives into the middle scalene muscle. The nerve is protected as the muscle is divided with scissors or the Harmonic scalpel. (See **Figure 5.2d**.)

The muscle is resected down to the first rib. At this point, the intercostal muscle is dissected away from the rib with a periosteal elevator. This dissection is carried beneath the rib up to the point where the brachial plexus crosses the first rib and then continued with finger dissection to the point beneath the subclavian artery. Similarly, the pleura is separated from the lower surface of the rib with finger dissection.

The posterior aspect of the rib is then divided within 1 cm of the transverse process using a Schumacher bone cutter or Raney rongeur. This allows mobilization of the rib and may facilitate further dissection of the intercostal muscles and pleura away from the rib. (See **Figure 5.2e**.)

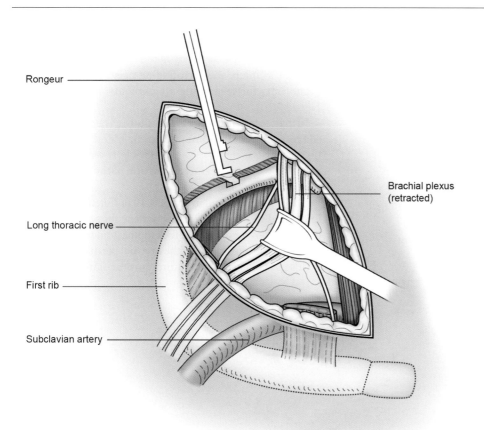

Rongeur

Brachial plexus
(retracted)

Long thoracic nerve

First rib

Subclavian artery

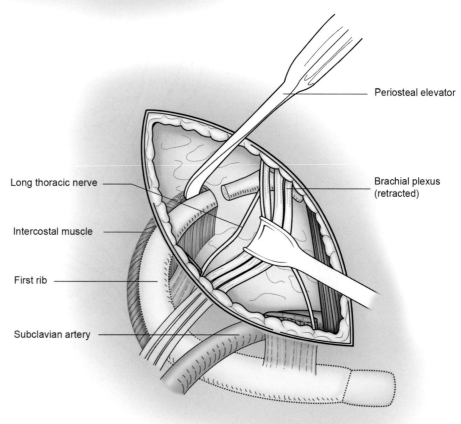

Periosteal elevator

Long thoracic nerve

Brachial plexus
(retracted)

Intercostal muscle

First rib

Subclavian artery

5.2e

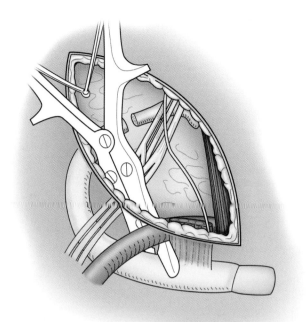

Finally, the rib is divided anteriorly beneath the subclavian artery using a Dale rongeur.

The resected rib segment is then extracted while taking care not to injure the surrounding nerve structures. At the same time, the remaining attachments are divided. (See **Figure 5.2f**.)

In patients with venous symptoms (i.e., arm swelling, congestion, venous compression, or blood clot), an additional incision inferior to the clavicle is required to allow resection of the most anterior portion of the first rib and the subclavius muscle.

The wound is closed in layers. A 10 Fr fluted drain is placed in the bed of the incision. The scalene fat pad is sutured to the lateral border of the sternocleidomastoid to return it to its normal position and to pad the brachial plexus. The platysma is closed with absorbable suture, as is the skin.

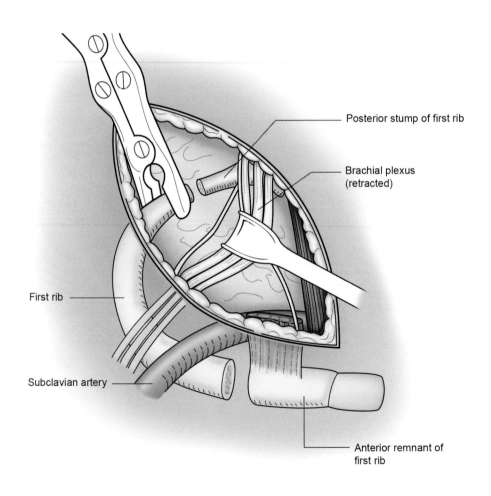

Posterior stump of first rib

Brachial plexus (retracted)

First rib

Subclavian artery

Anterior remnant of first rib

5.2f

FIRST RIB RESECTION: POSTERIOR APPROACH

Conceptual approach

The posterior approach to the resection of a first rib is most useful for the removal of a long residual rib segment following prior transaxillary or supraclavicular operation. It has the advantages of avoiding the reoperative planes of the prior surgery and allowing direct access to the residual rib segment. It has the disadvantage of requiring division of the trapezius and rhomboid muscles—where many patients find a nidus of pain and muscular spasm.

Execution

The patient is placed in lateral decubitus with an axillary roll, padded on bean bag and pillows. The arm rests on a Mayo stand or arm support. (See **Figure 5.3a**.)

The incision is centered over the T1 vertebral body, midway between the scapula and vertebral body. Dissection is carried down to the muscle layer where the trapezius and rhomboid muscles are divided. (See **Figure 5.3a**.)

The posterior superior serratus muscle is resected and the sacrospinalis is retracted. This allows identification of the first rib stump. (See **Figure 5.3b**.)

The stump of the first rib is dissected free of intercostal muscle with a narrow periosteal elevator or cautery. Once separated from the surrounding muscle and tissue, the rib remnant may be resected with a rongeur or transected using a rib shear. It is important to observe and protect the T1 nerve root during this process.

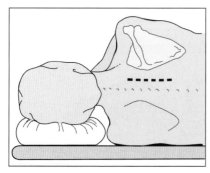

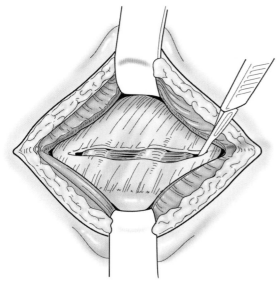

5.3a

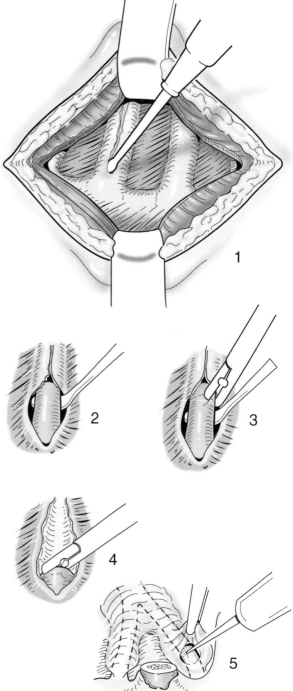

5.3b

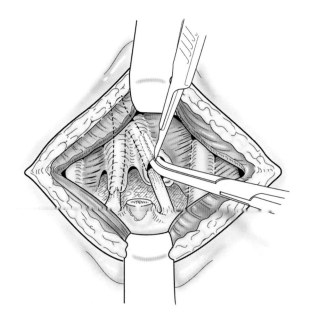

5.3c

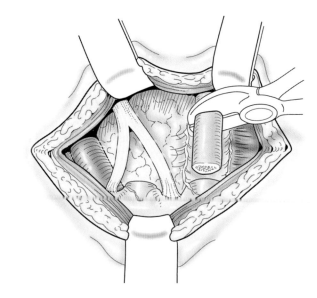

5.3d

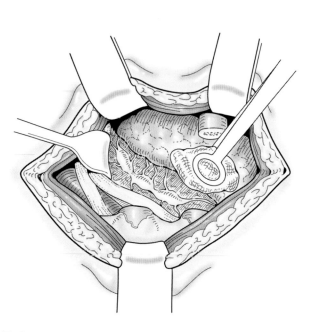

5.3e

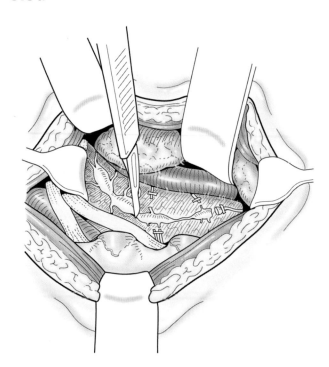

5.3f

The T1 nerve root is identified with a nerve stimulator. Once identified, neurolysis is performed by carefully clearing the nerve of investing scar tissue using magnification and micro scissors. With cephalad extension of the incision, neurolysis may be performed on the C7 and C8 nerve roots as well. (See **Figure 5.3c**.)

If sympathectomy is to be performed at the same time, the incision is extended caudad to allow exposure of the second rib. The rib is separated from the intercostal muscles and a 2 cm segment is resected (head and neck). (See **Figure 5.3d**.)

This allows mobilization of the pleura and exposure of the sympathetic chain (see **Figure 5.3e**).

The lower third of the stellate ganglion is divided (T1) sharply. The T1, T2, and T3 ganglia are removed sharply and branches are clipped (see **Figure 5.3f**).

Wound closure is accomplished by approximating the muscle layers with interrupted figure-eight absorbable sutures. A 10 Fr round fluted drain is placed at the bed of the incision. Skin is closed with skin clips.

Outcome

The result of surgical decompression for neurogenic TOS is greatly influenced by patient selection. Excellent surgeons will experience disappointing outcomes in poorly selected patients. A standardized protocol for evaluation and preparation of patients is essential.

Adjunctive use of video-endoscopy, fiber optic lights, and mechanical wound and limb retractors allows better visualization and safer execution of the surgery. Use of Seprafilm to reduce adhesions is done routinely. Assistance with pain management, psychological support, and physical therapy help from a care team improves outcomes.

The results of surgery for the vascular presentations of TOS are usually excellent. The prompt restoration of patency is essential to improving outcomes. If thrombolysis or thrombectomy is not performed promptly (within 7 to 10 days) restoration of vascular patency and resolution of symptoms are far less likely.

AN ALTERNATIVE APPROACH

Definition

Thoracic outlet compression syndrome (TOCS) is characterized by compression of the important neurovascular structures in the thoracic outlet, resulting in a complex of signs and symptoms of the upper extremity, shoulder girdle region, upper chest, and neck and head areas. These symptoms and signs include upper extremity pain, numbness, tingling, weakness, and other manifestations such as coldness, vasomotor, and sometimes nail-shape changes and swelling in the hands and fingers. Structures compressed include the brachial plexus (most common) and the subclavian vein and artery (less common). The compression is usually caused by either some congenital or acquired changes in the soft and osseous tissues located in this region, which result in the occurrence of some narrowing in this area and symptoms that follow.

It is now well known that at least 40%–50% of TOCS cases have associated distal nerve compression symptoms, such as cubital tunnel; carpal tunnel; pronator teres; and, less often, radial tunnel compression. These associated findings have been attributed to disturbance of the antegrade axonal transportation, causing the neural sheath and distal nerve to become more vulnerable to compression. However, when a combined procedure is indicated and correctly performed, it results in total decompression of the neurovascular structures, creating a larger space for their passage and less chance of recurrence.

Anatomy

Anatomically, there are three locations within the thoracic outlet region that are responsible for the development of compression of the neurovascular structures: (1) the interscalene triangular space; (2) the costoclavicular space; and, less commonly, (3) the subpectoralis minor space (see **Figure 5.4**).

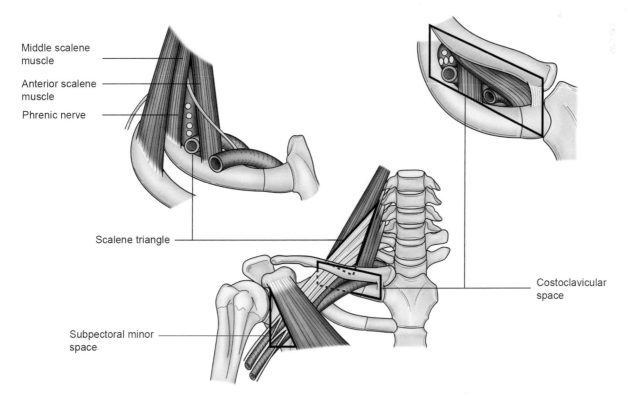

Middle scalene muscle

Anterior scalene muscle

Phrenic nerve

Scalene triangle

Subpectoral minor space

Costoclavicular space

5.4   Three anatomical spaces in the thoracic outlet region can be responsible for TOCS.

Etiology and incidence

Two tissue groups—soft tissue and osseous structures—are associated with the development of TOCS (see **Figure 5.5**). The soft tissue group is the main etiological factor and is responsible for 70%–80% of all cases of TOCS. This group includes congenital and acquired aberrant scalene muscle bundles and their sheath changes; abnormal bands and ligaments; and, rarely, tumors (schwannoma) (see **Figure 5.6**). The osseous group comprises less than 30% of all etiological factors in the development of the symptoms of TOCS. This group includes all bony structures in the thoracic outlet region, including the cervical rib, first rib, second rib, and some clavicular abnormalities that are either congenital or excessive callus formation following a fracture (see **Figure 5.7a through d**). Trauma to the neck, shoulder girdle, and upper extremity is often the factor that provokes the reporting of symptoms, with 70%–80% of patients with TOCS reporting such a history.

The nature of the trauma can be a repetitive or single blow that results in inflammation, swelling, thickening, and spasm in the scalene muscles and their sheaths. In addition, some muscle fiber changes also have been reported.[8] These changes may result in narrowing, especially at the interscalene triangle, with resultant initiation of the classic symptoms.

The incidence of TOCS has been reported to occur in 0.5%–0.7% of the population;[9,10] however, I believe the incidence to be much higher, specifically involving at least 1%–2% of the population. In my experience, nearly 40%–50% of new patients complained of upper extremity pain, numbness, and tingling. Approximately 50% of these patients presented with a history and physical examination that suggested evidence of TOCS. Age at presentation was most commonly in the range of 25 to 40 years old. The oldest patient seen was 69 and the youngest was 10 years old. The female to male ratio was about 4:1. There probably are additional patients who may have mild symptoms of arm pain and numbness and tingling but never seek help.

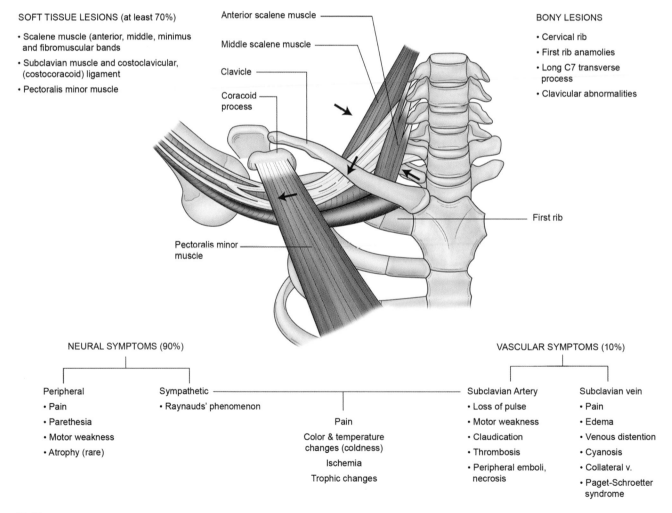

SOFT TISSUE LESIONS (at least 70%)

- Scalene muscle (anterior, middle, minimus and fibromuscular bands
- Subclavian muscle and costoclavicular, (costocoracoid) ligament
- Pectoralis minor muscle

Anterior scalene muscle

Middle scalene muscle

Clavicle

Coracoid process

Pectoralis minor muscle

First rib

BONY LESIONS

- Cervical rib
- First rib anamolies
- Long C7 transverse process
- Clavicular abnormalities

NEURAL SYMPTOMS (90%)

Peripheral
- Pain
- Parethesia
- Motor weakness
- Atrophy (rare)

Sympathetic
- Raynauds' phenomenon

Pain
Color & temperature changes (coldness)
Ischemia
Trophic changes

VASCULAR SYMPTOMS (10%)

Subclavian Artery
- Loss of pulse
- Motor weakness
- Claudication
- Thrombosis
- Peripheral emboli, necrosis

Subclavian vein
- Pain
- Edema
- Venous distention
- Cyanosis
- Collateral v.
- Paget-Schroetter syndrome

5.5 Summary of etiologic factors and symptomatology in TOCS.

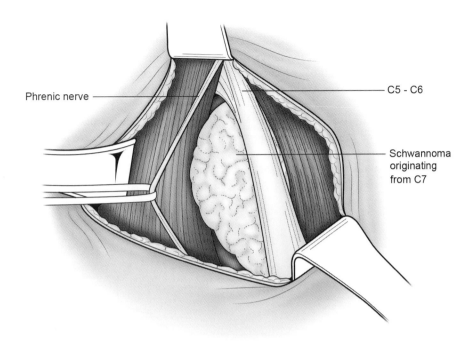

5.6 Schwannoma of left C7 root. Unresolved TOCS symptoms following transaxillary left first rib resection. The tumor was discovered during the scalenectomy. The patient had remarkable improvement of symptoms after removal.

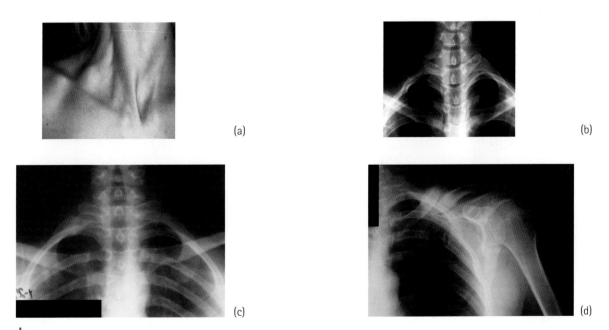

5.7a–d (a) A quite prominent tip of the right cervical rib on the right side of neck. (b) An X-ray of the same patient showing the cervical rib fused with the first rib. (c) Fractured right first rib while playing American football. (d) Fractured left clavicle after an injury during a wrestling match.

Symptomatology

There is a range in symptomatology depending on whether the upper brachial plexus (C5, 6, 7 nerve roots), the lower plexus (C8, T1), or the entire (so-called combined) brachial plexus is involved by the compression. (see **Figure 5.8a and b**).

The lower and combined types comprise nearly 90% of all TOCS cases. Depending on the level of involvement, the patient usually presents with upper extremity symptoms related to the ulnar or medial nerve distribution, in addition to possibly headaches, facial and jaw pain; earache and stiffness; and neck, shoulder, upper back, pectoral, and myofascial pain.

The symptoms increase in severity during daily activities. Upper extremity weakness, tiredness, heaviness, and pain are the most common complaints. Often these symptoms are magnified when activities involve the upper extremity remaining above the shoulder. Sleeping on the involved extremity often causes worsening of symptoms.

TOCS is classified into two groups: (1) neurogenic TOCS, which comprises at least 90% of all cases, and (2) true vascular TOCS, including both venous and arterial types, which involves about 10% or less of all cases. The venous type

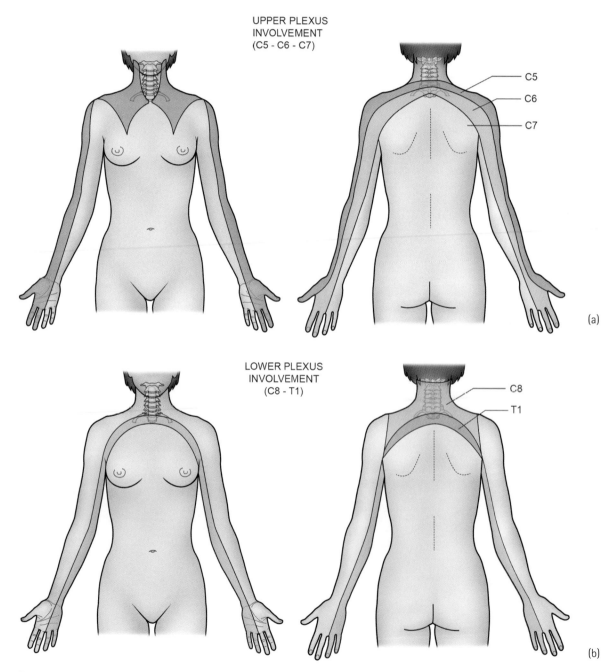

5.8a–b Pain distribution to the upper extremity, upper chest, and neck with upper (C5-C6-C7) and lower (C8-T1) plexus involvement.

occurs far more commonly than the arterial type, comprising nearly 80% of all vascular cases.

The compression on the subclavian vein most commonly occurs at the junction between the anterior scalene muscle insertion on the first rib, and the subclavius tendon and costoclavicular ligament insertion on the very medial part of the first rib. Subclavian vein thrombosis may occur in this area, producing an entity known as "effort thrombosis," or "Paget–Schroetter syndrome" (see **Figure 5.9a and b**).

Neurologists have classified neurogenic TOCS into two groups: (1) true neurogenic, which is often accompanied by abnormal electromyography and nerve conduction studies

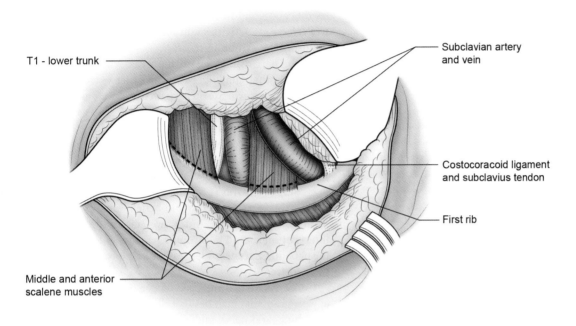

Right transaxillary first rib resection

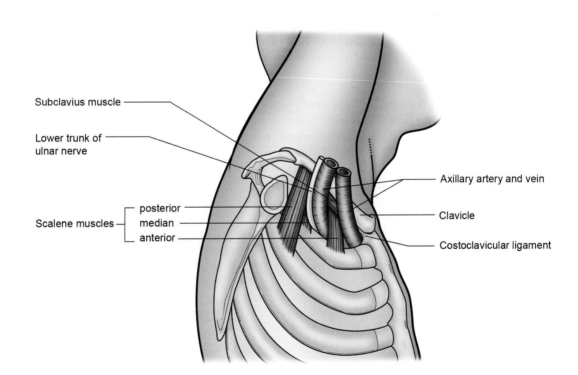

5.9a–b (a) Exposure of scalene muscles, subclavian vessels, lower trunk, and T1. T1, first thoracic root of brachial plexus. (b) Wider axillary view of important structures during right transaxillary first rib resection.

(EMG/NCS), and (2) disputed neurogenic TOCS, which is the more common presentation and which may fail to demonstrate positive findings on EMG/NCS. Routine cervical spine X-ray, magnetic resonance imaging, and vascular studies often do not reveal any abnormal findings.

The physician must rely on the patient's history, subjective complaints, and findings on physical examination. A negative finding on EMG/NCS does not rule out the presence of TOCS if the patient has a history of classic complaints and findings on physical examination. For this reason, I strongly believe that an accurate history of complaints and at least some positive physical findings are the gold standard in diagnosing TOCS.

Examination and diagnosis

The patient's involved extremity should be carefully examined for any temperature or color changes, venous distention, and any evidence of atrophy. It should also be determined if there are any associated peripheral nerve compression symptoms associated with carpal tunnel, cubital tunnel, pronator teres, and even radial tunnel compression.

Both the supraclavicular and infraclavicular areas should be examined for evidence of tenderness and, using compression and percussion, the presence of radiating Tinel's sign to the extremity, including to individual digits. Grip strength in both hands should be evaluated. The presence of bilateral upper back and pectoral myofasciitis should be investigated in addition to looking for any winging of the scapula.

Nearly 50% of patients will have complaints of coldness in the involved extremity. This is usually secondary to the compression of the brachial plexus, resulting in sympathetic overactivity and vasomotor changes with resultant coldness and color changes. In many cases, the diagnosis of TOCS is overlooked and the patient may be treated for reflex sympathetic dystrophy (regional pain syndrome).

Specific tests for TOCS, including neck tilting (reverse Adson's),[11] upper extremity hyperabduction (Wright's test), costoclavicular compression, and the elevated arm stress test, known as the "Roos" test or "EAST," should be performed. The Roos test is considered one of the most reliable. If the patient has no symptoms after 3 minutes of arm elevation, the result is considered normal. (see **Figure 5.10a through e**).

In 2008, medial antebrachial cutaneous nerve measurements for the diagnosis of neurogenic TOCS were reported by Machanic and Sanders and this has proven to be a fairly reliable technique to confirm the diagnosis of neurogenic TOCS.[12]

Generally, not much emphasis is given to the weakness of the extremity and associated myofascial trigger points in the upper back and pectoral area. The chance of alleviating upper extremity symptoms with surgery is about 80% or greater, but alleviation of the symptomatic myofascial trigger points only occurs in about 50% of patients, even when considering all existing treatment modalities.

Treatment

CONSERVATIVE

Although surgery for TOCS often provides relief by substantially reducing the arm and hand symptoms, the chronic upper back myofascial pain and upper extremity weakness remain the most important factors in preventing patients from returning to their original activities. In many cases, the myofascial pain and weakness are present well before the patient consults a physician seeking symptomatic relief. Job modification and work restriction, such as avoiding repetitive strenuous activities and limiting weight lifting are the mainstays for symptom relief.

As the patient may guard the weak symptomatic upper extremity, they may over use the other extremity, which carries an approximate 50% chance of developing a similar problem to the abnormal extremity.

Before planning any surgical intervention, the patient should follow a regimen of conservative measures, such as job modification, physical therapy, and medication. If the patient has a long history of complaints and physical findings compatible with TOCS that have been present for several months or years, limited or no benefit should be expected from physical therapy. Under those circumstances, surgical intervention should be strongly recommended, especially if the patient has some evidence of muscle atrophy and swelling in the extremity.

Conservative treatment involves a directed physical therapy program that includes first rib relaxation, scalene muscle stretching, and nerve-gliding exercises. This remains somewhat controversial, as many physicians are of the opinion that physical therapy can not cure patients with well-established TOCS.

Markedly painful myofascial trigger points can be treated with injections of long-lasting local anesthetics combined with a low dose of steroids. For example, depending on the size of the patient, 20–30 mL of 0.5% Marcaine and 2–3 mL of 10% Kenalog can be injected into multiple painful trigger points. Some patients may require repeat injections several weeks or a few months apart.

Other modalities include proper postural training, muscle relaxants, nonsteroidal anti-inflammatory agents, moist heat in chronic cases, and moist cold packs and cold spray in acute cases. In addition, ultrasound with phonophoresis and iontophoresis, and transcutaneous electrical nerve stimulation can be used for very symptomatic myofascial trigger points.

Anterior scalene muscle injection, which involves injecting the muscle about 3.8 cm above the clavicle using a 25-gauge needle with 5–7 mL of 0.5% Marcaine and 1 mL Celestone, or 1 mL of 10% Kenalog may also be tried depending on the location of the painful point.[9] If the injection is effective, the symptomatic relief is generally temporary, and so can be repeated within a few weeks.

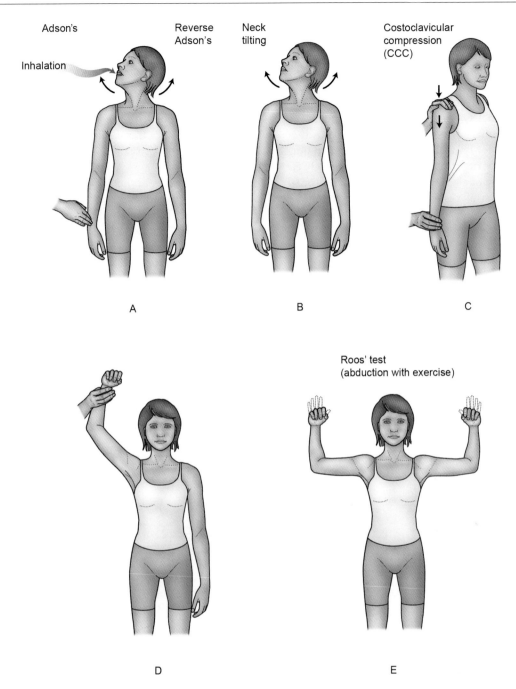

Adson's   Reverse   Neck
           Adson's   tilting   Costoclavicular
                                                 compression
Inhalation   (CCC)

A   B   C

                    Roos' test
                    (abduction with exercise)

D   E

5.10a–e Tests used for diagnosis of TOCS: (a) Adson's, reverse Adson's; (b) neck tilting (tilting the neck to the opposite side of the symptomatic extremity); (c) costoclavicular compression test; (d) Wright's test (hyperabduction); (e) the Roos elevated arm stress test (abduction with exercise up to 3 minutes).

SURGICAL

We no longer recommend nor do we employ anterior scalenectomy because of the high rate of recurrence, which approaches 60%. Transcervical first rib resection is more difficult, carries a higher risk of injury to the subclavian vein, and if the rib is not fully excised there is a high likelihood of recurrent symptoms of TOCS. In a true venous vascular TOCS, where the subclavian vein is compressed, complete division of the costocoracoid ligament and subclavius tendon is difficult and can be problematic (see **Figure 5.9a and b**). The T1 nerve root also is at risk for injury during this approach. For these reasons, some surgeons intentionally open the pleura and retract the lung for easier removal of the first rib. This may cause an increase in morbidity and a resultant longer recovery time.

For true venous vascular TOCS, some surgeons occasionally perform first rib resection via a video-assisted thoracoscopic surgery (VATS) approach. VATS removal of the scalene muscles carries a significant risk because of the possibility of injury to the brachial plexus and other important nerves in this area; therefore, thoracoscopic scalenectomy has not been attempted. Robot-assisted removal of the first rib is another minimally invasive approach that is currently used in only a few centers; it markedly increases the cost and almost assuredly carries with it a negative contribution margin.

Formerly, transaxillary removal of the first rib was the procedure of choice for lower TOCS cases; however, in our experience, it is very rare to see pure lower type TOCS. Usually, 90% or more of all TOCS cases present with combined upper and lower plexus involvement. In my opinion, the main indication for isolated transaxillary first rib resection is when there are changes in the bony structures within the thoracic outlet, such as fracture of the first rib and clavicular head with excessive callous formation (see **Figure 5.7c and d**); there is a symptomatic cervical rib of more than 2.5 cm; or there is a bifid first rib. Fused first and second ribs are associated with classic symptomatology. In addition, pure subclavian vein compression and recurrent subclavian vein thrombosis without any symptoms of concomitant brachial plexus compression may also be indications for this approach. The presence of any neurological symptoms may require transcervical scalenectomy under the same anesthetic.

My current knowledge and experience with TOCS, acquired over many years, has lead me to prefer a transcervical anterior and middle scalenectomy because soft tissue changes in the thoracic outlet comprise at least 70% or more of the etiological factors in the development of neurogenic TOCS (see **Figure 5.5**). Also, very large muscular and excessively overweight patients are ideal candidates for this type of intervention, since transaxillary first rib resection carries significant risk and also can be quite difficult to perform on these patients.

Following injuries to the neck, shoulder girdle, or to the upper extremity, changes may occur in the scalene muscles, such as swelling, inflammation due to scarring, spasm, and some thickening in those tissues that ensheathe the scalene muscles. Even fiber changes and increased connective tissue within the muscle have been reported.[8] Almost 90% of these cases involve the entire brachial plexus thus involving nerve roots from C5 to T1 to varying degrees. These kinds of injuries are quite common, but the development of TOCS symptoms remains relatively rare in these patients.

The beginning of TOCS symptoms following these types of injuries can be explained on the basis of preexisting congenital narrowing in the thoracic outlet, especially at the interscalene space, and the presence of congenital bands, muscles, cervical ribs, and thick scalene muscles and their

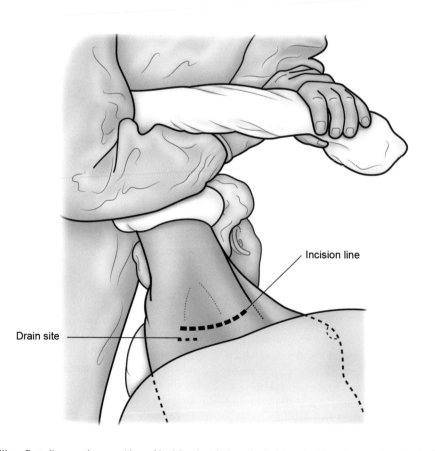

5.11 Right transaxillary first rib resection; marking of incision just below the hairline, holding the arm in wrist lock position.

sheaths. Following a traumatic injury such as major whiplash or repetitive strenuous injury, additional changes will take place in the thoracic outlet area. It is these changes that most likely serve as the triggering factor for the development of TOCS because they result in additional narrowing of the space with resultant pressure on the brachial plexus and, at times, on the subclavian vessels.[13]

Combined transaxillary first rib resection and transcervical anterior and middle scalenectomy

After performing more than 700 first rib resections and nearly 200 transcervical scalenectomies prior to 1989, and more than 850 transaxillary first rib resections combined with immediate transcervical anterior and middle scalenectomies in the following 22 years, I strongly believe if the patient's physical condition is suitable (i.e. they are not very muscular or obese) using this combined procedure provides total decompression of the thoracic outlet, creating a larger space for the neurovascular structures to easily pass through, and decreases the chance of developing recurrent symptoms.

Following transaxillary removal of the first rib, the scalenectomy can be accomplished with greater ease, since scalene muscle insertions to the first rib have already been divided as part of the first rib resection.

Technique of transaxillary first rib resection

Under general anesthesia, the patient is placed in the lateral decubitus position. With the wristlock position maintained by an assistant (see **Figure 5.11**), a curvilinear incision is made along the inferior aspect of the axilla and the dissection carried down on the chest wall below the axillary fat pad, specifically avoiding this lymphatically rich region. At the superior aspect of the operative field, the first rib and subclavian vein can be visualized. By gently reflecting the areolar tissue superiorly, adequate exposure of the first rib, subclavian vein, anterior scalene muscle, subclavian artery, lower cord of the brachial plexus, and the middle scalene insertion on the first rib can be achieved clearly (see **Figures 5.9a and b, and 5.12**).

Attention is then directed to the anterior portion of the first rib, which is removed first. Partial and, at times, nearly complete division of the pectoralis minor muscle facilitates exposure in this area. Then the anterior scalene muscle is divided just superior to the first rib by inserting a right angle clamp around the muscle and cutting with scissors (see **Figures 5.12 through 5.14**). Next, the subclavian vein is gently reflected superiorly and the subclavius tendon and costocoracoid ligament are divided just over the first rib by passing rib stripper a little beyond the costochondral

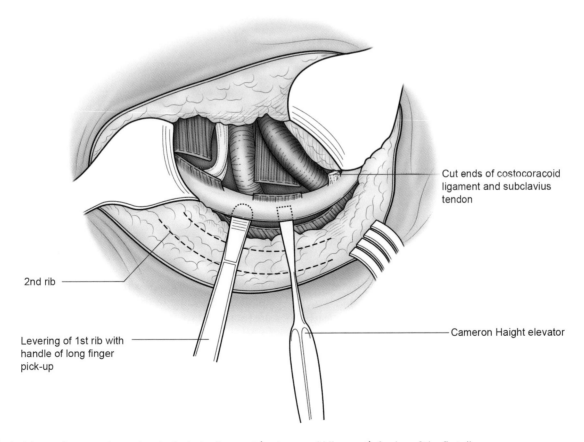

Cut ends of costocoracoid ligament and subclavius tendon

2nd rib

Levering of 1st rib with handle of long finger pick-up

Cameron Haight elevator

5.12   Incising scalene muscles and costoclavicular ligament (costocoracoid ligament), freeing of the first rib.

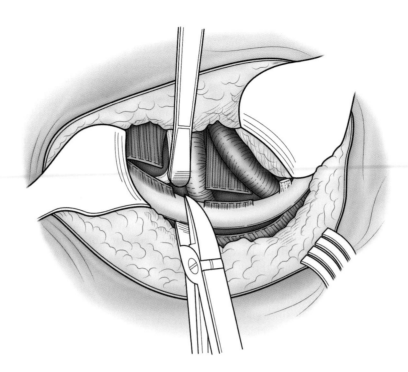

5.13 Cutting the right first rib near its middle area.

junction. This is important for the patient who has subclavian vein compression, especially one who has subclavian vein thrombosis. Then, the inferior border of the rib is cleared until passing beyond the costochondral junction. After clearing and dissecting of the posterior periosteum, the rib is cut with a special angled first rib cutter. Further dissection is carried out along both the upper and lower border of the first rib posteriorly, stripping off the periosteum (see **Figure 5.14**). The dissection is carried out approximately 1 cm beyond the costochondral junction and then this portion of the first rib is avulsed from the costochondral junction. If avulsion is not possible (it usually is possible in most cases), the first rib is cut at or very close to the costochondral junction. The tips are rongeured so no sharp edges remain.

Attention is then directed to the posterior portion of the rib (see **Figure 5.15**), and the middle scalene muscle insertion is divided, staying close to the rib. Next, the intercostal muscles are divided and stripped along the inferior border of the rib. Sometimes division and stripping the insertions of the first, and even second, digitations of the serratus anterior scalene muscle are needed, especially in patients who have prominent thick digitations.

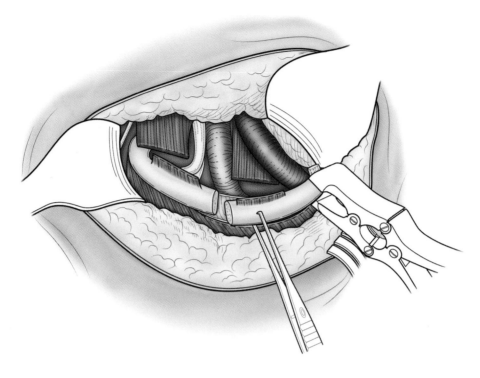

5.14 Removal of the anterior part of the first rib.

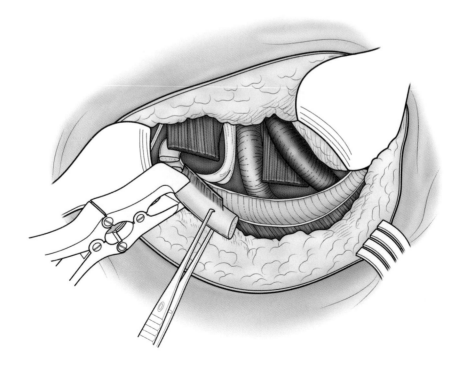

5.15 Removal of the posterior part of the first rib. The remaining posterior portion of the first rib is removed by using a first rib rongeur. Normally, no more than 1 cm of the first rib should remain.

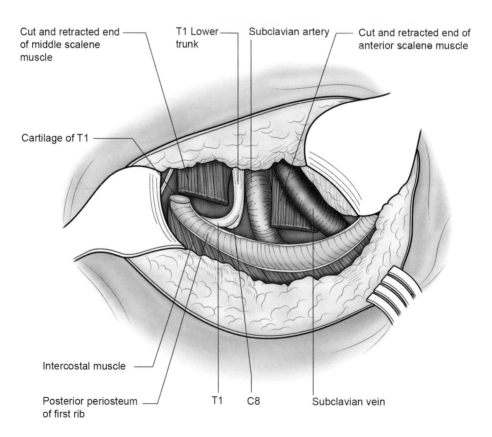

Intercostal brachial cutaneous nerve

Lower trunk

Subclavian artery

Remnant of first rib

Posterior periosteum of first rib

Intercostal muscle

Subclavian vein

5.16 Rongeuring of the very posterior portion of the first rib with first rib rongeur, first using Sauerbruch rongeur then smaller Weck rongeur.

Cut and retracted end of middle scalene muscle

T1 Lower trunk

Subclavian artery

Cut and retracted end of anterior scalene muscle

Cartilage of T1

Intercostal muscle

Posterior periosteum of first rib

T1

C8

Subclavian vein

5.17 View following about 90% resection of the right first rib. Visible important structures: lower trunk of brachial plexus, C8, T1, and subclavian artery and vein.

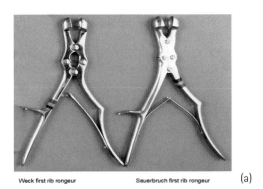

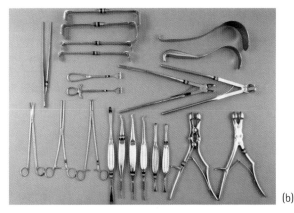

Weck first rib rongeur   Sauerbruch first rib rongeur   (a)

(b)

5.18a–b   (a) Weck and Sauerbruch rongeurs. (b) Major instruments used during a first rib resection.

This posterior part of the first rib is elevated with a Kocher clamp and further dissection is carried out posteriorly, as close as possible to the junction of the first rib to the transverse process of T1. Then the rib is cut and removed or, more appropriately, disarticulated. If rib remains attached to the transverse process, a rongeur is used to remove the piece that remains attached. Recall that the first rib inserts between the C8 and T1 nerve roots, both of which should be easily visible. No more than 1 cm of the posterior part of the first rib should remain (see **Figures 5.16, 5.17, and 5.18a and b**).

Technique of transcervical scalenectomy

Transcervical scalenectomy is usually performed in two stages to include both the anterior and the middle scalene muscle. With the patient in the supine position, the back and head are elevated nearly 40 degrees and a long piece of thick foam (20 × 10 cm) is placed under and across the shoulders to keep the neck moderately hyperextended and turned toward the opposite direction. The arms are kept crossed and taped on the lower anterior chest wall. The skin incision is made, ideally along a crease approximately 1.5–2.0 cm above the clavicle (see **Figure 5.19a**).

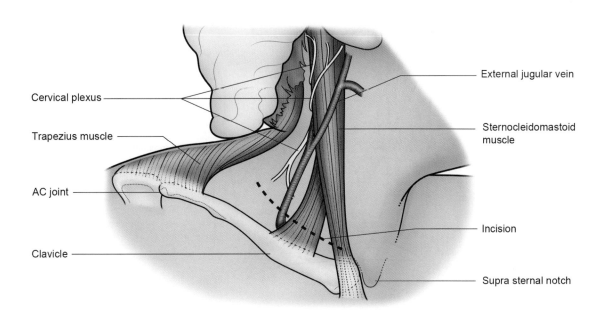

Cervical plexus

Trapezius muscle

AC joint

Clavicle

External jugular vein

Sternocleidomastoid muscle

Incision

Supra sternal notch

5.19a   Skin marking with detailed structures.

Next, proximal and distal full thickness skin flaps are elevated in a subplatysmal plane. Approximately two-thirds of the clavicular insertion of the sternocleidomastoid muscle is divided slightly superior to the clavicle and the prescalene fatty tissue is exposed. The omohyoid muscle is divided (see **Figure 5.19b and c**). The transverse cervical artery and accompanying vein are dissected, ligated, and divided. Next, the prescalene fatty tissue is divided longitudinally near its middle area by staying about 2 cm away from the internal jugular vein. The divided fatty tissue is elevated and reflected toward both sides, exposing the anterior scalene muscle, the upper trunk of the brachial plexus (C5-C6), and a portion of the middle scalene muscle. Next, the phrenic nerve is carefully exposed as it crosses the anterior scalene muscle from a lateral to medial direction, starting at C5 and extending to the lower medial side of the muscle. Careful dissection of the phrenic nerve, leaving some adipose tissue around the nerve, is quite important to keep its vascularity intact. A Silastic vascular loop is passed around the nerve for gentle intermittent traction and additional dissection of the nerve is carried out (see **Figure 5.20a and b**).

The scalenectomy is clearly facilitated following completion of the transaxillary first rib resection. The cut end of the anterior scalene muscle is gently pulled upward to expose the subclavian artery. Following further elevation of the muscle, additional dissection is carried out along the brachial plexus on the lateral side, the ascending cervical artery on the medial side, and the anterior scalene muscle sheath on the posterior

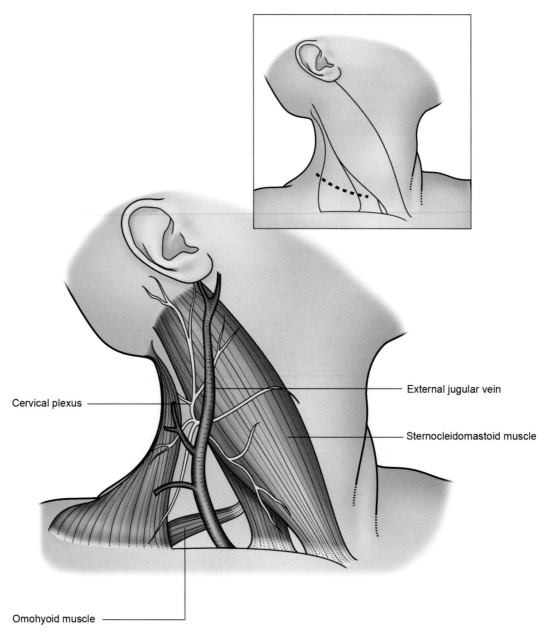

Cervical plexus

External jugular vein

Sternocleidomastoid muscle

Omohyoid muscle

5.19b Right transcervical anterior and middle scalenectomy: marking of incision and superficial anatomy. Inset shows incision mark.

aspect. When the junction between the phrenic nerve and the C5 nerve root is reached, additional dissection is carried out inferior to the junction, and the muscle is pulled down and away from the junction and cut with scissors, allowing it to be freed from the phrenic nerve (see **Figure 5.20a and b**).

Next, the exposed fibro fatty posterior sheath of the anterior scalene muscle is dissected and removed. Then full exposure of the C5, C6, and C7 nerve roots becomes apparent. At the inferior aspect of the operative field, the dorsal scapular artery (also called the "deep transverse cervical artery"), which is present in most cases, can be seen (see **Figure 5.20a and b**). To better visualize the inferior part of the brachial plexus (C8 and T1), this artery should be ligated and divided. If the scalenectomy is to be done as a primary operation

(see **Figure 5.20a and b**), the anterior scalene muscle is first divided at its middle portion and, while lifting the muscle, small cuts of the muscle are made until the subclavian artery becomes visible. After full exposure of the artery is achieved, while staying very close to the distal part of the anterior scalene muscle, further dissection is carried out and this portion of the muscle is removed. On the left side of the neck, care should be taken to avoid the thoracic duct, which terminates in the subclavian vein near the junction of the internal jugular vein. Removal of the proximal part of the anterior scalene muscle is performed as previously described above in the section on "Technique of transaxillary first rib resection".

The next step is the middle scalenectomy. The lateral part of the prescalene fat pad is exposed and even further lateral

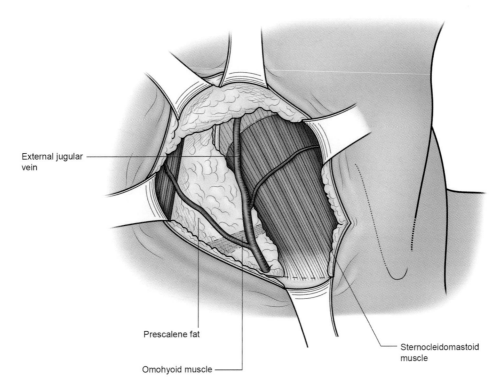

External jugular vein

Prescalene fat

Omohyoid muscle

Sternocleidomastoid muscle

5.19c Superficial anatomy after raising upper and lower flaps including skin and platysma muscle.

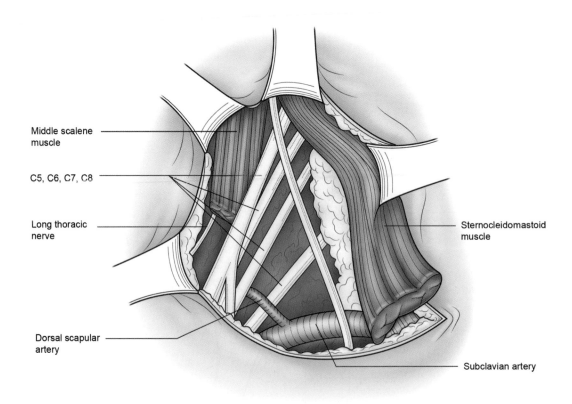

5.20a   Division of most of the clavicular head of the sternocleidomastoid muscle, mobilization of the phrenic nerve, and removal of the anterior scalene muscle.

5.20b   Completion of scalenectomy; 80%–90% of the anterior and about 50% of the middle scalene muscles (distal half) have been removed. C5, C6, C7, and C8 cervical roots of the brachial plexus; T1, first thoracic root of the brachial plexus.

dissection is required to expose the middle scalene muscle clearly. First, the long thoracic nerve should be exposed (see **Figure 5.20b**). This is usually located at the lateral border of the muscle and leaves the muscle at the junction of the middle and lower third.

Following first rib resection, the sheath of the middle scalene muscle is exposed, opened, and divided, allowing the lower end of the muscle to be clearly seen. The long thoracic nerve is visualized and preserved. If a dorsal scapular artery is present, it should be re-ligated and divided, as this will make dissection and removal of at least 50% of the muscle easier.

If the scalenectomy is the only procedure to be performed, first, the lower part of the middle scalene should be exposed and the long thoracic nerve located. Next, the inferior portion of the middle scalene is elevated and pulled proximally, then it is partially divided as low as possible near its insertion to the first rib. The first rib is exposed (see **Figures 5.21 through 5.23**).

During this part of the operation, some intermittent traction on the brachial plexus is carried out using a large right-angle clamp (see **Figures 5.21 through 5.23**). A few remaining tendinous insertions of the middle scalene along the concave medial edge of the first rib are divided.

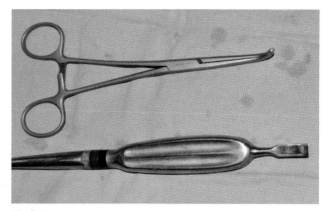

5.21   Long right-angle clamp and small rib scraper.

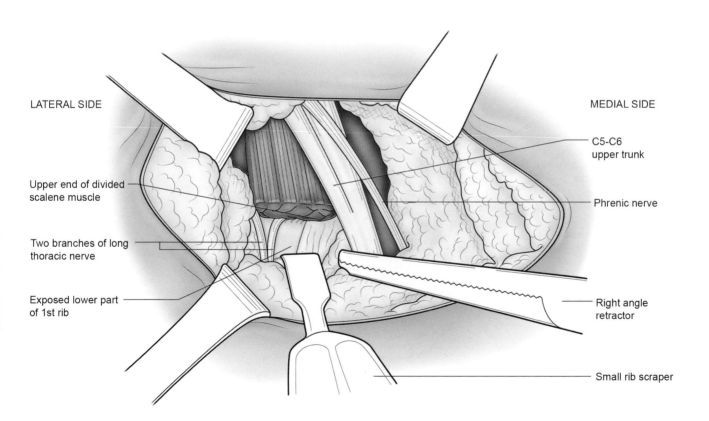

LATERAL SIDE

MEDIAL SIDE

Upper end of divided scalene muscle

Two branches of long thoracic nerve

Exposed lower part of 1st rib

C5-C6 upper trunk

Phrenic nerve

Right angle retractor

Small rib scraper

5.22   Lower division of middle scalene muscle, locating first rib, and scraping with rib scraper

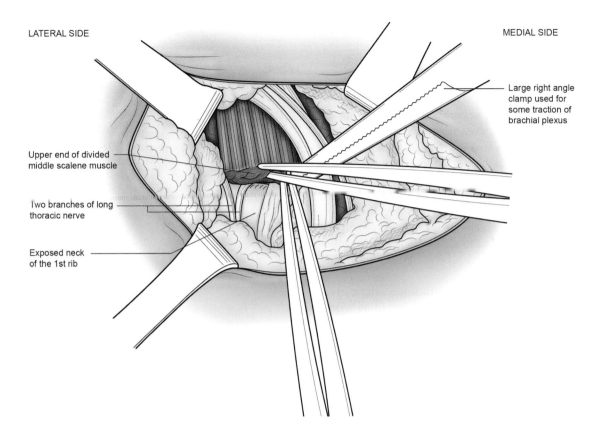

LATERAL SIDE

MEDIAL SIDE

Large right angle
clamp used for
some traction of
brachial plexus

Upper end of divided
middle scalene muscle

Two branches of long
thoracic nerve

Exposed neck
of the 1st rib

5.23   More scraping and removal of most of the scalene muscle and exposing the neck of the first rib.

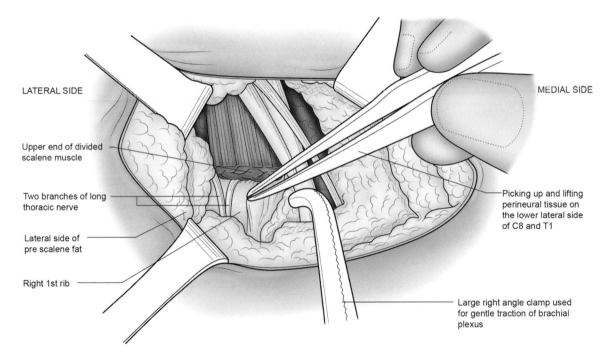

LATERAL SIDE

MEDIAL SIDE

Upper end of divided
scalene muscle

Two branches of long
thoracic nerve

Lateral side of
pre scalene fat

Right 1st rib

Picking up and lifting
perineural tissue on
the lower lateral side
of C8 and T1

Large right angle clamp used
for gentle traction of brachial
plexus

5.24   Picking up and gentle lifting of the perineural tissue on the lower medial side of the C8.

Attention is then directed to the lower part of the anterior scalenectomy site and the C8 and T1 nerve roots are exposed (see **Figure 5.24**). Next, the closed jaw of a large right-angle clamp is passed under the C8 and T1 nerve roots to ensure full freedom of the lower plexus from the first rib (see **Figures 5.25a through c, 5.26, and 5.27**). Two 6 mm Penrose drains are inserted at the lateral corner at the incision and through prescalene fat. These are usually removed 1–2 days postoperatively. The patient is given instructions on daily dressing changes, in addition to a series of postoperative exercises that are to be done for several months (see **Figure 5.28**).

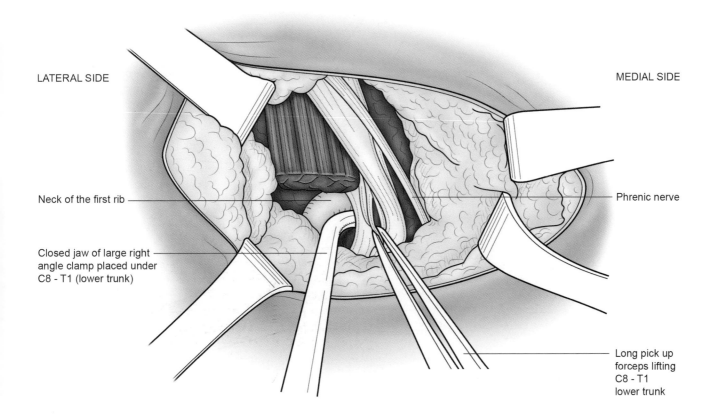

LATERAL SIDE

MEDIAL SIDE

Neck of the first rib

Phrenic nerve

Closed jaw of large right
angle clamp placed under
C8 - T1 (lower trunk)

Long pick up
forceps lifting
C8 - T1
lower trunk

5.25a   Passing the closed jaw of the large right-angle clamp under C8-T1.

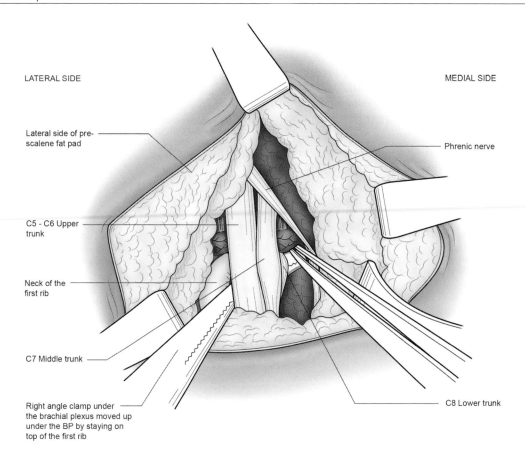

LATERAL SIDE

MEDIAL SIDE

Lateral side of pre-
scalene fat pad

Phrenic nerve

C5 - C6 Upper
trunk

Neck of the
first rib

C7 Middle trunk

Right angle clamp under
the brachial plexus moved up
under the BP by staying on
top of the first rib

C8 Lower trunk

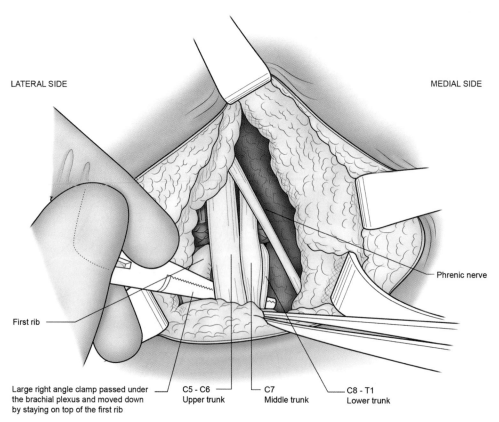

LATERAL SIDE

MEDIAL SIDE

Phrenic nerve

First rib

Large right angle clamp passed under
the brachial plexus and moved down
by staying on top of the first rib

C5 - C6
Upper trunk

C7
Middle trunk

C8 - T1
Lower trunk

5.25b–c Closed end of the right-angle clamp moved up and down under the brachial plexus by staying at the top of the first rib to ensure full freedom of the C8 and T1 from the first rib.

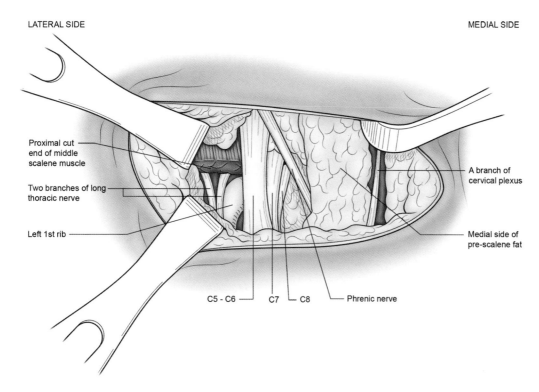

LATERAL SIDE

MEDIAL SIDE

Proximal cut end of middle scalene muscle

Two branches of long thoracic nerve

Left 1st rib

A branch of cervical plexus

Medial side of pre-scalene fat

C5 - C6   C7   C8   Phrenic nerve

5.26 Final view post anterior and middle scalenectomy.

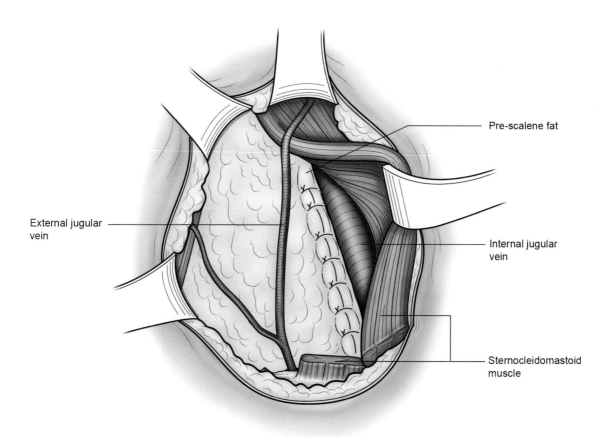

Pre-scalene fat

External jugular vein

Internal jugular vein

Sternocleidomastoid muscle

5.27 Suturing prescalene adipose tissue and covering the brachial plexus.

Exercises: repeat at least 4 times every 2 hours while awake

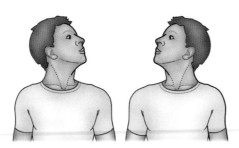

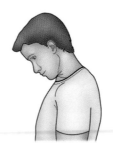

Point chin toward left shoulder and tilt neck toward ceiling; hold 3-5 seconds. Repeat pointing chin toward right side. Rest a few seconds.

Raise head up and bring it down.

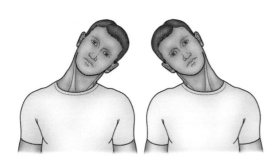

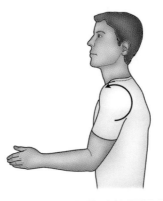

Bend neck to each side. Rest.

Breathe in, roll shoulders forward, then toward ears. Hold for a moment. Breathe out, roll shoulders back and down to start.

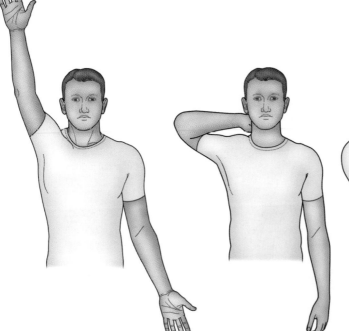

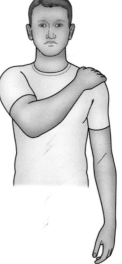

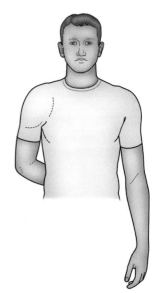

Lift arm up toward ceiling. Hold 3-5 seconds.

Put hand to back of neck then to top of the opposite shoulder blade.

Place hand behind back.

5.28 Postoperative exercises.

Summary

There are a few surgical procedures available for TOCS. The choice of the procedure for any particular patient depends on the history, symptomatology, and the physical findings, in addition to laboratory studies and the patient's overall condition.

For neurogenic TOCS, the most common presentation, in the absence of changes in the bony structures of the first rib, clavicle, or the presence of a cervical rib of no more than 2.5 cm, transcervical scalenectomy is our preferred procedure, especially with large, overweight patients.

For full decompression of the thoracic outlet, the combined approach of transaxillary first rib resection and scalenectomy is generally considered, especially for the smaller patient with or without bony changes.

If the patient has pure subclavian vein compression, without any neurological symptoms, the optimal procedure is transaxillary first rib resection.

If venous and neurogenic compression symptoms are present, the combined procedure can be considered, depending on the patient's size and condition. In the case of arterial TOCS (which is quite rare), the transaxillary approach is the first choice, but it can also be combined with the transcervical procedure.

Treatment of vascular TOCS

If subclavian vein thrombosis is present and if the occlusion has occurred within the past 2 or 3 days, thrombolytic agents can be infused to lyse the clot and the patient should be heparinized. In a timely fashion, transaxillary first rib resection should be performed to prevent the recurrence of compression. If the patient is very muscular or markedly obese, a transcervical scalenectomy would be the best choice in our opinion.

If the patient is seen several days after the occurrence of the thrombosis, the subclavian vein should be opened using thrombolytic agents, the patient should continue on a heparin infusion, and then be transitioned to Coumadin, which should be continued for 3–4 months. Depending on the patient's size, either transaxillary first rib resection or transcervical scalenectomy should be considered. If the patient has minimal or no symptoms, in our opinion, operation and first rib resection are not indicated.

Arterial TOCS is very rare. A transaxillary approach for removal of the offending structure, such as the cervical rib, first rib, or associated bands and muscles, should be performed. If the patient has the symptoms of neurogenic TOCS, transcervical scalenectomy should be performed under the same anesthetic.

Complications

The thoracic outlet has been classified as "tiger country" because of the potential for disaster due to the presence of multiple important structures such as the subclavian vessels,

the thoracic duct, and several major nerves (brachial plexus, phrenic, long thoracic, and intercostal brachial cutaneous nerves).[14]

There is a reported incidence of pneumothorax as high as 33%.[14] A 1% rate of subclavian artery injury, a 1%–2% rate of subclavian vein injury, and an incidence of major nerve injuries of the brachial plexus of 0.5%–1.0% and the long thoracic nerve of 1%–2% have also been reported.[8,15,16] Phrenic nerve injury is more common, with a reported rate of 6%–12%.[8,15]

After transaxillary first rib resection, patients commonly have relatively minor complaints of hypesthesia and paresthesia in the axilla and along the medial and posterolateral aspect of the upper arm. This usually results from the retraction on the second and third intercostal brachial cutaneous nerves. Generally, the discomfort improves within 3–4 months.

Very rarely, some degree of Horner's syndrome may occur because of injury to the stellate ganglion at the level of the T1. The stellate ganglion is usually not seen during transaxillary first rib resection. Also, dissection in the left neck can put the thoracic duct at risk for injury resulting in a chylous collection.

Recurrences

Recurrent symptoms usually occur when excessive scar tissue forms within the operative field, causing adhesions between the nerves and surrounding structures such as the remaining portions of scalene muscles, first rib, cervical rib, or chest wall. Recurrence may also become apparent following an insufficient procedure for TOCS.

We categorized patients into two groups based on the interval when the procedure was performed. The first group included recurrence after a single surgical intervention, whether it was a transaxillary first rib resection or transcervical scalenectomy, done between the mid-1970s and late 1989. In the second group, the recurrent symptoms occurred after a combined procedure from 1989 to 2002. In the first group, there were 938 patients with a recurrence rate of 30%–35%. In the second group, there were 538 patients who had the combined procedure, followed by active and passive range-of-motion exercises starting the day after surgery, with a recurrence rate of 5%–10% (**Table 5.1**[17]). With the improved technique and early postoperative exercises (similar to flexor tendon repair) the rate of recurrence was noted to drop from 30%–35% to 5%–10%. Since 2003, more than 350 patients who have had this combined procedure have had results that are as good as, if not better than, those reported in 2004 (**Table 5.2**).

It should be noted that many physicians do not start immediate (i.e., day after surgery) active and passive range-of-motion exercises with the neck and shoulder girdle. However, to decrease the chance of recurrence due to the possibility of scar tissue formation around the brachial plexus and vessels, and the harmful effect of this, it is very important to start postoperative exercises the day after surgery, and patients

Table 5.1   Results of combined first rib resection and scalenectomy (1989–2002)

Percent improvement	Description	Number of patients
70%–100%	Excellent (almost complete relief of symptoms)	36
50%–70%	Good (disappearance of all major symptoms)	24
30%–50%	Better (almost 50% improvement of all symptoms)	26
10%–30%	Fair (partial relief of symptoms)	9
Less than 10%	Very poor (no improvement)	5

Note: Results based on 100 respondents to a questionnaire, out of 532 surgeries.

Table 5.2   Results of combined first rib resection and scalenectomy (2003–2012)

Percent improvement	Description	Number of patients
70%–100%	Excellent (almost complete relief of symptoms)	50
50%–70%	Good (disappearance of all major symptoms)	9
30%–50%	Better (almost 50% improvement of all symptoms)	6
10%–30%	Fair (partial relief of symptoms)	7
Less than 10%	Poor (no improvement)	4

Note: Results based on 57 respondents to a questionnaire—who underwent a total of 76 operations, 19 of which were bilateral—out of 350 patients.

should be informed, both preoperatively and postoperatively, as to the importance of this.

Repetitive, strenuous activities of the upper extremity after previous TOCS surgery can also, in our opinion, result in recurrent symptoms. Again, the key to preventing the harmful effect of scar tissue is to start active and passive range-of-motion exercises with the neck and shoulder girdle on the first postoperative day.

If the recurrent symptoms are severe enough, a surgical procedure could be considered as a last resort, after job modification and a trial of physical therapy and medication. The operation would depend on what was previously performed and the findings on cervical spine imaging. If there is less than a 1 cm remnant of the posterior part of the first rib, a transcervical scalenectomy is generally the choice for external neurolysis of the brachial plexus and removal of the scalene muscle or remnants of muscles.

Results

Prior to 1989, our long-term results for first rib resection and scalenectomies as a one-stage procedure revealed an improvement rate of about 70%, with a 30%–35% recurrence rate.[16]

Between 1989 and the end of 2002, 532 patients had this combined procedure. Only 358 of these patients were located for questioning, and, of those, only 102 responded to a questionnaire. The results were subjective according to the patient's statements. Based on the patients' responses, 90%–95% reported improvement of their symptoms and the rate of recurrence was 5%–10% (see **Table 5.1**).[17,18]

From 2003 to 2012, more than 350 patients from a wide geographic area underwent the combined procedure and only 57 responded to the questionnaire. There were 19 bilateral combined procedures performed a few months apart for a total of 76 procedures. Again, a simple grading symptom was used and, according to the patients' own assessments, this revealed 95% improvement of symptoms (see **Table 5.2**). There were three recurrences—two occurred after motor vehicle accidents and one after excessive computer work.

The initial operations for decompression of the brachial plexus (such as first rib resection, scalenectomy, or combined procedure) are generally considered demanding, difficult, and high risk. The surgical procedures available for recurrent TOCS are even more difficult, demanding, and carry greater risk than the primary operations.[17,18]

REFERENCES

1. Cooper A. On exostosis. In: Cooper A, Travers B (eds.). *Surgical essays*. Edn. 3. London: Cox and Son; 1818; p. 128.
2. Peet RM, Henricksen JD, Anderson TP, Martin GM. Thoracic-outlet syndrome: evaluation of a therapeutic exercise program. *Proc Staff Meet Mayo Clinic.* 1956; 31: 281–7.
3. Clagett OT. Presidential address: Research and Prosearch. *J Thorac Cardiovasc Surg.* 1962; 44: 153–8.
4. Roos DB. Transaxillary approach for first rib resection to relieve thoracic outlet compression syndrome. *Annals of Surgery.* 1966; 163: 354–8.
5. Sanders RJ, Raymer S. The supraclavicular approach to scalenectomy and first rib resection: description of technique. *Journal of Vascular Surgery.* 1985; 2: 751–6.

6. Thompson RW, Schneider PA, Nelken NA, Skioldebrand CG, Stoney RJ. Circumferential venolysis and paraclavicular thoracic outlet decompression for "effort thrombosis" of the subclavian vein. *Journal of Vascular Surgery.* 1992; 16: 723–32.

7. Urschel HD JR, Razzuk MA. The failed operation for thoracic outlet syndrome: the difficulty of diagnosis and management. *Annals of Thoracic Surgery.* 1986; 42: 523–8.

8. Sanders RJ, Haug CE. *Thoracic outlet syndrome: a common sequela of neck injury.* Philadelphia: Lippincott; 1991.

9. Atasoy E. Thoracic outlet compression syndrome. *Orthop Clin North Am.* 1996; 27: 265–303.

10. Atasoy E. A hand surgeon's further experience with thoracic outlet compression syndrome. *J Hand Surg.* 2010; 35: 1528–38.

11. Adson AW, Coffey JR. Cervical rib: A method of anterior approach for relief of symptoms by division of the scalenus anticus. *Ann Surg.* 1927; 85: 839–57.

12. Machanic BI, Sanders RJ. Medial antebrachial cutaneous nerve measurements to diagnose neurogenic thoracic outlet syndrome. *Ann Vasc Surg.* 2008; 22: 248–54.

13. Brantigan CO, Roos DB. Etiology of neurogenic thoracic outlet syndrome. *Hand Clin.* 2004; 1: 17–22.

14. Leffert RD. Complications of surgery for thoracic outlet syndrome. *Hand Clin.* 2004; 1: 91–8.

15. Wehbé MA, Leinberry CF. Current trends in treatment of thoracic outlet syndrome. *Hand Clin.* 2004; 20: 119–121.

16. Atasoy E. Thoracic outlet syndrome: recurrent thoracic outlet syndrome. *Hand Clin.* 2004; 20: 99–105.

17. Atasoy E. Combined surgical treatment of thoracic outlet syndrome: transaxillary first rib resection and transcervical scalenectomy. *Hand Clin.* 2004; 20: 71–82.

18. Atasoy E. A hand surgeon's advanced experience with thoracic outlet compression syndrome. *Handchir Mikrochir Plast Chir.* 2013; 45: 131–50.

6

Tracheostomy

ABBAS E. ABBAS

HISTORY

Since early civilization, making a sharp cut into the easily palpable cervical trachea has been known as a quick method to either cut off or deliver air to the lungs. Indeed, a form of tracheotomy was first depicted on Egyptian hieroglyphs dating back to 3600 BC and was later described by the Greek Homerus of Byzantium and Hippocrates. The first anatomically correct description of the tracheostomy operation for treatment of asphyxiation was by Ibn Zuhr in the twelfth century, and the first recorded successful tracheostomy was by Antonio Musa Brassavola (1490–1554), who treated a patient suffering from a peritonsillar abscess by tracheotomy. However, it remained an operation with a high mortality rate, and there are only few cases reported before the 1800s. With the beginning of the nineteenth century, several surgeons began using this technique for both emergent and elective reasons. In 1852, Armand Trousseau reported a series of 169 tracheotomies, and after that, the indications for this procedure rapidly expanded to include the treatment of diphtheria, croup, and poliomyelitis, in addition to using it as an adjunct for tracheal intubation and administration of inhalational anesthesia.

The currently used technique for open tracheostomy was accurately described in 1909 by the American surgeon Chevalier Jackson (1865–1958), who emphasized the importance of postoperative care to reduce morbidity and mortality. More recently, percutaneous approaches based on the Seldinger technique have also become popular. These were first described by Sheldon and Pudenz in 1957. In 1985, Ciaglia described the technique of serial dilatations using a set of seven progressively larger sized dilators in order to establish the stoma for the tracheostomy tube. In 1989, Griggs et al. described a single-step dilator technique and, in 1997, Fantoni et al. described the retrograde percutaneous translaryngeal tracheostomy. Other techniques have since been described and each has its proponents and opponents.

SURGICAL ANATOMY

Understanding the surface anatomy of the trachea, shown in **Figure 6.1**, is essential when performing tracheostomy. In the neck, it is a superficial structure, allowing easy palpation of the superior thyroid notch, cricoid cartilage, tracheal rings,

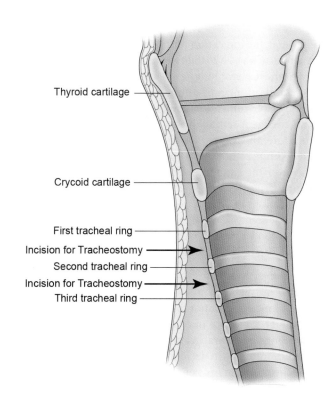

Thyroid cartilage

Crycoid cartilage

First tracheal ring
Incision for Tracheostomy
Second tracheal ring
Incision for Tracheostomy
Third tracheal ring

6.1 Surface anatomy. (With permission from Cook Medical, Bloomington, Indiana, United States.)

Notes: (1) Thyroid cartilage; (2) cricoid cartilage; (3) first tracheal ring; (4) second tracheal ring; (5) a third tracheal ring; (5) incision for tracheostomy.

and suprasternal notch. Also palpable are the innominate artery; the carotid artery; and, when present, a goiter. The adult trachea measures 10–13 cm, and its upper half lies above the suprasternal notch. However, in obese or kyphotic patients, most of the trachea may reside in the chest, making the cervical exposure of the trachea more difficult.

It is a D-shaped structure with anterior cartilaginous arch-like incomplete rings and a posterior flat membranous wall. In the neck, the trachea lies posterior to the strap muscles (the sternohyoid and sternothyroid muscles) and is crossed by the thyroid isthmus at the level of the second to fourth tracheal rings. It is shrouded by the pretracheal fascia, in which the inferior thyroid veins and sometimes a midline thyroid ima artery course. Inferior to the thoracic inlet, it dives posteriorly into the mediastinum, posterior to the thymus gland, innominate vein, and innominate artery. The esophagus is intimately adjacent to the membranous wall along its entire course.

The blood supply to the cervical trachea is segmental and is derived from branches of the inferior thyroid artery that form a longitudinal plexus running laterally alongside the cartilaginous–membranous junction. Also laterally, the recurrent laryngeal nerves run in the tracheoesophageal groove. It is therefore important to avoid any lateral dissection of the trachea during this procedure.

INDICATIONS FOR TRACHEOSTOMY

In general, the indication for tracheostomy is an obstructed proximal airway, an inability to safely maintain a patent airway, or the need for long-term positive-pressure ventilation. These indications range from the elective to the emergent. Although a cricothyroidotomy is more commonly performed in an emergent setting due to it being a simpler and faster procedure, this should always be converted to a tracheostomy within 24 hours if a surgical airway is still necessary. Whenever the situation allows, a tracheostomy should be the primary surgical airway in order to avoid the potential complications of cricothyroidotomy, specifically glottic and subglottic stenosis, which are more common when a cricothyroidotomy stoma is maintained longer than 48 hours.

Common indications include:

- Prolonged ventilatory support. It is recommended to perform tracheostomy if a patient continues to require mechanical ventilation beyond 7 days in order to avoid the high incidence of tracheal strictures associated with prolonged endotracheal intubation. (Clinical judgment comes into play in deciding the optimal time to perform tracheostomy in a patient requiring prolonged mechanical ventilation. Almost two-thirds of tracheostomies are currently performed for this indication.)
- Glottic or subglottic obstruction, either acquired or congenital.
- The need for pulmonary toilet in situations with excessive bronchial secretions or in cases of vocal cord paralysis.

- Patients with maxillofacial trauma, at risk for upper airway obstruction, may require a temporary tracheostomy until the airway is stabilized.
- As an adjunct to other surgical procedures on the upper aerodigestive tract, which have the potential to produce proximal airway edema and obstruction.
- Hypoventilation syndromes such as spinal cord injuries, phrenic nerve paralysis, and neuromuscular disorders affecting the diaphragm and chest wall.
- Smoke inhalation injury and airway burns.

Contraindications to tracheostomy include any medical condition contraindicating surgery such as uncontrolled coagulopathy or hemodynamic instability. Patients who require high levels of inspired oxygen, significant positive end-expiratory pressure or have high peak airway pressures may not tolerate a procedure possibly associated with a period of apnea until establishing an airway. Such patients should be stabilized and optimized before an elective tracheostomy.

The indications for percutaneous tracheostomy are the same as those already listed. However, relative contraindications to the percutaneous technique include emergent situations and being a member of the pediatric population.

PROCEDURE

There are two surgical options for creation of a tracheostomy: open and percutaneous. The decision on which one to use depends on several factors including surgeon preference.

Open technique (see **Figures 6.2 through 6.6**)

LOCATION FOR THE PROCEDURE
The procedure is typically performed in the operating theater.

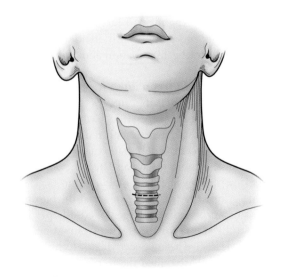

6.2   Incision for tracheostomy.

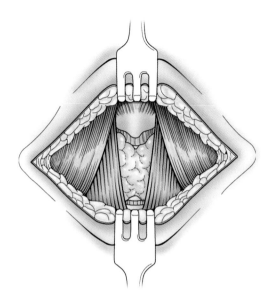

6.3 Exposure of the thyroid isthmus and underlying cervical trachea.

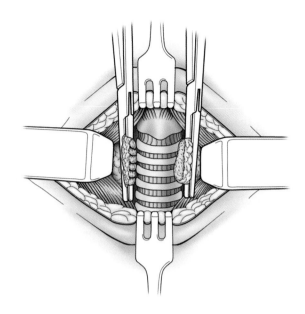

6.4 Division of the thyroid isthmus.

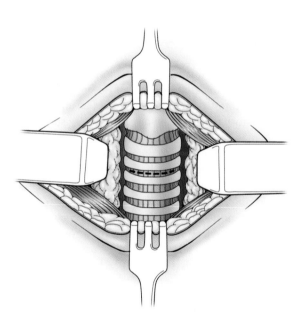

6.5 Tracheotomy incision.

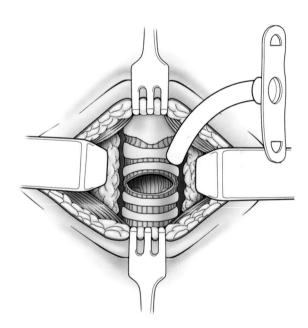

6.6 Insertion of tracheostomy tube.

POSITION

The ideal position is supine with the neck hyperextended, which is achieved by placing the patient on a shoulder roll. This maximizes delivery of the proximal trachea into the neck and allows excellent exposure of the tracheal cartilages.

THE TUBE (see **Figure 6.7**)

In general, the components of the tracheostomy tube include a hollow cannula of different lengths and diameters, a loading dilator, and the option for a balloon cuff. Selection of the tracheostomy tube depends on patient factors (age, body-mass index, sex, size of the airway) and whether a cuffed tube is necessary. Male patients have wider airways than females and obese patients may require an extra-long tube due to the thicker skin flap. When placed for postoperative ventilator support, a cuffed tube is necessary to allow positive-pressure ventilation. In general, a 6–8 mm standard tube is feasible in most adult patients.

The selected size of the appropriate tube type is opened on the field, and the cuff is tested before insertion. Tubes with different diameters and lengths should also be immediately available in the operating room. The circulating nurse should be ready to immediately open a different size should the need arise while inserting the tube.

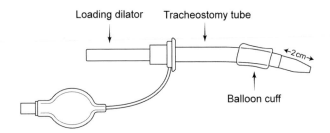

6.7 Components of the standard tracheostomy tube. (With permission from Cook Medical, Bloomington, Indiana, United States.)

Notes: (1) Tracheostomy tube; (2) loading dilator; (3) balloon cuff.

INCISION

A 3–4 cm incision is made in a transverse or longitudinal fashion. A transverse incision is less likely to cause significant scarring and is the preferred incision. It should be placed 2 cm above the sternal notch. A longitudinal incision, in contrast, has the advantage of easier exposure of multiple levels of the trachea. It can easily be extended superiorly or inferiorly. Regardless of the orientation of the incision, it should be centered perfectly along the midline or, in cases of tracheal deviation, on the trachea itself.

DISSECTION

Throughout this phase, it is critical to maintain perfect hemostasis. The incision is carried down through the skin, subcutaneous tissue, and platysma. The plane of dissection then shifts to the midline longitudinally to divide the fascia between the strap muscles. The two strap muscles on each side (superficial sternohyoid and deeper sternothyroid) are elevated and carefully retracted off the trachea. Either a handheld or self-retaining retractor may be used for this purpose. This exposes the underlying pretracheal fascia, thyroid isthmus, and inferior thyroid veins. If large or extensive, these veins can be ligated or divided with a thermal vessel sealant. Otherwise, they can be retracted off the trachea. The pretracheal fascia is then divided longitudinally, exposing the tracheal rings.

MANAGING THE THYROID ISTHMUS

Usually, this is only a few millimeters in length and can be easily separated from the trachea and retracted cephalad. If long and bulky, the isthmus can be divided between hemostat clamps after dissecting the central portion off the trachea. Care is taken to avoid lateral dissection so as to not injure the recurrent laryngeal nerve in the tracheoesophageal groove. Once the isthmus is divided, the cut ends are oversewn with a running 3-0 absorbable suture and the clamps removed.

TRACHEOTOMY

Once the upper tracheal rings are exposed, an incision in the trachea—a tracheotomy—is made. The preferred location for this incision is between the second and third cartilaginous rings. Before this is done, it is important to alert the anesthesiologist to deflate the cuff of the endotracheal tube. To avoid the catastrophic complication of an airway fire, it is also mandatory to stop using any heat energy source at this time, such as an electric cautery. A tracheal hook is placed around the inferior edge of the cricoid cartilage to deliver and stabilize the anterior tracheal wall as it is being opened.

The incision is made using a scalpel between the second and third rings. More proximal tracheostomies are prone to subglottic stenosis, while more distal ones may erode into the innominate artery. A simple incision through the inter-cartilaginous space is adequate to allow passage of the tube. A 2-0 Prolene staystitch is placed at each end of the incision and used to retract the trachea. Other more elaborate superior- or inferior-based H-shaped or U-shaped flaps have been described but have also been associated with increased incidence of anterior tracheal wall weakness, granulation tissue, and strictures. One such technique is the Bjork flap, created by dividing the second and third tracheal rings laterally then connecting the two ends superiorly. The flap is then sutured to the inferior edge of the neck incision. This may facilitate exchange of the tracheostomy tube.

Once the tracheotomy is made, the endotracheal tube cuff is reinflated while the stoma is widened with a two- or three-pronged or a hemostat. The endotracheal tube is then visualized and the anesthesiologist is asked to deflate the cuff once more and retract it until the distal tip is seen at the superior aspect of the stoma. Should there be any difficulty in placing the tracheostomy tube, the anesthesiologist can simply advance the tube and reinflate the cuff. It is therefore important for the anesthesiologist to not completely remove the endotracheal tube until the tracheostomy tube is in a good position.

The inner cannula is removed and replaced by the obturator within the lumen of the tube. Sterile tubing is then used to connect the tube to the circuit. The two tracheal staystitches can then be sewn to the inferior skin incision and can be removed a week later. In the event of accidental postoperative decannulation, these stitches may provide a means to retract the trachea and replace the tube. The tracheostomy tube flange system is secured to the skin with 2-0 sutures. The skin incision itself does not require closure or dressing. Finally, but only after confirming adequate ventilation with chest rise, end-tidal carbon dioxide, appropriate tidal volume, and oxygenation, can the endotracheal tube be completely removed and discarded.

Percutaneous technique

Several techniques have been described for this procedure, which minimizes the dissection of the pretracheal tissue. All of these techniques rely on the Seldinger principle and over-wire dilation of a tract from the skin of the neck to the tracheal lumen, followed by passage of a tracheostomy tube over a dilator and through the tract. The entire procedure is usually done under endoscopic guidance, using a flexible bronchoscope through the endotracheal tube. The most commonly used percutaneous tracheostomy system at the author's institution is the one-step dilational method using the commercially available Ciaglia Blue Rhino kit (Cook Medical, Bloomington, Indiana, United States).

LOCATION FOR THE PROCEDURE

The procedure is performed either in the operating room or in the intensive care unit, depending on personal and institutional preference. Regardless, an open tracheostomy set should be immediately available.

TECHNIQUE (see **Figures 6.8 through 6.12**)

- The same skin incision as described for the open procedure is made and carried down to the pretracheal tissue.
- The bronchoscopist guides the withdrawal of the endotracheal tube such that the tip is just below the cords and transillumination is seen through the incision.
- An introducer needle is passed below the second tracheal ring and aspiration of air confirms intratracheal location.
- A guidewire is advanced into the tracheal lumen, followed by removal of the needle and sheath.
- The tract between the skin and the tracheal lumen is then dilated over the guidewire.
- In females, a size 6 cuffed Shiley tube is loaded onto a 26 Fr dilator, while in males, a size 8 cuffed Shiley tube is loaded onto a 28 Fr dilator.
- The tracheostomy tube is then advanced under bronchoscopic vision into the lumen.
- Next, the bronchoscope is passed through the tracheostomy tube to identify the carina, thus confirming intratracheal position.
- The tube is secured to the skin as described in the "Open procedure" section.

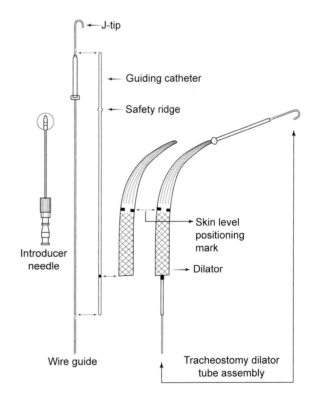

6.8 Components of the percutaneous Ciaglia Blue Rhino kit. (With permission from Cook Medical, Bloomington, Indiana, United States.)

Notes: (1) J-tip; (2) safety ridge; (3) skin level positioning mark; (4) introducer needle; (5) wire guide; (6) guiding catheter; (7) dilator; (8) tracheostomy dilator tube assembly.

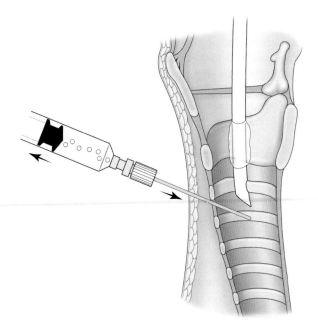

6.9 Verify entrance into the tracheal lumen by aspirating air into the syringe. (With permission from Cook Medical, Bloomington, Indiana, United States.)

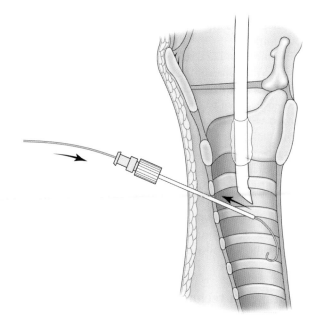

6.10 Wire is passed through the needle and into the tracheal lumen. (With permission from Cook Medical, Bloomington, Indiana, United States.)

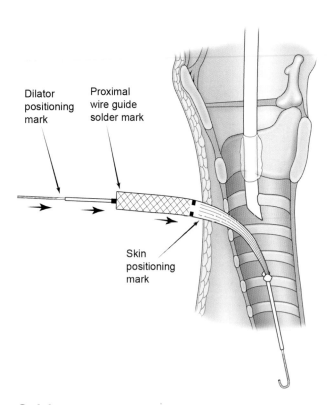

6.11 Advancing the dilator over the wire. Care is taken not to overadvance past the skin level marked on the dilator. (With permission from Cook Medical, Bloomington, Indiana, United States.)

Notes: (1) Proximal wire guide solder mark; (2) dilator positioning mark; (3) skin positioning mark.

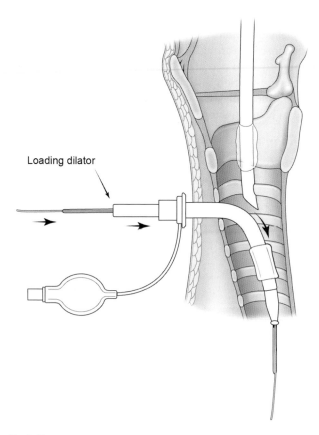

6.12 Loading the dilator tracheostomy tube assembly. The tracheostomy tube is loaded onto the loading dilator and advanced into the trachea. (With permission from Cook Medical, Bloomington, Indiana, United States.)

Note: (1) Loading dilator.

Comparison of percutaneous and open tracheostomy

Along with the development of percutaneous approaches in other surgical procedures, there is a perception that a percutaneous tracheostomy is less invasive. However, this is not a procedure with a shorter incision. The main technical difference between the two techniques is that the percutaneous one relies on rigid dilation of a stoma into the trachea rather than a sharp incision. The biggest advantage of the percutaneous tracheostomy procedure is, in the author's opinion, the ability to perform it at the bedside in the intensive care unit, thus eliminating the need for transporting critically ill patients to the operating room. A secondary benefit of this may be reduced hospital costs.

Numerous randomized studies and meta-analyses have been performed to compare open and percutaneous tracheostomy. Few have shown any convincing difference in important short-term and long-term outcomes. There has been a suggestion in some of these studies of a tendency of lower incidence of wound infections and chronic strictures with the percutaneous approach. Also suggested was lower overall cost for percutaneous tracheostomy, especially when performed in the intensive care unit. As for overall safety, none has shown statistically significant differences between the two techniques.

POSTOPERATIVE CARE

When the tract between the skin and tracheal lumen is fully matured, it becomes a simple matter to remove and reinsert the tracheostomy tube for either cleaning or replacement. However, until the tract matures, it is essential to avoid accidental dislodgement of the tube. It is also important to use meticulous care in keeping this tube patent and clear of the encrustations that can develop from airway secretions and could lead to obstruction of the tube. The frequent and careful removal and cleaning of the inner cannula in addition to humidification of inspired oxygen help to prevent this deposition of encrusted secretions.

The time needed for maturity of the tract depends on the technique performed for the tracheostomy. For the open procedure, it usually takes about 4 or 5 days while the percutaneous technique may require up to 2 weeks to mature. Timing of the initial tracheostomy tube change therefore differs accordingly.

OUTCOME

Although rare, a tracheostomy procedure is accompanied by risks of many of the same postoperative complications associated with other surgical operations. Wound infection is extremely uncommon but, when identified, should be aggressively treated with drainage and systemic antibiotics. Early postoperative bleeding from the wound is usually related to superficial skin vessels and can be controlled by hemostatic agents at the bedside. However, a deeper source related to the thyroid gland or vessels is a potentially hazardous complication that can cause intratracheal aspiration of blood and asphyxiation. Similarly, a peritracheal hematoma can cause compression and obstruction of the airway. It is therefore essential to ensure hemostasis during the procedure. However, there should be a low threshold for surgical reexploration of the field for persistent or significant postoperative bleeding.

Long-term complications are usually related to the prosthetic tube. They include ischemic necrosis of the wall of the trachea, leading to erosion and fistulization into the surrounding structures. This can lead to the rare but dreaded complication of tracheoinnominate fistula (TIF), which is frequently fatal. Even minor hemoptysis after 48 hours of tracheostomy should be considered a sentinel bleed for TIF until proven otherwise. Other causes include site infection, coagulopathy, and malignant tumor invasion. When suspected, the patient should be carefully evaluated with rigid tracheobronchoscopy after withdrawing the tube to ensure visualization of the entire wall of the trachea. This should be done only in the operating suite with adequate preparation for immediate surgical intervention if necessary. If massive hemoptysis occurs at the bedside, tamponade of the bleeding can be attempted by overinflating the cuff and, if unsuccessful, digital extratracheal compression via the stoma can be performed. In the operating room, the rigid bronchoscope can be used to tamponade the innominate artery against the sternum. Surgical exploration is then performed with median sternotomy and ligation of the innominate artery. There is little evidence to suggest that this may lead to significant neurological or vascular compromise unless the patient has known vascular disease. An attempt at revascularization is therefore usually unnecessary. Prevention of this complication is much easier than its treatment by avoiding placing the tracheostomy too low and avoiding overinflation of the tracheal cuff. Most modern tracheostomy tubes are designed with lower cuff pressures to prevent ischemia of the adjacent tracheal wall.

Other long-term complications include extensive granulation tissue, tracheal stenosis, tracheomalacia, and tracheoesophageal fistula.

FURTHER READING

Ciaglia P, Firsching R, Syniec C. Elective percutaneous dilatational tracheostomy: a new simple bedside procedure: preliminary report. *Chest.* 1985; 87: 715–19.

De Leyn P et al. Tracheotomy: clinical review and guidelines. *Eur J Cardiothorac Surg.* 2007; 32(3): 412–21.

Fantoni A, Ripamonti D. A non-derivative, non-surgical tracheostomy: the translaryngeal method. *Intensive Care Med.* 1997; 23: 386–92.

Griggs WM, Worthley LIG, Gilligan JE, Thomas PD, Myburg JA. A simple percutaneous tracheostomy technique. *Surgery.* 1990; 170: 543–5.

Grillo HC et al. A low pressure cuff for tracheostomy tubes to minimize tracheal injury: a comparative clinical trial. *J Thorac Cardiovasc Surg.* 1971; 62(6): 898–907.

Jackson C. Tracheotomy. *The Laryngoscope.* 1909; 19: 285–90.

Sheldon CH, Pudenz RH, Freshwater DB, Cure BL. A new method for tracheostomy. *J Neurosurg.* 1955; 12: 428–31.

Stoller JK. The history of intubation, tracheotomy, and airway appliances. *Respir Care.* 1999; 44: 595–601.

Susarla SM et al. Percutaneous dilatational tracheostomy: review of technique and evidence for its use. *J Oral Maxillofac Surg.* 2012; 70(1): 74–82.

Walts PA et al. Techniques of surgical tracheostomy. *Clin Chest Med.* 2003; 24(3): 413–22.

7

Tracheal resection

PETER GOLDSTRAW

HISTORY

Early attempts at tracheal resection were timid, limited to 2 cm or less of the trachea and frequently less than circumferential. More extensive resections were attempted, exploring the use of various prostheses and homograft techniques. The results with such techniques were poor, adversely affected by failure of healing and granulation tissue ingrowth. The modern era of tracheal surgery began when Hermes. C. Grillo and colleagues undertook a series of cadaveric studies to establish the length of trachea that could be safely resected with end-to-end anastomosis. These studies were confirmed by a surgical series in which he and F. Griffith Pearson developed and expanded surgical techniques. These pioneers established the general principles of this surgery; the length of trachea that could be safely resected; and the ancillary measures required, allowing tension-free anastomosis. Although some have tried to extend these limits by developing newer prosthetic materials, these have not proven to be safe.

PRINCIPLES

Segmental resection of the trachea is appropriate for benign or malignant conditions affecting the trachea from the cricoid cartilage to the carina. Below this level, carinal resection and reconstruction is possible. Such conditions include fibrous stricture following intubation or tracheostomy; benign tumors of the airways such as carcinoid tumors; and malignant tumors, chiefly squamous carcinoma and adenoid cystic carcinoma. To be suitable for resection, the disease process has to be limited to a length of trachea that can be safely resected, and the patient must be sufficiently fit to tolerate such surgery safely. As a general rule, 50% of the trachea can be resected and repaired by end-to-end anastomosis. This length may be slightly greater in a young child and slightly less in an older person. As one approaches these limits, various release procedures are helpful to enable end-to-end anastomosis without undue tension.

A cervical approach allows resection of airway pathology affecting the distal larynx, the cervical trachea, and all but the distal 2–3 cm of the intrathoracic trachea. If this segment is involved, a thoracic approach is to be preferred, allowing carinal reconstruction, if necessary. The approach used will be influenced somewhat by the pathology. The length of airway to be resected can be more reliably determined for benign pathology. The margins of resection for malignant disease are less predictable and the surgeon will have to plan to allow for wider resection if necessary.

The choice of relieving procedure will, to some extent, also be influenced by the incision used.

In planning the surgical approach, consideration must be given to the alternatives available to allow continued ventilation during resection and reconstruction. The use of cardiopulmonary bypass has been tried in the past but has been rendered obsolete by alternatives that do not require heparinization.

Prophylactic antibiotics should be given for any operation on the airway, and anaerobic cover be added if there is severe obstruction or necrotic tumor.

As the surgeon will understandably restrict the length of resection to the minimum, the use of frozen section examination is recommended when undertaking airway resection for tumors, especially adenoid cystic carcinoma with its propensity for microscopic intramural extension.

For patients who are unfit for surgery, or whose disease is too extensive to permit resection, there are many alternative techniques. The appropriate technique will vary depending on the site, length, and pathology of the stricture, and include radiotherapy and a wide range of surgical procedures that achieve disobliteration and the maintenance of a safe airway by the use of temporary and permanent stents. These techniques are beyond the scope of this chapter. The long-term results of such therapy are less satisfactory than those achieved by an operation and the opinion of an appropriate surgical specialist should be sought before denying the patient an operation.

PREOPERATIVE ASSESSMENT

The severity of airway narrowing can be assessed clinically, by spirometry and lung function testing and by radiology. The extent of disease, particularly its intramural and extramural components, is aided by computed tomography. However, bronchoscopy remains the most critical evaluation, and the use of the rigid bronchoscope under general anesthesia has the advantages of a wide field of view, temporary breath holding, and the ability to take multiple large biopsies. In the emergency situation, its use can prove lifesaving, allowing measures to achieve rapid relief of critical stenosis. Using the rigid bronchoscope, the surgeon can accurately measure the length of the trachea; the extent of the segment that would require resection; and the relationship of its proximal and distal margins from such key landmarks as the carina, larynx, and any tracheostome. This is best done by marking the bronchoscope with thin strips of adhesive applied at the level of the upper incisors. The assessment of any dynamic, malacic component is aided by examining the airway with the patient coughing at the end of the evaluation.

Basic oncological principles apply when evaluating the feasibility of airway reconstruction for malignant disease. Distant metastases and extensive nodal disease should be excluded. Mediastinoscopy may be of value but local, mediastinal extension does not carry the same import as when evaluating lung cancer, as long as resection is deemed feasible.

Patient fitness must be assessed carefully. A greater level of fitness is necessary if a thoracic approach is needed, especially if concurrent pulmonary resection is contemplated. It is less of an issue if a cervical approach is judged suitable. Lung function testing is not representative of the patient's fitness in the presence of severe airway obstruction! Psychological and cerebral status may affect the patient's ability to cooperate with the physiotherapist in the postoperative period, and to tolerate the neck flexion necessary to safeguard the anastomosis.

Tracheal resection should not be undertaken as an emergency procedure. Surgical disobliteration will allow measured evaluation, accurate staging of malignant disease, discontinuation of steroid medication, and clearance of distal infection. The patient can then be brought to elective surgery fully appraised of the risks and benefits of surgery, and in the best physical and psychological state. The surgeon can plan the surgery carefully and ensure expert anesthetic support and the availability of frozen section pathology services.

OPERATIONS

Segmental resection of the trachea by a cervical approach

1. Following induction of anesthesia, it is helpful to repeat the bronchoscopic assessment using a rigid bronchoscope. This will allow the anesthetist to assess the size of endotracheal tube that can be negotiated through the strictured area. The surgeon can assess the location of the stricture relative to the skin incision by inserting a narrow-bore needle percutaneously into the lumen and viewing its relationship to the stricture through the bronchoscope. Ventilation during tracheal mobilization is safer if an endotracheal tube can be placed across the stricture. If this is not possible, the airway is precarious and intermittent obstruction may be encountered. A size 5.5 or 6.0 Fr armored endotracheal tube can usually be negotiated through the stricture into the distal, normal trachea. The patient is positioned supine, with the neck extended by a sandbag under the shoulders and the head secured in a ring. (See **Figure 7.1.**)

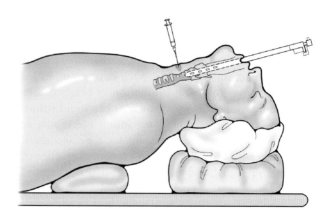

7.1

2. A curved, collar incision is made, centered on the tracheostomy scar, or midway between the thyroid cartilage and the suprasternal notch, extending between the lateral borders of the sternomastoid muscle on each side. The incision is deepened through platysma muscle using the diathermy, dividing superficial veins. The sternomastoid muscles are mobilized laterally from the suprasternal notch to the level of the thyroid cartilage. The trachea is identified in the midline and mobilized along its anterior aspect for the full length of the incision. The strap muscles may be divided but are usually reflected laterally. If necessary, the isthmus of the thyroid gland is divided between transfixion sutures. (See **Figure 7.2**.)

3. One must now decide where to make the initial incision into the trachea. It is usually preferable to make the distal transection first, as this allows one to speedily transfer ventilation to an endotracheal tube inserted into the distal trachea, if this is thought to be necessary. However, if the proximal margin of resection is easier to define, one can easily start at this point. The limits of the stricture may be apparent from external examination of the trachea, but if this proves difficult, identification of this important point is aided by temporarily withdrawing the endotracheal tube over a flexible bronchoscope. The light is visible through the tracheal wall, and the precise point at which to make the first incision can be identified by passing a fine-gauge needle into the lumen under endoscopic control. The trachea is mobilized circumferentially at this level. Care must be taken to avoid the recurrent laryngeal nerves. Some experts would favor dissection to identify these nerves.

However, the surrounding inflammatory response can make this difficult and it is usually preferable to avoid damage to the nerves by keeping the dissection close to the diseased tracheal wall. The contralateral nerve is at greater risk and extreme care is needed when dissecting between the trachea and the esophagus around the far side of the trachea.

The anterior wall of the trachea is incised with a pointed blade and circumferential division undertaken using scissors. Stay sutures of 2-02 monofilament are inserted into the anterior wall of the distal trachea to prevent retraction of the distal lumen. Ventilation is not interrupted, as the cuff of the tube should lie distal to this level. A longitudinal incision is then made along the anterior wall of the trachea, until the normal lumen is identified at the other limit of resection. (See **Figure 7.3**.)

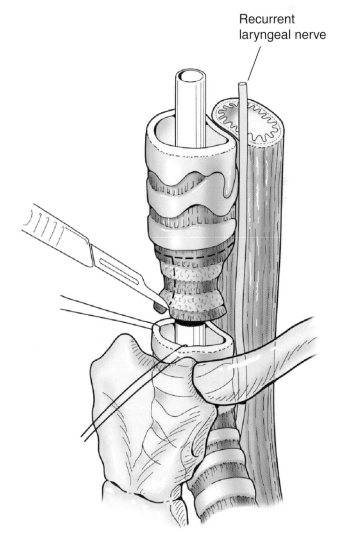

Recurrent laryngeal nerve

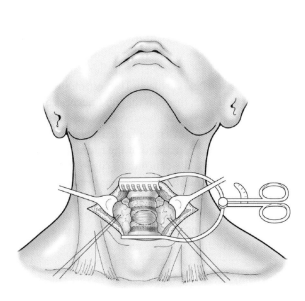

7.2

7.3

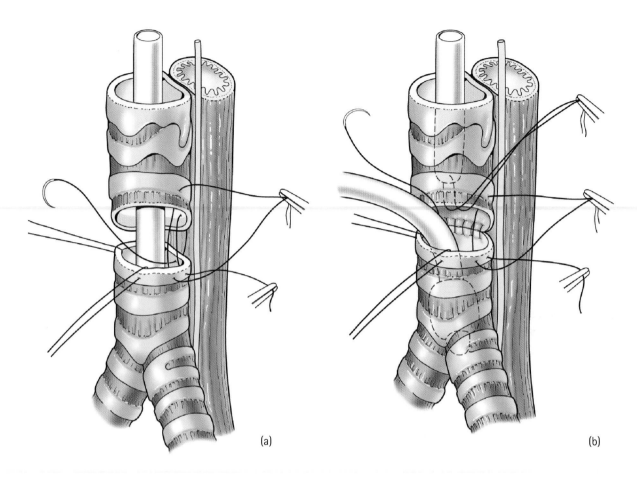

(a)

(b)

7.4a–b

4. The endotracheal tube can be retracted anteriorly while the whole circumference of the diseased segment is mobilized. If this step is difficult or prolonged, the endotracheal tube should be withdrawn into the larynx. A suture into its tip facilitates retrieval into the trachea. Ventilation is then transferred to an endotracheal tube inserted into the distal lumen across the operating field. A Bain's circuit is less intrusive for connecting this tube to the ventilator. This distal endotracheal tube is often in an unstable position and it is as well to delegate an assistant to focus entirely on maintaining satisfactory ventilation. Liaison with the anesthetist is essential during this type of ventilation. Care is necessary to keep close to the tracheal wall while undertaking this circumferential mobilization, avoiding damage to the esophagus and the recurrent nerves. Once the length of the tracheal defect is known, the surgeon should assess if further mobilization or release procedures are necessary to allow apposition of the tracheal ends without tension (see later). Mobilization of the distal airway should be limited to the anterior and posterior aspects of the trachea, preserving the lateral, vascular tissues. (See **Figure 7.4a and b.**)

5. An end-to-end anastomosis is performed using continuous monofilament material, such as 3-0 Prolene on a 17 mm needle. The anastomosis is reinforced at each quadrant with interrupted sutures of 2-0 Prolene, which, ideally, should pass through the cartilages of the trachea and not penetrate the lumen of the trachea. The first interrupted suture is placed at the near posterior cornu of the tracheal cartilage. The continuous suture runs, over and over, through the full thickness of the posterior tracheal wall to the opposite cornu, where the second stay suture is inserted. Each of the stay sutures should be inserted just ahead of the running suture to avoid damage to the continuous suture. Once the posterior wall of the anastomosis has been completed, the sandbag beneath the shoulders is removed. Traction of the two stay sutures approximates the ends of the trachea and the continuous suture is drawn tight. The continuous suture continues around the far wall of the trachea to the anterior aspect of the anastomosis. A further stay suture is inserted at this point. The standing suture at the near side of the posterior wall is then used to run in an over-and-over full thickness fashion around the nearside of the trachea to the anterior wall. The

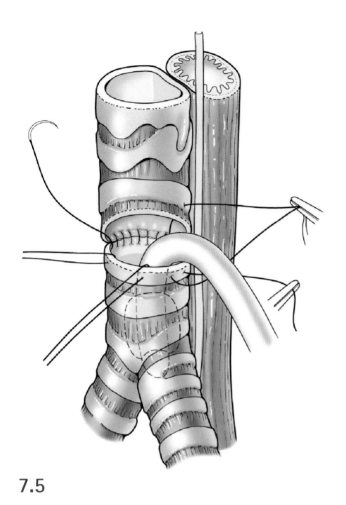

7.5

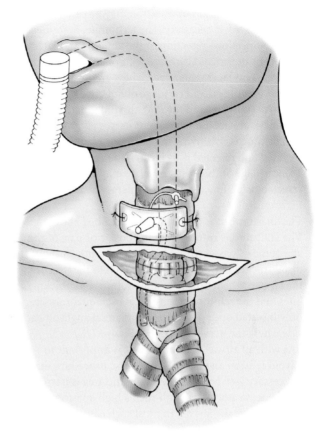

7.6

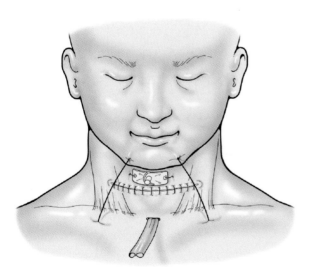

7.7

fourth stay suture is inserted at the anterior quadrant, ahead of the continuous suture. The continuous suture is tied, and the four stay sutures are tied to complete the anastomosis. If an endotracheal tube has been inserted into the distal lumen, at some point during the anastomosis, it will become intrusive. The translaryngeal tube is retrieved into the trachea to continue ventilation, and the distal tube is removed. (See **Figure 7.5**.)

6. Postoperative problems with sputum clearance are uncommon, but if this occurs, there can be great difficulty inserting a minitracheostomy tube. It is best to insert such a tube, above or below the anastomosis, as a routine. (See **Figure 7.6**.)

7. A corrugated drain is inserted and the strap muscles are approximated in the midline. The skin is closed with continuous subcuticular suture. The chin is fixed to the presternal skin using strong monofilament sutures with the neck in moderate flexion. (See **Figure 7.7**.)

Resection of the cricoid cartilage

8. The proximal margin of resection may be extended
   into the larynx if necessary. The technique, described
   by Pearson, allows resection of the anterior and lateral
   aspects of the cricoid cartilage with preservation of
   the recurrent laryngeal nerves. These are protected
   by dividing the cricoid cartilage obliquely, avoiding
   the posterior plate and the cricothyroid junction, the
   landmark at which the recurrent nerves enter the larynx.

   The mucosa overlying the posterior plate can be
   elevated and resected if, as is often the case, it is fibrotic.
   The cartilage of the posterior plate may also be partially
   resected using fine rongeurs to enlarge the lumen. (See
   Figure 7.8.)

9. The anastomosis is performed as described above.
   The continuous suture along the posterior part of the
   anastomosis passes through the membranous wall of the
   distal trachea and superiorly is limited to the mucosa of
   the larynx, which is usually quite robust. Full thickness
   bites and the reinforcing sutures at each quadrant are
   only inserted once past the posterolateral angle on each
   side where the nerves enter. (See **Figure 7.9**.)

10. As with all airway anastomoses, it is important to
    avoid tension and a laryngeal release procedure may be
    necessary (see below). The subglottic area is narrow,
    and edema associated with such a high anastomosis
    may involve the larynx. In most such cases, therefore,
    the author prefers to protect the upper airway by
    inserting a T-tube at the end of the procedure, leaving
    the proximal limb extending above the vocal cords. It

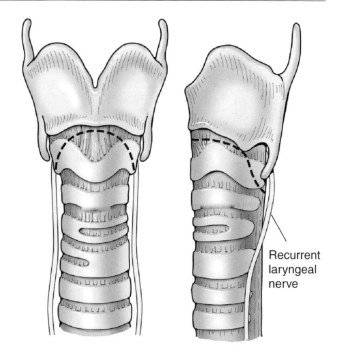

Recurrent
laryngeal
nerve

7.8

is best to bring the T-tube through the trachea above
or below the anastomosis. A minitracheostomy tube is
thus unnecessary. A corrugated drain is led through a
stab incision and the chin is fixed in slight flexion. (See
Figure 7.10.)

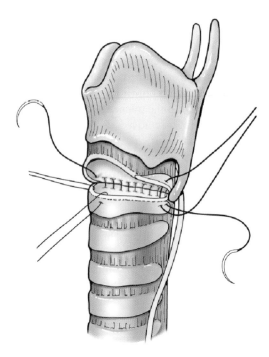

7.9

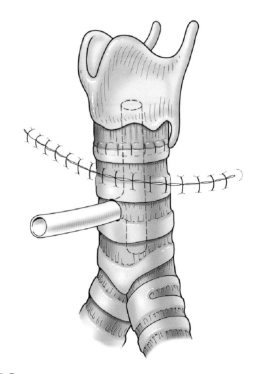

7.10

Release procedures

It is important to limit circumferential mobilization of the airway to the segment to be resected and a cuff at each end for anastomosis. This minimizes ischemic injury that may result in complete dehiscence or defects in the anastomosis leading to the formation of granulation tissue, a process often attributed to tissue reaction to suture material. However, tension on the anastomosis is equally undesirable. The early cadaveric studies undertaken by Grillo have shown the various release procedures that can allow more extensive airway resection to be undertaken without undue tension. However, individual surgeons will have to judge from their own experience when tension on the anastomosis is excessive, requiring a release procedure, and even when it is prudent to limit any further resection and accept an incomplete resection.

11. When tension is considered excessive, there are several steps that can be taken that will sequentially assist approximation of the anastomosis. First, check that the maximum flexion of the neck has been achieved. Freeing the anterior wall of the proximal and distal segments will allow the airway to slide a few millimeters without adding to the ischemic injury. Mobilizing the posterior wall is more effective but also more hazardous. Grillo has emphasized the importance of preserving the lateral vascular pedicles, although this seems less imperative given the good results of slide tracheoplasty. When a thoracic approach has been used, one can provide release by mobilizing the pulmonary hilum and freeing the pulmonary ligament. Additional length is achieved by incising the pericardial attachments of the pulmonary vessels. When carinal resection has been undertaken, a Barclay reconstruction (see later) may be necessary. When a cervical approach is used, a laryngeal release can be added, the method now preferred being the supralaryngeal release described by Montgomery. A second, circumferential, skin incision is made over the hyoid bone. Its anterior surface is cleared of platysma and the attachment of stylohyoid divided. The three thin muscular attachments to the superior surface of the hyoid, mylohyoid, geniohyoid, and genioglossus are divided, exposing the pre-epiglottic space. The lesser cornu is divided, freeing the pharyngeal muscles attached to it and releasing the sling of the digastric muscle. Heavy scissors are used to divide the body of the hyoid bone from the greater cornu on each side, immediately anterior to the sling of the digastric muscle, allowing the central portion to slide inferiorly. (See **Figure 7.11**.)

If a laryngeal release is judged to be necessary when undertaking a thoracic approach to the trachea or carina, it is logistically easier to perform this step prior to thoracotomy.

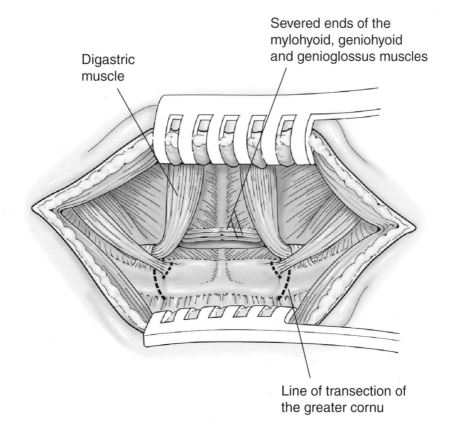

Digastric muscle

Severed ends of the mylohyoid, geniohyoid and genioglossus muscles

Line of transection of the greater cornu

7.11

Resection of the lower trachea

A right thoracotomy through the fourth intercostal or the bed of the fifth rib provides access to the intrathoracic trachea, the main carina, the whole of the right bronchial tree, and the left main bronchus to its lobar division. If the airway will accommodate a double-lumen endobronchial tube, this facilitates dissection prior to airway division.

12. The mediastinal pleura is incised over the lower trachea, the azygos vein is divided and its ends transfixed, and the hilum of the right lung is circumnavigated, freeing the hilar structures and dividing the pulmonary ligament. Lymph nodes around the affected segment of the airway will be resected and, in malignant cases, more extensive nodal evaluation is required. During this maneuver, bronchial and mediastinal vessels will be encountered. While one should divide as few as possible, it is important to accurately define the anatomy and the extent of disease. (See **Figure 7.12**.)

13. The airway is now ready to be divided. However, before doing so it should be decided how best to continue ventilation.

- Use the existing endotracheal tube, withdrawing it temporarily while resecting the airway and working around it while undertaking the anastomosis. The bulkiness of an endobronchial double-lumen tube makes this difficult. However, if the strictured area could only accommodate a narrow endotracheal tube, this should be left full length so that it can be advanced into the distal trachea or left main bronchus to continue ventilation during the anastomosis.

- The tube, whether endobronchial or endotracheal, is withdrawn and ventilation continued using an armored small caliber tube across the operating field into the distal trachea or left main bronchus. This prevents blood spilling into the left lung but is obtrusive and has to be removed at some stage during the anastomosis. This method is the one of choice when undertaking a Barclay reconstruction (see later).

- The tube, endotracheal or endobronchial, is withdrawn. A nasogastric tube is inserted through the original tube into the distal trachea or left main bronchus and used to provide ventilation using a Venturi injector. The nasogastric tube is sutured in place to prevent it flailing around. Hemostasis is important to limit the amount of blood insufflated into the left lung. This is probably the method of choice for uncomplicated segmental resection of the lower trachea or carinal reconstruction.

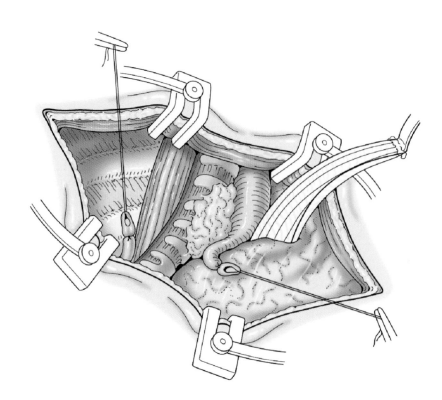

7.12

If the surgeon forewarns the anesthetist, pre-oxygenation will allow sufficient apnea time for the surgeon to transect the trachea, decide on the length of resection, and restore ventilation using one of these techniques. As always, the surgeon should resect to macroscopically normal airway, supplementing this assessment with frozen section histology in malignant cases. (See **Figure 7.13**.)

14. The anesthetist should flex the neck, supporting it with a pillow, before the surgeon begins the anastomosis. The anastomosis is similar to that described for segmental resection in the neck. A continuous suture commences at the far, posterior horn of the tracheal cartilage, continuing around the front wall to the posterior cornu at the near side. The standing end is then continued across the membranous wall and tied at the right posterior cornu. Reinforcing sutures are used at each quadrant, inserted ahead of the continuous suture to avoid damaging this suture. (See **Figure 7.14**.)

The mediastinal pleura is closed over the repair, a drain is inserted, and the thoracotomy is closed. The patient is rolled into the supine position with the neck fixed in moderate flexion. A minitracheostomy tube, a corrugated drain, and the neck-restraining sutures are inserted.

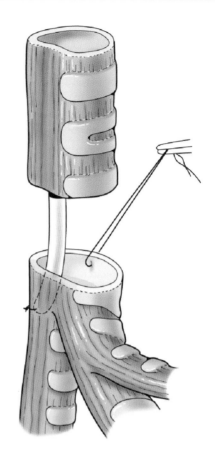

7.13

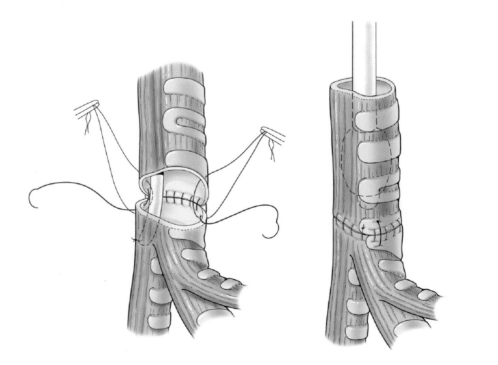

7.14

Carinal resection and reconstruction

15. Resection of the carina is undertaken using a right thoracotomy approach, providing continued ventilation by the Venturi method described above. Reconstruction is achieved by first recreating a new carina using the medial third of the circumference of both main bronchi, and anastomosing this double-barreled lumen to the distal trachea as described above. (See **Figure 7.15**.)

16. A variation of this technique allows resection of the right main bronchus and anastomosis of the intermediate bronchus and the left main bronchus to recreate the carina. If the right upper lobe bronchus can be preserved, it can be subsequently anastomosed to the side of the trachea, a centimeter above the main anastomosis. A small semicircular defect is created in the cartilage of the lateral wall of the trachea, at its junction with the membranous part of the tracheal wall. (See **Figure 7.16**.)

17. After carinal resection, elevation of the left main bronchus is limited by the aortic arch. If more extensive resection of the trachea or left main bronchus is necessary, this double-barreled reconstruction is not possible. The reconstruction described by Barclay allows an end-to-end anastomosis in such circumstances. In this, the right main bronchus, or the intermediate bronchus, is anastomosed to the distal trachea while the left lung is ventilated using a small armored endotracheal tube across the operative field. (See **Figure 7.17**.)

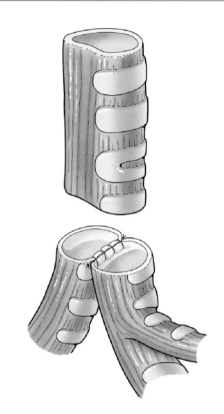

7.15

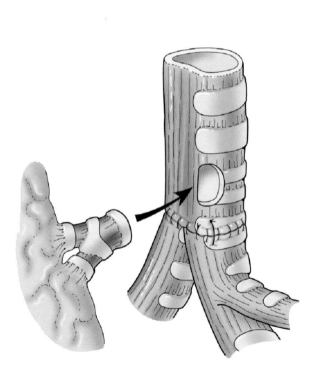

7.16

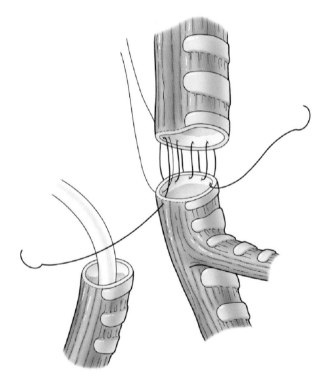

7.17

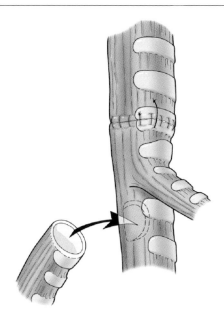

7.18

18. The left main bronchus is then anastomosed to the medial aspect of the intermediate bronchus after creating a small semicircular defect in the cartilage at its junction with the membranous portion of the airway (see **Figure 7.18**).

The mediastinal pleura is closed over the repair and the thoracotomy closed. The patient is rolled into the supine position with the neck held flexed. A minitracheostomy tube, a corrugated drain, and the neck-restraining sutures are inserted.

Slide tracheoplasty

This operation was originally devised to cope with congenital funnel (stove-pipe) trachea involving greater than 50% of the total tracheal length. It was accepted at that time that this was the maximum length of trachea that could be resected with end-to-end anastomosis. Various on-lay grafts using periosteum or rib had been tried with varied success. The concept of the slide tracheoplasty is simple—one halves the length of the trachea and doubles its circumference. The initial success of this operation infers that the trachea in this condition has an unusual circumferential blood supply. However, the operation has since been used successfully in long, benign, acquired strictures in adults.

The operation is usually undertaken through a cervical approach, allowing access to the whole of the trachea to the level of the carina. If the stenotic segment extends onto one of the main bronchi, especially when associated with an aberrant left pulmonary artery, the procedure can be undertaken through a right thoracotomy. Ventilation is difficult when operating on such tight stenoses in a tiny patient, but the operation is possible with intermittent apnea with the advantage that cardiopulmonary bypass has been avoided.

19. Once the full extent of the stenotic area has been exposed circumferentially, the trachea is divided transversely at the midpoint of the stenosis. The posterior wall of the distal segment is incised longitudinally until a normal caliber airway has been reached. The anterior wall of the upper segment is incised over a similar length. The ends of each segment may be trimmed slightly to create more of a pointed end on each flap. The proximal segment of trachea is drawn behind the distal segment, then the anastomosis begins on the posterior aspect of the distal segment, spirals around each side of the reconstructed airway, and is completed anteriorly. (See **Figure 7.19**).

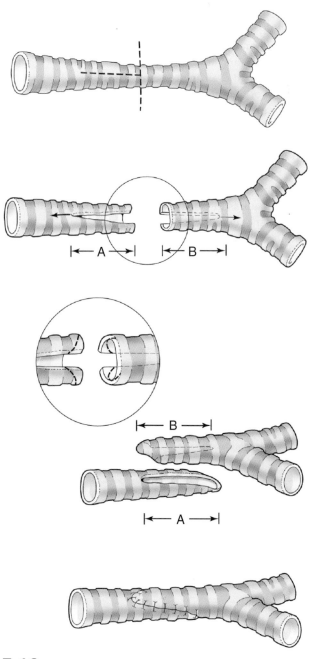

7.19

POSTOPERATIVE MANAGEMENT

After most airway reconstructions, the patient can usually be extubated at the end of the procedure. If a supralaryngeal T-tube is inserted, the closing minutes of the operation can be conducted using Venturi ventilation through the transverse limb of the tube. If there is any need to continue assisted ventilation, a laryngeal mask is preferred, thus avoiding an endotracheal tube across the anastomosis. Sputum clearance is facilitated by the minitracheostomy tube or T-tube. Prophylactic antibiotics are continued for 3–4 days.

Once speech has been assessed and adequate laryngeal function seems assured, the patient is allowed nourishing fluids, usually from the first postoperative morning. The use of a drinking straw is helpful until the patient becomes used to the neck-restraining sutures. A normal oral diet is usually established within 24 hours. A supralaryngeal T-tube may require more caution, but it is surprising how well patients swallow without any aspiration.

The wound drainage ceases over the first 24 hours, but removal of the drain is delayed until the eighth day when the minitracheostomy tube and neck-restraining sutures are also removed. The patient should be warned to protect the anastomosis from undue neck extension for a few weeks, particularly when sleeping. A U-shaped pillow is helpful. By the time they return to the clinic at 3–4 weeks, they will have lost the cautious approach and be moving their necks normally.

In situations in which a T-tube is considered necessary, the patient returns for endoscopic review under general anesthesia after 6 weeks. The tube is removed and healing and laryngeal function are assessed. If there is any concern, a clean T-tube is inserted for a further period, usually 6 weeks, and the assessment repeated.

Other postoperative problems are rare, but dysrhythmias can occur.

OUTCOMES

Postoperative mortality and morbidity depend on comorbid conditions, patient fitness, the length of airway resected, and the complexity of the reconstruction. Emergency resection can be avoided by the measures described previously.

Most benign lesions, and almost all postintubation strictures, can be resected, unless complicated by previous failed surgery or laser treatment. The perioperative mortality for such surgery is usually less than 2%. Good to excellent functional results are obtained in 90%–95% of patients.

The perioperative mortality for surgery in malignant cases, in which more extensive resections are required, is higher, in the region of 5%–6%. It is difficult to give estimates of prognosis after resection of malignancy, as, even in large series, the numbers in subgroups become small. The natural history of adenoid cystic carcinoma is often one of slow progression. Such patients can live for several years after radiotherapy alone, and asphyxia can be prevented by disobliteration techniques, stenting, and brachytherapy. In one series, mean survival after treatment of presumably more advanced disease by radiotherapy alone was 6.4 years, compared with 9.8 years after complete resection and 7.5 years after incomplete resection and radiotherapy. As in other cancer procedures, the surgeon should strive for complete resection but it is clearly unjustified to imperil the patient by striving for this if wider excision will complicate the reconstruction and add appreciably to perioperative risk. Such a delicately balanced decision requires experience. There are fewer statistics on survival after resection of squamous carcinomas, but survival in the region of 35% at 5 years has been reported.

Anastomotic problems, such as dehiscence or stricture, occur in less than 5% of operations performed in experienced units.

FURTHER READING

Barclay RS, McSwann N, Welsh TM. Tracheal reconstruction with the use of grafts. *Thorax*. 1957; 12: 177–80.

Goldstraw P. Endobronchial stents. In: Hetzel M ed. *Minimally invasive techniques in thoracic medicine and surgery*. 1st edn. London: Chapman and Hall, 1994.

Grillo HC. Development of tracheal surgery: a historical review. Part 1: techniques of tracheal surgery. *Annals of Thoracic Surgery*. 2003; 75: 610–19.

Grillo HC, Wright CD, Vlahakes GJ, MacGillivray TE. Management of congenital tracheal stenosis by means of slide tracheoplasty or resection and reconstruction, with long-term follow-up of growth after slide tracheoplasty. *Journal of Thoracic and Cardiovascular Surgery*. 2002; 123: 145–52.

Kutlu CA, Goldstraw P. Tracheo-bronchial sleeve resection using a continuous anastomosis: results of 100 consecutive cases. *Journal of Thoracic and Cardiovascular Surgery*. 1999; 117: 1112–17.

Maddaus MA, Toth JLR, Gullane PJ, Pearson FG. Subglottic tracheal resection and synchronous laryngeal reconstruction. *Journal of Thoracic and Cardiovascular Surgery*. 1992; 104: 1443–50.

Shankar S, George PJ, Hetzel MR, Goldstraw P. Elective resection of tumors of the trachea and main carina after endoscopic laser therapy. *Thorax*. 1990; 45: 493–5.

Tsang V, Murday AJ, Gillbe C, Goldstraw P. Slide tracheoplasty for congenital funnel-shaped tracheal stenosis. *Annals of Thoracic Surgery*. 1989; 48: 632–5.

8

Mediastinoscopy and mediastinotomy

JENNIFER L. WILSON AND ERIC VALLIÈRES

HISTORY

Recognition of advanced lung cancer by using a novel cervicomediastinal exploration technique was first described in 1954 by Dwight Harken. The publications of Eric Carlens in Sweden and F. Griffith Pearson in Canada, in 1959 and 1964, respectively, helped popularize the procedure. Today, mediastinoscopy remains an excellent minimally invasive technique to evaluate the mediastinal lymph nodes (see **Figure 8.1**) as well as anterosuperior mediastinal masses to histologically distinguish benign, malignant, and infectious processes.

Although the design of the modern mediastinoscope remains very similar to the original, the advancement to video mediastinoscopy, which was first described in 1989 by Lerut, has significantly improved visualization, teaching, safety, dissection, and reproducibility. In addition to permitting access to paratracheal and pericarinal superior mediastinal lymph nodes (stations 2R, 2L, 4R, 4L, and 7), due to superior visualization, video mediastinoscopy also allows access to the central N1 stations. Although there are no randomized controlled trials comparing video with the nonvideo original approach, several retrospective reviews suggest that video mediastinoscopy results in better nodal access and sampling.

The para-aortic (station 5) and aortopulmonary (station 6) lymph nodes are not accessible by conventional cervical mediastinoscopy (CM); to that effect, in 1966, McNeill and Chamberlain developed a technique known as "anterior mediastinotomy," the so-called Chamberlain procedure, to access these nodes. In the 1980s, the extended cervical mediastinoscopy (ECM) approach was described, where one accesses the station 5 and 6 lymph nodes through the CM incision by advancing the mediastinoscope over the aortic arch, medial to the left common carotid artery.

Ongoing methods of lymph node sampling continued to evolve and, in 1999, the first dedicated endobronchial ultrasound (EBUS) bronchoscopy system became commercially

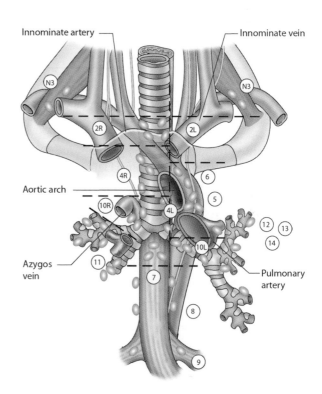

8.1 Mediastinal lymph node stations. Note: Station 4R is to the right of the trachea and station 4L includes nodal tissue overlying the trachea and to the left of the trachea.

available. This allows ultrasound-guided needle biopsy aspirates of lymph node stations 2, 4, 7, 10, 11, and 12. Furthermore, transesophageal endoscopic ultrasound (EUS) was developed, which allows needle biopsy aspirates of lymph node stations 4L, 5, 7, 8, and 9.

Hürtgen described another novel technique in 2003: video-assisted mediastinal lymphadenectomy (VAMLA).

This technique allows even better nodal sampling of stations 2R, 2L, 4R, 4L, and 7. The following year, Kuzdzał et al. described transcervical extended mediastinal lymphadenectomy (TEMLA), which allows near complete mediastinal lymphadenectomy, removing most lymph nodes in stations 1, 2R, 2L, 3a, 4R, proximal 4L, 5, 6, 7, and 8.

In summary, many complementary techniques exist for complete histologic evaluation of the mediastinum. To date, cervical video mediastinoscopy remains the gold standard for the mediastinal nodal staging of lung cancer. All lung cancer surgeons should be proficient at this technique and at anterior mediastinotomy, which allow access to the para-aortic and aortopulmonary lymph nodes. Here, these two most commonly employed techniques will be described, along with two emerging techniques, VAMLA and TEMLA. Other techniques of mediastinal lymph node sampling, such as ECM, EBUS, EUS-guided biopsy, as well as video-assisted thoracoscopic surgery (VATS) and percutaneous biopsy, while beyond the scope of this chapter, can also be useful mediastinal staging methods.

PRINCIPLES AND JUSTIFICATION

Accurate clinical staging of patients with lung cancer is imperative to offer patients appropriate therapy and imaging alone is insufficient. Results of the American College of Surgeons Oncology Group Z0050 trial in 2003 demonstrated that computed tomography (CT) plus fluorodeoxyglucose positron emission tomography (FDG PET) correctly identified N2/N3 disease in 53% of patients, which was significantly superior to CT alone (32%). In the study, FDG PET had a sensitivity of 61%, specificity of 84%, positive predictive value of 56%, and negative predictive value of 87%. In addition, the sensitivity of positron emission tomography (PET) for M1 disease was 83% and the specificity was 90%. Integrated CT/PET scans have improved imaging accuracy; however, in patients who are otherwise potential candidates for resection, enlarged lymph nodes on CT that are FDG PET avid do require at least cytological confirmation of involvement for accurate staging.

CM is an excellent procedure to access and biopsy several mediastinal lymph node stations. CM is better known as a modality used for lung cancer staging, but it is also very helpful to evaluate the etiology of mediastinal lymphadenopathy for conditions such as sarcoidosis and lymphoma in which cytology or smaller needle biopsies may not provide sufficient diagnostic tissue.

The proficiency and use of mediastinoscopy to clinically stage patients with lung cancer varies among surgeons. In a U.S. survey of 729 hospitals, preoperative mediastinoscopy was only performed in 27.1% of patients and node biopsy was successful in only 46.6% of these procedures. The fact that nodal tissue was sampled in less than half of mediastinoscopies is disappointing and may be related to the fact that non-thoracic-trained general surgeons performed many of these procedures. To support this theory, Wei et al.

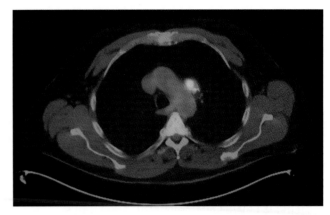

8.2 Left upper lobe lung cancer with PET-positive station 6 lymph node.

demonstrated that nodal tissue was sampled 100% of the time when mediastinoscopy was performed by a thoracic surgeon in a single center retrospective review of 1907 cases.

The false-negative rate of mediastinoscopy in identifying the presence of N2 nodal involvement is reported to be around 8%. However, one must recognize that about half of the missed involved nodes are located outside of the mediastinoscopy range.

As a consequence, thorough mediastinal lymph node sampling is imperative during lung resection and remains the standard of care.

Anterior mediastinotomy can be used to biopsy and diagnose anterior mediastinal masses on the right or left hemithorax. In situations where the involvement of station 5/6 mediastinal lymph nodes is suspected radiographically (see **Figure 8.2**), a left anterior mediastinotomy may allow direct biopsy to rule in or out such involvement. Alternatively, one may prefer a VATS approach for such biopsies, though this approach requires double lumen intubation and patient repositioning. In this scenario, a CM should be completed first, as a significant proportion of patients with involved stations 5 and 6 will also have involvement of the central superior mediastinal nodes and, if these are positive on frozen section analysis, one does not need to perform the mediastinotomy.

PREOPERATIVE ASSESSMENT AND PREPARATION

Mediastinotomy and CM can be safely performed in an ambulatory surgical setting. There are very few absolute contraindications to CM or mediastinotomy. The only absolute contraindication to CM is the presence of an aortic arch aneurysm and the only absolute contraindication to mediastinotomy is the presence of an internal mammary artery cardiac bypass graft. If the aortopulmonary window (AP window) needs to be sampled and the patient has an internal mammary graft or coronary artery bypass graft, a VATS approach is recommended.

In addition, patients with severe kyphosis or fused cervical vertebrae may not be able to extend their neck adequately for CM. Relative contraindications to CM include severe atherosclerotic disease of the aortic arch and right innominate and/or vertebral arteries, as this can put the patient at risk for an embolic stroke. Superior vena cava obstruction historically was considered a contraindication to CM, but this has been shown to be safe in experienced hands. Similarly, experience allows the possibility of safely performing repeat CM and mediastinotomy, which may be technically challenging due to scarring and fibrosis. Patients with large thyroid masses or prior irradiation that require CM may also be more challenging and, in these cases, CM and mediastinotomy should be performed by experienced surgeons.

MEDIASTINOSCOPY

Anesthesia and patient positioning

The patient is placed in the supine position. General endotracheal anesthesia is induced and the endotracheal tube is taped to the side of the patient's mouth to prevent dislodgement during the procedure. The use of a laryngeal mask airway has also been shown to be safe. Maximal cervical extension is very important. This may be accomplished by placing a roll beneath the shoulders while maintaining support of the head (see **Figure 8.3**). At times, one may have to drop the head of the operating table to maximize such extension. Both arms are tucked at the patient's side. The neck, chest, and upper abdomen are prepped and draped into the surgical field in case one needs to proceed to an emergent sternotomy in the very rare case of massive hemorrhage.

Equipment

- Standard surgical equipment: scalpel, forceps, Metzenbaum scissors
- Video (Lerut) mediastinoscope (see **Figure 8.4**)
- Insulated combined suction and cautery device connected to a foot pedal
- Mediastinoscopy biopsy forceps, straight and up biting
- Sternal saw (in the room)

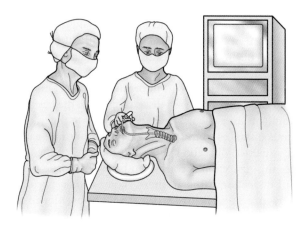

8.3 Patient positioning for CM.

8.4 Standard CM equipment: video mediastinoscope, biopsy forceps, and protected suction cautery.

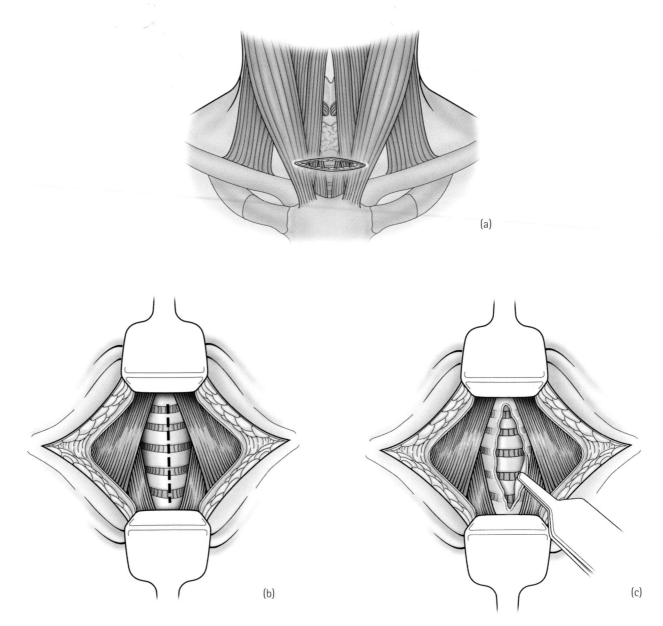

8.5a–c (a) Skin incision, (b) dissection between the strap muscles, and (c) pretracheal fascia.

Operation

A 2 cm transverse skin incision is made approximately 1.5 fingerbreadths above the sternal notch in the midline (see **Figure 8.5a**). Electrocautery is used to transect soft tissues and the platysma muscle transversally. Once the strap muscles are reached, the dissection is then carried out vertically in between the muscles overlying the trachea. Vertical dissection avoids injury to the anterior jugular veins laterally. Intermittent gentle blunt up-and-down finger dissection over the trachea is helpful to reorient oneself periodically during the procedure, as well as to palpate and identify the thyroid isthmus.

Once the pretracheal fascia is identified inferior to the thyroid isthmus, it is grasped and incised sharply with scissors (see **Figure 8.5b and c**). A right-angle retractor is then placed in the pretracheal space, gently lifting upward. Simultaneously, gentle pressure on the anterior wall of the trachea pushes the airway posteriorly, which allows dissection of the pretracheal plane under direct vision. One should aim to carry this visualized dissection below the level of the innominate artery, which crosses anteriorly to the trachea at various distances from the thoracic inlet. In some patients, this visualized dissection will reach the level of the carina. Once this dissection is completed beyond the field of view, blunt dissection using an index finger is then performed (see **Figure 8.6**). The finger pad should be positioned anteriorly and blunt digital dissection into the mediastinum is performed by advancing the finger into the mediastinum with care to maintain position directly over the trachea. The

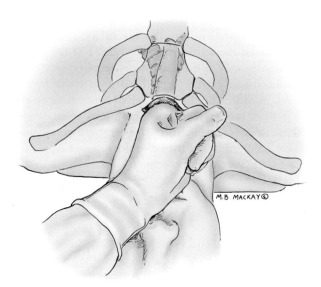

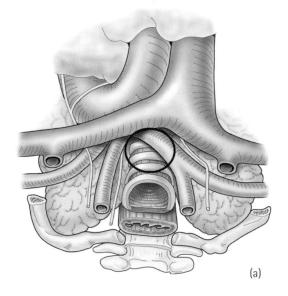

(a)

8.6 Blunt dissection with the index finger.

right innominate artery will be palpated at this time (see **Figure 8.7a**). The video mediastinoscope is then inserted into the tract, visualizing the trachea at all times to maintain orientation.

A combination of blunt and electrocautery dissection is performed overlying the trachea, advancing caudad to the subcarinal space. Identifying the subcarinal space is useful to accurately recognize the mediastinal anatomy. The right pulmonary artery is identified over the subcarinal space and is protected during dissection (see **Figure 8.7b**). Once the subcarinal space is identified, the scope is withdrawn slightly and the azygos vein is identified to the right of the trachea, traveling vertically in the tracheobronchial angle (see **Figure 8.8a**). an alternative is to initiate the dissection along the right paratracheal wall and pursue down to the right tracheobronchial angle until the azygos vein is identified.

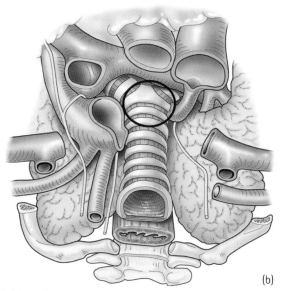

(b)

8.7a–b Anatomy: (a) right innominate artery and (b) right pulmonary artery crossing anterior to the trachea.

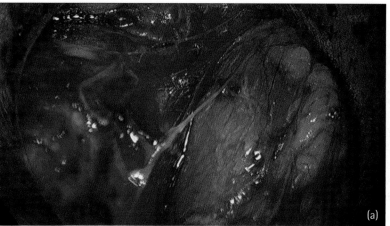

(a)

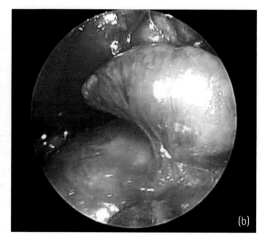

(b)

8.8a–b Video mediastinoscopy photos: (a) azygos vein and (b) lymph node.

The order of lymph node sampling may vary depending on the clinical scenario. It is important to dissect under direct vision with care to protect surrounding structures and to use cautery judiciously. The mediastinal parietal pleura is often seen in the right paratracheal area, particularly in individuals with emphysematous lungs: movements of the underlying lung are usually seen with each breathing cycle. When lymph node stations are identified, it is wise to bluntly dissect them free of surrounding tissues before biopsy (see **Figure 8.8b**). This can help distinguish nodal tissue from vascular structures. When nodes are sampled or dissected using electrocautery and cupped mediastinal biopsy forceps, hemostasis should be achieved before moving to the next station to optimize visualization and safe dissection. The use of cautery should be avoided in the left paratracheal and tracheobronchial angle zones so as to minimize the risks of left recurrent laryngeal nerve (RLN) injury.

The highest mediastinal lymph node station at 2R can be identified and sampled above the innominate artery. The station 4R lymph node packet can be identified above the azygos vein. Importantly, one should remember that, as per the latest iterations of the mediastinal nodal map, station 4R extends across the midline all the way to the left side of the trachea. Below the azygos vein, the right upper lobe bronchus can often be identified and station 10R can be sampled. The subcarinal (station 7) space often has crossing bronchial vessels that require coagulation. When these vessels are unusually large, a clip applier can be useful. The esophagus lies directly posterior to the subcarinal nodes and therefore cautery should be used judiciously in that area. Finally, station 2L lymph node and 4L lymph node packets are bluntly dissected without using electrocautery.

Temporarily packing the biopsied areas with unfolded gauze or a cut sheet of an absorbable hemostatic agent can be useful during dissection. The absorbable hemostatic agents may be left in place permanently, though they may, over time, cause an impressive local fibrotic reaction that may render the hilar dissection difficult at the time of a delayed resection (beyond 2 weeks). Once hemostasis is achieved, the wound is closed in layers using absorbable sutures. Reapproximation of the strap muscles is optional. The platysma and skin are closed with absorbable sutures and thin adhesive strips are placed as the only dressing.

Postoperative care

There is no need for obtaining a routine chest radiograph after CM unless one is concerned of having punctured the pleura. In general, these procedures are performed in an ambulatory setting and patients are discharged from the recovery area. The patient's voice should be assessed in the postanesthesia care unit to assess for RLN injury. Patients are instructed to call the office if they become hoarse after the procedure.

Outcome

The safety, high sensitivity and specificity, and very low morbidity and mortality (<0.25) of video CM has consistently been proven in the literature. Complications, which are rare and have been reported to occur in 1% or fewer of patients, include major hemorrhage, RLN paralysis, esophageal perforation, tracheobronchial injury, mediastinitis, cerebrovascular accident. RLN nerve palsy and wound infection are reported in less than 1% of patients. CM is safely performed in the outpatient setting.

Further reading

Adebibe M, Jarral OA, Shipolini AR, McCormack DJ. Does video-assisted mediastinoscopy have a better lymph node yield and safety profile than conventional mediastinoscopy? *Interactive Cardiovascular and Thoracic Surgery.* 2012; 14(3): 316–19.

Harken DE, Black H, Clauss R, Farrand RE. A simple cervicomediastinal exploration for tissue diagnosis of intrathoracic disease; with comments on the recognition of inoperable carcinoma of the lung. *New England Journal of Medicine.* 1954; 251(26): 1041–4.

Louie BE, Kapur S, Farivar AS, Youssef SJ, Gorden J, Aye RW, Vallières E. Safety and utility of mediastinoscopy in non-small cell lung cancer in a complex mediastinum. *Annals of Thoracic Surgery.* 2011; 92(1): 278–82.

Park BJ, Flores R, Downey RJ, Bains MS, Rusch VW. Management of major hemorrhage during mediastinoscopy. *Journal of Thoracic and Cardiovascular Surgery.* 2003; 126(3): 726–31.

Wei B, Bryant AS, Minnich DJ, Cerfolio RJ. The safety and efficacy of mediastinoscopy when performed by general thoracic surgeons. *Annals of Thoracic Surgery.* 2014; 97(6): 1873–83; discussion 1883–4.

MEDIASTINOTOMY

Anesthesia and patient positioning

General anesthesia with a single lumen endotracheal tube is preferred. Local anesthesia, however, may suffice in situations where one is to biopsy a large mediastinal mass with associated cardiovascular or airway compromise. If the awake patient does not tolerate the supine position hemodynamically or due to respiratory compromise, they may maintain the seated position. The entire chest and upper abdomen are prepped into the surgical field.

Equipment

- Standard surgical equipment: scalpel, forceps, suture ligatures and ties for control of the internal mammary vessels if needed
- Weitlander or other soft tissue retractor
- Video (Lerut) mediastinoscope if stations 5 and 6 are to be sampled (see **Figure 8.4**)

Operation

Preoperative CT imaging is extremely helpful in identifying the most optimal incision location, especially in cases of large anterosuperior mediastinal masses. In the majority of cases, as well as for access to the station 5 and 6 lymph nodes, the left-side 2nd intercostal space is used. Identifying the 2nd intercostal space can be accomplished by palpation. This is done by counting ribs and by palpating the sternal–manubrial junction (angle of Louis). Local anesthetic is injected into the soft tissues and a transverse 3–6 cm incision is made 1 cm lateral to the sternum overlying the 2nd intercostal space (see **Figure 8.9**). The pectoralis major muscle fibers are split parallel without division. The intercostal muscles are then divided over the rib superficial to the pleura. Medially, it is important to dissect carefully to avoid inadvertent injury to the internal mammary vessels (see **Figure 8.9a**). Historically, a segment of the second rib was removed to facilitate dissection; however, it is very rare in our practice to remove a portion of the rib, and it is done only if necessary to facilitate exposure. During this dissection, the internal mammary vessels can be preserved but, at times, suture ligation is required to facilitate exposure and avoid avulsion injury during the procedure (see **Figure 8.9b**). One may then proceed extrapleurally or transpleurally depending on the process being targeted.

In the case of large mediastinal masses, the tissue in question is often immediately visible and/or palpable at this time. Aspiration of the mass with a 25-gauge needle to rule out major vasculature can be helpful if the anatomy is severely altered. Biopsies are then taken using mediastinoscopy forceps and/or sharp dissection with a scalpel (see **Figure 8.10**). To evaluate the AP window and para-aortic lymph nodes (stations 5 and 6), a video mediastinoscope

(a)

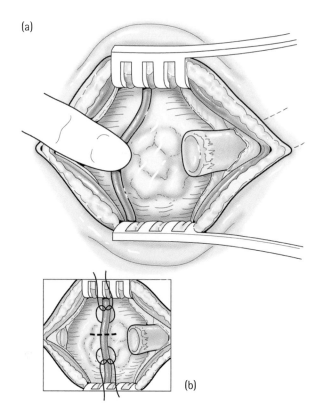

(b)

8.9a–b Mediastinotomy incision: (a) visualization of the left internal mammary artery and (b) division of the left internal mammary artery

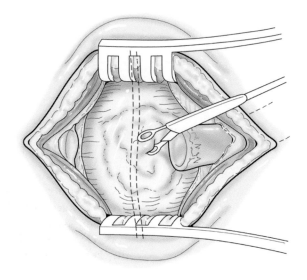

8.10 Biopsy of station 5 and 6 lymph nodes.

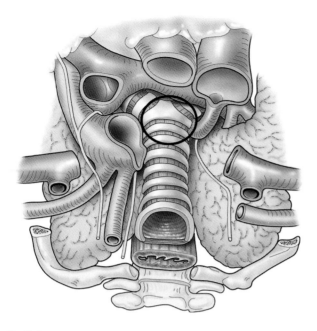

8.11 Video mediastinoscopy through an anterior mediastinotomy to evaluate stations 5 and 6; RLN is shown.

can be used to facilitate lymph node identification and biopsy (see **Figure 8.11**). Aspiration with a 25-gauge needle can be helpful if anatomy is altered to rule out major vasculature prior to biopsy. During biopsy, one should be careful not to injure the left phrenic and RLNs. In the presence of a bulky left hilar or AP window mass when resectability is questionable, if CM has been performed, simultaneous bimanual palpation via the CM under the aortic arch via the CM and left anterior mediastinotomy incisions may improve the evaluation (see **Figure 8.12a and b**).

In the absence of parenchymal lung injury, a drainage tube is not necessary. When the pleural space has been entered and the lung remains uninjured, a red rubber catheter can be temporarily used to evacuate air during closure. This is accomplished by closing the musculofascial layer around the tube in a tunneled fashion using absorbable 0 suture. The catheter is then removed in a coordinated way by asking the anesthetist to give a breath while tightening the suture line and closing the final defect as the tube is removed. The wound is then closed in layers using absorbable 2-0 and 3-0 sutures. Thin adhesive strips and a simple absorbent dressing are placed over the incision.

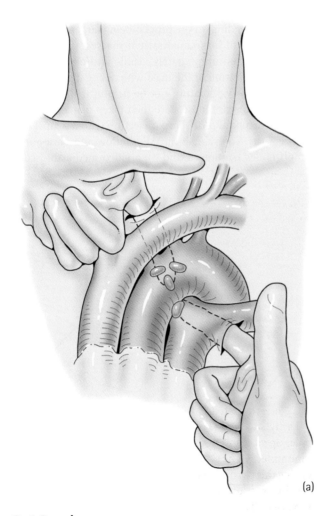

(a)

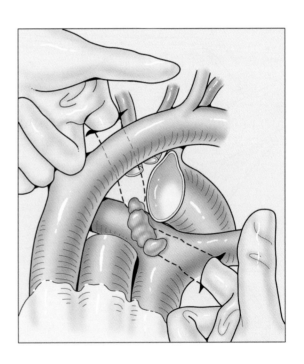

(b)

8.12a–b Bimanual palpation to evaluate stations 5 and 6.

Postoperative care

A chest X-ray is routinely obtained in the recovery unit to rule out effusion and significant pneumothorax. In general, patients are discharged the same day as the procedure.

Outcome

As with mediastinoscopy, mediastinotomy is safe, highly sensitive and specific, and can be performed in the outpatient setting with extremely low morbidity and mortality.

Further reading

Cerfolio RJ, Bryant AS, Eloubeidi MA. Accessing the aortopulmonary window (#5) and the paraaortic (#6) lymph nodes in patients with non-small cell lung cancer. *Annals of Thoracic Surgery.* 2007; 84(3): 940–5.

McNeill TM, Chamberlain JM. Diagnostic anterior mediastinotomy. *Annals of Thoracic Surgery.* 1966; 2(4): 532–9.

Okada M, Tsubota N, Yoshimura M, Miyamoto Y, Matsuoka H. Prognosis of completely resected pN2 non-small cell lung carcinomas: What is the significant node that affects survival? *Journal of Cardiovascular Surgery.* 1999; 118(2): 270–5.

Patterson GA, Piazza D, Pearson FG, Todd TR, Ginsberg RJ, Goldberg M, Waters P, Jones D, Ilves R, Cooper JD. Significance of metastatic disease in subaortic lymph nodes. *Annals of Thoracic Surgery.* 1987; 43(2): 155–9.

Vallières E, Page A, Verdant A. Ambulatory mediastinoscopy and anterior mediastinotomy. *Annals of Thoracic Surgery.* 1991; 52(5): 1122–6.

TRANSCERVICAL EXTENDED MEDIASTINAL LYMPHADENECTOMY

Anesthesia and patient positioning

The patient receives general anesthesia with a single lumen endotracheal tube (a double lumen tube may be used if the patient is also scheduled to undergo lobectomy) and is placed in the supine position. The entire chest and upper abdomen are prepped into the surgical field.

Equipment

- Specialized sternal retractor that mounts onto the operating room table and allows upward retraction of the manubrium
- Thirty-degree video thoracoscope
- Nineteen-centimeter Wolf mediastinoscope (Richard Wolf GmbH, Knittlingen, Germany)

Operation

A 5–8 cm collar incision is made above the sternal notch and the anterior jugular veins are divided. Skin flaps are raised to the level of the thyroid cartilage superiorly and sternum inferiorly. Strap muscles are divided in the midline and retracted. The right middle thyroid veins are divided. The right carotid artery and brachiocephalic artery are fully mobilized and the RLN is protected. Next, the left carotid artery is mobilized and the left RLN is visualized and protected.

A sternal retractor is placed under the manubrium and mounted on the operating table with a traction system allowing sternal elevation. Next, the upper thymic poles are separated from the thyroid and retracted upward. This allows the superior surface of the innominate vein to be dissected free. Kuzdal, who initially described the technique, stresses the importance of mobilizing the carotid arteries, brachiocephalic artery, left internal jugular vein, and bilateral innominate veins to improve mediastinal exposure.

At this time, the lymphadenectomy is begun starting with station 1. This is accomplished by removing *en bloc* the tissue anterior to the trachea, posterior to the upper poles of the thymus, and superior to the left innominate vein between the RLNs bilaterally. Next, the right paratracheal space is exposed by elevating the confluence of the innominate veins, retracting the trachea to the left, and opening the tissue below and above the brachiocephalic artery. The 2R lymph nodes can be accessed above the artery and the 4R lymph nodes can be accessed between the artery and the tracheal wall. These nodes are removed to the level of the azygos vein *en bloc* bordered by the innominate vein, vena cava, vertebral column, mediastinal pleura, trachea, ascending aorta, and right main bronchus.

Next, the left paratracheal space is dissected by retracting the trachea to the right and the left common carotid artery to the left and upward. Lymph nodes 2L and 4L are removed with care to avoid the RLN. A 19 cm Wolf mediastinoscope is used for removing stations 7 and 8. Station 6 lymph nodes are dissected by opening the space between the left common carotid artery and left innominate vein. The left vagus is protected at this time. The vein is retracted upward and the anterior surface of the aortic arch is exposed, allowing station 6 to be removed to the level of the AP window and station 5. The station 5 lymph nodes are best visualized using a 30-degree laparoscopic camera, which is inserted between the left innominate vein and the common carotid artery. Station 5 lymph nodes are removed to the level of the left pulmonary artery. The left vagus nerve is an important landmark during dissection of the station 5 lymph nodes and can be used as a guide to avoid injury to the accessory hemiazygos vein.

Lastly, station 3 is dissected by retracting the upper thymic poles upward and to the left, allowing blunt dissection of the innominate vein confluence. A cloth-tipped dissector is used during this portion of the case for blunt dissection and downward retraction of the brachiocephalic vein and superior vena cava. This allows removal of the station 3 nodes. After hemostasis is achieved, the wound is closed without a drain.

Postoperative care

Length of hospital stay has not been well described, as, in many series, TEMLA is performed in conjunction with a pulmonary resection.

Outcome

In a retrospective review of 256 patients that underwent TEMLA for non-small-cell lung cancer, a mean of 38.9 lymph nodes (range 15–85) were removed during the procedure. Permanent RLN palsy was reported in only 0.8% of patients, while a temporary RLN palsy was reported in 2.3% of patients. Mediastinal scarring has been well described and authors have recommended pulmonary resection in the early postoperative period if it is planned.

Further reading

Kuzdzał J, Zieliński M, Papla B, Szlubowski A, Hauer Ł, Nabiałek T, Sośnicki W, Pankowski J. Transcervical extended mediastinal lymphadenectomy: The new operative technique and early results in lung cancer staging. *European Journal of Cardiothoracic Surgery*. 2005; 27(3): 384–90.

Kuzdzał J, Zieliński M, Papla B, Urbanik A, Wojciechowski W, Narski M, Szlubowski A, Hauer L. The transcervical extended mediastinal lymphadenectomy versus cervical mediastinoscopy in non-small cell lung cancer staging. *European Journal of Cardiothoracic Surgery*. 2007; 31(1): 88–94.

Zieliński M. Transcervical extended mediastinal lymphadenectomy: Results of staging in two hundred fifty-six consecutive patients with non-small cell lung cancer. *Journal of Thoracic Oncology*. 2007; 2(4): 370–2.

VIDEO-ASSISTED MEDIASTINAL LYMPHADENECTOMY

Anesthesia and patient positioning

The patient receives general anesthesia with a single lumen endotracheal tube (a double lumen tube may be used if the patient is also scheduled to undergo lobectomy) and is placed in the supine position. The entire chest and upper abdomen are prepped into the surgical field.

Equipment

Video mediastinoscope with two-bladed speculum design (Richard Wolf GmbH).

Operation

The mediastinoscope is inserted in the same fashion as has been described for standard cervical video mediastinoscopy as noted in an earlier section of this chapter. Radical mediastinal lymphadenectomy is performed, completely excising stations 1, 2R, 2L, 4R, 4L, and 7. Dissection of each station is done similarly to that described in detail for conventional video CM, as noted earlier in this chapter, with the exception that the mediastinoscope blades can be separated, allowing bimanual lymphadenectomy.

Postoperative care

VAMLA is typically an outpatient procedure.

Outcome

In a retrospective review of 37 patients, RLN injury was reported in one patient by Hürtgen et al. in 2005. In addition, increased mediastinal scarring has been reported.

Further reading

Hürtgen M, Friedel G, Toomes H, Fritz P. Radical video-assisted mediastinoscopic lymphadenectomy (VAMLA): Technique and first results. *European Journal of Cardiothoracic Surgery*. 2003; 21(2): 348–51.

Hürtgen M, Friedel G, Witte B, Toomes H, Fritz P. Systematic video-assisted mediastinoscopic lymphadenectomy (VAMLA). *Thoracic Surgical Science*. 2005; 2: Doc02.

Leshber G, Holinka G, Linder A. Video-assisted mediastinoscopic lymphadenectomy (VAMLA): A method of systematic lymphnode dissection. *European Journal of Cardiothoracic Surgery*. 2003; 24(2): 192–5.

9

Anterior mediastinal lesions

ANTONIO D'ANDRILLI, ERINO ANGELO RENDINA, AND FEDERICO VENUTA

The mediastinum is a virtual three-dimensional space located between the lungs, above the diaphragm, posteriorly to the sternum, and anteriorly to the spine. The thoracic inlet (or outlet) is open toward the neck. Due to its complexity, the great number of anatomical structures and the list of disorders that may affect them, the mediastinum is classically divided into compartments. The classification is extremely useful to drive a differential diagnosis for a given mediastinal mass. The classical anatomical classification of the mediastinum reports four compartments: anterior, superior, middle, and posterior. The anterior and the superior compartments are often unified in a single region (the anterosuperior compartment) since most of the disorders affecting one of them usually involve, or might involve, the other. The anterior compartment is bounded anteriorly by the posterior aspect of the sternum and posteriorly by the pericardium. The superior compartment is that territory above an imaginary line drawn from the sternomanubrial junction and the inferior border of the fourth thoracic vertebra. The union of these two regions corresponds to what Shields called the "prevascular zone."[1] This space contains mediastinal fat, the thymus, and lymph nodes. Since germ cell tumors can arise within this region, germ cell remnants are theoretically assumed to be present; however, they are seldom found in a nonneoplastic state. In addition, ectopic parathyroids are occasionally found, sometimes embedded within the thymus. Also, it is in these compartments that the thyroid gland can descend as a retrosternal goiter.

The most common tumors in this region are thymoma, lymphoma, germ cell tumor, and parathyroid adenoma.

THYMOMA

Tumors of the thymus gland are known as "thymomas." Although these lesions are relatively rare, they account more than 50% overall making them the most common anterior mediastinal masses.[2,3] They can present both as small, round, encapsulated lesions or huge infiltrating masses involving the surrounding structures. Calcifications can be found in approximately 10%–20% of the cases.

Thymomas are often associated with a variety of *parathymic syndromes*. The most frequent is myasthenia gravis (MG), which has been reported in up to 45% of these patients. The presence of this condition in association with an anterior mediastinal mass is usually pathognomonic for a thymoma.

Although thymoma may occur at all ages, this disease is more frequent in those aged between 40 and 70 years. Patients with MG tend to be slightly younger, with a peak between 30 and 60 years. Only 10%–15% of the patients with MG are found to have thymoma.[4]

Therefore, in adult patients with MG and a typical presentation on computed tomography (CT) scan, the diagnosis of thymoma appears very likely. In such cases, a biopsy to confirm diagnosis is generally considered not necessary and surgical resection based on clinical findings is justified when feasible without induction therapy.

At younger ages, without MG, if the mediastinal lesion has no typical radiographic features, histological confirmation is required, particularly for large infiltrating masses.

Fine needle or core biopsy should be preferred as a first step; however, these procedures frequently yield insufficient material, with subsequent need for surgical sampling through anterior mediastinotomy or (more rarely) thoracoscopy. The average sensitivity of needle biopsy has been reported as high as 60% compared with approximately 90% of surgical approach; however, the ability to accurately determine the exact histology of thymoma on a limited biopsy has been reported as low.[5]

Management of stage I and II thymic tumors

Surgical resection is the gold standard of thymoma treatment, resulting in high overall and disease-free survival rates in patients with stage I and II disease.

In a review including a series with more than 100 patients, Detterbeck and Parsons reported 5-year survival rates ranging from 80% to 100% after resection of stage I thymoma, with an average rate of 91%.[4] An average 5-year survival of 80% was reported for stage II thymoma, with a higher variability in results among the series (range 42%–100%). Average overall 10-year survival rates were 87% (range 75%–100%) for stage I and 67% for stage II. The average recurrence rate was 3% after resection of stage I tumor and 11% for stage II thymoma.

Complete resection is the norm and is expected for stage I tumors. For stage II lesions an average complete resection rate of 87% has been reported, but wide variation among different studies exists.[6]

Recommendation for total thymectomy is made even when the thymoma involves only a limited portion of the gland, although no definitive evidence has been demonstrated to support this recommendation.

PREOPERATIVE ASSESSMENT FOR THYMOMA

1. The tumor usually is first detected on a chest radiograph. The extent of the tumor can be well evaluated by conventional chest CT and magnetic resonance imaging (MRI). An exact histological diagnosis is very important to differentiate thymomas from other malignant thymic tumors, especially when the lesion appears to be locally invasive. CT-guided biopsy, anterior mediastinotomy, or rarely a thoracotomy is used for this purpose. (See **Figure 9.1**.)

ANESTHESIA FOR THYMOMA

If airway compromise is present, awake endotracheal intubation should be considered. Otherwise, general anesthesia can be induced in the usual manner. A double lumen endotracheal tube is indicated for procedures where a partial lung resection may be indicated. Central venous pressure should be carefully monitored if the venous return is impaired. A thoracic epidural catheter is placed for intraoperative and postoperative pain management. In cases of MG, the anesthesia should be managed accordingly with careful attention paid to the appropriate use of neuromuscular blocking agents.

OPERATION FOR THYMOMA

Preparation for tumor resection

2. An extended total thymectomy, including the tumor in conjunction with resection of any invaded adjacent structure, is the ultimate goal. The anterior mediastinum is entered through a full median sternotomy. The intact part of the thymus is first dissected along with pericardium if involved. When the mediastinal pleura is invaded by the tumor, the pleura is incised and taken with the specimen. If invasion into the lung is present, partial resection is performed with a linear stapler. Thus, the thymus and the tumor can be freed from the surrounding structures, except for the SVC and brachiocephalic veins if they are involved. The right and left brachiocephalic veins should be dissected sufficiently distal to the tumor invading site and encircled with cotton umbilical tape. The SVC is also mobilized and encircled with tape, either inside or outside the pericardium, depending on the extent of tumor invasion to the SVC. The azygos vein above the pulmonary hilum and the internal mammary vein are separated and divided between the ligatures. The phrenic nerve is sacrificed if absolutely necessary to achieve a complete resection. (See **Figure 9.2**.)

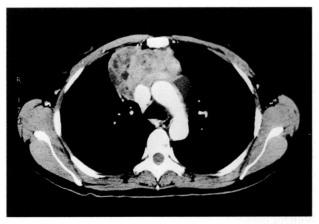

9.1

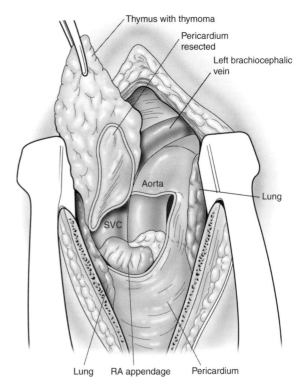

9.2

Reconstruction of the left brachiocephalic vein and the superior vena cava

3. In general, reconstruction is first performed between the left brachiocephalic vein and the right atrium, followed by reconstruction between the right brachiocephalic vein and the SVC. After heparin sodium is intravenously administered, the left brachiocephalic vein is occluded distally with an atraumatic vascular clamp and ligated proximally, and then divided. An anastomosis between the distal stump of the left brachiocephalic vein and the appendage of the right atrium is performed using a ringed Gore-Tex 8.0 mm graft secured with a 5-0 monofilament polypropylene suture by a simple continuous technique. (See **Figure 9.3a and b.**)

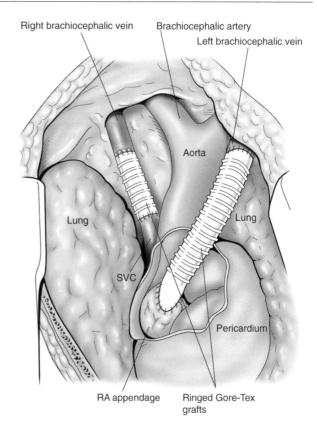

9.4

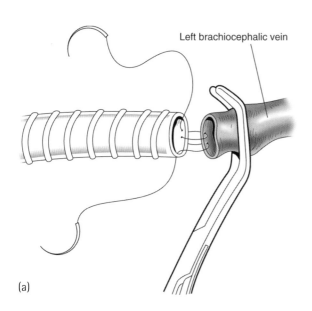

(a)

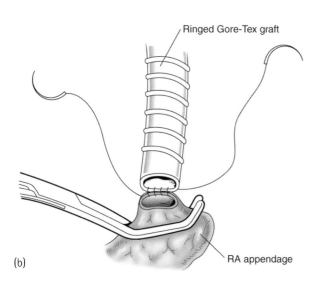

(b)

9.3a–b

4. The right brachiocephalic vein is occluded distally and the SVC proximally, and both veins are divided on the tumor side. Thus, the thymus, including the tumor, is completely removed. The SVC is reconstructed in the same manner as the left brachiocephalic vein using a ringed Gore-Tex 10.0 mm graft. Some surgeons believe that one brachiocephalic vein is adequate to return blood from the upper half of the body to the heart. Reconstruction of the right brachiocephalic vein can be abandoned without major complications, except for transient swelling in the right upper extremity. In this instance, effort should be made to leave the azygos vein intact. (See **Figure 9.4.**)

Complications

Major complications are rarely encountered. Occlusion of the graft, particularly that used for the left brachiocephalic vein, sometimes occurs, because it is long and could be compressed by the sternum and ascending aorta. When both veins are reconstructed, however, occlusion of only one graft may not cause a problem. Postoperative respiratory failure may be related to the severity of the associated MG and complicated if the phrenic nerve was sacrificed. As patients with MG have a relatively early stage thymoma, this ominous combination is quite rare.

Table 9.1 Masaoka thymoma staging system[7]

Stage	Definition
I	Macroscopically encapsulated tumor, with no microscopic capsular invasion
IIA	Microscopic transcapular invasion into surrounding fatty tissue or mediastinal pleura
IIB	Macroscopic transcapular invasion into the capsule
III	Macroscopic invasion into neighboring organs
IVA	Pleural or pericardial metastases
IVB	Lymphogenous or hematogenous metastasis

OUTCOME FOR THYMOMA

The clinical staging system for thymomas devised by Masaoka, which is based on the local extension of the tumor, has been shown to best reflect the prognosis, and the significance of staging by this system has been validated by several other institutions.[7] A brief description of Masaoka's criteria is presented in **Table 9.1**.

Among 194 consecutively treated patients with thymoma who underwent a complete resection or subtotal resection at our institution, the 10-year and 20-year survival rates were, respectively, 99% and 90% for stage I disease, 94% and 90% for stage II tumors, 88% and 56% for stage III disease, 30% and 15% for stage IVA lesions, and 0% and 0% for stage IVB tumors.[8] In addition, the 10-year and 20-year survival rates for patients with stage III disease were, respectively, 97% and 75% when no involvement of the great vessels was present, and 70% and 29% when these vessels were involved. Thus, involvement of the great vessels was the single independent prognostic factor in patients with stage III disease, by multivariate analysis.

The TNM [tumor node metastasis] Classification of Malignant Tumors staging system has been also proposed for thymoma with limited acceptance, particularly because prognosis and treatment strategies for this tumor are mainly influenced by the T status, which is well described by the Masaoka system, while mediastinal node involvement (N factor) has a minor significance.

Pathologic classification has been reported as an additional factor potentially influencing prognosis and it should be considered for tumor management.[9]

The World Health Organization (WHO) classification was originally proposed in 1999 and it is now the most widely adopted.[10] This system has several similarities to the previously used Müller-Hermelink classification[11] and recognizes six different types of thymic tumor (see **Table 9.2**): A, AB, B1, B2, B3, and C.

However, although currently considered the most detailed pathologic system, its clinical relevance in predicting long-term outcome and guiding clinical management is controversial. Studies assessing its prognostic significance by multivariate analysis generally indicate the WHO pathologic category to be an independent prognostic factor, although clinical stage always represents the most significant factor for prognosis.[12] There is general evidence that histologic type C is related to worse survival, and that type B3 is predictive of intermediate survival, while no clear correlation with prognosis has been defined for other subtypes due to conflicting and nonhomogeneous results across studies.[7]

Table 9.2 WHO/Histogenetic thymic tumor classification

WHO	Histogenetic
A	Medullary thymoma
AB	Mixed thymoma
B1	Predominantly cortical thymoma
B2	Cortical thymoma
B3	Well-differentiated thymic carcinoma
C	Thymic carcinoma (histologic types listed below)
	Epidermoid keratinizing (squamous cell) carcinoma
	Epidermoid nonkeratinizing carcinoma
	Lymphoepithelioma-like carcinoma
	Sarcomatoid carcinoma
	Clear cell carcinoma
	Basaloid carcinoma
	Mucoepidermoid carcinoma
	Undifferentiated carcinoma

ADJUVANT THERAPY

Only limited data are available in the literature to assess the role of adjuvant therapy after resection of early stage (I and II) thymoma. Little or no role has been generally reported for adjuvant chemotherapy at this stage.

In two large retrospective studies, Ströbel et al. and Singhal et al. showed no evidence of increased survival rates with adjuvant RT in completely resected and margin-negative stage I and II thymomas.[13,14] Based on the findings of these two studies one could conclude that no additional treatment is required if a complete resection of early stage thymoma is accomplished.

In the largest published series, of 1320 patients with thymoma from 115 centers, Kondo and Monden showed that prophylactic mediastinal radiotherapy was not effective in preventing recurrences in patients with radically resected stage II and III thymomas.[15]

Management of stage III thymic tumors

Thymic tumors invading the surrounding structures such as the pericardium, great vessels (SVC, innominate veins and arteries, aorta, and pulmonary artery), lung, diaphragm, and chest wall are classified as Masaoka stage III. These tumors often provide a major surgical challenge, mainly due to the need for extended resections and even complex reconstructive procedures.

The brachiocephalic veins, SVC, lung, pericardium, right atrium, and diaphragm can be safely resected with or without reconstruction increasing the complete resection rate.[16,17,18] Also, resection and reconstruction of the aorta and the main pulmonary artery may be indicated in selected cases to achieve complete resection.[19]

Extended and technically demanding operations can be justified at this stage, since, if complete tumor removal is accomplished, survival rates can be achieved that are comparable to those of patients with stage I and II disease.[20]

Regnard and colleagues[21] reported a 75% 10-year survival rate after radical resection of stage III thymoma.

Since these tumors have been documented to be chemoresponsive, attempts have been made in recent years to increase their resectability rate by the administration of preoperative induction chemotherapy.[20,22]

An average recurrence rate of 26% was reported from literature data of stage III patients treated between 1980 and 2002.[23]

The average 5-year survival of stage III tumor patients was 78% after induction chemotherapy plus surgery, compared with 65% after surgery alone.[23] However, most series using induction chemotherapy have excluded patients with thymic carcinoma, while series of resection alone have generally included these patients.

Management of stage IV thymic tumors

Current treatment strategies for Masaoka stage IV thymic tumors include different strategies for stage IVA and IVB.

Stage IVA tumors presenting with pleural or pericardial dissemination are generally treated by a multimodal approach including surgery, chemotherapy, and sometimes radiotherapy.[24] At stage IVB, chemotherapy is the recommended treatment without surgical resection though resection. has been considered in selected cases.[25]

Chemotherapy has been promoted for stage IVA, usually as an induction agent but also in an adjuvant fashion in association with resection with the aim of increasing progression-free survival.

Several surgical options have been proposed: partial or complete pleurectomy associated with thymectomy or, in selected cases, pleuropneumonectomy.[26] Pleurectomy is a viable option allowing encouraging long-term survival (43% at 5 years) when associated with either induction or adjuvant chemotherapy.[27] Pleuropneumonectomy has been proposed as a possible option in selected cases with extensive and confluent pleural disease invading the lung and precluding gross tumor removal with pleurectomy.[26] Although this approach may look excessively aggressive, the biologic behavior of this tumor that usually is consistent with long-term survival even in the presence of recurrence seems to support the rationale for such an operation. Induction chemotherapy is generally administered to improve results. Irradiation has been beneficial in an adjuvant setting.

Residual microscopic or macroscopic infiltration after resection of stage IV thymoma is a frequent finding regardless of the surgical option that has been adopted. Some additional local treatments have been therefore experimentally proposed for these patients.

LYMPHOMA OF THE MEDIASTINUM

Many histologic subtypes of lymphoma can arise in the chest, but only few of these present with isolated mediastinal localization. Those with potential primary mediastinal presentation include: Hodgkin lymphoma, large B-cell lymphoma, lymphoblastic lymphoma, and pulmonary mucosa-associated lymphoid tissue lymphoma. Although marked geographic variability is reported in the incidence of lymphoma subtypes, Hodgkin lymphoma generally represents about 10%–15% of the total number of new cases, with stable numbers over the last decade, while non-Hodgkin lymphoma subtypes account for about 85%–90%, with a progressive increase over the last years.[28]

Clinical presentation may be similar among different subtypes, as most of these neoplasms generally appear as large invasive anterior mediastinal masses with possible involvement of the surrounding structures.

Possible symptoms are attributable to compression from the enlarging neoplasm and can include chest pain, cough, dyspnea, wheezing, stridor, dysphagia, and signs referable to superior vena cava syndrome. Pericardial effusion is sometimes present and can be occasionally responsible for cardiac tamponade. Asymptomatic presentation is infrequent but is more frequently observed in patients with Hodgkin lymphoma and large B-cell lymphoma as opposed to other types.

Surgery has a limited role in the management of lymphoma, since the treatment is almost exclusively based on chemotherapy with or without radiotherapy. Thus, surgery usually plays only a diagnostic role, as adequate tissue sampling is crucial for a precise histological definition and subsequent treatment.

Correct histological diagnosis can sometimes be achieved by less invasive approaches such as percutaneous fine needle aspiration (FNA) or core biopsy (generally under CT guidance) or by more invasive surgical procedures for biopsy, including anterior mediastinotomy, mediastinoscopy, and videothoracoscopy.[29,30]

Surgical biopsy

Although more invasive than percutaneous procedures, surgical approaches, including anterior mediastinotomy, mediastinoscopy, and videothoracoscopy, certainly represent the most effective diagnostic options for patients with mediastinal lymphoma. These techniques establish definitively a specific histologic diagnosis and provide adequate tissue for phenotyping avoiding more extended surgical approaches such as thoracotomy and sternotomy.[30]

Anterior mediastinotomy is the most commonly used procedure for lesions presenting in a retrosternal location. We reported the possibility of safely and effectively performing a biopsy using this approach under local anesthesia.[31]

Mediastinoscopy is the procedure of choice when the tumor is present in the paratracheal or subcarinal region. Videothoracoscopy may also be a valid alternative.

GERM CELL TUMORS

Germ cell tumors, though exceedingly rare, represent 10%–20% of all anterior mediastinal masses. These tumors comprise three histologic categories: (1) mature teratoma, (2) seminomatous germ cell tumor, and (2) nonseminomatous germ cell tumor.[32] A specific staging classification has been proposed for these tumors[33] (see **Table 9.3**).

Mature teratoma

Mature teratomas account for about 60%–70% of all mediastinal germ cell tumors.[32] Although reported at all ages, the majority of these tumors occur in infancy and childhood with equal distribution between the sexes.

Histologically, they are characterized by mature tissue derived from all three germinal layers. They also may include the presence of bone, cartilage, fat, and squamous and glandular epithelia.

These lesions generally present at CT scan as a multilocular, well-circumscribed, partially cystic anterior mediastinal mass containing fluid and fat density.[34] Calcification is present in about half of patients, with occasional identification of bone or teeth. Occasionally, undifferentiated fetal tissue can be identified. These mature teratomas can grow more rapidly and may rarely degenerate into non-germ-cell tumors, such as sarcoma and epithelial cancer.[33–5] Serum tumor markers, including alpha-fetoprotein (α-FP) and beta-human-chorionic gonadotropin (β-hCG), usually are not elevated.[35]

Mature teratomas are not responsive to chemotherapy or RT. Therefore, in the presence of an anterior mediastinal mass with typical CT findings and normal serum tumor markers, surgical resection without biopsy can be justified.

Since most teratomas present as a large anterior mediastinal mass, median sternotomy is usually the optimal surgical approach. For tumors presenting in a more lateral location, a thoracotomy incision is preferred. Excision of smaller masses through a minimally invasive thoracoscopic approach has been also reported.[36] In selected patients with large masses extending bilaterally with possible involvement of deep structures such as the pulmonary hilum, a bilateral thoracosternotomy, the so-called clamshell incision, has been used.

Despite the benign behavior of these tumors, adhesion to surrounding structures may be present. Therefore, careful dissection is required to preserve crucial mediastinal structures such as great vessels and phrenic nerves.

After complete resection of these tumors, excellent long-term survival rates have been reported, with no local or distant recurrences.[35]

Although the coexistence of malignant components in a mature teratoma has been reported only rarely, the risk of dissemination has been pointed out in patients with intraoperative rupture of cystic tumors.[37]

Table 9.3 Germ cell tumor staging (Moran and Suster[33])

Stage	Definition
I	Well-circumscribed tumor with or without focal adhesions to the pleura or pericardium but without microscopic evidence of invasion into adjacent structures
II	Tumor confined to the mediastinum with macroscopic and/or microscopic evidence of infiltration into adjacent structures (such as pleura, pericardium, and great vessels)
III	Tumor with metastasis
IIIA	Metastasis to intrathoracic organs (the lymph nodes, lung, etc.)
IIIB	Extrathoracic metastases

Seminomatous germ cell tumors

Primary mediastinal seminomatous germ cell tumors represent almost half of all malignant primary mediastinal neoplasms, which are exceedingly rare. They generally occur in young adult males between 20 and 40 years of age. Growth of these tumors is usually slow and the onset of related symptoms (pain, cough, dyspnea) is therefore frequently late.[38] Typically these lesions present as a lobulated but homogeneous mass with occasional infiltration into the surrounding structures.

Serum tumor markers are usually normal; however, mildly elevated levels (<10 mg/mL) of β-hCG have been found in about 10% of patients.

To plan the most appropriate treatment strategy, histological confirmation is required. A percutaneous FNA can be generally sufficient to achieve diagnosis. Alternatively, anterior mediastinotomy or video-assisted thoracic surgery (VATS) allows effective biopsy if the percutaneous procedure has proved unsuccessful.

It has been shown that a residual mass after chemotherapy frequently does not contain viable tumor cells. For this reason, surgical resection may be not indicated in this situation and only clinical and radiographic follow-up is recommended.

RT is considered rarely in case of failure of second-line chemotherapy. Alternatively, surgical resection has been proposed in selected cases after ineffective chemotherapy though these tumors usually are quite radiosensitive and thus a course of radiation therapy may be warranted.

Nonseminomatous germ cell tumors

Nonseminomatous germ cell tumors account for more than 50% of all germ cell tumors.[39] They are comprised of three histologic subtypes, alone or in combination: (1) yolk sac tumor, (2) embryonal carcinoma, and (3) choriocarcinoma. In some cases, they can be mixed with mature teratoma; seminoma; or other malignancies, such as sarcoma, adenocarcinoma, and neuroectodermal tumors.[40]

These tumors are rapidly growing; usually occur in males from 20 to 40 years of age; and present as heterogeneous, generally large masses, sometimes with evidence of necrosis or hemorrhage. Infiltration into adjacent structures including the lung; the SVC; innominate veins; the pericardium; and, occasionally, other great vessels and the heart can be visible on CT scan. Although pleural and pericardial effusion are not rare, they are usually not related to the presence of pleural metastases.

Serum tumor markers (α-FP and β-hCG) are significantly elevated in almost all cases, and a marked increase in their value, in association with typical features on CT scan, is diagnostic of primary malignant nonseminomatous germ cell tumors (PMNSGCTs) even without biopsy. In the Indiana University experience, only 5% of these neoplasms showed normal serum markers.[39]

Cytological or histologic confirmation, possibly with CT-guided FNA or a surgical approach (anterior mediastinotomy or VATS) may be required before treatment in patients with normal or only marginally elevated tumor markers.

Although these tumors are histologically and serologically identical to their counterparts originating in the testis or in the retroperitoneum and are treated with similar protocols, their long-term prognosis is significantly poorer. An average 5-year overall survival of 49% is reported for PMNSGCTs compared with 80% for tumors originating in the testis and 63% for those originating in the retroperitoneum.[41]

Also, the possible presence of immature teratomatous elements in PMNSGCTs has been found responsible for degeneration into more aggressively behaving, chemotherapy-refractory non-germ-cell cancer.

However, based on the results of historical series reporting poor prognosis for patients treated by surgery alone, cis-platinum-based chemotherapy has become the first-line therapeutic approach.

The prognostic impact of marker elevation has still not clearly been defined. In the Indiana University experience, the presence of rising markers had a significantly negative effect on survival, while elevated but not rising markers did not.[42] In the study, surgery showed a higher cure rate for patients with rising markers than second-line chemotherapy.

The role of surgery was also assessed in the 28-year experience of the Memorial Sloan Kettering Cancer Center:[41] Fifty-seven patients with nonseminomatous germ cell tumor undergoing surgical resection after platinum-based chemotherapy were included. About half of these patients had limited disease (stage I–II). Preoperative tumor markers normalized after chemotherapy in 79% of the patients. The most common surgical approach in this series (performed in 38.6% of cases) was anterolateral thoracotomy with partial sternotomy ("hemi-clamshell incision"). An R0 resection was achieved in 91% of patients, with a major morbidity of 17.5% and no postoperative mortality. The median overall survival was 31.5 months. Factors correlated with better survival on univariate analysis included: necrosis and teratoma versus residual tumor at final pathology, R0 resection, normalization or reduction of marker levels after chemotherapy, stage I–II, and surgery after the year 2000. Normalized or decreased serum markers after chemotherapy were the strongest predictors of improved survival.

At present, in some centers, surgery is offered only to those patients who show normalized serum tumor markers after chemotherapy, otherwise more intensive or second-line chemotherapeutic regimens are administered.[43] Others[44] proceed directly to surgery after chemotherapy if the patient is operable, regardless of marker status.

PARATHYROID TUMORS

Tumors of the parathyroids arise in different sites, including the mediastinum, since these glands may have variable locations other than the neck. This reflects their embryogenetic derivation from the third and the fourth branchial pouches.

The inferior parathyroids originate from the third branchial pouch and are those with the most variable location, since they may migrate with the thymus in the superior mediastinum and can drop areas of parathyroid tissue along this course. In a surgical series of 112 patients, inferior parathyroids were found in a mediastinal location in 60% of cases.[45]

Ectopic presentation of the inferior parathyroids in the superior mediastinum may involve the anterior compartment in a parathymic location, or may be adjacent to vascular structures such as the innominate veins and arteries, SVC, aorta, and even left pulmonary artery.

Superior parathyroids, more rarely, can migrate in the posterior mediastinum (generally in a periesophageal location) because of the negative intrathoracic pressure.

Most patients with parathyroid adenoma present symptoms related to hypercalcemia.

After a diagnosis of hyperparathyroidism has been established, imaging for localization uses technetium-99m-sestamibi scanning, generally associated with CT scanning and MRI.

Surgical exploration of the neck, following a diagnosis of hyperparathyroidism without imaging studies, has been reported to be a viable option with a success rate of 96%.[46]

Surgical resection of pathologic glands is the only curative option for patients with hyperparathyroidism. The intraoperative use of rapid serum PTH measurement has significantly improved the success rate of surgery, allowing confirmation of appropriate resection during the operation.[47–49] The success rate of surgery with this management has been reported to be as high as 99%.

Exploration of the mediastinum is indicated when preoperative imaging shows the presence of ectopic glands in this location. Mediastinal parathyroids have been found in 10%–20% of cases with primary hyperparathyroidism.[46]

Even if imaging has not been done preoperatively mediastinal exploration is indicated at the initial operation if four glands are unable to be located in the absence of an obvious adenoma.

Excision of a mediastinal parathyroid adenoma can be accomplished through the standard collar-type cervical incision in most cases.[50] This approach provides good exposure, especially of the glands that lie adjacent to the thymus. However, lesions in the upper paraesophageal and peritracheal location have also been successfully removed through such an incision.[47]

More recently, minimally invasive videothoracoscopic approaches have been successfully employed for the removal of mediastinal parathyroid adenoma.[51–54] Transcervical thymectomy using the Cooper thymectomy retractor has also been used with great success in removing glands aberrantly located in the thymus.

REFERENCES

1. Shields TW. Primary tumors and cysts of the mediastinum. In: Shields TW, ed. *General Thoracic Surgery*, Philadelphia: Lea and Febiger; 1989: 1096–123.

2. Davis RJ Jr, Oldham HN Jr, Sabiston DC Jr. Primary cysts and neoplasms of the mediastinum: Recent changes in clinical presentation, methods of diagnosis, management, and results. *Ann Thorac Surg.* 1987; 44: 229–37.

3. Mullen B, Richardson JD. Primary anterior mediastinal tumors in children and adults. *Ann Thorac Surg.* 1986; 42: 338–45.

4. Detterbeck FC, Parsons AD. Thymic tumors: A review of current diagnosis, classification, and treatment. In: Patterson GA, Pearson FG, Cooper JD, Deslauriers J, Rice TW, eds. *Pearson's Thoracic and Esophageal Surgery*, 3rd edition, Philadelphia: Elsevier; 2008: 1589–614.

5. Moran CA, Suster S. On the histologic heterogeneity of thymic epithelial neoplasms: Impact of sampling in subtyping and classification of thymomas. *Am J Clin Pathol.* 2000; 114: 760–6.

6. Detterbeck FC. Evaluation and treatment of stage I and II thymoma. *J Thorac Oncol.* 2010 Oct; 5(10 Suppl 4): S318–22.

7. Masaoka A, Monden Y, Nakahara K, Tanioka T. Follow-up study of thymomas with special reference to their clinical stages. *Cancer.* 1981; 48: 2485–92.

8. Ricci C, Rendina EA, Pescarmona EO, Venuta F, Di Tolla R, Ruco LP, Baroni CD. Correlations between histological type, clinical behaviour, and prognosis in thymoma. *Thorax.* 1989; 44: 455–60.

9. Rendina EA, Pescarmona EO, Venuta F, Nardi S, De Rosa G, Martelli M, Ricci C. Thymoma: A clinico-pathologic study based on newly developed morphologic criteria. *Tumori.* 1988 Feb 29; 74(1): 79–84.

10. Detterbeck FC. Clinical value of the WHO classification system of thymoma. *Ann Thorac Surg.* 2006; 81: 2328–34.

11. Müller-Hermelink HK, Marino M, Palestro G, Schumacher U, Kirchner T. Immunohistological evidences of cortical and medullary differentiation in thymoma. *Virchows Arch A Pathol Anat Histopathol.* 1985; 408: 143–61.

12. Kondo K, Yoshizawa K, Tsuyuguchi M, Kimura S, Sumitomo M, Morita J, Miyoshi T, Sakiyama S, Mukai K, Monden Y. WHO histologic classification is a prognostic indicator in thymoma. *Ann Thorac Surg.* 2004; 77: 1183–8.

13. Ströbel P, Bauer A, Puppe B, Kraushaar T, Krein A, Toyka K, Gold R et al. Tumor recurrence and survival patients treated for thymomas and thymic squamous cell carcinomas: A retrospective analysis. *J Clin Oncol.* 2004; 22: 1501–9.

14. Singhal S, Shrager JB, Rosenthal DI, LiVolsi VA, Kaiser LR. Comparison of stages I–II thymoma treated by complete resection with or without adjuvant radiation. *Ann Thorac Surg.* 2003; 76: 1635–41, discussion 1641–2.

15. Kondo K, Monden Y. Therapy for thymic epithelial tumors: A clinical study of 1,320 patients from Japan. *Ann Thorac Surg.* 2003; 76: 878–84.

16. Venuta F, Rendina EA, Kepletko W, Rocco G. Surgical management of stage III thymic tumors. *Thoracic Surg Clin.* 2011; 21: 85–91.

17. D'Andrilli A, Venuta F, Rendina EA. Surgical approaches for

invasive tumors of the anterior mediastinum. *Thorac Surg Clin.* 2010; 20: 265–84.

18. D'Andrilli A, De Cecco CN, Maurizi G, Muscogiuri G, Baldini R, David V, Venuta F, Rendina EA. Reconstruction of the superior vena cava by biologic conduit: Assessment of long-term patency by magnetic resonance imaging. *Ann Thorac Surg.* 2013; 96: 1039–45.

19. Fujino S, Tezuka N, Watarida S, Katsuyama K, Inoue S, Mori A. Reconstruction of the aortic arch in invasive thymoma under retrograde cerebral perfusion. *Ann Thorac Surg.* 1998; 66: 263–4.

20. Kim ES, Putnam JB, Komaki R, Walsh GL, Ro JY, Shin HJ, Truong M et al. Phase II study of a multidisciplinary approach with induction chemotherapy, followed by surgical resection, radiation therapy, and consolidation chemotherapy for unresectable malignant thymomas: Final report. *Lung Cancer.* 2004; 44: 369–79.

21. Regnard JF, Magdeleinat P, Dromer C, Dulmet E, de Montpreville V, Levi JF, Levasseur P. Prognostic factors and long-term results after thymoma resection: A series of 307 patients. *J Thorac Cardiovasc Surg.* 1996; 112: 376–84.

22. Lucchi M, Ambrogi MC, Duranti L, Basalo F, Fontanini G, Angeletti CS, Mussi A. Advanced stage thymomas and thymic carcinomas: Results of multimodality treatments. *Ann Thorac Surg.* 2005; 79: 1840–4.

23. Venuta F, Rendina EA, Longo F, De Giacomo T, Anile M, Mercadante E , Ventura L, Osti MF, Francioni F, Coloni GF. Long-term outcome after multimodality treatment for stage III thymic tumors. *Ann Thorac Surg.* 2003; 76: 1866–72.

24. Huang J, Rizk NP, Travis WD, Seshan VE, Bains MS, Dycoco J, Downey RJ, Flores RM, Park BJ, Rusch VW. Feasibility of multimodality therapy including extended resections in stage IVA thymoma. *J Thorac Cardiovasc Surg.* 2007; 134: 1477–84.

25. Ishikawa Y, Matsuguma H, Nakahara R, Suzuki H, Ui A, Kondo T, Kamiyama Y et al. Multimodality therapy for patients with invasive thymoma disseminated into the pleural cavity: The potential role of extrapleural pneumonectomy. *Ann Thorac Surg.* 2009; 88: 952–7.

26. Wright CD. Pleuropneumonectomy for the treatment of Masaoka Stage IVA thymoma. *Ann Thorac Surg.* 2006; 82: 1234–9.

27. de Bree E, van Ruth S, Schotborgh CE, Baas P, Zoetmulder FA. Limited cardiotoxicity after extensive thoracic surgery and intraoperative hyperthermic chemotherapy with doxorubicin and cisplatin. *Ann Surg Oncol.* 2007; 14: 319–26.

28. Jemal A, Siegel R, Ward E, Murray T, Xu J, Thun MJ. Cancer statistics, 2007. *CA Cancer J Clin.* 2007; 57: 43–66.

29. Moonim MT, Breen R, Fields PA, Santis G. Diagnosis and subtyping of de novo and relapsed mediastinal lymphomas by endobronchial ultrasound needle aspiration. *Am J Respir Crit Care Med.* 2013; 188: 1216–23.

30. Rendina EA, Venuta F, De Giacomo T, Ciriaco PP, Pescarmona EO, Francioni F, Pulsoni A, Malagnino F, Ricci C. Comparative merits of thoracoscopy, mediastinoscopy, and mediastinotomy for mediastinal biopsy. *Ann Thorac Surg.* 1994; 57: 992–5.

31. Rendina EA, Venuta F, De Giacomo T, Ciccone AM, Moretti MS,

Ibrahim M, Coloni GF. Biopsy of anterior mediastinal masses under local anesthesia. *Ann Thorac Surg.* 2002; 74(5): 1720–2, discussion 1722–3.

32. Kesler KA. Germ cell tumors of the mediastinum. In: Patterson GA, Pearson FG, Cooper JD, Deslauriers J, Rice TW, eds. *Pearson's Thoracic and Esophageal Surgery*, 3rd edition. Philadelphia: Elsevier; 2008: 1615–21.

33. Moran CA, Suster S. Primary germ cell tumors of the mediastinum: I. Analysis of 322 cases with special emphasis on teratomatous lesions and a proposal for histopathologic classification and clinical staging. *Cancer.* 1997; 80: 681–90.

34. Strollo DC, Rosado de Christenson ML, Jett JR. Primary mediastinal tumors: Part I; Tumors of the anterior mediastinum. *Chest.* 1997; 112: 511–22.

35. Allen MS. Benign mediastinal germ cell tumors. In: Wood DE, Thomas Jr CR, eds. *Mediastinal Tumors: Update 1995*, Berlin: Springer-Verlag; 1995: 41–2.

36. Shintani H, Funaki S, Nakagiri T, Inoue M, Sawabata N, Minami M, Kadota Y, Okumura M. Experience with thoracoscopic resection for mature teratoma: A retrospective analysis of 15 patients. *Interact Cardiovasc Thorac Surg.* 2013; 16: 441–4.

37. Chang CC, Chang YL, Lee YC. Cystic malignant teratoma with early recurrence after intraoperative spillage. *Ann Thorac Surg.* 2008; 86: 1971–3.

38. Weidner N. Germ-cell tumors of the mediastinum. *Semin Diagn Pathol.* 1999; 16: 42–50.

39. Strollo DC, Rosado de Christenson ML, Jett JR. Primary mediastinal tumors: Part I; Tumors of the anterior mediastinum. *Chest.* 1997; 112: 511–22.

40. Kesler K, Rieger K, Hammoud Z, Kruter LE, Perkins SM, Turrentine MW, Schneider BP, Einhorn LH, Brown JW. A 25-year single institution experience with surgery for primary mediastinal nonseminomatous germ cell tumors. *Ann Thorac Surg.* 2008; 85: 371–8.

41. Sarkaria IS, Bains MS, Sood S, Sima CS, Reuter VE, Flores RM, Motzer RJ, Bosl GJ, Rusch VW. Resection of primary mediastinal non-seminomatous germ cell tumors: A 28-year experience at Memorial Sloan-Kettering Cancer Center. *J Thorac Oncol.* 2011; 6: 1236–41.

42. Kruter L, Kesler K, Yu M, Hammoud ZT, Rieger KM, Einhorn LH. The predictive value of serum tumor markers for pathologic findings of residual mediastinal masses after chemotherapy for primary mediastinal nonseminomatous germ cell tumors [abstract]. *Proc Am Soc Clin Oncol.* 2008; 5087.

43. Vuky J, Bains M, Bacik J, Higgins G, Bajorin DF, Mazumdar M, Bosl GJ, Motzer RJ. Role of post chemotherapy adjunctive surgery in the management of patients with nonseminoma arising from the mediastinum. *J Clin Oncol.* 2001; 19: 682–8.

44. Hartmann JT, Nichols CR, Droz JP, Horwich A, Gerl A, Fossa SD, Beyer J et al. Prognostic variables for response and outcome in patients with extragonadal germ-cell tumors. *Ann Oncol.* 2002; 13: 1017–28.

45. Wang C-A. Parathyroid re-exploration: A clinical and pathologic study of 112 cases. *Ann Surg.* 1977; 186: 140–5.

46. Udelsman R. Six hundred fifty-six consecutive explorations for primary hyperparathyroidism. *Ann Surg.* 2002; 235: 665–70.

47. Peeler BB, Martin WH, Sandler MP, Goldstein RE. Sestamibi

parathyroid scanning and preoperative localization studies for patients with recurrent/persistent hyperparathyroidism or significant comorbid conditions: Development of an optimal localization strategy. *Am Surg.* 1997; 63: 37–46.

48. Russell CF, Edis AJ, Scholz DA, Sheedy PF, van Heerden JA. Mediastinal parathyroid tumors: Experience with 38 tumors requiring mediastinotomy for removal. *Ann Surg.* 1981; 193: 805–9.

49. Hall BL, Moley J. Mediastinal parathyroid tumors. In: Patterson GA, Pearson FG, Cooper JD, Deslauriers J, Rice TW, eds. *Pearson's Thoracic and Esophageal Surgery*, 3rd edition. Philadelphia: Elsevier; 2008.

50. Wharry LI, Yip L, Armstrong MJ, Virji MA, Stang MT, Carty SE, McCoy KL. The final intraoperative parathyroid hormone level: How low should it go? *World J Surg.* 2014; 38: 558–63.

51. Smythe WR, Bavaria JE, Hall RA, Kline GM, Kaiser LR. Thoracoscopic removal of mediastinal parathyroid adenoma. *Ann Thorac Surg.* 1995; 59: 236–8.

52. Conn JM, Goncalves MA, Mansour KA, McGarity WC. The mediastinal parathyroid. *Ann Surg.* 1991; 57: 62–6.

53. Medrano C, Hazelrigg SR, Landreneau RJ, Boley TM, Shawgo T, Grasch A. Thoracoscopic resection of ectopic parathyroid glands. *Ann Thorac Surg.* 2000; 69: 221–3.

54. Demmy TL, Krasna MK, Dtterbeck FC, Kline GG, Kohman LJ, DeCamp MM Jr, Wain JC. Multicenter VATS experience with mediastinal tumors. *Ann Thorac Surg.* 1998; 66: 187–92.

10

Resection of posterior mediastinal lesions

JOSEPH B. SHRAGER

INTRODUCTION

The posterior mediastinum is bounded anteriorly by the posterior pericardium and extends posteriorly to the chest wall and laterally to include the costovertebral sulci. Important structures that it contains include the descending thoracic aorta, inferior vena cava and azygous veins, the sympathetic chains and origins of the intercostal nerves at their nerve roots, and the esophagus and associated vagi. Most anatomic systems consider only lesions that are caudal to the fourth thoracic vertebral body to be within the posterior mediastinum, with more cephalad lesions resting within the superior mediastinum.

The majority of posterior mediastinal masses in adults are benign. They can be classified in a clinically useful way according to whether they are cystic or solid on radiographic evaluation. Cystic masses in this region typically represent *bronchogenic cysts* or *esophageal duplication cysts*, whereas solid masses are most commonly *benign neurogenic tumors* (see **Figure 10.1**) (e.g., schwannomas, neurofibromas, or ganglioneuromas). These neural tumors usually arise from the sympathetic chain or the proximal intercostal nerves, but often the precise anatomical origin does not become clear until operation. Occasionally, one comes across a patient with a pheochromocytoma or paraganglioma, which arise from the randomly located mediastinal paraganglionic cells and may secrete hormones. At initial office evaluation, one should be alert to the presence of hypertension or palpitations, which should dictate measurement of urine metanephrines. Esophageal leiomyomas (benign intramuscular tumors within the esophageal wall) are also generally grouped among the posterior mediastinal lesions. The approach to these lesions and to esophageal duplication cysts differs somewhat from the approach to lesions that are unassociated with the esophagus.

In the modern era, posterior mediastinal masses most often come to light as asymptomatic, incidentally identified,

radiographic abnormalities. They do less commonly, however, present with signs of infection (in the case of infected cysts), dysphagia, chest pain, cough or dyspnea, or neurological changes (e.g., Horner's syndrome from tumors involving the upper sympathetic trunk; lower extremity symptoms from dumbbell paravertebral tumors) resulting from mass effect on adjacent structures.

At present, because of the applicability of low morbidity, minimally invasive approaches to the vast majority of posterior mediastinal masses, most authors recommend resection, even when lesions are asymptomatic. I believe that the recommendation about whether to proceed with resection of a posterior mediastinal mass needs to be individualized. Clearly, a symptomatic lesion is best managed by resection, except in unusual circumstances. When an asymptomatic lesion has all of the radiographic characteristics of a benign

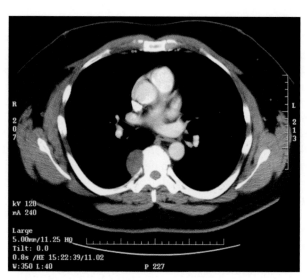

10.1 Computed tomographic image of a typical benign neurogenic tumor in the costovertebral sulcus.

cyst or tumor (i.e., smooth margins, simple-appearing cyst material, minimally positron emission tomography [PET] positive if PET has been done), the age and general medical condition of the patient are the key considerations. Since these lesions do generally grow—albeit at a fairly slow rate—it is likely that a young patient will eventually develop symptoms due either to impingement on surrounding structures or infection of a cyst. In patients under the age of approximately 60, then, who are otherwise good surgical candidates, even asymptomatic lesions are best managed by resection. For older patients, or those who have substantial comorbidities, it is perfectly reasonable to follow these benign-appearing, asymptomatic lesions with serial radiographic studies and operate only if they begin to grow dramatically, the patient develops symptoms, or a change in radiographic appearance suggests malignancy. In any case, there is no urgency to remove these cysts and tumors promptly. The significance of the very few reports of development of malignancy within a benign posterior mediastinal mass is probably overstated.

SURGICAL PRINCIPLES

Video-assisted thoracoscopic surgery (or robotics) versus thoracotomy

Resection of posterior mediastinal masses may be accomplished by means of either minimally invasive approaches or thoracotomy. The original, simplest, and probably the least costly minimally invasive approach remains video-assisted thoracoscopic surgery (VATS).[1] Robotic approaches are simply VATS approaches that make use of the robot as an "instrument," which may provide both certain advantages and certain disadvantages. The procedure, apart from the incisions, is essentially the same whether one uses a minimally invasive approach or thoracotomy, and the goal is, of course, complete resection. With some exceptions, minimally invasive approaches are considered preferable to thoracotomy in this setting; it has been well established by now that both VATS and robotics result in less postoperative pain and quicker functional recovery than thoracotomy.[2] Some surgeons may still argue that minimally invasive approaches may be more likely to leave a patient with microscopic residual disease. In my own experience and that of many others, however, recurrence of these lesions is very rare after VATS/robotic excision. Given the low recurrence rate and the fact that these masses are almost always benign, the risk–benefit ratio favors VATS/robotics in nearly all cases, in my opinion.

There are, however, several *circumstances in which thoracotomy is indicated from the outset*. A suggestion of malignancy (in particular, frank invasion of surrounding structures) on preoperative radiography I believe mandates exploration and resection by thoracotomy; in this situation, the potential consequences of positive margins justify the more aggressive approach. This, however, is quite rare for posterior mediastinal masses. The presence of active infection within a cyst is a relative indication for thoracotomy, in that this usually causes substantial obliteration of normal tissue planes and thereby renders VATS/robotic dissection more difficult and possibly hazardous given the more limited instrumentation and angles that can usually be achieved by these approaches. Solid masses larger than approximately 6 cm also call for an open approach, in my opinion: such lesions are typically more difficult to mobilize safely from underlying structures than smaller lesions, they are more likely to be malignant (though this is still rare), and their removal between the ribs is likely to necessitate substantial rib spreading, which may negate the benefit of pure VATS/robotics. Another approach is to attempt VATS/robotics for these larger lesions, but to have a low threshold to convert to thoracotomy if difficulty is encountered. If the dissection can be completed by VATS, one can then typically remove larger tumors by resecting a small portion of rib without sacrificing an intercostal nerve. It is likely that this will result in less pain and earlier recovery than a standard thoracotomy with rib spreading, but this has never been studied to my knowledge.

Other preoperative issues

A patient with a centrally located cyst should undergo bronchoscopy to rule out the rare occurrence of a communication with the bronchial tree. This may be suggested on computed tomography (CT) scans by the presence of an air–fluid level. If a communication is identified, strong consideration should be made to proceed with thoracotomy rather than VATS. *When a cyst arises from or abuts the esophagus*, the possibility of a communication between the cyst and the esophageal lumen should be similarly investigated. To rule out this also-rare phenomenon, I obtain a barium contrast study during the preoperative workup, followed by intraoperative esophagoscopy at the commencement of the operation. If a communication is identified, I prefer thoracotomy. Although there are individuals who would still be comfortable proceeding with a minimally invasive approach, with endoscopic suturing after excision of an esophageal duplication cyst with a communication, safe reapproximation of the esophageal mucosa is the paramount consideration in these cases, and, in my view, this is still most reliably carried out through an open approach.

Preoperative investigation with esophagoscopy should also be done to confirm the presence of intact overlying mucosa in cases of suspected *leiomyoma* of the esophagus. If the mucosa is intact, the possibility of malignancy is essentially ruled out. Simultaneously, endoscopic ultrasonography may be performed to establish the depth to which the esophageal wall is involved. With a preoperative diagnosis of probable leiomyoma, VATS is the approach of choice in our practice.

So-called *dumbbell neurogenic tumors* (tumors that invade the neural foramen and have a spinal canal component) are special cases. Any solid mass in the costovertebral sulcus that cannot be clearly separated on CT imaging from the neural foramen should be evaluated by means of magnetic resonance imaging. Although invasion of the neural foramen by tumor is not in itself an indication for thoracotomy, it does necessitate a combined approach with neurosurgical involvement for the intraspinal portion of the procedure. Several versions of such an approach have been described, including a posterior approach via costotransversectomy or extension of a posterior midline incision into a posterolateral thoracotomy, through which both the intraspinal and intrathoracic components of the tumor can be resected.[3–6] I prefer to perform the the operation using the following approach: under a single anesthetic, the neurosurgeons first resect the intraspinal component (laminectomy and intervertebral foraminotomy), then the patient is repositioned to lateral decubitus and we carry out the remainder of the procedure (via VATS or robotics). Failure to diagnose a dumbbell tumor preoperatively and plan an appropriate combined operation with neurosurgeons may lead to inadvertently cutting through tumor from within the chest. This has the potential to result acutely in tumor hemorrhage within the spinal canal and spinal cord compression, with disastrous consequences. In the long-term, the positive margin of resection will result in local recurrence unless recognized and managed appropriately.

Patients with functioning paragangliomas or pheochromocytomas, if hypertensive, should receive approximately 2 weeks of alpha-adrenergic blockade and volume loading, followed by beta blockade. In these cases, before incision, clear discussion should be undertaken between the surgeon and the anesthesiologist about the intraoperative anesthetic and plan for control of the patient's blood pressure.

There is, in the vast majority of cases, no advantage to preoperative needle biopsy of posterior mediastinal lesions, although this can usually be readily performed either transthoracically, or, in the case of periesophageal masses, transesophageally at the time of endoscopic ultrasound. Only in cases of invasion suggestive of malignancy might a biopsy alter the therapeutic approach. For example, extremely large or invasive-appearing tumors that turn out to be sarcomas may be best treated by preoperative chemotherapy and/or radiation. It is therefore appropriate to obtain a needle biopsy in the unusual cases in which these features are present.

Although VATS/robotics are often excellent approaches to posterior mediastinal lesions, it must be emphasized that one should never hesitate to convert a minimally invasive procedure to a thoracotomy if required. Accordingly, informed consent to undergo thoracotomy should be sought before operation from all patients being treated for posterior mediastinal lesions, even when VATS or robotics is the intended approach. Further, any patient with a tumor encroaching on the neural foramen should understand preoperatively that there is a very rare possibility of spinal cord compromise from the operation, as well as of cerebrospinal fluid (CSF) leak.

SURGICAL TECHNIQUES

I will describe the VATS approaches to these tumors, which are very similar to robotic approaches—simply using different tools to access and manipulate the pathology. It is possible that the "wrists" at the end of robotic instruments afford slightly greater facility over currently available VATS instruments in dissecting posterior mediastinal tumors. However, whether this advantage outweighs the disadvantages of robotics—for example, the increased cost, the loss of tactile sense, and the need for surgeons to undergo a second learning curve—is unclear.

VATS resection of neurogenic tumors of the posterior mediastinum

Resection of a solid neurogenic tumor of the posterior mediastinum that *does not* invade the neural foramen proceeds as follows.[7] The figures are drawn from intraoperative photographs of several separate VATS operations that the author has performed.

STEP 1: INTUBATION AND ENDOSCOPY
The patient is intubated with a double-lumen endotracheal tube to allow single-lung ventilation. Preoperative bronchoscopy (for cystic lesions adjacent to airways) or esophagoscopy (for lesions abutting the esophagus) is performed as indicated (see "Other preoperative issues" section).

STEP 2: PATIENT POSITIONING AND PLACEMENT OF PORTS
The patient is placed in lateral decubitus and stabilized with a bean bag so that the operating table can safely be tilted as much as 45 degrees anteriorly. With this degree of tilt, the lung will almost always fall away from the field of vision; thus, there is rarely a need to place an additional port for a lung retractor or to use carbon dioxide (CO_2) gas insufflation. The lack of need for CO_2 allows one to employ a reusable, metal introducer port for the camera and to avoid altogether the more costly, commercially provided, disposable ports.

The port for the camera is placed through an incision that is generally slightly posterior to the anterior axillary line, in the same rib space or one rib caudal to the craniocaudal level of the mass (see **Figure 10.2**); if it is placed much more anteriorly than the anterior axillary line, the view of these posterior lesions may be obscured by the lung. I prefer a 5 mm, 30-degree camera, which keeps the incision very small and provides less risk of traumatizing the intercostal nerve, yet provides excellent optics. The 30-degree lens provides much greater versatility and visualization around to the "far side" of lesions than a 0-degree lens.

The two "working" incisions are approximately 1.5 cm long (to allow a variety of instruments to be passed without difficulty) and are made at least two rib spaces cephalad and caudal, to the camera port. In general, the more caudal working incision is placed 5–8 cm more posteriorly than the camera port, while the more cephalad working incision is

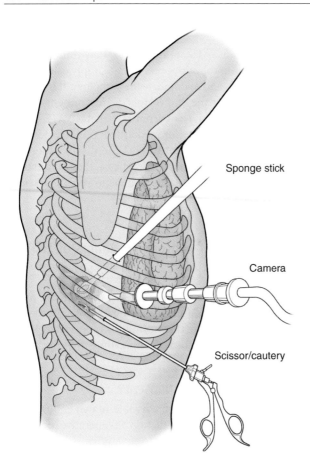

10.2 Placement of the skin incisions and camera port.

made 1–3 cm more anteriorly than the camera port (robotic approaches require these to be farther apart still). Sometimes, placement of an alternative cephalad working port positioned posterior to the scapula is advantageous, although I try to avoid this, since the rib spaces are so narrow here that intercostal nerve trauma is, I believe, more likely. The main working instruments are an endoscopic scissors-cautery, a ring clamp, an endoscopic peanut dissector, a Maryland dissector, a long right-angle clamp, a hook-cautery, and an endoscopic clip applier.

STEP 3: INCISION OF PLEURA

The parietal pleura/mediastinal pleura is incised with a margin of approximately 1 cm circumferentially around the mass (see **Figures 10.3 and 10.4**). In straightforward cases, this dissection can be done with the hook-cautery, which will both create the lift away from underlying critical structures (esophagus, vagus, intercostal bundle, azygous vein) and incise the pleural tissue. In cases where the planes are less clear, such as with an infected mediastinal cyst, the pleura can be tented up by initial blunt dissection using a right-angle clamp or the Maryland dissector to first clearly separate it from the underlying structures. This separation then allows the safe use of the electrocautery which provides both hemostasis and division of the pleura. This dissection and all subsequent work are facilitated by placing gentle

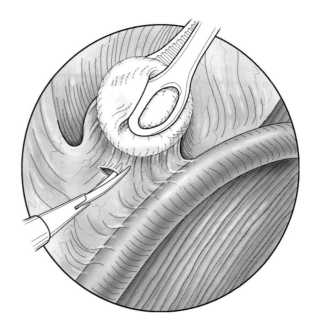

10.3 The pleura is incised circumferentially, approximately 1 cm from the tumor.

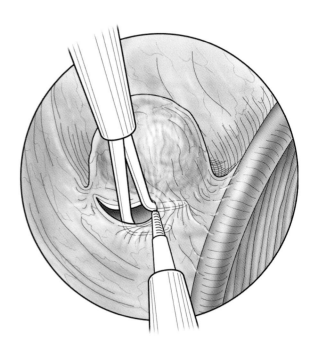

10.4 The pleura is incised circumferentially, approximately 1 cm from the tumor.

traction on the mass with a sponge stick or, for smaller lesions, by grasping the entire mass within a ring clamp to allow manipulation. In some cases, I have placed a figure-of-eight suture through the mass to provide the needed counter traction. This sort of manipulation must be minimized in the case of a functioning paraganglioma/pheochromocytoma to avoid a significant spike in blood pressure.

STEP 4: DISSECTION OF SOFT TISSUE ATTACHMENTS

Once the pleura has been incised circumferentially, the soft tissue attachments are further dissected bluntly with the endoscopic peanut dissector. Attachments that are relatively thick or vascular are controlled with the hook-cautery when remote from surrounding structures, or by double-clipping and division when closer to danger (see **Figure 10.5**). Often, one needs to use cautery to dissect the tumor and associated periosteum cleanly off the surface of one or two ribs above or below the tumor. By dissecting in a progressively shrinking circular motion around the tumor, dividing all attachments to the mass, one moves progressively closer to the source of the tumor, which is most commonly from the anterior primary ramus of the spinal nerve or its associated intercostal nerve near the neural foramen. Once all attachments other than those to the intercostal bundle have been divided, gentle dissection first at the lateral/anterior margin of the tumor, just inferior to the associated rib, will identify the nerve (or sympathetic chain) that is the source of the lesion.

STEP 5: DIVISION OF SOURCE INTERCOSTAL BUNDLE

Usually, the next step is to mobilize, doubly clip, and divide the entire source intercostal bundle lateral to the tumor (including nerve, artery, and vein). The mobilization of the bundle is facilitated by use of a long, thin periosteal freer/elevator. Once the bundle lateral to the tumor has been divided, further blunt and cautery dissection is performed until the nerve root emerging from the neural foramen, medial/posterior to the tumor, and the associated intercostal vessels here, are the last remaining attachments. If the tumor originates from the sympathetic chain, the chain is clipped above and below the tumor, and the intercostal bundle, which is typically uninvolved, is spared. Occasionally, even with a tumor that originates from the intercostal nerve root/nerve, the associated intercostal vessels can be dissected free of the tumor and be spared rather than being divided (see **Figure 10.6**).

STEP 6: REMOVAL OF SPECIMEN

In most cases, the "live" end of the intercostal bundle, posterior/deep to the tumor, is the final structure to be gently dissected and isolated. Once a few millimeters of the nerve are clearly seen, it is doubly clipped and divided at least 2 mm medial/posterior to the point where the tumor tapers into normal nerve. The associated artery and vein are, in some cases, more easily clipped and divided simultaneous with the nerve; in other cases, they may be clipped and divided separately, or they may require no division at all at this level if uninvolved (see **Figure 10.6**). The mass is removed in an endoscopic bag.

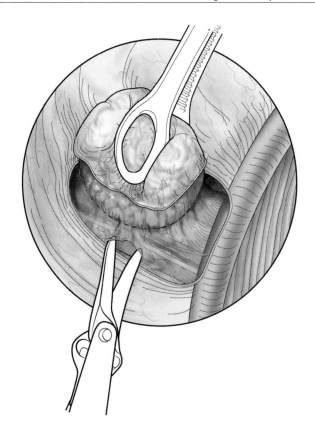

10.5 As additional attachments are dissected, one often encounters some more vascular attachments that require division with the hook-cautery.

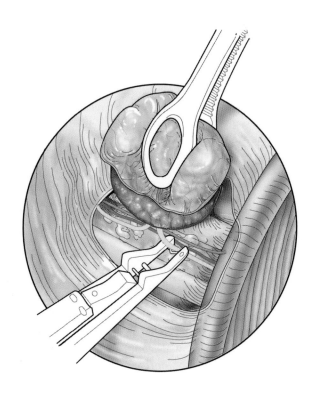

10.6 The final step is isolation and division of the associated intercostal bundle medial/posterior to the tumor.

STEP 7: DRAINAGE

A 24 Fr chest tube is positioned posteriorly at the apex.

POTENTIAL PROBLEMS AND THEIR AVOIDANCE

Care must be taken to ensure that only very gentle traction is exerted on a mass adjacent to the neural foramen. Overzealous traction can cause tearing of the nerve root proximal to the extraspinal extent of the dura, and this tearing can lead to a CSF leak, which most often becomes evident only postoperatively (in the form of persistent, clear chest-tube output). The diagnosis of CSF leakage can be confirmed by measuring the beta$_2$-transferrin level in the fluid. If CSF leakage is confirmed, reoperation with a neurosurgeon is mandatory; the site of the leak is repaired and buttressed with vascularized tissue.

Overzealous retraction at the final stages of the operation may also cause complete disruption of the tumor's attachment at the neural foramen, including its blood supply. This blood supply could potentially retract into the foramen, causing bleeding that could threaten the spinal cord with compression by an intraspinal hematoma. Tamponade with hemostatic agents should never be employed for bleeding at the neural foramen, as this may simply trap blood within the spinal canal, promoting dangerous hematoma formation there. Careful use of pinpoint, bipolar electrocautery at the bony margins of the foramen and intraoperative watchful waiting are the only ways to manage this unusual problem of oozing around the foramen. If hemostasis cannot be achieved with these measures, a neurosurgical consultation should be obtained. In the event of oozing from the vicinity of a foramen that is not easily controlled, there should be no hesitation in converting a VATS/robotic procedure to an open procedure.

In a minority of patients, clipping and division of an intercostal nerve results in substantial intercostal neuralgia after the procedure; the possibility that this may occur must be discussed with the patient preoperatively. Many patients who undergo division of a lower thoracic intercostal nerve that supplies an upper abdominal dermatome notice minor postoperative bulging of the ipsilateral abdomen in the area supplied by that nerve for a few months postoperatively.

VATS resection of a benign cyst of the posterior mediastinum

Resection of a benign cystic mass of the posterior mediastinum closely resembles resection of a neurogenic tumor (see steps in "VATS resection of neurogenic tumors of the posterior mediastinum" section). One starts by incising the pleura circumferentially, then dissecting and dividing attachments progressively, circumferentially, until the cyst has been completely mobilized. The procedures are typically simpler since there is no intercostal bundle with which one has to deal.[8]

POTENTIAL PROBLEMS AND THEIR AVOIDANCE

In the initial stages of dissection of a benign cyst of the posterior mediastinum, care should be taken *not* to rupture the cyst; initial mobilization from surrounding structures is far easier when the cyst wall remains under tension. However, I generally *intentionally* rupture a larger cyst, but only after I have completed 70%–80% of the circumferential dissection with the cyst wall intact. Intentional rupture of a large cyst toward the end of the dissection provides a much better view of the deepest extent of the field (e.g., for subcarinal bronchogenic cysts), facilitating the last steps of complete removal.

Occasionally, a portion of the cyst wall is found to be inseparable from an important mediastinal structure such as the esophagus or the membranous wall of the airway, and, in this situation, the cyst cannot be removed safely in its entirety. This is more common in the case of active or recent infection of the cyst. In these situations, I resect all of the nonadherent portion of the cyst wall and ablate the residual adherent cyst wall with electrocautery or argon beam to destroy any potential remaining secretory tissue. In one difficult case, I was forced to leave approximately 35% of the wall of a bronchogenic cyst in place—and this cyst has never recurred. It is my recommendation, however, that if more than approximately 35% of a cyst must be left in place, conversion to thoracotomy should be considered to allow resection of as much of the wall as possible and prevent recurrence.

Resection of esophageal leiomyomata and duplication cysts

In addition to the steps described in the "VATS resection of neurogenic tumors of the posterior mediastinum" section, there are three special maneuvers that facilitate resection of esophageal intramural masses, such as leiomyomata and duplication cysts.

1. After incising the pleura, the longitudinal esophageal muscle fibers that overlie the mass are separated as shown (see **Figure 10.7**) with endoscopic scissors or with the hook-cautery in the line of the fibers, extending about 1 cm proximal and distal to the mass. These fibers often are markedly attenuated as a result of the expansion of the mass.
2. Blunt dissection with an endoscopic peanut dissector allows careful, progressive mobilization of the mass, first from the muscle layer and then from the underlying mucosa (see **Figure 10.8**). Gentle traction on the mass aids exposure during this portion of the procedure. A figure-of-eight suture is often placed into the tumor to facilitate this retraction if the ring clamp, as shown, does not provide a secure grasp. Having an assistant place the endoscope within the esophageal lumen to distend and illuminate the mucosa also may be helpful at this stage. Once the mass has been completely resected, it is sent for pathologic examination. Even horseshoe-type

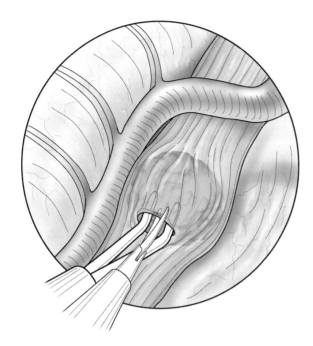

10.7 The attenuated longitudinal muscle fibers are divided in the line of the fibers to expose the submuscular mass.

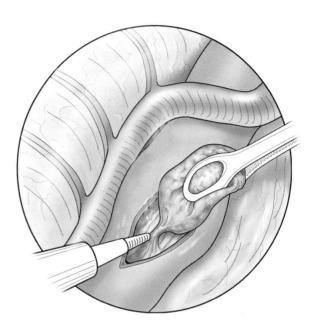

10.8 The mass is dissected bluntly away from the underlying mucosa.

leiomyomata can usually be successfully resected by this technique.

3. After resection, the esophagus is distended by insufflating air from above through the endoscope while the distal esophagus is occluded with a sponge stick (see **Figure 10.9**). The air-filled esophagus is then submerged in saline, and the area of the resection is examined for air leakage.

POTENTIAL PROBLEMS AND THEIR AVOIDANCE

The muscular defect in the esophageal wall must be closed after resection to ensure that an esophageal diverticulum does not develop. Such closure may be accomplished by means of thoracoscopic (or robotic) suturing.

Frequently, duplication cysts are more adherent to the underlying esophageal mucosa than leiomyomas, and trans-illumination of the esophageal wall helps define the plane at which blunt dissection should be performed. Where the cyst wall becomes difficult to separate from the mucosa, a small amount of the wall may be left in place if, in the surgeon's judgment, attempting to remove all of it might lead to a breach in the mucosa. In my opinion, if the mucosa is breached, a thoracotomy should be performed to ensure precise mucosal and muscle layer repair. In this situation, an intercostal muscle flap is also recommended. All patients should have a contrast study to ensure mucosal integrity prior to advancing the diet on postoperative day 2.

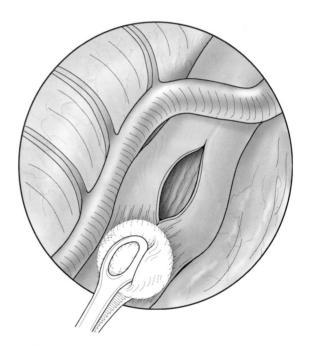

10.9 Following removal of the mass, the mucosa is tested for integrity by submerging in saline while insufflating air from above with an endoscope and occluding the esophagus distally with a sponge stick.

RESULTS

There should be essentially zero recurrences if the principles and techniques described here are followed in the resection of benign posterior mediastinal masses and cysts. Patients are generally discharged on postoperative day 2 but are frequently ready to leave on postoperative day 1. The severe complications mentioned of spinal cord compression, CSF leak, and esophageal leak should never occur when attention is paid to the details of the procedure. The most common ill effect, in my experience, is intercostal neuralgia when the intercostal nerve requires clipping and division. Since there is no known way to prevent this when the nerve must be sacrificed, patients need to be informed of the possibility, and this possibility needs to be weighed in the decision about whether to proceed with surgical resection or follow these lesions radiographically.

REFERENCES

1. Demmy TL, Krasna MJ, Detterbeck FC et al. Multicenter VATS experience with mediastinal tumors. *Ann Thorac Surg.* 1998; 66: 187–92.

2. Cerfolio RJ, Bryant AS, Minnich DJ. Operative techniques in robotic thoracic surgery for inferior or posterior mediastinal pathology. *J Thorac Cardiovasc Surg.* 2012; 143: 1138–43.

3. Osada H, Aoki H, Yokote K et al. Dumbbell neurogenic tumor of the mediastinum: a report of three cases undergoing single-staged complete removal without thoracotomy. *Jpn J Surg.* 1991; 21: 224–8.

4. Rzyman W, Skokowski J, Wilimski R et al. One step removal of dumb-bell tumors by postero-lateral thoracotomy and extended foraminectomy. *Eur J Cardiothorac Surg.* 2004; 25: 509–14.

5. Shadmehr MB, Gaissert HA, Wain JC et al. The surgical approach to "dumbbell tumors" of the mediastinum. *Ann Thorac Surg.* 2003; 76: 1650–4.

6. Vallières E, Findlay JM, Fraser RE. Combined microneurosurgical and thoracoscopic removal of neurogenic dumbbell tumors. *Ann Thorac Surg.* 1995; 59: 469–72.

7. Venissac N, Leo F, Hofman P et al. Mediastinal neurogenic tumors and video-assisted thoracoscopy: always the right choice? *Surg Laparosc Endosc Percutan Tech.* 2004; 14: 20–22.

8. Martinod E, Pons F, Azorin J et al. Thoracoscopic excision of mediastinal bronchogenic cysts: results in 20 cases. *Ann Thorac Surg.* 2000; 69: 1525–8.

11

Thymectomy

LARRY R. KAISER

HISTORY

Over the past few decades, complete removal of the thymus gland has been shown to improve the clinical course of patients with myasthenia gravis (MG), though many neurologists continue to be hesitant about referring patients for thymectomy. However, the precise relationship between the thymus gland and the onset of MG has not been completely elucidated. Alfred Blalock performed a thymectomy via median sternotomy in 1936 for a woman with thymoma and MG and noted an improvement in her myasthenic symptoms. He subsequently reported on a series of patients without thymoma who underwent thymectomy, noting similar improvement in the clinical course of the disease. In this report of 20 thymectomies, he observed improvement in 13 of 17 survivors.[1] Recently a prospective randomized trial to assess the role of surgery on the clinical course of MG has been reported that demonstrated superiority of thymectomy over medical management with respect to clinical outcome over a 3 year period.[2] This study confirmed what already has been known based on a number of carefully controlled cohort studies comparing thymectomy with standard medical management. Essentially, all of these studies have shown a significantly greater incidence of remission in the operated group versus in those treated with medication alone.[3,4,5]

PRINCIPLES AND JUSTIFICATION

The presence of MG constitutes the most common indication for the performance of elective thymectomy. The other main indication is the presence of a mass within the thymus gland. Approximately 15% of patients with MG have thymoma, while approximately 35% of patients with thymoma have MG. Patients presenting with a thymoma should be thoroughly evaluated for symptoms of MG, and, likewise, those presenting with MG should have a computed tomography (CT) scan of the chest to evaluate the anterior mediastinum. The relationship between MG and the thymus gland has been well established, though the precise mechanism for the improvement of symptoms following thymectomy has not been established. Ten percent of patients with autoimmune MG are found to have a thymoma, a situation that may play a role in disease initiation through multiple mechanisms including, but not limited to, expression of self-antigens by thymoma cells and impaired negative selection of autoreactive T lymphocytes.[6] Approximately 90% of patients with generalized MG have measurable circulating acetylcholine receptor (AChr) antibodies. It has been well established that MG is an autoimmune disorder of the neuromuscular junction, with inflammatory destruction of the neuromuscular endplate membrane as the acute event. On a chronic basis, the membrane appears to reform, though with decreased amounts of AChr. The effect at the neuromuscular junction appears to be due solely to the autoantibodies that primarily target the 67 to 76 portion of the alpha subunit of the AChr, known as the "main immunogenic region" (MIR).

Following thymectomy, up to 40% of patients with MG can be expected to achieve a complete response, as measured by no requirement for medication. The time course of the improvement may vary, and continued resolution of symptoms may occur for up to 18 months following thymectomy. Further improvement would not be expected to occur after this time period. An additional 30%–40% of patients will achieve a partial response, usually manifested by a significant reduction in the amount and type of medication required for symptom control. A small percentage of patients fail to achieve any symptomatic relief from their disease. Patients should understand the time to achieving maximal response may vary, and there is no immediate resolution of symptoms. They should be aware of the response rate, so that an informed decision regarding thymectomy may be made. With the development and refinement of minimally invasive approaches to thymectomy, the risk–benefit ratio seems to be tilted toward the performance of thymectomy, even in the older patient or those with minimal symptoms. In the past, when a median sternotomy was required for thymectomy, many neurologists were hesitant about referring patients for such an extensive operation. However, especially with the transcervical approach, such hesitation is no longer warranted.

PREOPERATIVE ASSESSMENT AND PREPARATION

Put simply, any patient with MG is a candidate for thymectomy, but this principle certainly does not imply that all patients with the disease are referred for resection. No laboratory test or other diagnostic maneuver exists that will predict the response to thymectomy—this only can be assessed following the procedure. This unpredictability is probably one of the reasons that many neurologists refer only the occasional patient for thymectomy, despite the recognition that many patients will have a beneficial response. Much of this reluctance is predicated on the "size" and perceived magnitude of the operation—namely, a median sternotomy, which is the procedure most commonly employed for thymectomy. Less invasive approaches to thymectomy—specifically, the transcervical approach as presented in this chapter—should go a long way toward addressing many of these concerns.

Specific preoperative testing prior to thymectomy is limited to CT scanning of the chest and measurement of pulmonary function. The CT scan of the chest is used to assess for the presence of a thymoma, a finding that could dictate the operative approach. The key finding, in addition to whether or not a thymoma is present, is an assessment of size and whether the mass appears to be encapsulated or invasive. The definitive assessment of invasion can only be made at the time of operation, but often a fairly reliable assumption regarding encapsulation can be made. A CT scan of the chest should be obtained in all patients following a diagnosis of MG to specifically exclude a thymoma, a finding present in up to 30%–40% of these patients. A measurement of forced vital capacity (as a minimum) should be made to ascertain whether any involvement of respiratory muscles exists, a finding that could have implications following general anesthesia and the operation. Respiratory muscle involvement, if severe, could be predictive of a postoperative mechanical ventilation requirement and would clearly mandate the need for more intensive preoperative preparation.

Prior to thymectomy, patients should be managed with optimal medical therapy following establishment of the specific diagnosis of MG. First-line therapy in MG usually consists of pyridostigmine, an anticholinesterase inhibitor, given as a single agent. The majority of patients experience significant relief of symptoms following initiation of this drug, and in most patients, it is the only drug needed. Corticosteroids, most commonly prednisone, are the most commonly used immunosuppressive agents for treating the symptoms of MG and may be necessary in the occasional patient who responds less than optimally to pyridostigmine. Other immunosuppressants, such as azathioprine, may also be used. Prior to operation, depending on the judgment of the referring neurologist, plasmapheresis may be performed, which usually consists of three plasma exchanges carried out during the week preceding the operation. This procedure significantly reduces the level of circulating anti-AChr antibodies. Depending on venous access, this procedure may be done on an outpatient basis. Following plasmapheresis, patients usually report feeling better than they have done in many months. Plasmapheresis should be performed for patients with reduced vital capacity, though this procedure becomes less important when the thymectomy is performed via the transcervical approach.

ANESTHESIA

General anesthesia can be performed safely in patients with MG following optimal preparation and adequate monitoring of neuromuscular transmission during and following the surgical procedure. Patients are requested to take their medication on the morning of the operative procedure just as they would normally. Due to the decreased number of AChrs or their functional blockade by antibodies directed against them, the use of succinylcholine or other nondepolarizing muscle relaxants is avoided. Other types of muscle relaxants can be used in smaller amounts as part of a balanced technique of anesthesia. It is important that an anesthesiologist experienced in the care of patients with MG be part of the team in order to avoid postoperative problems. Neuromuscular transmission should be monitored during the operation by peripheral nerve stimulation to aid in titrating the dose of muscle relaxants and to ensure complete reversal of neuromuscular block at the conclusion of the procedure. A detailed discussion of anesthetic technique is beyond the scope of this chapter but may be found in the paper by Baraka.[7]

OPERATION

The standard operation for thymectomy in patients with MG consists of a median sternotomy with total removal of all thymic tissue. This operation is essentially the same operation as described for excision of an anterior mediastinal mass in Chapter 9, "Anterior mediastinal lesions," so a detailed description will not be provided in this chapter. The critical factor for thymectomy in the patient with MG is the complete removal of the thymus gland. Some have argued that aberrant rests of thymic tissue are so common that more radical operations are justified.

My preferred operation for thymectomy is the extended transcervical approach, using the technique originally described by Joel Cooper.[8] This less invasive approach is contraindicated only when a large thymoma (>4 cm) is present or hyperextension of the neck is unable to be achieved. Otherwise, cervical thymectomy is the approach that we have now used in over 200 patients.

2. The patient is positioned supine with an inflatable bag behind the scapulae and with the neck hyperextended. A transverse skin incision is made just at the level of the sternal notch and deepened through the platysma. Superior and inferior subplatysmal flaps are raised so as to maximize the operative field and allow for the placement of skin retractors. Dissection is carried along the midline, separating the right and left strap muscles, specifically, the sternohyoid and sternothyroid muscles. The sternothyroid muscle is elevated, and the dissection proceeds along the posterior surface of the muscle. (See **Figure 11.2.**)

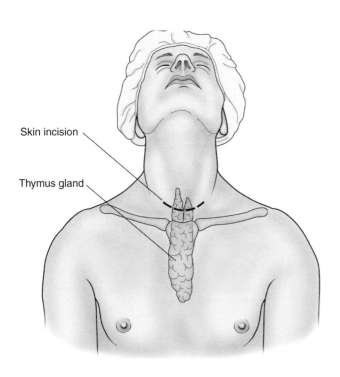

Skin incision

Thymus gland

11.1

1. Masaoka first described the extended transsternal thymectomy where not only the gross thymus but also the surrounding adipose tissue in the anterior mediastinum is removed (see **Figure 11.1**).

This procedure removes all thymic tissue as well as adipose tissue from the lower poles of the thyroid (superior extent) to the diaphragm (inferior) and from the phrenic nerve to phrenic nerve (posterior). A modification of this procedure, the maximal thymectomy, was advocated by Jaretzki and others and involves a cervicomediastinal approach with both a cervical incision and median sternotomy. The extent of this procedure exceeds that of the extended thymectomy by including the cervical region, the aortopulmonary window, and the lateral region of the phrenic nerves. The pericardium is taken along with both pleural reflections. As might be expected, the incidence of complications following this procedure exceeds that reported for other procedures, including phrenic and recurrent laryngeal nerve injuries, as well as postoperative respiratory failure.

Despite the assumption made by advocates for the more extensive procedures, it seems likely that in a patient with multiple aberrant rests of thymus, any procedure will remove all thymic tissue, especially since many of these areas are visible only microscopically. Indeed, results with a less invasive approach, transcervical thymectomy, are equivalent to those achieved with the "extended" approaches, with significantly less morbidity and shorter hospital stay.

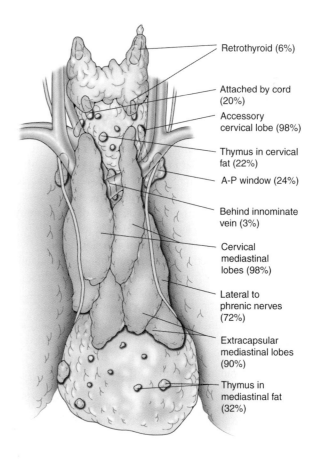

Retrothyroid (6%)

Attached by cord (20%)

Accessory cervical lobe (98%)

Thymus in cervical fat (22%)

A-P window (24%)

Behind innominate vein (3%)

Cervical mediastinal lobes (98%)

Lateral to phrenic nerves (72%)

Extracapsular mediastinal lobes (90%)

Thymus in mediastinal fat (32%)

11.2

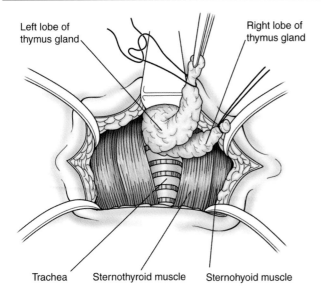

11.3

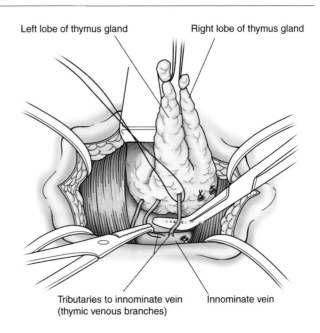

11.4

3. The lobe of the thymus gland is identified anterior to the inferior thyroid vein. The gland can be distinguished from adjacent fat by its salmon pink color and by the presence of a capsule. Once the gland is identified, it is freed up laterally and medially and the dissection proceeds superiorly while applying downward retraction on the gland. This maneuver allows for complete dissection of the gland up to its origin, where a small vein usually is found. The vein is clipped, and the gland is mobilized anteriorly and freed away from adjacent structures. A silk ligature is placed at the apex of the lobe of the gland to be used as a "handle" to facilitate the mobilization. Dissection then proceeds toward the mediastinum until the innominate vein is encountered. Both lobes of the gland are freed away from surrounding structures in a similar manner. Locating one lobe of the gland leads to the other lobe, as the dissection proceeds caudad. The gland is always located anterior to the inferior thyroid veins, and the veins are dissected away from the gland and left intact. (See **Figure 11.3.**)
4. Both lobes of the gland are lifted anteriorly, and, using blunt dissection with peanut sponges, the gland is separated away from the innominate vein. As this maneuver proceeds, individual thymic venous branches come into view. These are individually ligated and divided. The number of branches varies but usually at least two or three are identified and must be divided to mobilize the gland away from the vein. Care must be taken to avoid avulsing one of these venous branches, since bleeding is difficult to control in the limited operative field. The gland usually courses anterior to the innominate vein, but, in the occasional patient, either a lobe or the entire gland may pass posterior to the vein. This anatomical variant needs to be recognized and dealt with appropriately so as not to leave any residual

gland. Using ball sponges on ring forceps, the gland is separated away from the sternum anteriorly. (See **Figure 11.4.**)
5. The Cooper thymectomy retractor (Teleflex, Inc (Pilling), Morrisville, North Carolina) is put in place to further define the operative field and allow for better visualization of the anterior mediastinum. This retractor attaches to the operating table, and the L-shaped blade is placed behind the sternal notch and lifted. The inflatable bag is deflated so that an optimal view of the mediastinum is provided. If the neck is able to be well extended, the entire thymus gland may be visualized, and the mediastinum is viewed down to the diaphragm, with appropriate downward traction applied to the pericardium. (See **Figure 11.5.**)

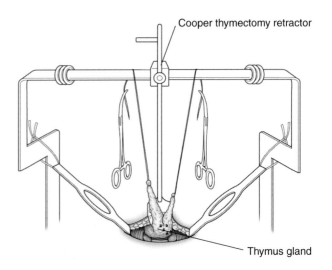

11.5

6. Once the retractor is in place, additional skin retraction is provided by an army-navy retractor placed on each side of the incision, held in place by Penrose drains attached to the arms of the Cooper retractor. The gland is completely dissected away from the pericardium down to its inferior extent by blunt dissection with ball sponges. Likewise, the gland is completely separated from the sternum anteriorly. The gland is bluntly dissected away from the right pleural reflection and reflected from right to left. Care is taken to avoid entry into the pleural space, but if a rent is made in the pleura, the lung is simply reexpanded at the time of closure by placing a red rubber tube through the pleural rent while the anesthesiologist inflates the lungs. The gland is easily distinguished from pleural fat by the difference in appearance and texture. The gland readily separates from the pleural reflection with blunt dissection. Once the gland is freed off the right pleural reflection, the left lobe is likewise freed. Often there is a tongue of gland that tracks down into the aortopulmonary window, and this extension needs to be followed to its termination to ensure complete removal of the gland. All of the dissection in this area is done bluntly, taking care to avoid any significant traction on the phrenic nerve. The gland is then reflected from inferiorly up into the neck, sweeping off any residual pericardial attachments, some of which may need to be divided sharply. Following this,

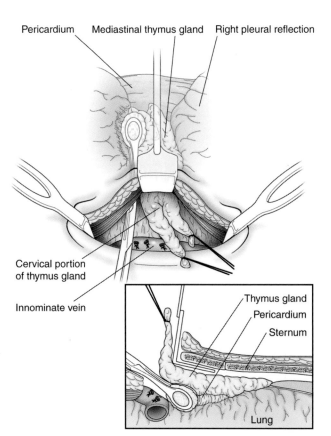

Pericardium   Mediastinal thymus gland   Right pleural reflection

Cervical portion of thymus gland

Innominate vein

Thymus gland
Pericardium
Sternum

Lung

11.6

the gland is delivered into the neck and removed. With the retractor still in place, a thorough inspection is made to ensure hemostasis, as no drains are left. Both pleural reflections should be assessed for integrity. The retractor is then removed. The neck is closed in layers in the usual fashion, first reapproximating the strap muscles in the midline followed by a subcuticular skin closure. (See **Figure 11.6.**)

POSTOPERATIVE CARE

With careful neuromuscular monitoring, the patient should be easily awakened and extubated prior to transfer to the postanesthesia recovery area. A chest radiograph should be obtained to ensure that both lungs are fully inflated in case any entry into the pleural space had been made. Preoperative medications are resumed as soon as the patient is fully awake and able to take fluids by mouth. Patients are observed for several hours in the recovery area prior to discharge. Routinely in our experience, patients are discharged home on the day of the procedure, though, early in our experience, they were discharged on the morning of the first postoperative day. Mild analgesics are prescribed for postoperative discomfort, and patients usually return to full activity within 1 week.

OUTCOME

The goal of thymectomy in MG is the induction of remission or improvement of symptoms with less reliance on medication. Complete remission, as defined by no symptoms off all medication, can be expected in 40%–50% of patients undergoing thymectomy, but the time that it takes to achieve this rate may be somewhat prolonged. Patients may see continued improvement for up to 18 months following their operation, and some patients may not go into remission until months or even years later. Our data and that from Cooper's group suggest that results obtained following transcervical thymectomy do not differ from those obtained via the transsternal route, either the extended or the maximal approach.[9]

REFERENCES

1. Blalock A, McGehee HA, Ford FR et al. The treatment of myasthenia gravis by removal of the thymus gland: preliminary report. *JAMA.* 1941; 117: 1529–33.
2. Wolfe GI, Kaminski HJ, Aban IB et al. Randomized trial of thymectomy in Myasthenia Gravis. *N Engl J Med.* 2016; 375: 511–22.
3. Bril V, Kojic J, Ilse WK et al. Long-term clinical outcome after transcervical thymectomy for myasthenia gravis. *Annals of Thoracic Surgery.* 1998; 65: 1520–2.

4. Jaretzki A III, Wolff M. "Maximal" thymectomy for myasthenia gravis: surgical anatomy and operative technique. *Journal of Thoracic and Cardiovascular Surgery.* 1988; 96: 711–16.

5. Masaoka A, Yamakawa Y, Niwa H et al. Extended thymectomy for myasthenia gravis patients: a 20-year review. *Annals of Thoracic Surgery.* 1996; 62: 853–9.

6. Ha JC, Richman DP. Myasthenia gravis and related disorders: Pathology and molecular pathogenesis. *Biochim Biophys Acta.* 2015 Apr; 1852(4): 651–7.

7. Baraka A. Anesthesia and critical care of thymectomy for myasthenia gravis. *Chest Surgery Clinics of North America.* 2001; 11: 337–61.

8. Cooper JD, Al-Jilaihawa AN, Pearson FG et. al. An improved technique to facilitate transcervical thymectomy for myasthenia gravis. *Ann Thorac Surg.* 1988 Mar; 45(3): 242–7.

9. Shrager JB, Nathan D, Brinster CJ et al. Outcomes after 151 extended transcervical thymectomies for myasthenia gravis. *Ann Thorac Surg.* 2006 Nov; 82(5): 1863–9.

12

Right-sided pulmonary resections

LARRY R. KAISER

HISTORY

Evarts Graham performed the first successful pneumonectomy for lung cancer in 1933.[1] Pulmonary resection was also applied to patients with tuberculosis before effective drugs were developed. Lobectomy became the standard procedure as a radical resection for lung cancer in the 1950s. Cahan described procedures of mediastinal and hilar lymph node dissection for pneumonectomy and lobectomy in 1951 and 1960. Bronchoplasty and arterioplasty were introduced to lung cancer surgery in the 1970s. Techniques for locally advanced lung cancer invading great vessels and/or the heart were described in the 1960s and were applied as clinical practice in the 1980s. Limited resection—that is, segmentectomy or partial resection of the lung—were examined as potential operations for lung cancer. However, the results of a randomized controlled trial revealed that local and/or regional recurrence occurred more frequently in the limited resection group than in the conventional lobectomy group and this translated into a survival difference. Video-assisted thoracoscopic surgery (VATS) lobectomy has been introduced as an option for early stage lung cancer and, in many centers, is the procedure of choice for a majority of pulmonary resections.

PRINCIPLES AND JUSTIFICATION

Right-sided pulmonary resections include pneumonectomy, lobectomy with or without bronchoplastic procedures, segmentectomy, and partial (wedge) resection. These procedures are common and applicable to lung malignancies, inflammatory lesions, and congenital anomalies. Most of the inflammatory diseases can be controlled pharmacologically, and lung cancer has become the most common reason to proceed with pulmonary resection. Bronchoplastic procedures are performed on the right side much more frequently than on the left because of asymmetric anatomy of the

tracheobronchial tree and the pulmonary artery, specifically because of the position and angulation of the right upper lobe orifice in relation to the carina. That being said, bronchoplastic procedures on the left side are feasible but often involve resection and reconstruction of the pulmonary artery in order to preserve pulmonary parenchyma and avoid a pneumonectomy.

PREOPERATIVE ASSESSMENT AND PREPARATION

The size, extent, and location of the lesion are the most important factors in deciding what procedure to choose. Computerized tomography (CT) provides good information concerning the extent of the locoregional disease in addition to identifying the presence of distant metastatic disease. Thoracic CT images the primary tumor, nodal involvement, intrapulmonary metastases, and pleural involvement with or without effusion or pleural dissemination. Malignant effusion and intrapulmonary metastases, if seen on CT scan, render the patient inoperable and contraindicate curative resection of a lung cancer. A tissue diagnosis should be confirmed histologically or cytologically, either with a percutaneous needle aspiration biopsy or bronchoscopy. Upper mediastinal lymph node metastases can be documented histologically, either by mediastinoscopy or endobronchial ultrasound guided biopsy if the thoracic CT shows enlarged lymph nodes.

ANESTHESIA

Smoking should cease at least 4 weeks prior to surgery to decrease bronchial secretion and to reduce the likelihood of postoperative pulmonary complications. This often is difficult for the patient who has been a long-term smoker. In cases of an inflammatory lesion or a lung cancer with airway obstruction, secretions from the lesion and/or obstructed bronchi must be controlled during the operation. The face-down prone position prevents secretions from flowing into the opposite healthy lung. However, the face-down position limits the operative procedure. More commonly, operations are performed in the lateral decubitus position under anesthesia, with a separate ventilation tube to suction secretions during the operative procedure. Inhalation anesthesia stimulates the bronchial glands and increases secretion. Instead of inhalation anesthesia, intravenous anesthesia with epidural anesthesia is used in cases where significant secretions are expected. Epidural analgesia, instituted at the time of operation usually is continued until after the chest drain has been removed.

OPERATION

Incision and exploration

Pneumonectomy and lobectomy may be performed through a standard posterolateral thoracotomy. However, with recent advances including the introduction of VATS and the development of surgical instruments, skin incisions have become smaller than those formerly used for standard thoracotomy. Although some doctors recommend VATS lobectomy even for cases of lung cancer, open remains the most common procedure used to perform radical resection with systematic nodal dissection for lung cancer.

Exposure of the hilum

1. Exposure of the hilum of the lung is the first step of pulmonary resection. The reflection of the mediastinal pleura is opened from anterior to posterior beyond the right main bronchus. In the case of lung cancer located in the hilum, intrapericardial division of pulmonary vessels may be required depending on the extent, or lack thereof, of hilar invasion. (See **Figure 12.1**).

Pneumonectomy

In cases of lung cancer involving the main bronchus, right pulmonary artery, pulmonary veins, or left atrium, pneumonectomy has to be a consideration to achieve a curative resection, though an assessment should always be made as to whether a bronchoplastic procedure with or without a vascular resection might be feasible.

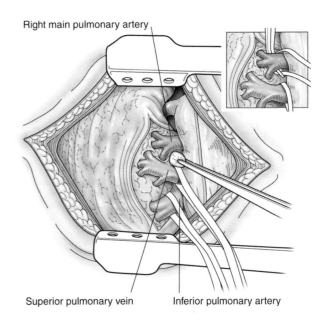

Right main pulmonary artery

Superior pulmonary vein   Inferior pulmonary artery

12.1

DISSECTION OF THE PULMONARY LIGAMENT

2. In cases of lung cancer located in the lower or middle lobe, lower mediastinal lymph node dissection is required. After opening the pleura along with pulmonary ligament at the reflection, fatty tissue including lymph nodes is divided from the esophagus and the vagus nerve until the lower border of the inferior pulmonary vein is exposed. Retracting the lower lobe cephalad provides adequate exposure. (See **Figure 12.2**).

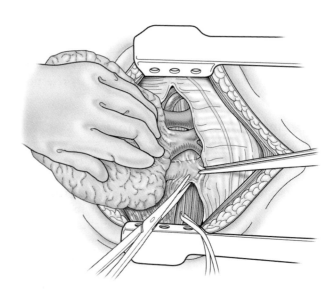

12.2

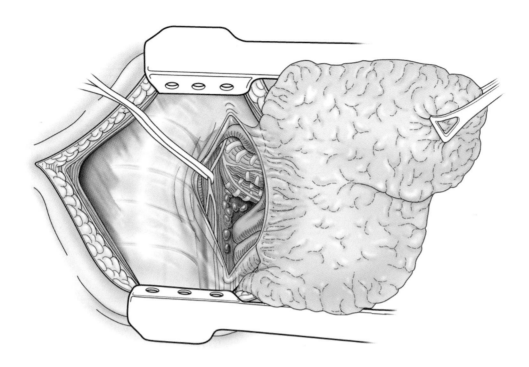

12.3

SUBCARINAL LYMPH NODE DISSECTION

3. The subcarinal lymph node space is triangle shaped, with the nodes located posterior to the right pulmonary artery, left atrium, and both pulmonary veins. Therefore, early dissection of the subcarinal lymph node improves the exposure of the inferior pulmonary vein as well as the mainstem bronchi. The dissection is begun by elevating the lymph node mass off the pericardium using clips on the many small vessels encountered during the dissection. The nodal mass may be grasped with ring forceps to provide counter traction. Clips should be used liberally. Vagal branches going toward the lung are clipped and divided. Ideally, the entire nodal mass is removed as a package, with clips placed to minimize bleeding. (See **Figure 12.3**).

DIVISION OF THE INFERIOR PULMONARY VEIN

4. The inferior pulmonary vein is exposed after the inferior mediastinal and subcarinal lymph node dissection has been completed. The vein should be encircled and the adventitia of the vein exposed to perform complete lymph node dissection and to confirm the reflection of the pericardium around the vein. The vein will be divided by a stapler or, after double ligation, with a suture ligature. (See **Figure 12.4**).

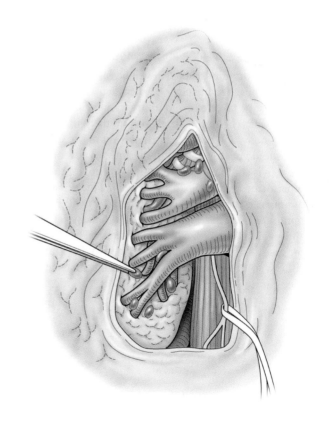

12.4

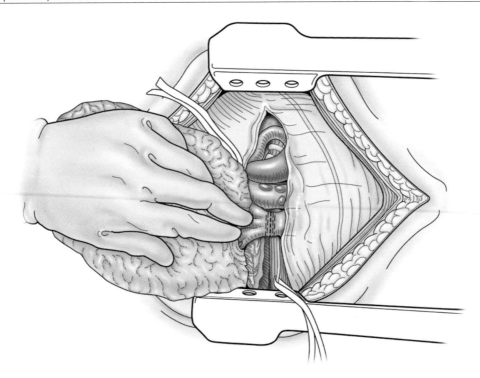

12.5

5. If the incision line crosses the pericardium, the pulmonary veins and artery should be divided within the pericardium (see **Figure 12.5**).

DIVISION OF THE SUPERIOR PULMONARY VEIN

6. The superior pulmonary vein will be easily exposed by incising the overlying pleura. When encircling the vein, care must be taken to avoid injury to the pulmonary artery, which lies immediately behind the vein. The soft tissue and lymph nodes located in front of the superior vein should be dissected until the anterior adventitia of the vein is completely exposed. If dissection of the vein is performed in the subadventitial plane the possibility of injury to the adjacent pulmonary artery will be minimized. Recently, the superior pulmonary vein has almost always been divided with a stapler. However, in the case of a tumor invading or located in the hilum, either a suture or suture ligation technique may be used. (See **Figure 12.6**).

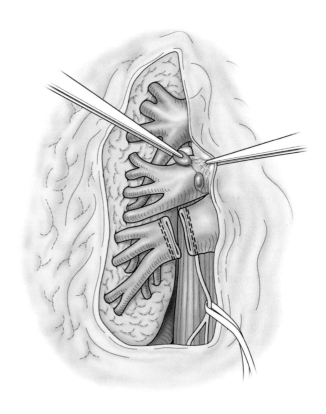

12.6

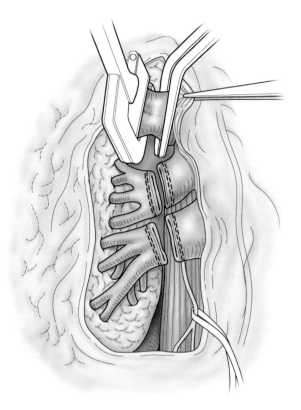

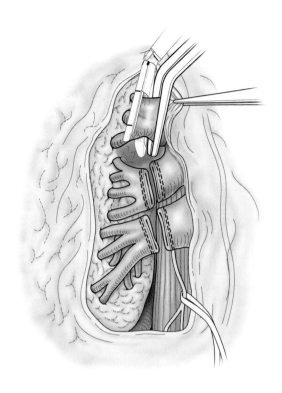

12.7a–b

DIVISION OF THE RIGHT PULMONARY ARTERY

7. The right pulmonary artery and superior vena cava are connected by a fibrous membrane at the bifurcation of the upper and lower branches of the pulmonary artery. This membrane is a part of the pericardium. Division of this membrane makes central dissection of the anterior aspect of the right pulmonary artery easy. As the posterior wall of the right pulmonary artery is covered by a fibrous portion of the pericardium attaching the trachea and both main bronchi, this fibrous portion should be divided from the bronchus to expose the artery completely. This is particularly important for very proximal lesions where safe division of the artery requires obtaining adequate length. The safest move to execute division of the pulmonary artery employs the use of a vascular stapler. When the stapler is used to divide the pulmonary artery, ideally a vascular clamp should be placed, in case of the very rare occurrence of the stapler cutting without laying down staples. After the artery is cut, the central stump should be dissected from neighboring structures to render the stump free from tension to avoid tearing near the staples. (See **Figure 12.7a and b**).

MEDIASTINAL LYMPH NODE DISSECTION

8. To expose the superior mediastinum, the mediastinal pleura is opened longitudinally from the azygos vein to the apex of the thorax and horizontally at the apex. The

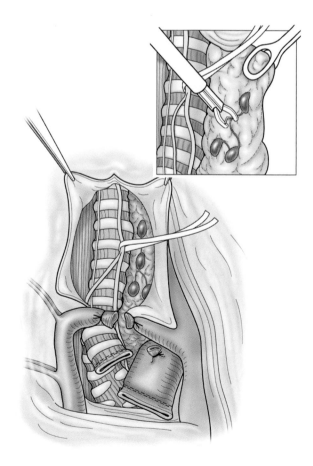

12.8

azygos vein may be divided to facilitate the dissection, especially if lymph nodes are enlarged secondary to the tumor, but rarely is this necessary. The entire contents of the space bordered by the trachea posteriorly, the superior vena cava anteriorly, the right subclavian artery superiorly, and the azygous vein inferiorly should be removed with the liberal use of hemoclips and electrocautery. The dissection may be facilitated by grasping the nodal mass with ring forceps. The subcarinal space is then entered and the lymph nodes removed, taking care to clip any bronchial arterial branches. (See **Figure 12.8**).

DIVISION OF THE RIGHT MAIN BRONCHUS

9. If there is enough length of the bronchus to obtain a grossly negative margin, mechanical closure with a stapler is preferred. If the tumor encroaches proximally or if there is a question of the proximal extent of an endobronchial lesion, open division with suture closure should be carried out. Even though stapled closure of the bronchus is used so commonly, it remains important to know how to suture the open bronchial stump for those instances when a stapled closure is not feasible. Covering of the stump of the bronchus with a pericardial fat pad or with an intercostal muscle should be considered in those patients who have received preoperative chemotherapy and/or radiotherapy. In the case of intense chemoradiotherapy, use of a pedicled flap of gastrocolic omentum may provide additional protection to that provided by pericardial fat or intercostal muscle. (See **Figure 12.9**).

Upper lobectomy

The right upper lobe is a common site for lung cancer, although the reason for the predilection of that location is not clear. Therefore, right upper lobectomy with systematic nodal dissection is considered by some to be the prototypical resection for lung cancer surgery.

DIVISION OF THE SUPERIOR PULMONARY VEIN

10. The upper lobe of the right lung should be pulled posteriorly to expose the anterior hilum of the lung. After incising the pleura of the hilum, the superior pulmonary vein is dissected and encircled. Care must be taken to avoid injuring the pulmonary artery that lies immediately posterior and may be injured when attempting to encircle the vein. The bifurcation between the tributary of the vein from the upper lobe and the middle lobe should be identified so as to ensure preservation of the middle lobe vein. On occasion, there may be more than a single middle lobe vein and simply elevating the middle lobe with a lung clamp will aid in identifying venous drainage of the lobe. Once the middle lobe venous drainage is identified, the upper lobe vein usually may be ligated and divided with a vascular stapler, providing exposure to the pulmonary artery. If division and closure of the vein with sutures is preferred, a proximal suture ligature is placed with individual ligation of distal venous branches to ensure an adequate venous stump following division of the vein. (See **Figure 12.10a and b**).

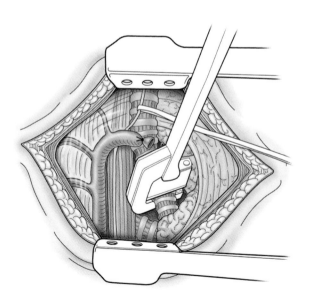

12.9

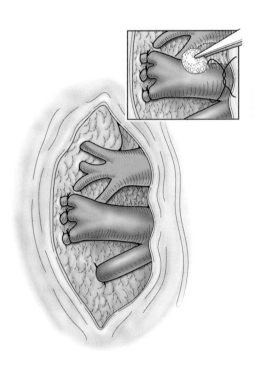

12.10a–b

DIVISION OF THE SUPERIOR PULMONARY ARTERY

11. Lying just superior and posterior to the vein is the right main pulmonary artery. The artery is dissected circumferentially and followed proximally, where it is observed as it courses posterior to the superior vena cava. The artery is easily encircled with a finger once the appropriate plane of dissection is entered. For an open thoracotomy, proximal control of the artery is usually established in this fashion if there is even a suggestion that the dissection may be difficult. It is not necessary to encircle the right main pulmonary artery in every case but one cannot be too safe in taking the extra precaution of having proximal control. The artery is dissected distally and the apical-anterior arterial branch is identified. This usually occurs as a common trunk but the individual segmental branches may arise separately from the main artery, with the branch to the anterior segment coming off the artery as the most proximal branch. An arterial branch should be completely dissected free circumferentially prior to trying to pass a right-angle clamp around the vessel. To do this, the thin connective tissue overlying the artery is grasped with forceps and lifted to allow a cut by the scissors. Once the correct plane on the artery is reached, closed blunt-tipped scissors are used to gently push the artery away while continuing to hold the incised tissue. This rapidly creates the plane of dissection and frees up the adjacent arterial branch. If an attempt to pass the right angle clamp is met with any resistance, further dissection should be performed rather than trying to force the clamp around the vessel and potentially perforating the back wall. The so-called truncus anterior of the pulmonary artery may be stapled with the vascular stapler and divided, or the branches individually ligated and divided as illustrated. At this point, the upper lobe bronchus is readily identified and may be encircled and divided if the surgeon prefers. The azygous vein is an important landmark, as it crosses to the superior vena cava just superior to the origin of the right upper lobe bronchus. (See **Figure 12.11**).

DISSECTION OF THE UPPER MEDIASTINUM

Superior mediastinal lymph node dissection is performed as described in the "Pneumonectomy" section. The lymph node packet surrounded by the trachea, azygous vein, superior vena cava, and the right subclavian artery should be removed *en bloc*, using clips to maintain hemostasis. Care should be taken to avoid injury to the right recurrent laryngeal nerve at the superior extent of the dissection. The subcarinal space is exposed by retracting the lung anteriorly and incising the overlying pleura. Bronchial arterial branches commonly course through this space and should be carefully identified and clipped while removing the nodal packet.

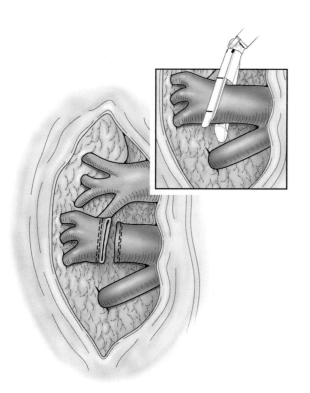

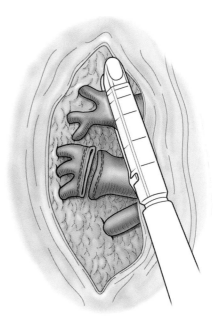

12.11

DIVISION OF THE FISSURE

12. There is little need to dissect directly into a fissure and thus create air leaks. Often, the major fissure is fairly complete and presents no difficulty, but the minor fissure, important in separating the middle lobe from the upper lobe, is rarely complete. Dissecting posteriorly at the bifurcation of the upper lobe bronchus and the bronchus intermedius allows one to elevate the lymph node that always resides in that bifurcation. Using a finger placed within the bifurcation, the parenchyma is thinned and usually a window may be developed, allowing for placement of the linear stapler and completion of the posterior portion of the major fissure. The middle lobe arterial branch is readily visualized from the anterior aspect of the hilum and, to facilitate division of the fissure and separation of the middle lobe from the upper lobe, the branch should be mobilized for a short distance. The arterial branch to the posterior segment of the upper lobe at times may be seen through this anterior exposure, or an additional anterior segmental branch may be identified. Once the artery is identified from this anterior approach and the middle lobe artery is seen, the minor fissure, which, as mentioned, is usually incomplete, may be divided with the application of a linear stapler.

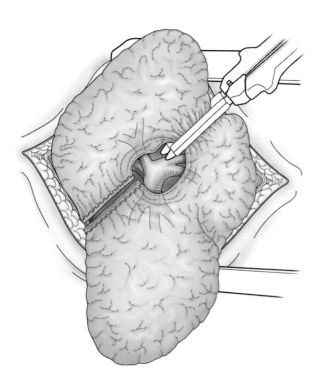

12.12

The posterior segmental branch of the artery is ligated and divided within the fissure. With the lung again retracted anteriorly, the origin of the upper lobe bronchus is well seen and a stapler is used to close the bronchus. The bronchus is taken as close as possible to its origin without compromising the lumen of the right mainstem bronchus. The bronchus is divided and the upper lobe removed if the minor fissure has been divided. If the minor fissure remains, it is completed with a firing of the linear stapler. To obtain definitive staging information, a complete mediastinal lymph node dissection should be performed.

Following division of the minor fissure and removal of the right upper lobe, the middle lobe is left without an attachment, since the oblique fissure is usually relatively complete. Postoperatively, this situation may predispose to torsion and infarction of the middle lobe. To prevent this very significant complication, the middle lobe is "reattached" to the lower lobe, either by placement of several absorbable sutures placed in a figure-of-eight fashion or by placing a row of staples between the two lobes. The middle lobe must be properly oriented prior to attaching it to the lower lobe. (See **Figure 12.12**).

Right middle lobectomy

If the major fissure is well developed and the pulmonary artery can be visualized easily within the fissure, the overlying pleura is incised. If the artery is not visible, the fissure must be divided in order to identify the artery. Within the fissure, the middle lobe arterial branch is identified as it originates from the main pulmonary artery, usually just opposite the branch to the superior segment of the lower lobe (see **Figure 12.13**). Most commonly there is a single arterial branch to the middle lobe, but occasionally two branches are identified. The arterial supply to the middle lobe is ligated with silk ligatures and divided. Once the arterial supply is divided, the middle lobe bronchus may be seen lying deep to the artery and slightly inferior, as viewed from within the fissure. The middle lobe bronchus is dissected back to its origin from the bronchus intermedius, stapled, and divided. Alternatively, the bronchus may be divided and closed with interrupted sutures of braided or monofilament absorbable material of size 3-0 or 4-0.

With the lung retracted posteriorly, the anterior hilar pleura over the superior pulmonary vein is incised. The middle lobe venous tributary or tributaries most commonly drain into the superior pulmonary vein but can drain into the inferior vein on rare occasions (see **Figure 12.14**). To ensure that a tributary is coming from the middle lobe, the lobe may be grasped with a lung clamp and retracted laterally (upward toward the incision). This will avoid division of small branches coming from the upper lobe. The venous branch is then divided after ligating with silk ligatures and securing with a suture ligature.

Once the bronchovascular structures have been divided, the minor fissure is completed with a firing of the linear stapler. The anterior portion of the major fissure is probably well developed and is easily completed and the lobe removed.

An alternative technique for middle lobectomy likely to be more useful and versatile is also illustrated. This technique does not rely on the pulmonary artery being visible within the fissure and does not require extensive dissection in the fissure to identify the artery. The lung is retracted posteriorly. The hilar pleura overlying the superior pulmonary vein is incised and the middle lobe vein identified. The vein is ligated and divided. Immediately posterior and slightly superior to the vein lies the middle lobe bronchus (see **Figure 12.15**). The bronchus should be followed back to its origin at the bronchus intermedius. The middle lobe arterial branch lies just posterior and slightly superior to the middle lobe bronchus but may not be visible prior to dividing the bronchus. The bronchus is encircled with a right-angle clamp, staying close to the bronchial wall to avoid damage to the adjacent arterial branch (see **Figure 12.16**). The bronchus is divided with a scalpel using a right-angle clamp as a guide. The bronchial stump is closed with interrupted sutures. Alternatively,

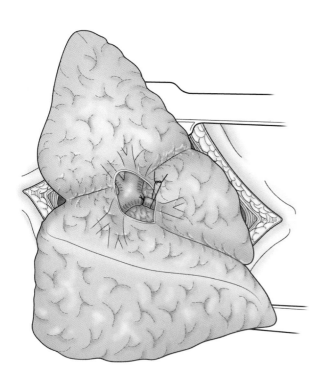

12.13

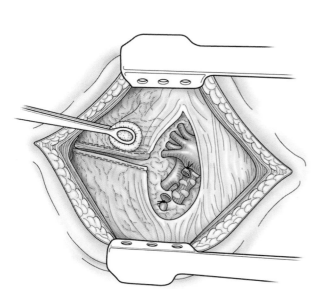

12.14

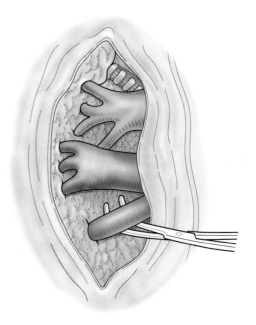

12.15

a stapler may be applied to close the middle lobe bronchus.

Following division of the bronchus, the middle lobe arterial branch is easily seen and is ligated and divided (see **Figure 12.17**). Once the bronchus, artery, and vein are divided, the minor fissure and the portion of the oblique fissure in contact with the middle lobe are divided with several firings of the linear stapler, and the lobe is removed. A mediastinal lymph node dissection is then completed in order to obtain the most accurate and complete staging information.

Lower lobectomy

Due to the close proximity of the bronchovascular structures of the middle lobe, resection of the right lower lobe provides several unique challenges and is one of the more difficult lobectomies. Similar to middle lobectomy, the pulmonary artery must be identified within the fissure in order to complete the resection and in those cases where the fissure is poorly developed a direct attack through the parenchyma often proves to be quite unsatisfying often resulting in bleeding and air leaks. The chest is entered through either a standard posterolateral thoracotomy incision (5th intercostal space) or a vertical axillary muscle sparing incision (4th space). If disease is noted within the fissure or if the hilum is involved, it is safest, in my opinion, to obtain control of the proximal right main pulmonary artery. The hilar pleura is incised anteriorly and superiorly with the lung retracted posteriorly and the proximal pulmonary artery is encircled just lateral to the superior vena cava.

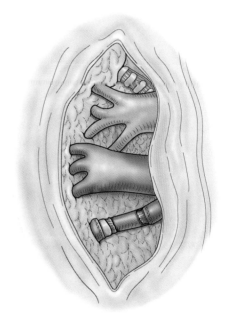

12.17

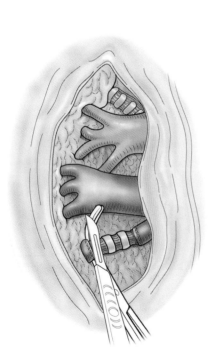

12.16

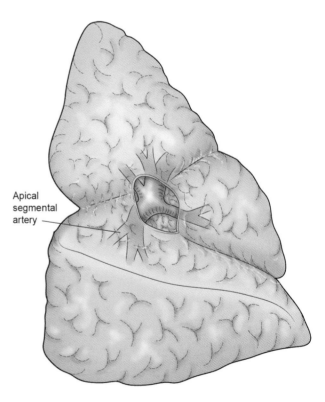

Apical segmental artery

12.18

If the fissure is reasonably well developed, the pleura overlying the pulmonary artery is incised and the dissection is carried down onto the plane of the artery (see **Figure 12.18**). The branch to the superior segment of the lower lobe is first identified and the middle lobe arterial branch is most commonly found arising from the opposite aspect of the artery, just across from the superior segmental origin. With the lung retracted anteriorly, the pleura overlying the bifurcation formed by the upper lobe bronchus and bronchus intermedius is incised, and a linear stapler encompassing the parenchyma within the fissure may be inserted from just above the superior segmental arterial branch through the area of the bifurcation. This move is possible since there are no vascular structures present posterior to the origin of the superior segmental arterial branch. On the superior aspect of the artery, just opposite the superior segment, the posterior segmental branch—the so-called recurrent branch (posterior segmental)—to the upper lobe arises and is easily visualized. The posterior aspect of the major fissure is then divided and completed.

The relationship of the superior segmental branch to the middle lobe arterial branch determines whether the lower lobe artery may be divided as a complete trunk or whether the superior segmental branch and basal arterial trunk need to be taken separately (see **Figure 12.19**). As illustrated in **Figure 12.19** the superior segmental branch must be taken separately to avoid damage to the middle lobe arterial supply. The dotted line (see inset, **Figure 12.19**) indicates the position for division of the basal segmental trunk. This is usually a 1–2 cm trunk and should be double ligated with a suture ligature or divided with a linear vascular stapler. The simplest stapling maneuver uses the endoscopic linear stapler with a vascular cartridge for closure and division. The stapler may be placed obliquely to include the superior segment branch

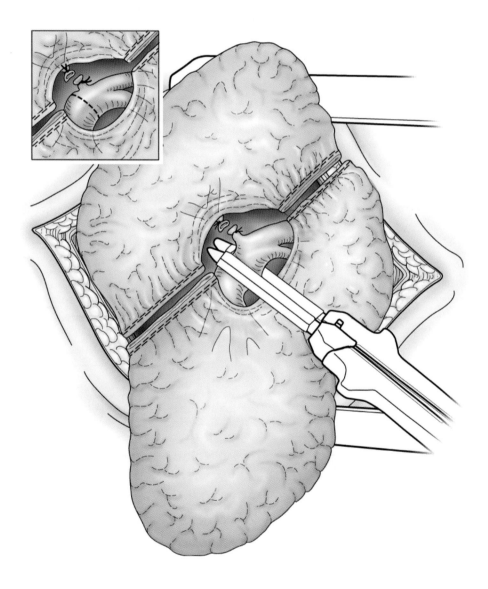

12.19

while avoiding the middle lobe artery.

Dividing the pulmonary artery reveals the bronchus that lies just deep (medial) to the artery. With the artery retracted superiorly, the origin of the middle lobe bronchus may be visualized and the location for division of the lower lobe bronchus established (see **Figure 12.20**). The middle lobe artery lies superficial and superior to the middle lobe bronchus. Care must be taken to avoid compromising the origin of the middle lobe bronchus when stapling or dividing the lower lobe bronchus (see inset, **Figure 12.20**). The bronchus may be either closed with a stapler or divided with a scalpel then closed with interrupted absorbable sutures.

With the lung retracted toward the apex of the chest, the inferior pulmonary ligament is divided up to the level of the inferior pulmonary vein (see **Figure 12.21**). An inferior pulmonary ligament lymph node (level 9) should be excised for staging purposes. The inferior pulmonary vein is dissected, encircled, and divided with a vascular stapler (see inset, **Figure 12.21**). Alternatively, the vein may be clamped, divided, and sutured with a running monofilament thread, or doubly ligated prior to division. At minimum, a tie and a suture ligature are placed to secure the vein. The anterior aspect of the major fissure is now easily completed with a firing of the linear stapler that allows the lobe to be removed.

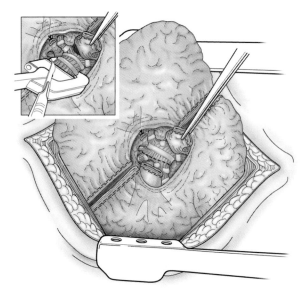

12.20

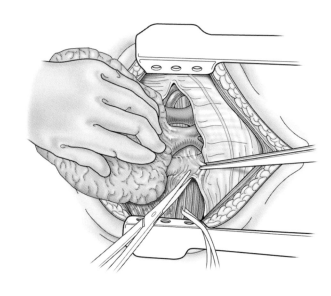

12.21

Middle and lower lobectomy (bilobectomy)

Occasionally, the location of a lesion will mandate removal of the middle and lower lobes, a procedure that can be accomplished *en bloc* because of the common origin of these lobes from the bronchus intermedius. A tumor originating in the bronchus intermedius usually requires removal of both lobes but a lower lobe lesion that involves the external aspect of the lobar bronchus may also mandate taking the middle lobe. Where an indication exists for bilobectomy, the vascular supply for each lobe is isolated and divided as described for each individual lobectomy. Once the pulmonary arterial branches have been divided, the point of division of the bronchus becomes obvious; the bronchus should be divided above the origin of the middle lobe bronchus, just distal to the origin of the upper lobe bronchus (see **Figure 12.22**). Morbidity and mortality for bilobectomy exceed those for lobectomy alone, so this resection should not be performed solely for ease or convenience. The middle lobe should never just be assumed to be expendable. The bronchial stump placed so close to the upper lobe bronchus may be at somewhat increased risk for breakdown compared with other bronchial closures. Indeed, a postoperative air leak may be prolonged following bilobectomy, especially if the remaining right upper lobe is not large enough to fill the entire space. The residual space, which precludes complete visceral and parietal pleural apposition, facilitates the air leak.

POSTOPERATIVE CARE

Lung resection not only changes ventilation but also changes the circulatory condition of the patient because of a decrease of the pulmonary vascular bed. Two major issues exist during the postoperative care of patients with a pulmonary resection. First, the patient is adapting to the change of ventilation and circulation. The second issue is prevention of postoperative complications. The management of bronchial toilet and limiting fluids to avoid overload are important for a good recovery.

Early rehabilitation

On the first postoperative day, the patient should sit on a chair beside the bed and take a meal. The patient should also walk around the ward with or without oxygen, depending on his or her condition.

Bronchial toilet

Oxygen and inhalation drugs used during the operation increase the secretion of sputum after surgery. Expectoration of sputum is the best method to clean the bronchial tree. However, some patients have difficulty in expectorating sputum, which may lead to pulmonary consolidation and, at times, pneumonitis. There should be no hesitation in performing a therapeutic bronchoscopy if the chest radiograph demonstrates lobar consolidation.

REFERENCE

1. Graham EA, Singer JJ. Successful removal of an entire lung for carcinoma of the bronchus. *JAMA*. 1933; 101: 1371–4.

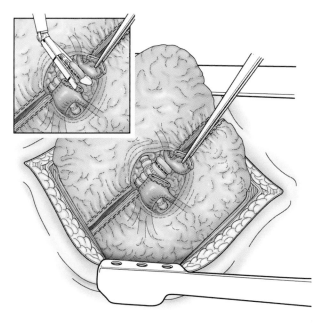

12.22

13

Left-sided pulmonary resections

REZA MEHRAN AND JEAN DESLAURIERS

PRINCIPLES AND JUSTIFICATION

The most common indication for left-sided pulmonary resection is lung cancer. Surgery may also be indicated for the management of less common malignancies affecting the lung or for benign diseases such as bronchiectasis.

The objective of any type of resection done for lung cancer is the complete removal of both the tumor and the draining lymph nodes. Indeed, the main difference between resecting lung for carcinoma and resecting lung for benign diseases is the need in cancer procedures to include draining nodes and sometimes adjacent tissues such as the chest wall, which may be directly invaded by the neoplasm. For lung cancer, limited resections such as wedge resections, or "segmentectomies," are therefore only used under special circumstances. Incomplete or "debulking" procedures also play no role in the management of lung cancer.

For most patients with early stage lung cancer, lobectomy is the procedure of choice. If the tumor cannot be completely resected by lobectomy, pneumonectomy must be considered if the patient's pulmonary reserve allows it. Left-sided sleeve resections are done infrequently not only because no bronchus intermedius exists on that side but also because left pneumonectomy is better tolerated than right pneumonectomy. Pulmonary arterioplasties have also become standard procedures in some centers. When the tumor involves—either directly or through adjacent nodes—the hilum of the lung, the pulmonary vascular pedicle, or the aortopulmonary window, mobilization and ligation of blood vessels may have to be done from within the pericardium.

PREOPERATIVE ASSESSMENT AND PREPARATION

Evaluation of physiological status

The evaluation of patients prior to left-sided pulmonary resection is somewhat different depending on whether the indication for surgery is lung cancer or a benign process. Regardless of the underlying pathology, proper evaluation of cardiopulmonary function and of other risk factors for morbidity must be carried out. All of these patients should have a thorough history taken and a physical examination. Of particular interest to the surgeon are smoking history, possible occupational exposure, grade of dyspnea, weight loss, and associated comorbidities.

The evaluation of pulmonary function should be complemented by spirometric studies and analysis of arterial blood gases. If the patient has clinical or physiological evidence of impaired pulmonary function (forced expiratory volume in 1 second [FEV1] <2.0 L/s), additional information must be obtained, especially when a strong possibility of pneumonectomy exists. This information is best obtained through exercise testing with measurements of oxygen (O_2) saturation, arterial blood gases, and maximal oxygen consumption (VO_2 max). A VO_2 max lower than 15 mL/kg/min is a warning that postoperative pulmonary complications are likely to occur. Prediction of postoperative pulmonary function through the use of isotope perfusion lung scanning also can be useful. Very often, however, numbers only tell part of the story and experience and clinical judgment are just as important when deciding if a given individual has enough pulmonary reserve to withstand lung resection. Adjustment of bronchodilators, cessation of smoking, and a short period of rehabilitation will often improve the patient's endurance and reduce the likelihood of complications. Oral corticosteroids should be avoided as much as possible and replaced with inhaled steroids if necessary.

In addition, time and effort also must be spent to evaluate the cardiac function if the patient has a history of coronary heart disease or an abnormal electrocardiogram. For most, an exercise test is all that will be required. If the test is positive, either clinically or electrocardiographically, a thallium isotope scan should be done, and we recommend that all these patients are seen preoperatively by a cardiologist. One area that is frequently overlooked is the carotid arterial system, and in cases of possible compromised circulation, complementary investigation must be done. Similarly, all other comorbidities, such as diabetes mellitus, should be looked at carefully and their treatment optimized prior to operation.

In several cases, the planning of the actual surgery is done at the time of the bronchoscopic examination. Indeed, no patient should undergo any kind of pulmonary resection without prior bronchoscopy. Whether the examination should be done by the surgeon or by an experienced "medical" bronchoscopist remains controversial and may vary from center to center.

Resectability of the tumor

In addition to deciding whether the patient needs surgery and if he or she can withstand pulmonary resection, determination of whether the tumor is technically resectable is necessary. Anatomically, the extent of disease and therefore the type of resection likely to be required are best determined through the interpretation of computed tomography (CT) images and bronchoscopy findings.

1. With specificity in the range of 70%–80%, CT scan can accurately predict the need for chest wall resection. CT scanning is also useful to assess the status of mediastinal nodes. Obviously, bronchoscopic examination is of paramount importance to determine the feasibility of standard lobectomy, sleeve resection, and pneumonectomy. (See **Figure 13.1a**.)

   Due to an overall CT diagnostic accuracy of less than 80% to assess lymph node status, many surgeons almost routinely perform a cervical mediastinoscopy

before resecting a lung cancer. This examination allows for palpation, inspection, and biopsy of mediastinal nodes and is more sensitive and specific than either CT or magnetic resonance imaging to detect metastatic nodes. This is especially important for left-sided lesions, since the level 2 and level 4 nodal stations may be more easily sampled at mediastinoscopy than at thoracotomy because of the position of the aortic arch. When planning to operate on the left side, one must also take into account the predilection for left lower lobe lesions to spread to contralateral lymph nodes that can only be sampled via mediastinoscopy.

Endobronchial ultrasound can also be used to stage the mediastinum. The procedure is less invasive than mediastinoscopy and can reach lymph node stations unreachable by mediastinoscopy, such as the hilar nodes. The procedure, however, still requires general anesthesia and takes longer to perform than a mediastinoscopy. (See **Figure 13.1b**.)

Accurate pretreatment staging of the mediastinum has now become an important priority because most patients with clinical N1 or N2 disease should undergo induction systemic therapy. On the left side, upper lobe tumors can metastasize to the aortopulmonary or anterior mediastinal nodes in up to one-third of cases. Since these nodes are not accessible by cervical mediastinoscopy, an anterior second space exploration (Chamberlain procedure) or an extended cervical mediastinoscopy is often added to standard mediastinoscopy.

Positron emission tomography (PET) scanning is very useful to detect abnormal adenopathy and is used for the staging of almost all patients with lung cancer in North America.

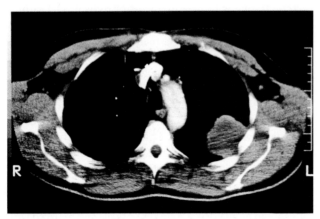

13.1a

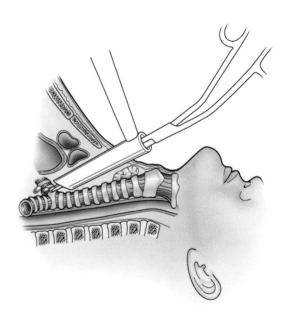

13.1b

The drawback of PET in detecting metastatic mediastinal adenopathy is the false-positive rate, which can be as high as 20% if the patient lives in a geographical area endemic for granulomatous disease. All patients with detectable "hot" mediastinal lymph nodes should therefore undergo surgical staging to confirm the nature of these nodes.

Another issue that must be considered is the need for a tissue diagnosis. Many surgeons feel that if CT scan and bronchoscopy demonstrate a potentially resectable tumor in a fit patient, preoperative biopsy is not indicated because the results of the biopsy are unlikely to alter the decision to operate. In contrast, those who are advocates of preoperative biopsy (often done by fine needle aspiration) point out that having a diagnosis before operation can help streamline the investigation as well as avoid reliance on frozen section analysis at the time of surgery. Indeed, transthoracic needle biopsy (TTNB) can be done with very low morbidity, and in most series, it has a very high diagnostic accuracy (90%–95%). The concern that TTNB may spread tumor cells and adversely affect outcome is not substantiated.

Preparation for surgery

One of the most important steps in the preparation for surgery is the need to have a clear discussion with the patient and the relatives not only of what will happen during or after the operation but also of the risks involved, most common complications, and chances of prolonged survival. Ideally, patients should discontinue cigarette smoking, but this goal is difficult to achieve because of time constraints and the possible increase in patient stress regarding the upcoming operation.

As previously alluded to, a 6-week period of rehabilitation with supervised exercise has been shown to decrease morbidity in high-risk (borderline pulmonary reserve) patients undergoing lung resection for carcinoma. During that time, medication and nutrition are optimized, and the patient's endurance is improved, as evidenced by increased distances during the 6-minute walking test. Unfortunately, most centers do not follow this approach because they do not have the infrastructure to implement and supervise such programs.

The surgeon's preparation is also important, and he or she must be able to perform bronchoplasties instead of pneumonectomies in selected cases. The surgeon must also be able to deal with invasive tumors that may require intrapericardial ligation of blood vessels or concomitant chest wall resection for their complete removal.

PAIN MANAGEMENT, ANESTHESIA, AND THE CONCEPT OF ENHANCED RECOVERY AFTER THORACIC SURGERY

All patients are seen preoperatively by an anesthesiologist and are admitted on the day of surgery. Since it is common practice to use epidural analgesia during the postoperative period, the catheter is inserted before operation (awake patient) so that continuous analgesia can be delivered throughout the operation. All patients have an arterial line (radial artery) for monitoring, a central venous line that can be used for massive fluid infusion, and a Foley catheter. All procedures require a general inhalation anesthetic, most often given through the use of a disposable double-lumen tube. These tubes come in right-sided and left-sided models, and their position is verified with a pediatric flexible bronchoscope. If any problems occur during the operation, the tube can easily be repositioned with the bronchoscope. Single lung ventilation also can be achieved with the use of a Fogarty catheter used as a bronchial blocker advanced and inflated in the mainstem bronchus of the operated side. Our policy is to give the first dose of antibiotics and 5000 units of heparin (subcutaneously) prior to incising the skin.

The practice of analgesia for thoracic surgery described has not changed over the last three decades and is still used in most centers in North America. With regard to optimal pain management, the epidural catheter has many drawbacks and its efficacy is very dependent on a number of factors, such as the anatomy of the patient and the skill of the anesthesiologist. It takes time to put one in and the insertion of an epidural indwelling catheter can easily use 1 hour of precious operative time. The epidural is kept in place traditionally for at least 3 days. During this time, patients need a Foley catheter, which increases the risk for urinary tract infection. Urinary tract infections are now considered a preventable outcome by Medicare in the United States and fall into the same category as pressure ulcers. Finally, once an epidural catheter is in place, the use of other narcotics, parenterally or orally, by the surgical team is contraindicated, and all titrations are managed by the anesthesia pain team.

To most efficiently manage the patient and improve her or his overall outcome, care maps and clinical pathways are now available that not only address issues of deep vein thrombosis (DVT) prophylaxis and early ambulation but also streamline the management of common complications after surgery. These changes form the principles of a new concept called "enhanced recovery after thoracic surgery," or "ERATS." The treatment of frequent complications is automated by having established order sets for atrial fibrillation, myocardial infarction, and pneumonia that can be immediately initiated by the nursing staff. Care maps have also started to address the management of pain and new concepts have emerged replacing the use of epidural analgesia with better multilevel pain management that is entirely controlled by the surgeon and provides outcomes that are better in many respects than the standard of care centered on epidural analgesia.

ERATS starts by addressing pain issues before the actual surgery. Patients are taught about pain and what to expect from the treating team; the objective is to appease their anxiety associated with pain issues. The visual analog scale and the use of patient-controlled analgesia (PCA) are reviewed. Patients learn that they may be discharged home with a chest tube if the air leak lasts more than 2 days. The day before the surgery, patients are started on gabapentinoids, which are known to decrease the narcotic requirements after surgery. Arterial lines are replaced with noninvasive monitoring connected to LiDCO devices, which measure constantly the cardiac output and the volume status of the patients. This allows the anesthesiologist to titrate the fluid infusions to exactly what the patient needs.

At the time of surgery, intercostal spaces are injected with very long acting local anesthetics such as preparations of liposomal bupivacaine (Exparel). The thoracotomy is preferably performed via a muscle-sparing non-rib-cutting method (see next section). On closure, additional local anesthesia is injected by the surgeon around the costotransverse joints under direct vision. The chest tube site is also infiltrated. At the end of the operative procedure, the anesthesiologist administers anti-inflammatory drugs, such as Ketorolac supplemented by intravenous acetaminophen. Postoperatively, all patients are continued on oral anti-inflammatory drugs, Tylenol, and oral synthetic narcotics such as Tramadol, around the clock. Patients are also put on PCA. Chest tubes are removed when there is no drainage of air, blood, or chyle (i.e., no A, B, or C). The volume of drainage is not a factor in removing the chest tube anymore. ERATS maneuvers not only allow a more effective usage of operating room time but also permit the optimization of the postoperative time in the hospital. With ERATS, patients with simple thoracotomies can often be discharged within 48 hours of the surgical procedure. Epidural regional analgesia is still useful under special circumstances, such as complex thoracotomies with chest wall resection, pleurectomy, decortication, or bilateral procedures.

OPERATION

Position, incision, and exploration

2. The posterolateral incision is used by most surgeons because it provides considerable exposure to the entire pleural space. This incision is versatile and allows the surgeon the possibility of modifying the operative strategy, if required. The patient is in the lateral decubitus position with the arm extended anteriorly and superiorly, gliding the scapula away from the fifth intercostal space. The head of the patient is supported, and a roll is inserted in the axilla to spread the intercostal spaces at the site of the incision. The table is maximally flexed at the lumbar area to push the pelvis away from the incision and spread the ribs even further. The legs are supported with pillows, and the patient is immobilized on a bean bag. (See **Figure 13.2a**.)

A posterolateral thoracotomy, which follows initially the posterior and inferior edges of the scapula, is then performed. The incision is carried down to the latissimus dorsi, which is incised with the cautery. The serratus anterior is preserved because it is a functional cough muscle as well as a potential source for a transposition flap in the future. The muscle is retracted anteriorly. The ribs and intercostal spaces are counted, and for most cases, the pleural space is entered in the fifth intercostal space. We almost never remove a rib and neither do we divide the posterior sixth rib to increase mobility, as advocated by some surgeons. (See **Figure 13.2b**.)

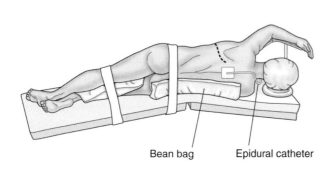

Bean bag   Epidural catheter

13.2a

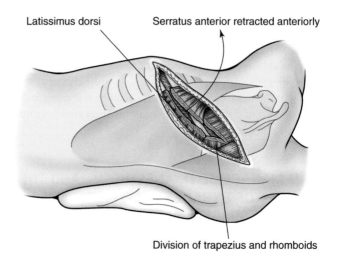

Latissimus dorsi   Serratus anterior retracted anteriorly

Division of trapezius and rhomboids

13.2b

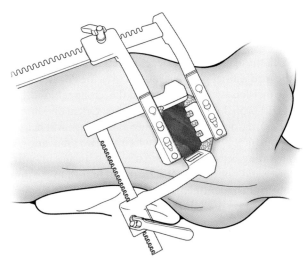

13.2c

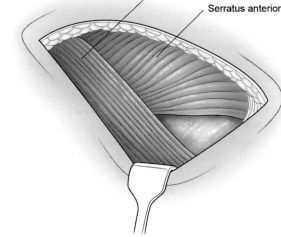

Latissimus dorsi

Serratus anterior

13.2d

In the technique of muscle-sparing thoracotomy, no muscle is divided. The latissimus dorsi muscle is reflected anteriorly after it is elevated from the overlying skin and subcutaneous tissue. The incision is centered over the tip of the scapula. The fifth intercostal space is entered. One retractor distracts the ribs, the other keeps the muscles out of the field of view. (See **Figure 13.2c and d.**)

The first stages of the operation involve the freeing of the lung, if there are any adhesions, and a thorough exploration of the lung itself, as well as all surfaces of the pleura, and mediastinum. Any suspicious lesion should be sampled, and in lung cancer operations, routine sampling of nodes located in predetermined areas should be carried out. On the left side, sampling of hilar lymph nodes (level 10), aortopulmonary nodes (level 5), and subcarinal nodes (level 7) should be done prior to deciding which procedure should be carried out. Careful inspection and palpation of the tumor itself also can help in deciding the extent of resection that will be needed.

Sometimes, the resectability of large central tumors can only be determined by opening the pericardium and palpating the pulmonary artery (PA) and veins from inside the pericardium. In some cases, the decision to undertake resection requires considerable experience and judgment because once one is committed to resection, it may not be possible to abort the procedure.

General techniques of dissection and division of lung structures

Although the PA and/or its branches are usually taken first, followed by the pulmonary veins and bronchus, anatomical and pathological considerations can bring about variations in the order of mobilization and division of lung structures. Some surgeons believe that the pulmonary veins must be ligated first to avoid potential spillage of tumor cells, but this

concept has never been validated. One possible disadvantage of dividing the pulmonary vein first is that it may bring some degree of hypertension not only in the pulmonary arterial system but also in the bronchial arteries, which, in turn, may increase blood loss throughout the operation. Depending on the type of lesion being dealt with and its location, the operator must be able to conceive and execute the most appropriate strategy. Often in difficult cases, for instance, it is easier to divide the bronchus first then ligate and divide the vascular pedicle.

3. The main elements of the left lung pedicle are located underneath the mediastinal pleura, which must be opened to reach them. Within the interlobar fissure, each branch of the PA can be found after opening the deep recess of the visceral pleura. The mobilization of the main PA or of any of its branches involves the opening of the adventitia of the blood vessel, dissection of its lateral borders, and use of a Lahey clamp to complete the mobilization posteriorly. The main PA is usually controlled with a vascular stapler, while the individual branches are doubly ligated with 2-0 silk ties and divided against a clamp applied as far back as possible within the parenchyma. When one is using ligatures, it is important to leave a long enough stump so as to prevent "dislocation" of the ties when the vessel is cut. In cases where dissection appears to be hazardous, it is always wise to get proximal control of the left main PA. In cases of pneumonectomy, one may have to enter the pericardium to get such control. Pulmonary veins are handled in the same general way as the PA.

If an arterial injury should occur, it is important to digitally control the site of the tear and apply a vascular clamp more proximally. We have seen many cases where a small tear became a large one because clamps were put blindly, hurriedly, and with great panic. Once the hemorrhage is controlled, the operative field must be properly exposed so that the vascular wound can be adequately and safely repaired. Currently, most surgeons use a stapling device to close the bronchus. These have been shown to be safe and, indeed, are very convenient for inexperienced surgeons. Sound surgical principles to avoid bronchial dehiscence include careful dissection with attention to trying to preserve the bronchial vascular supply, and parallel stapling or simple interrupted suture closure using resorbable sutures and covering of the suture line with autologous tissue in cases where the bronchus appears to be at risk of dehiscence. (See **Figure 13.3a through d**.)

Lobectomy

UPPER LOBECTOMY

4. With the apex of the lung gently retracted inferiorly, the mediastinal pleura is incised over the PA, and the incision is extended around the left upper lobe (LUL) bronchus and into the fissure. Often, dividing the posterior part of the fissure at this stage will help by opening up the space between the two lobes and providing better exposure to arterial branches to both lower and upper lobes. Each arterial branch to the upper lobe is then identified, ligated, and divided. We prefer to

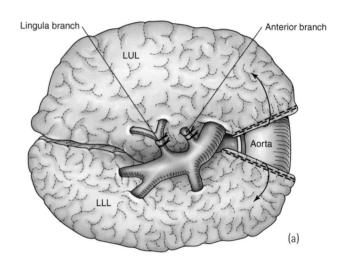

(a)

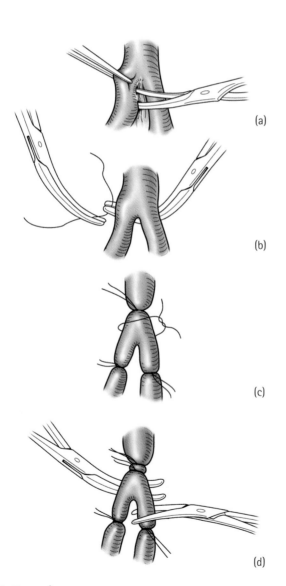

(a)

(b)

(c)

(d)

13.3a–d

13.4a

ligate and divide the most distal branch (lingula) first and then move proximally, because in this fashion it is easier to gain access to the apical dorsal branch (most proximal branch). This branch should be handled with great caution because it has a very short length, and it is often surrounded by nodes. If it cannot be safely mobilized, it is advisable to loop and clamp the main PA before accidental lacerations occur. The lung is then retracted posteriorly, and the superior pulmonary vein is isolated, stapled, and divided. While doing so, it is important to make sure that the inferior vein is not included in the suture line because, on occasion, both veins will have a common origin from a single trunk. Obviously, the division of both veins while doing an upper lobectomy will lead to catastrophic consequences. (See **Figure 13.4a through c.**)

An umbilical tape is then placed around the LUL bronchus to allow for traction, and a stapling device is used to secure the bronchus at its origin. The inferior pulmonary ligament is then released to allow the lower lobe to move up and fill the space previously occupied by the upper lobe. (See **Figure 13.4d and e.**)

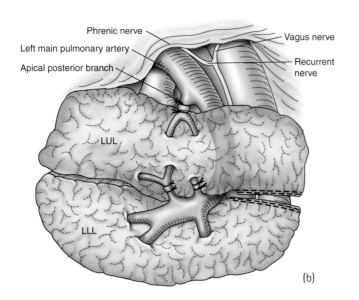

(b)

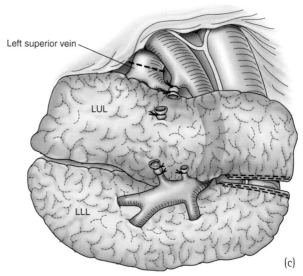

(c)

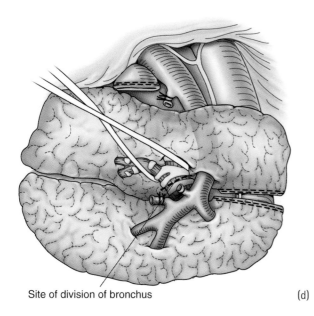

Site of division of bronchus   (d)

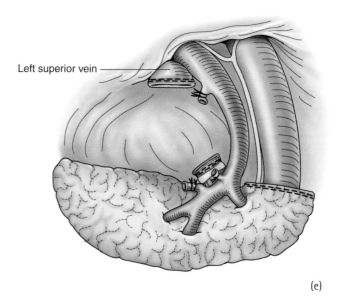

(e)

13.4b–e

When performing an LUL sleeve resection, the arteries and superior pulmonary vein are ligated and divided as they are in a standard left upper lobectomy. The PA is then mobilized and retracted away from the upper lobe bronchus. A sleeve resection of the main bronchus is accomplished by dividing it on each side of the takeoff of the upper lobe bronchus. A circumferential anastomosis is then carried out between the proximal mainstem bronchus and lower lobe bronchus using interrupted 3-0 polyglycolic sutures. If necessary, the repair can be buttressed through the use of parietal pleura or intercostal muscle. (See **Figure 13.4f through i.**)

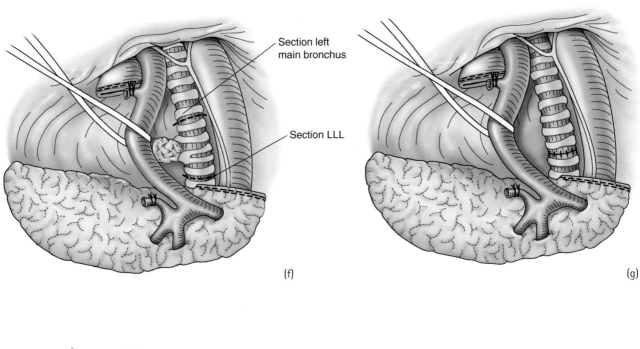

Section left
main bronchus

Section LLL

(f)

(g)

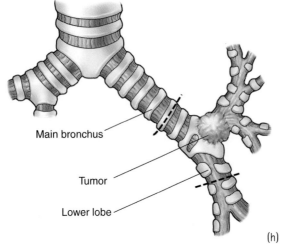

Main bronchus

Tumor

Lower lobe

(h)

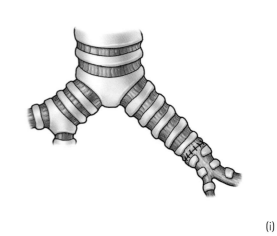

(i)

13.4f–i

LOWER LOBECTOMY

5. The procedure is similar to that of left upper lobectomy. The interlobar fissure is first exposed, with the assistant retracting the upper lobe superiorly and anteriorly. The visceral pleura is then opened, and both branches of the PA going to the lower lobe (basal and apical) are identified, dissected, and ligated. Before ligating the basal artery, it is important to clearly identify the arterial branch of the PA going to the lingula so that it can be preserved. (See **Figure 13.5a.**)

The inferior pulmonary ligament is then mobilized and the inferior pulmonary vein identified and stapled. At this stage, both anterior and posterior portions of the fissure are divided, and the lower lobe bronchus is freed right up to the origin of the upper lobe where it is stapled and divided. For proximal endobronchial lesions of the lower lobe, a sleeve resection can be done by reattaching the upper lobe to the mainstem bronchus. However, this type of bronchoplasty is seldom done. (See **Figure 13.5b through e.**)

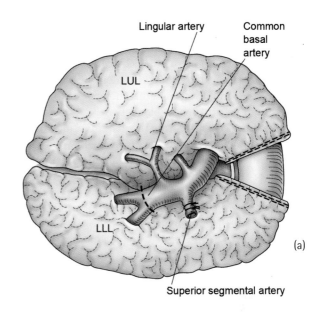

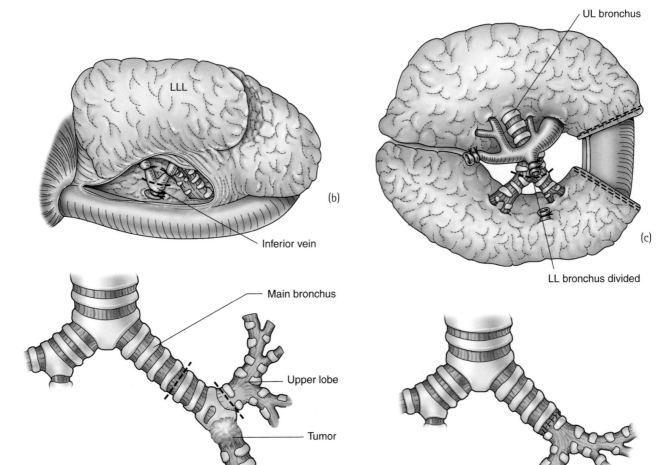

13.5a–e

LEFT LOBECTOMY WITH CHEST WALL RESECTION

Occasionally, lung cancer locally invades the chest wall, which must then be resected *en bloc* with the involved lobe. If this type of resection has been anticipated through the review of the CT scan or because the patient presents with chest pain, the pleural space is entered one or two intercostal spaces below the area where the tumor is invading the ribs. The chest wall dissection and resection is then done prior to exposure of the hilum or suturing of blood vessels. Ribs should be divided at least 2 cm away from the margins of the tumor. It is also recommended to remove one rib below and one rib above the site of involvement. This technique is facilitated by lifting the scapula away from the ribs. When the chest wall is completely freed, it falls down into the pleural space along with the rest of the lung, and the lobectomy can be carried out. The chest wall is only repaired when the scapula does not cover the defect, and in such cases, a prosthetic mesh is used.

Intraoperative maneuvers useful to decrease complications after lobectomy

One of the most common complications of lobectomies is a persistent air leak (>5 days) with or without residual space. This problem is commonly due to incomplete lung reexpansion; and, indeed, air leaks tend to be minimal when the lung is completely reexpanded because the parenchyma is in contact with the parietal pleural where it creates an inflammatory reaction that tends to seal the air leak.

When full reexpansion appears possible, prolonged air leaks can be prevented by careful suturing of parenchymal tears or by the use of staples, reinforced staples, or biological glues over suture lines and fissures. When full reexpansion does not appear possible—for example, after combined left lower lobectomy and lingulectomy—one can reduce the "boundaries" of the pleural space through the use of a pleural tent (after upper lobectomy) or pneumoperitoneum (after left lower lobectomy). This latter technique has never been popular but can at times be very useful. A small catheter is inserted intraoperatively through the diaphragm into the peritoneal cavity. This catheter is brought out through a separate skin incision adjacent to the chest tube, and it is attached to a three-way stopcock. If a residual space is present despite proper pleural space drainage, air can be injected into the peritoneal cavity to elevate the hemidiaphragm and help collapse the pleural space.

Pneumonectomy

STANDARD PNEUMONECTOMY

6. With the lung retracted posteriorly and inferiorly, the mediastinal pleura is opened and the left main PA identified. During this dissection, care must be taken not to injure the phrenic or the vagus nerves. If necessary, the ligamentum arteriosum can be divided to increase the length of the main artery available for dissection and division. To get around this artery, one can use a Lahey clamp or finger dissection. Once freed, the artery is stapled proximally, clamped distally, and divided (see **Figure 13.6a**).

   The superior pulmonary vein is then identified in the anterior hilum when it is stapled and divided. Sometimes, it is easier to divide the superior vein first to gain access to the main PA. The inferior vein is then located at the base of the hilum after division of the inferior pulmonary ligament and it is mobilized, stapled, and divided. An umbilical tape is then passed around the left main bronchus, which is freed posteriorly and anteriorly up to the carina, where the stapler is applied and the bronchus divided. During this dissection, great care must be taken not to injure the esophagus, which is located immediately posterior to the bronchus. Sometimes, we ask the anesthetist to withdraw the double-lumen tube in the trachea to increase the mobility of the carina. We seldom recover the left main bronchus because its stump retracts underneath the aortic arch, which acts as autologous tissue. This situation is different than on the right side, where the pneumonectomy stump is free in the pleural space (see **Figure 13.6b through** f).

On occasion, it may be advantageous to divide the bronchus before ligating the pulmonary blood vessels (bronchus-first technique). If this technique is done, one has to be careful in freeing the bronchus which is very close to the superior vein (anteriorly), the PA (superior border), and the lower vein (lower border). Dividing the bronchus first is particularly helpful to gain access to the superior vein and main PA in cases of completion pneumonectomies.

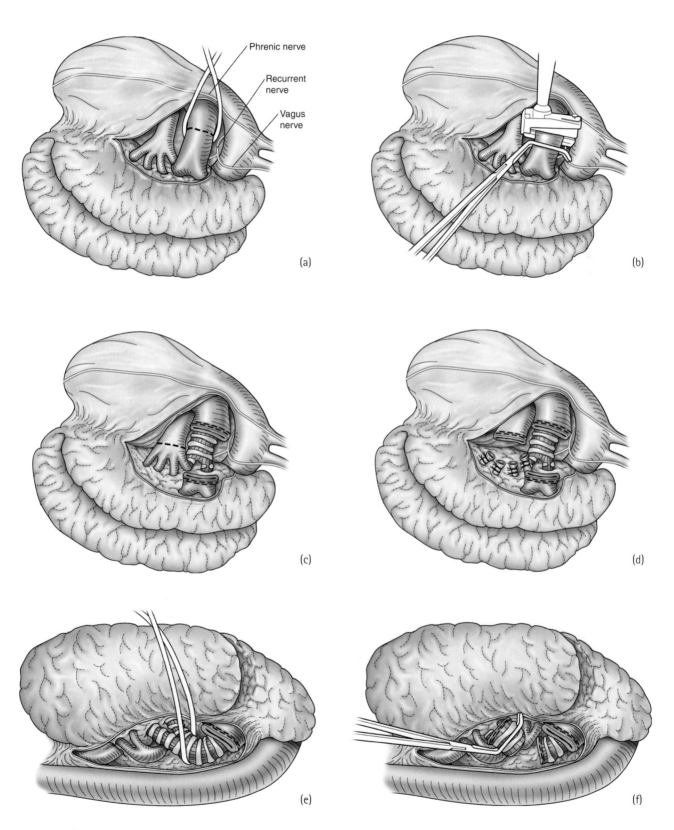

Phrenic nerve

Recurrent nerve

Vagus nerve

(a)

(b)

(c)

(d)

(e)

(f)

13.6a–f

INTRAPERICARDIAL PNEUMONECTOMY

7. The opening of the pericardium greatly facilitates access to the main pulmonary blood vessels, especially when the tumor is centrally located and/or is very large. The pericardium is usually opened anterior to the phrenic nerve, and the incision is carried upward to the aorta. The PA is mobilized first and, to improve access, the pericardial incision is carried right up to its reflection over the PA. This maneuver will lead the operator directly to the adventitia of the artery, which can be opened, and the PA is fully mobilized and stapled. Once the artery has been secured, the access to the pulmonary veins becomes much easier. (See **Figure 13.7**.)

In cases of intrapericardial pneumonectomy, we try to divide only one of the two pulmonary veins within the pericardium in the hope of preventing postpneumonectomy cardiac herniation (the vein that is divided extrapericardially will anchor the heart and prevent its herniation). Once the lung has been removed, it is also important to close the pericardium to prevent herniation of the heart, which is fatal in the majority of cases. This goal is accomplished with interrupted nonabsorbable sutures. A PTFE patch can be used to close defects that cannot be closed primarily.

Segmental resections of the left lung

The most commonly resected segments of the left lung are the lingula and apical segment of the lower lobe. Indications for this type of operation include lung cancer in compromised individuals and bronchiectasis or tuberculosis limited to one segment.

The principles of pulmonary segment resection are similar to those of lobectomy, although the surgery is done in two rather than three phases. The first step is the identification of the artery and bronchus (bronchovascular pedicle), while the second step consists of retrograde dissection starting at the hilum and following the plane of the intersegmental vein, which must stay with the remaining lung. Most surgeons now use staplers to divide the intersegmental plane rather than the more classic finger dissection while the anesthetist inflates the lung.

8. The lingula consists of two segments (superior and inferior), which are usually resected together. In principle, lingulectomy is an easy operation. The interlobar fissure is opened, and the arterial branch to the lingula (the most distal branch) is first identified and ligated. The bronchus is then identified and stapled, and the segment is removed. The venous drainage is through a common trunk, which is the lower part of the superior vein. This trunk is easily mobilized and divided (see **Figure 13.8a**).

    The surgical pedicle to the apical segment is also made up of a bronchus and an arterial branch. The artery is first mobilized from the fissure then ligated and divided. The bronchus can also be reached through the fissure, divided, and closed (manually or with a stapler). For this segment, no clear venous branch can be identified, so that, on freeing the segment from the basal segments, each collateral or secondary vein is freed, clipped, and divided (see **Figure 13.8b and c**).

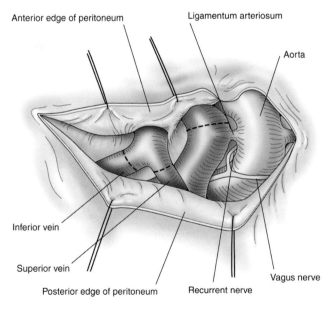

Anterior edge of peritoneum   Ligamentum arteriosum

Aorta

Inferior vein

Superior vein

Posterior edge of peritoneum   Recurrent nerve   Vagus nerve

13.7

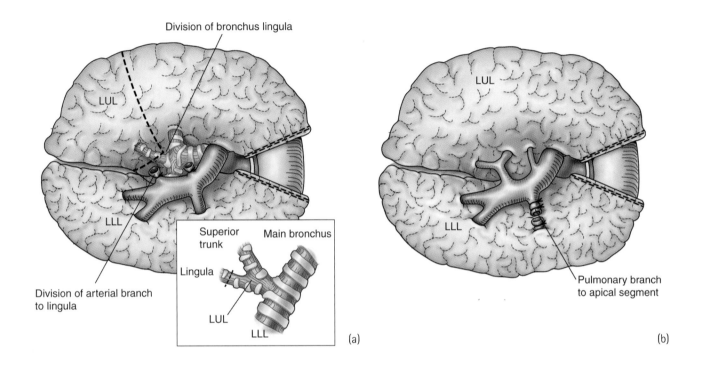

Division of bronchus lingula

LUL

LLL

Division of arterial branch
to lingula

Superior
trunk   Main bronchus

Lingula

LUL

LLL

(a)

LUL

LLL

Pulmonary branch
to apical segment

(b)

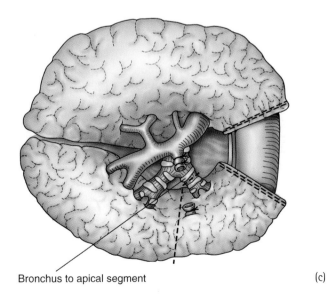

Bronchus to apical segment

(c)

13.8a–c

Video-assisted thoracoscopic surgery (VATS)

VATS is a minimally invasive procedure that allows pulmonary resection and node dissection without the need for rib spreading. Avoiding rib spreading is thought to improve the outcome of many perioperative variables, such as pain and return to work. Taking standard thoracotomy as a benchmark, it appears that this advantage holds true. VATS is technically challenging and difficult to teach.

VATS is practiced in many different ways. As long as there is no muscular or rib division, it is classified as a minimally invasive procedure. Some surgeons use a four port technique with carbon dioxide (CO_2) insufflation using typical laparoscopic instruments, while others prefer an open port technique using long modified open instruments. Some even prefer an 8 cm long minithoracotomy, the so-called access port, and use standard open instruments to dissect the lung.

As far as the steps inside the chest are concerned, they are very similar to those of the open thoracotomy technique. The vein is divided first followed by the artery and then the bronchus. Difficulty arises when the fissure is incomplete, which limits the access to the artery in the fissure. This has led to the development of the "fissureless" technique, whereby the bronchus is divided after the vein is. Then the lung in the area of the fissure is stapled simultaneously with the artery.

The extraction of the lung requires the use of a heavy and solid bag (Anchor bag). Since the principle of minimally invasive surgery is to avoid rib spreading, the maximum size of the tumor should be less than 5 cm. Morcellation is not used in thoracic surgery, as the anatomy of the tumor is important to the pathologist for the determination of the stage of the tumor.

Robotic-assisted thoracic surgery (RATS)

Recently, another technique has become available to surgeons for lobectomy, which involves the assistance of the da Vinci robot. In terms of steps and what is performed inside the chest, the procedure is the same as when done in an open fashion. The use of the robot has certain advantages, mainly in the form of increasing the dexterity of the surgeon and offering better visibility inside the chest. However, the robot also has a number of limitations, one of the major ones being that it is no better than VATS. In fact, a number of perioperative variables do worse with the use of the robot, such as the length of surgery and cost. A particular disadvantage of the robot is that the surgeon is not at the bedside of the patient. The person at bedside manipulating the nondocked instruments, such as the stapler or the suction, often are nonsurgeons, and in the event of a bleeding catastrophe, by the time the surgeon gets control of the bleeding, the patient may be a candidate for blood transfusions.

Nonetheless, many surgeons continue to use the robot and advocate its safety and advantage compared with VATS or the open technique. The port placement of RATS varies slightly with those of VATS. The issue is to avoid arm "collisions," and the ports must be placed and specially spaced so as to prevent the robotic arms interfering with each other outside the body of the patient.

The most commonly used port placement is a five-port design centered around the eighth intercostal space. Each port is spaced about 9 cm from the previous one. The first port, a 5 mm port, is positioned just outside the erector spinae muscle; the next one, 9 cm away, is a 8 mm robot port; next there is a 12 mm camera port, followed by another 8 mm robot port; finally, a 12 mm assistant port is placed around the tenth intercostal space. The rest of the procedure is performed in a similar fashion to the open thoracotomy approach.

The use of the robot requires all members of the surgical team to have a good knowledge of the procedures of docking and undocking and troubleshooting of the equipment, obtained through simulation and practice in a laboratory.

The robot seems particularly advantageous when dissecting the nodal stations, as the extra dexterity offered by the robot makes this part of the surgery easier than when done by VATS.

POSTOPERATIVE CARE

Tube drainage

After lobectomy or segmentectomy, one or two chest tubes are left in the pleural space. If two tubes are used, one is placed anteriorly and at the apex, and the second one is positioned inferiorly and posteriorly. The chest tubes are connected to an active suction system usually with −20 cm of water suction. They are removed when there is no longer an air leak and when the amount of fluid drainage is below 300 mL/24 h. For those applying the concepts of ERATS, as mentioned earlier, the chest tube is removed when there is no A, B, or C and the volume of fluid is not a factor in deciding when the chest tube needs to be removed.

Most surgeons do not drain pneumonectomy spaces because drainage through a water seal system can lead to an extreme mediastinal shift and overexpansion of the remaining lung. Instead of drainage, we recommend aspirating 1000–1200 mL of air from the space to position the mediastinum just past the midline to the left. Other options are to leave a chest tube that is either removed when the patient is turned over onto his or her back or is clamped until the following morning. Finally, a chest tube can be inserted and hooked to a "balanced drainage" system. Using balanced drainage allows a moderate shift of the mediastinum. The chest tube is removed the day after the surgical procedure.

Analgesia

The methods used to control postoperative pain have changed considerably over the years, but their purpose has remained the same. They must provide proper analgesia so that the patient can have more efficient breathing and coughing. To do so, a proper balance must be reached between too much analgesia, which will sedate the patient, and not enough, which will make the patient uncooperative.

The most commonly used technique is that of epidural analgesia, with the drugs being administered at the lumbar or thoracic level. For most patients, this method provides good pain control, although side effects such as nausea, itching, urinary retention, and even drowsiness are common. The epidural catheter is inserted prior to operation and left for 3–4 days postoperatively. When the catheter is removed, the patient is started on narcotics given subcutaneously or by mouth.

When epidural catheters are not used, the pain management follows the principles mentioned earlier. Patients are continued on gabapentinoids. Patients receive PCA, which is complemented by anti-inflammatory drugs, Tylenol, and oral narcotics. When the epidural is not used, the urinary catheter can be removed the day after surgery

DVT prophylaxis and pulmonary toilet

All patients are given heparin subcutaneously as a prophylaxis against DVT. Patients are also given antibiotics for 2–3 doses after operation. O_2 is given to titrate saturation at 92% or higher. Although bronchodilation drugs can be added, the best way to improve respiratory efficacy is through active physiotherapy and use of incentive spirometry, which are started the evening of the operation. If mucous and sputum retention do occur, we do not hesitate to perform bedside bronchoscopy or even insert a minitracheotomy for the sole purpose of suctioning. After left-sided resections, it is possible to have vocal cord paralysis because of accidental or deliberate trauma to the recurrent nerve. One must be aware that these patients are more likely to have respiratory and coughing difficulties. If this becomes a problem, the left vocal cord can be stiffened by the injection of Teflon, adipose tissue, or other material under the care of a head and neck surgeon and speech pathologist.

Although arrhythmias are a common problem after pneumonectomy (incidence of 15%–20%), it is generally not recommended to use prophylactic antiarrhythmic medication prior to surgery.

OUTCOME

Early

The accepted mortality rate for left pneumonectomy is in the range of 5%–6%, and most causes of death are respiratory. These problems include infectious complications, pulmonary embolism, and postpneumonectomy pulmonary edema. Fatal cardiovascular events are relatively uncommon. Risk factors for mortality after pneumonectomy include age of the patient; preoperative cardiopulmonary compromise; extent

of resection; and associated comorbidities, such as diabetes.

For lobectomy, whether upper, lower, or associated with sleeve resection, the operative mortality is in the neighborhood of 2.5%–3.0%. Common complications include prolonged air leaks, arrhythmias, and respiratory events. Bronchopleural fistulae (BPF) are uncommon if bronchial closure is handled with care. The incidence is less than 3% after pneumonectomy and less than 1% after lobectomy. Once the diagnosis is made, BPF can be treated in a variety of ways. BPF are seldom a cause of death, although they usually are associated with prolonged morbidity.

Late

When treating lung cancer, long-term results reflect the stage of disease rather than the extent of operation. Since pneumonectomies are done for higher stages of disease, 5-year survival results are worse than those seen after lobectomy and are in the range of 20%–25%. By comparison, 5-year survival after sleeve resections of the left lung is approximately 50%. The use of adjuvant treatments, either as induction or postoperatively, does not change those results. In most series, patients with squamous cell carcinoma do better than those with adenocarcinoma.

CONCLUSION

In general, operation on the left lung can be done quite safely if the operating surgeon follows a systematic, carefully thought-out approach for the mobilization of bronchovascular pedicles. As a whole, they are technically easier than similar procedures on the right side, and they are better tolerated. Indeed, the incidence of major morbidity or mortality is less after left pneumonectomy than after right pneumonectomy. Special attention must be given to preserve the recurrent laryngeal nerve, which is much more accessible to trauma on the left side than on the right side.

FURTHER READING

Backhus L, Puneet B, Bastawrous S, Mariam M, Michael M, Varghese T Jr. Radiographic evaluation of the patient with lung cancer: surgical implications of imaging. *Curr Probl Diagn Radiol*. 2013 May–Jun; 42(3): 84–98.

Jones NL, Edmonds L, Ghosh S, Klein AA. A review of enhanced recovery for thoracic anaesthesia and surgery. *Anaesthesia*. 2013 Feb; 68(2): 179–89.

Kokkonouzis I, Strimpakos AS, Lampaditis I, Tsimpoukis S, Syrigos KN. The role of endobronchial ultrasound in lung cancer diagnosis and staging: a comprehensive review. *Clin Lung Cancer*. 2012 Nov; 13(6): 408–15.

Stringer W, Casaburi R, Older P. Cardiopulmonary exercise testing: does it improve perioperative care and outcome? *Curr Opin Anaesthesiol*. 2012 Apr; 25(2): 178–84.

14

Extrapleural pneumonectomy

YIFAN ZHENG, WILLIAM G. RICHARDS, JULIANNE S. BARLOW, ADRIENNE CAMP, AND RAPHAEL BUENO

HISTORY

The incidence of malignant pleural mesothelioma (MPM) worldwide is expected to increase in the next two decades.[1] The paradigm for treatment of this aggressive disease has evolved to include combined multimodality therapies, which offer the prospect of improved outcomes for selected patients with clinically localized disease.[2]

The extrapleural pneumonectomy (EPP) operation consists of the *en bloc* resection of parietal pleura, lung, ipsilateral pericardium, and hemidiaphragm, and the subsequent reconstruction of the defects left from the excised pericardium and diaphragm. This operation was first described in the 1940s for an infectious empyema[3] and is now used to treat some malignancies such as MPM, as well as, on occasion, destroyed lung from chronic infections. As part of a multimodality treatment regimen, this operation is performed with curative intent in carefully selected MPM patients. A less extensive resection, known as "pleurectomy and decortication" (PDC) is preferred for patients who have earlier stage disease. PDC, extended PDC, or partial pleurectomy may be performed and is often reserved for patients who have disease confined to one hemithorax but are unable to tolerate an EPP.[4]

PRINCIPLES AND JUSTIFICATION

The initial EPPs performed in patients with MPM in the 1970s and 1980s were associated with mortality rates as high as 30%–40%.[5] As a consequence, most surgeons either preferred to perform what they thought was a less aggressive operation—pleurectomy or partial pleurectomy—usually as a palliative approach to relieve dyspnea, or, more likely, avoided surgery altogether. However, persistent focus on improving the surgical outcome at a small number of specialized institutions in the early 1990s resurrected this procedure and established new patient-selection strategies, decreased operative times, improved surgical techniques, and focused pre- and postoperative management regimens, resulting in reducing mortality to as low as 3.4%–5.2%.[6,7] This initial success has led to additional institutions progressively developing surgical programs for MPM and wider acceptance of this approach in the medical community. Though morbidity rates remain high, ranging from 38% to 59%, the range of mortality rates dropped substantially to 3% from 12% as surgeons gained more experience with the procedure and especially with managing early postoperative complications.[8–13]

PREOPERATIVE EVALUATION AND PATIENT SELECTION

Successful application of multimodality treatment approaches depends critically on patient selection. Through the collective experiences of specialty centers for this rare disease, a standardized staging system for surgical patients has been established and continues to evolve.[14] In addition, because clinical staging of MPM is challenging for a variety of reasons, a number of predictive clinical and molecular biomarkers have been established to assist with selecting appropriate MPM patients for surgery. These include histology, lymph node status (negative better than positive), hemoglobin, sex >, tumor volume, and the gene ratio prognostic molecular test.[7,15–19]

Patients with MPM often present with nonspecific symptoms such as chest pain and shortness of breath. Evaluation begins with a thorough history and physical, noting risk factors such as asbestos exposure and smoking history. Imaging evaluation includes chest computed tomography and magnetic resonance imaging (MRI) to evaluate the extent of disease invasion. MRI is particularly helpful in determining diaphragmatic or great vessel involvement. If there is extensive invasion into the chest wall, abdominal cavity, mediastinum, or contralateral hemithorax, radical resection is contraindicated. Imaging may show pleural effusion or pleural nodularity. Cytologic diagnosis may be obtained from sampling the pleural fluid but is often inconclusive. Instead, histologic diagnosis by thoracoscopic pleural biopsy is recommended to establish a definitive diagnosis, since differentiating adenocarcinoma from mesothelioma may, at times, be challenging. As the extent of invasive disease is not always apparent on imaging, thoracoscopic and laparoscopic exploration allows for direct evaluation of disease spread and is recommended to patients if there are radiologic concerns for chest wall or diaphragmatic invasion.[20] A single thoracoscopic incision should be made in the line of a future thoracotomy. Partial pleurectomy or insufflation of talc at the time of diagnosis is discouraged. Additionally, a staging cervical mediastinoscopy is performed, and if the findings are negative—that is, no metastatic disease found in the lymph nodes—the preparation continues for an EPP.

Once a pathological diagnosis is established, a diagnosis of the histological subtype must also be rendered. The epithelioid subtype of MPM is more common and is associated with better prognosis than biphasic subtypes (mixed), while the sarcomatoid subtype has the worst prognosis.[7] The decision to perform an EPP should be weighed carefully and this operation should be recommended to patients with the best chances for survival, so that the associated risks are justified. However, while diagnosis by pleural biopsy is reliable, it is not always accurate for differentiating subtypes, particularly when the final pathology is nonepithelial.[21]

As diagnosis and extent of disease are determined, the ability of the patient to tolerate pneumonectomy is evaluated. The following selection criteria are based on the experience of Brigham and Women's Hospital, which has reached an annual volume of 90 to 100 major surgical resections for MPM including approximately 30 to 50 EPPs. To be eligible for an EPP, a patient must have good performance status, usually indicated by a Karnofsky score of greater than 70. The patient must also have normal cardiac, liver, and renal function. This preoperative evaluation is critical to the patient's tolerance of the operation, as well as the ability to tolerate hyperthermic intraoperative chemotherapy should operation be offered.[22] A pulmonary function test is obtained usually in conjunction with a quantitative ventilation/perfusion scan to ensure that patients meet the minimum criteria of 1 L of predicted postoperative FEV_1 and favorable distribution of perfusion.

Each patient being considered for an EPP has a Doppler echocardiogram to evaluate for pulmonary hypertension and further evaluation is obtained as warranted by the results and age of the patient. Usually, an exercise stress test or echocardiogram is also advised. When there is a question as to operability based on findings of cardiac disease or pulmonary hypertension, catheterization and/or a pulmonary exercise test for determination of mixed venous oxygen saturation is obtained. Pulmonary hypertension is a concerning contraindication to proceeding with an EPP.

As the recommendation for an EPP is based on the performance status of the patient and the extent of disease, there is no absolute age restriction for undergoing the operation. However, the surgery is rarely recommended to patients older than 70 years of age, particularly when considering the morbidity and mortality risks. In fact, age over 70 to 75 years is an independent risk factor for mortality after EPP. One should also consider that a left-sided EPP is better tolerated than one done for right-sided disease and some criteria may be relaxed for left-sided MPM.

Preoperatively, patients are treated with a bowel preparation and undergo lower extremity ultrasonography to assess for deep venous thromboses.

OPERATION

Prior to beginning the operation, a thoracic epidural catheter is placed for optimal pain control. Central venous access is obtained, a pulmonary artery catheter is placed, an arterial line is established, and a Foley catheter is inserted into the bladder. Standard monitoring also includes telemetry and pulse oximetry. Antibiotic prophylaxis is administered and pneumatic compression boots are placed to guard against venous stasis of the lower extremities. General anesthesia is then induced and the patient is intubated with a single lumen endotracheal tube and fiber-optic bronchoscopy is performed to examine the airway. If no abnormalities are found, the single lumen endotracheal tube is replaced with a double lumen endotracheal tube or a selected balloon bronchial blocker is placed in the main bronchus of the operative side. A nasogastric tube is also placed for identification of the esophagus during dissection and for postoperative decompression of the stomach. Finally, the patient is repositioned as appropriate for the side of surgery in a lateral decubitus position.

Right extrapleural pneumonectomy[20]

1. The patient is positioned in a left lateral decubitus position and the right chest is prepared and draped in a sterile fashion. An extended right posterolateral thoracotomy is made along the sixth rib. Electrocautery is used to divide through the subcutaneous tissue and the serratus anterior and latissimus dorsi muscles. Next, the sixth rib is identified, the periosteum stripped, and the rib is resected in a subperiosteal fashion with a bone cutter, from the level of the anterior chondrocostal cartilage to that of the spinous muscles. (See **Figure 14.1**.)

2. Extrapleural dissection is begun with blunt manual dissection, establishing a plane along the anterolateral thoracic wall and proceeding toward the apex. Care should be paid to avoid injuring the subclavian vessels, and packing sponges can be placed to control bleeding from the chest wall as the dissection progresses. The trick is to keep the lung initially inflated, particularly in patients with early disease, to avoid getting into the pleural space. Then, work should continue in all directions from the incision to enlarge the extrapleural plane and concentration be put on developing long fronts of dissection. Once the entire area of incision is cleared from the chest wall, retractors are then placed anteriorly and posteriorly and the extrapleural dissection is continued. The apex is released and dissected down to the hilum from both anterior and posterior approaches. The dissection then continues medially to mobilize the lung and tumor away from the superior mediastinum, being careful not to injure the superior vena cava or azygos vein. The dissection proceeds posteriorly and it is important to remember that, just anterior to the vertebral bodies, the posterior dissection needs to move to a more shallow plane to leave the azygos vein and its branches intact. The same approach applies anteriorly to spare the internal mammary arteries as the dissection nears the pericardium. (See **Figure 14.2**.)

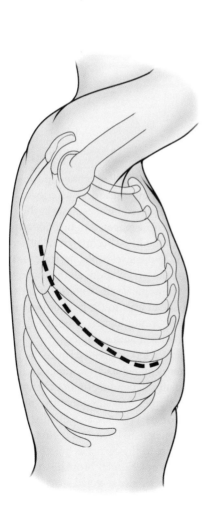

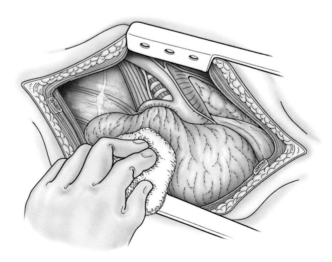

14.1

14.2

3. Continue the dissection inferiorly toward the lateral attachments of the diaphragm to the chest wall. This part of the dissection is performed with the surgeon's fingertips. It is easy to feel the cleavage plane between the tumor, the diaphragm, and the peritoneum, which should stay intact. If any opening is made in the peritoneum, it should be closed primarily. Once the lateral attachments of the diaphragm are freed, one can use a sponge stick to dissect the peritoneum away, extending this dissection along the inferior vena cava. The diaphragm is also freed from its medial and pericardial attachments, leaving the crus intact for diaphragmatic reconstruction. (See **Figure 14.3.**)

4. The pericardium is opened anteriorly and the pericardial space is evaluated for disease invasion. If any disease is detected here, elsewhere in the mediastinum, or into the chest wall, the EPP operation is aborted.

   The pericardial incision is made in line with the diaphragm posteriorly, allowing the identification and preservation of the inferior vena cava. There is a plane between the pericardium and the diaphragm that is extrapleural, which allows for safer dissection. The pericardium is then dissected and cut to the level of the pulmonary veins. (See **Figure 14.4.**)

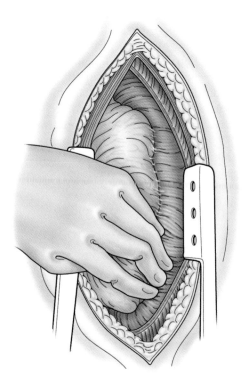

14.3

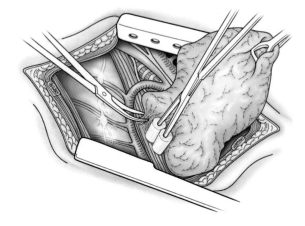

14.4

5. The separation of the EPP specimen in the same dissection plane then continues posteriorly. The nasogastric tube placed by anesthesia at the start of the operation is now palpated to help identify the esophagus, and the EPP specimen is dissected away from the esophagus to the level of the pericardium and this allows cutting the pericardium all the way to the level of the inferior pulmonary vein. Anteriorly, the pericardial incision is made at least to the level of the superior pulmonary vein, if not higher, so both veins are easily exposed for division with a stapler.

6. The pulmonary artery is divided (once the pulmonary artery catheter is pulled back) intrapericardially or extrapericardially, depending on the anatomy, with an endovascular stapler, and subsequently, the superior and inferior pulmonary veins are also divided in a similar manner. The mainstem bronchus is circumferentially dissected as close to the carina as possible, TA closed with a surgical stapler under bronchoscopic observation and divided. The *en bloc* resected specimen is sent to the pathology laboratory for analysis, which will confirm whether the bronchial stump margin of the resected specimen is negative for tumor.

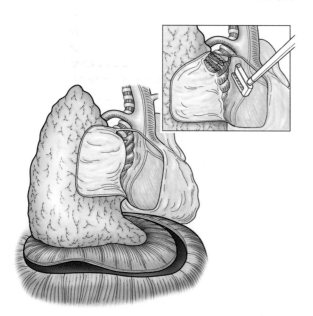

14.5

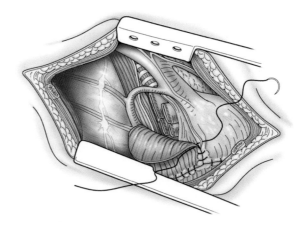

14.6

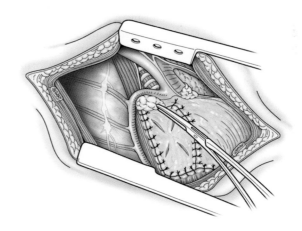

14.7

7. Next, a lymphadenectomy is completed from regional levels 4, 7, 8, 9, and 10. Meticulous hemostasis is achieved with electrocautery or the argon beam coagulator. The hemithoracic cavity is filled with warm saline and the airway pressure is increased to 30 mmHg while the saline pool is observed for evidence of air bubbles indicating a leak in the closure of the bronchial stump. If possible, the stump should be buttressed with muscle or omentum at the conclusion of the case.

    It is at this point in the procedure that intraoperative heated chemotherapy is administered if the patient is an appropriate candidate. This is beyond the scope of this chapter; for more information on this treatment, see Sugarbaker et al.[22] Prior to the chemotherapy, we generally perform a manual scrub with hydrogen peroxide and then several liters of pulse irrigation using saline and water. Argon coagulation is then used to aid in hemostasis and the destruction of possible remaining tumor cells.

    After ensuring coagulation of all bleeding sites and removal of all macroscopic tumor, areas that may require radiation therapy are marked with clips. (See **Figure 14.5**.)

8. The reconstruction portion of the operation consists of recreating the excised pericardium and diaphragm specifically to prevent the liver and the heart from herniating and causing hemodynamic problems. The diaphragm is reconstructed with a 1–2 mm Gore-Tex Soft Tissue Patch (W. L. Gore and Associates, Inc., Newark, Delaware, United States) secured to the chest wall and the mediastinum with interrupted Prolene sutures (Ethicon U.S., LLC, Somerville, New Jersey,

United States). Medially, the patch is secured to the pericardium and the crural fibers of the diaphragm. (See **Figure 14.6**.)

9. The pericardial defect is repaired with a 0.1 mm Gore-Tex patch to prevent herniation of the heart. This patch is sutured to the pericardial and diaphragmatic edges with interrupted 2-0 Prolene stitches (approximately eight) taking care to avoid making it too tight. The pericardial patch is fenestrated to allow drainage of fluid and to prevent cardiac tamponade. Care must be given not to narrow the vena-caval exit and to have no tied suture in contact with the heart lest it erode into a coronary artery. (See **Figure 14.7**.)

10. A final check is made for hemostasis and the chest cavity is irrigated with saline. Considerations may be given to place a fat, muscle or pericardial flap to cover the bronchial stump. A 12 Fr Rob-Nel red rubber catheter (Covidien, Medtronic, Dublin, Ireland, and Fridley, Minnesota, United States) is then placed percutaneously into the operative hemithorax. The ribs are reapproximated and closed with braided absorbable sutures and the incision is irrigated. The muscles and subcutaneous tissues are reapproximated with absorbable sutures in the standard fashion, and the skin is closed with a subcuticular suture. Prior sites of access for diagnostic biopsies are resected down to muscle and closed. Dressings are applied and the patient is returned to a supine position. A three-way stopcock is connected to the red rubber catheter and 750–1000 mL of air is evacuated from the chest to help maintain the mediastinal structures in a midline position.[23] In the intensive care unit (ICU) this catheter is used for pressure monitoring. A 24 Fr Blake drain (Ethicon U.S., LLC) is placed percutaneously into the contralateral side to help equalize the intrathoracic pressure and a completion bronchoscopy is performed as a final evaluation of the bronchial stump. The patient is then awoken from anesthesia, extubated, and taken to recovery in the ICU. (See **Figure 14.8**.)

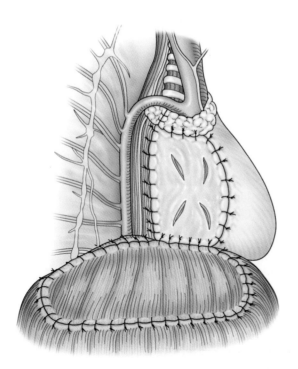

14.8

Left extrapleural pneumonectomy

1. Many of the operative steps in the left EPP are the same as when the procedure is performed in the right hemithorax. This section will emphasize the procedural differences between the two sides. First, the patient is positioned in a right lateral decubitus position for access in a left EPP. The thoracotomy is made at the level of the sixth rib, the left hemithorax is entered, and the extrapleural dissection is completed in the same fashion as described for the right side.

2. Particular attention should be paid during the dissection in the mediastinum to avoid injuring the left vagus and left recurrent laryngeal nerves. As the dissection is continued along the aorta, care is taken to avoid injury of the intercostal branches of the aorta and the thoracic duct.

3. The circumferential dissection in the extrapleural plane continues until the diaphragm is reached. The pericardium is opened and the pericardial space is inspected. The EPP is aborted if disease is detected in the mediastinum or invading into the chest wall. The diaphragm and hilar structures are then resected in a manner similar to that used on the right side.

4. Once the *en bloc* resected specimen has been sent to pathology for evaluation, a lymphadenectomy is performed of the lymph node levels resected on the right as well as the lymph nodes of levels 5 and 6.

5. After a check for hemostasis, the diaphragm is reconstructed. Surgeons' opinions vary on whether a pericardial reconstruction is needed on the left side. One school of thought reasons that the reconstruction is not necessary because the risk of herniation with torsion and compromise of venous return is not high on the left. However, it is our practice to perform the pericardial reconstruction on the left to prevent constrictive pericarditis, which can occur from development of a fibrous covering around the heart.[24] The chest is closed in the same manner as previously described for the right side and the patient is awakened, extubated, and taken to the ICU.

POSTOPERATIVE CARE

After EPP, patients are usually extubated in the operating room and managed in the ICU for about 3 days before being transferred to the intermediate care unit. On arrival to the ICU, pain control is evaluated and titrated via use of the preoperatively placed thoracic epidural, which is used for 3–5 days before transitioning to oral pain medications. A portable chest X-ray is obtained to evaluate all drain and line placements and to assess the position of the mediastinum. The red rubber catheter placed during the operation may be used to aspirate or introduce air as necessary to maintain central positioning of the mediastinum.[23]

If the patient received hyperthermic intraoperative

chemotherapy, an intravenous hydration protocol is begun. If no intraoperative chemotherapy regimen was given, the patient is fluid restricted to 1 L per day for the first few postoperative days so as to reduce the risk of developing pulmonary edema. Active diuresis may be given, particularly if the patient endures frequent oxygen desaturations secondary to excessive fluid resuscitation or retention. The patient is kept on bed rest for the first 2 postoperative days to ensure mediastinal stability. On postoperative day 2 the patient is first encouraged to dangle his or her legs and then to get up and walk once the pulmonary artery catheter is removed. When not ambulating, deep venous thrombosis prophylaxis is provided with pneumatic compression boots and subcutaneous heparin injections, and chest physiotherapy by trained nursing staff is encouraged to help clear airway secretions. Bronchoscopy is performed as required to help maintain airway patency.

Drains and tubes are removed as the need for them diminishes throughout the postoperative course. The nasogastric tube placed during the operation is removed on postoperative day 2. The red rubber catheter and contralateral chest drain are usually removed on postoperative day 3–5, depending on the stability of the fluid collection in the chest. Diet advancement occurs gradually with return of bowel function and the patient is then transitioned to oral pain medications and the epidural catheter is removed.

Postoperative management is also directed toward early detection and/or prevention of complications. Routine radiographic imaging, such as daily chest X-ray, is used to screen for pneumonia or shifts in the position of mediastinal structures. The nasogastric tube is used to decompress the stomach and prevent aspiration. Lower extremity ultrasounds are obtained weekly starting on postoperative day 7 to assess for deep venous thromboses and to prevent the secondary complication of pulmonary embolism by early diagnosis and treatment of these thromboses. Patients are usually discharged from the hospital after a stay of 10–14 days, but may be discharged as early as 7 days after operation.

COMPLICATIONS

Intraoperative complications

The main intraoperative complications are bleeding and damage to the vital structures encountered during the operation. Bleeding is a common complication and hemostasis is meticulously evaluated throughout the procedure. The argon beam coagulator is available, in addition to electrocautery, to control bleeding from the chest wall. Careful dissection technique, with attention paid to avoiding major blood vessels, needless to say, is critical if major blood loss is to be avoided. However, if any postoperative radiographs demonstrate rapid fluid accumulation in the operated hemithorax, reoperation to identify the source and control the bleeding should be performed expeditiously. Hemothorax may require evacuation to avoid infection or persistent fluid loss.

Another structure that may be injured during the EPP is the thoracic duct, particularly as the dissection approaches the posterior mediastinum. If a milky fluid that turns out to have an elevated triglyceride level is noted in the chest drain contents postoperatively, a chylothorax may be present and, if the technical expertise is available, may be treated with percutaneous embolization of the thoracic duct. If embolization fails, the patient is taken to the operating room for ligation of the thoracic duct.

The recurrent laryngeal nerve is a structure that if injured during the operation leads to increased aspiration risk because of the inability to completely appose the vocal cords to protect the airway. This is due to the fact that the paralyzed vocal cord remains in the abducted position and cannot meet the other vocal cord to completely close the glottis opening. Careful dissection is critical to avoid injuring this nerve, particularly during a left EPP when the dissection approaches the vagus nerve along the transverse aortic arch, where the recurrent laryngeal nerve originates. If a breathy cough or any voice changes are noted in the postoperative period, immediate evaluation of the vocal cords should be performed with direct laryngoscopy, as these could be signs of vocal cord paresis or paralysis. This complication is treated with vocal cord medialization and a swallow evaluation prior to permitting an oral diet.

Postoperative complications

The EPP operation is associated with a high postoperative incidence of morbidity.[8,9,11] The most common postoperative complication is atrial fibrillation. There is currently no guaranteed method to prevent this complication from occurring, but every patient is placed on a prophylactic beta-blocker regimen postoperatively. Other cardiac complications include cardiac tamponade and the constrictive pericarditis referenced earlier. A fenestrated patch is used to reconstruct the excised pericardium and care is taken to ensure that the patch placement is not too constricting. The fibrous rind that is deposited over the heart causing constrictive pericarditis has not been encountered with pericardial reconstruction. If cardiac tamponade does occur, reoperation is necessary to loosen the pericardial patch and evaluate for potential causes of the tamponade, including bleeding.

Cardiac arrest is a rare complication, but if it occurs, emergent reopening of the thoracotomy incision is required, followed by open cardiac massage because the empty hemithorax allows the mediastinum to easily shift and render chest compressions ineffective. The pericardial patch is removed to facilitate resuscitation efforts. Another rare complication is patch disruption. It requires having the patient be rotated to the contralateral decubitus position and urgent reoperation.

Much of the postoperative care is directed toward preventing pulmonary complications. Even so, complications such as pulmonary edema, atelectasis, and pneumonia can occur. Use of a diuretic and fluid restriction are used to treat pulmonary edema, which, if it occurs, usually presents within the first

4 postoperative days. Chest physiotherapy and bronchoscopy are used to maintain airway patency and reexpand lung parenchyma. Antibiotic therapy is immediately begun if there is clinical suspicion of pneumonia.

If there is indication of infection in the operated hemithorax, treatment can be difficult because of the prosthetic patches in place. We routinely maintain an intravenous antibiotic regimen for 5 postoperative days as prophylaxis against infectious complications.

The specific operative procedure for treating an empyema of the operated hemithorax depends on when it occurs in the postoperative period and if there are other associated complications. An empyema that occurs in the first 30 days after operation without an associated bronchopleural fistula requires treatment with antibiotics and probably a thoracoscopic operation to remove the prosthetic patch and irrigate the thoracic cavity. An empyema with associated bronchopleural fistula from bronchial stump breakdown is treated with an open window thoracostomy and staged removal of the prosthetic patches. Waiting until after 2–3 weeks of dressing changes to perform the patch removal allows the mediastinum to fix into place. Finally, if a patient following EPP presents with empyema after the 30-day postoperative period, she or he is also managed with an open window thoracostomy but the prosthetic patches are excised without staging.

OUTCOME

In recent years, particularly at high volume institutions, EPP outcomes have improved as improved criteria for patient selection and refinements in operative technique and perioperative care have been used. In this age of multimodality treatments for cancer, the EPP has found some success as part of the treatment regimen for MPM. The patients with MPM who benefit the most from an EPP are those with the pure epithelioid subtype who have no systemic disease, no nodal involvement, and have negative resection margins.[21] The mortality rate at high volume institutions has decreased to as low as 3.4%, but this operation is still associated with an overall morbidity rate as high as 60%.[6,8,9,11] With close monitoring and aggressive management, efforts will continue to be made to further decrease the morbidity from this radical operation. The EPP has proven to be a challenging operation that requires not only an experienced surgical team but also an experienced postoperative critical care team.

REFERENCES

1. "Mesothelioma Cancer Trends." The Mesothelioma Center, n.d. Web. June 20, 2014 www.asbestos.com/mesothelioma/mesothelioma-trends/
2. Weder W, Stahel RA, Bernhard J, Bodis S, Vogt P, Ballabeni P, Lardinois D et al. Swiss Group for Clinical Cancer Research. Multicenter trial of neo-adjuvant chemotherapy followed by extrapleural pneumonectomy in malignant pleuralmesothelioma. *Annals of Oncology.* 2007; 18(7): 1196–202.
3. Sarot IA. Extrapleural pneumonectomy and pleurectomy in pulmonary tuberculosis. *Thorax.* 1949; 4(4): 173–223.
4. Rice D, Rusch V, Pass H, Asamura H, Nakano T, Edwards J, Giroux DJ et al. International Association for the Study of Lung Cancer International Staging Committee and the International Mesothelioma Interest Group. Recommendations for uniform definitions of surgical techniques for malignant pleural mesothelioma: a consensus report of the International Association for the Study of Lung Cancer International Staging Committee and the International Mesothelioma Interest Group. *Journal of Thoracic Oncology.* 2011; 6(8): 1304–12.
5. Butchart EG, Ashcroft T, Barnsley WC, Holden MP. Pleuropneumonectomy in the management of diffuse malignant mesothelioma of the pleura: experience with 29 patients. *Thorax.* 1976; 31(1): 15–24.
6. Sugarbaker DJ, Jaklitsch MT, Bueno R, Richards W, Lukanich J, Mentzer SJ, Colson Y et al. Prevention, early detection, and management of complications after 328 consecutive extrapleural pneumonectomies. *Journal of Thoracic and Cardiovascular Surgery.* 2004; 128(1): 138–46.
7. Rusch VW, Venkatraman ES. Important prognostic factors in patients with malignant pleural mesothelioma, managed surgically. *Annals of Thoracic Surgery.* 1999; 68(5): 1799–804.
8. Shapiro M, Swanson SJ, Wright CD, Chin C, Sheng S, Wisnivesky J, Weiser TS. Predictors of major morbidity and mortality after pneumonectomy utilizing the Society for Thoracic Surgeons General Thoracic Surgery Database. *Annals of Thoracic Surgery.* 2010; 90(3): 927–34.
9. Patel RL, Townsend ER, Fountain SW. Elective pneumonectomy: factors associated with morbidity and operative mortality. *Annals of Thoracic Surgery.* 1992; 54(1): 84–8.
10. Wada H, Nakamura T, Nakamoto K, Maeda M, Watanabe Y. Thirty-day operative mortality for thoracotomy in lung cancer. *Journal of Thoracic and Cardiovascular Surgery.* 1998; 115(1): 70–3.
11. Bernard A, Deschamps C, Allen MS, Miller DL, Trastek VF, Jenkins GD, Pairolero PC. Pneumonectomy for malignant disease: factors affecting early morbidity and mortality. *Journal of Thoracic and Cardiovascular Surgery.* 2001; 121(6): 1076–82.
12. Algar FJ, Alvarez A, Salvatierra A, Baamonde C, Aranda JL, López-Pujol FJ. Predicting pulmonary complications after pneumonectomy for lung cancer. *European Journal of Cardiothoracic Surgery.* 2003; 23(2): 201–8.
13. Mansour Z, Kochetkova EA, Santelmo N, Meyer P, Wihlm JM, Quoix E, Massard G. Risk factors for early mortality and morbidity after pneumonectomy: a reappraisal. *Annals of Thoracic Surgery.* 2009; 88(6): 1737–43.
14. Pass HI, Giroux D, Kennedy C, Ruffini E, Cangir AK, Rice D, Asamura H et al. International Association for the Study of Lung Cancer (IASLC) Staging Committee and Participating Institutions. Supplementary prognostic variables for pleural mesothelioma: a report from the IASLC staging committee. *Journal of Thoracic Oncology.* 2014; 9(6): 856–64.
15. Gill RR, Richards WG, Yeap BY, Matsuoka S, Wolf AS, Gerbaudo

VH, Bueno R, Sugarbaker DJ, Hatabu H. Epithelial malignant pleural mesothelioma after extrapleural pneumonectomy: stratification of survival with CT-derived tumor volume. *American Journal of Roentgenology.* 2012; 98(2): 359–63.

16. Taioli E, Wolf AS, Camacho-Rivera M, Flores RM. Women with malignant pleural mesothelioma have a threefold better survival rate than men. *Annals of Thoracic Surgery.* 2014; 98(3): 1020–4.

17. Gordon GJ, Rockwell GN, Godfrey PA, Jensen RV, Glickman JN, Yeap BY, Richards WG, Sugarbaker DJ, Bueno R. Validation of genomics-based prognostic tests in malignant pleural mesothelioma. *Clinical Cancer Research.* 2005; 11(12): 4406–14.

18. De Rienzo A, Dong L, Yeap BY, Jensen RV, Richards WG, Gordon GJ, Sugarbaker DJ, Bueno R. Fine-needle aspiration biopsies for gene expression ratio-based diagnostic and prognostic tests in malignant pleural mesothelioma. *Clinical Cancer Research.* 2011; 17(2): 310–16.

19. Sugarbaker DJ, Richards WG, Gordon GJ, Dong L, De Rienzo A, Maulik G, Glickman JN et al. Transcriptome sequencing of malignant pleural mesothelioma tumors. *Proceedings of the National Academy of Sciences of the United States of America.* 2008; 105(9): 3521–6.

20. Chang MY, Sugarbaker DJ. Extrapleural pneumonectomy for diffuse malignant pleural mesothelioma: techniques and complications. *Thoracic Surgery Clinics.* 2004; 14(4): 523–30.

21. Bueno R, Reblando J, Glickman J, Jaklitsch MT, Lukanich JM, Sugarbaker DJ. Pleural biopsy: a reliable method for determining the diagnosis but not subtype in mesothelioma. *Annals of Thoracic Surgery.* 2004; 78(5): 1774–6.

22. Sugarbaker DJ, Gill RR, Yeap BY, Wolf AS, DaSilva MC, Baldini EH, Bueno R, Richards WG. Hyperthermic intraoperative pleural cisplatin chemotherapy extends interval to recurrence and survival among low-risk patients with malignant pleural mesothelioma undergoing surgical macroscopic complete resection. *Journal of Thoracic and Cardiovascular Surgery.* 2013; 145(4): 955–63.

23. Wolf AS, Jacobson FL, Tilleman TR, Colson Y, Richards WG, Sugarbaker DJ. Managing the pneumonectomy space after extrapleural pneumonectomy: postoperative intrathoracic pressure monitoring. *European Journal of Cardiothoracic Surgery.* 2010; 37(4): 770–5.

24. Byrne JG, Karavas AN, Colson YL, Bueno R, Richards WG, Sugarbaker DJ, Goldhaber SZ. Cardiac decortication (epicardiectomy) for occult constrictive cardiac physiology after left extrapleural pneumonectomy. *Chest.* 2002; 122(6): 2256–9.

15

Biportal fissureless video-assisted thoracoscopic surgery lobectomy

ALESSANDRO BRUNELLI

HISTORY

The first reports, from Italy and North America, regarding video-assisted thoracoscopic surgery (VATS) lobectomy performed according to modern technical and oncologic principles were published simultaneously.[1,2]

It took several years and significant technological improvements (dedicated VATS instruments and high definition [HD] video systems, among others) to facilitate the diffusion of this technique. Yet, a recent report from the Society of Thoracic Surgeons (STS) database showed that only about 30% of all lobectomies were performed by VATS, and in Europe this proportion was less than 10%.[3] Despite favorable outcomes and comparable oncologic results, there are still barriers that slow down adoption of this approach.

The Cancer and Leukemia Group B (CALGB) 39802 trial of the American Society of Clinical Oncology has defined VATS lobectomy by the presence of the following criteria: no rib spreading, one 4–8 cm utility incision, one to three additional ports, video guidance, individual dissection and transection of the hilar structures, and standard node sampling or dissection.[4] These criteria have set standards allowing for comparative analyses and pooling of data from different centers.

Several papers have now confirmed the validity of VATS lobectomy as a safe, economically and oncologically sound technique. However, the surgeon must use their wisdom and employ an evidence-based approach to recognize its limitations and applicability in all lung resections and all thoracic patients.

PRINCIPLES AND JUSTIFICATION

VATS anatomic lung resections are governed by the same principles as those for open surgery. When VATS lung resections are performed for malignant disease, preoperative surgical staging of the mediastinum with positron emission tomography and endobronchial ultrasound or mediastinoscopy are of paramount importance. What matters is not the ability to perform a VATS procedure but the ability to offer the correct treatment with it. The computed tomography scan remains a useful tool to map the hilar structures, define their anatomic relationship, and provide additional information regarding any potential intraoperative challenges. The slightest hint of being out of one's depth should encourage the wise surgeon to revert to the procedure with which they are most comfortable. Therefore, in the modern era of VATS, a quality measure should be the number of planned conversions versus unplanned ones.

A recent consensus statement from 50 VATS lobectomy experts states that VATS lobectomy is indicated for tumors of a size less than 7 cm and for N0/N1 disease. VATS lobectomy is contraindicated when there is the suspicion of chest wall involvement and relatively contraindicated if tumor invades hilar structures.[5]

Clearly, the inability to ventilate one lung and to provide a complete resection remains the main contraindications for VATS resections.

In experienced centers, previous chest surgery, the presence of bulky lymph nodes, endobronchial pathology, pericardial or diaphragmatic invasion, or neoadjuvant chemo radiotherapy are no longer absolute contraindications.

The importance of remaining safe and oncologically sound cannot be emphasized enough against the urge to record a successful VATS resection.

In a recent large multicenter study analyzing the occurrence of intraoperative major complications during VATS lobectomy, the conversion rate was 5.5% (49% for complications, 29.0% for technical reasons, and 22.0% for oncologic causes). Twenty-three percent of the in-hospital mortalities were related to the major intraoperative complications.[6] Vascular injuries were reported in 2.9% and led to conversion in nearly 80.0% of cases. The probability for conversion for non-oncological reasons decreased with experience (2.4% every ten cases). This information may represent a reference to assess quality of surgical care and can be used during preoperative counseling.

PREOPERATIVE ASSESSMENT AND PREPARATION

Preoperative evaluation for VATS anatomic lung resection follows the same principles as for the open approach. The American College of Chest Physicians functional algorithm is used.[7]

A preliminary cardiologic evaluation is performed in all patients.

Those patients with low cardiologic risk or with optimized cardiologic performance may proceed with the rest of functional workup. Forced expiratory volume in 1 second (FEV1) and diffusion capacity of the lung for carbon dioxide (D_{LCO}) are systematically measured in all patients. Patients deemed at low cardiologic risk and with both predicted postoperative forced expiratory volume in 1 second (ppoFEV1) and predicted postoperative diffusion capacity of the lung for carbon dioxide (ppoD_{LCO}) greater than 60% are regarded at low risk for surgery (risk of mortality lower than 1%). Patients with either ppoFEV1 or ppoD_{LCO} between 30% and 60% should undergo a low technology exercise test as a screening test. If the performance on the low technology exercise test is satisfactory, patients are regarded at moderate risk (morbidity and mortality rates may vary according to the values of split lung functions, exercise tolerance, and extent of resection). A cardiopulmonary exercise test is indicated when ppoFEV1 or ppoD_{LCO} are lower than 30% or when the performance at the stair climbing test or shuttle walk test is not satisfactory (i.e., altitude reached at stair climbing test <22 m or a shuttle walk distance <400 m). A maximal oxygen consumption (VO_2 max) of less than 10 mL/kg/min or 35% predicted indicates high risk for mortality when undergoing a major anatomic resection.

However, current functional algorithms are based on data that included patients operated on through an open approach. Several reports have now shown a reduction in morbidity rates in patients operated on through VATS.[8–11] This is probably explained by the minimal impact of this operation on the chest wall mechanics. This effect is even more evident in patients with compromised pulmonary function. For instance, in patients with an FEV1 of less than 60% or a D_{LCO} of less than 60%, FEV1 and D_{LCO} remained associated with complications only in patients undergoing thoracotomy but not thoracoscopy.[12]

Similarly, in patients submitted to lobectomy and with FEV1 of less than 60% registered in the STS database, those operated on through thoracotomy had an increased pulmonary complication rate compared with VATS patients. No significant difference was noted in patients with an FEV1 of more than 60% predicted.[13]

These findings are confirmed by a recent investigation showing lower respiratory complications and shorter hospital stay after VATS lobectomy compared with thoracotomy in chronic obstructive pulmonary disease patients.[14]

A recent analysis from the STS database[15] showed that patients with a ppoFEV1 of less than 40% had significantly lower morbidity and mortality rates after VATS lobectomy than their case-matched counterparts operated on through thoracotomy (21.9% vs. 12.8% and 0.7% vs. 4.8%, respectively). Similarly, patients with a ppoD_{LCO} of less than 40% had also reduced morbidity and mortality rates after VATS compared to thoracotomy. (10.4% vs. 14.9% and 2% vs. 5.2%, respectively).

In addition to these important findings, other studies have shown better preservation of pulmonary function compared to preoperative values in patients undergoing VATS lobectomy compared to thoracotomy.[16,17]

A recent study from the European Society of Thoracic Surgeons database has showed that low aerobic capacity (VO_2 max) before surgery is not associated with increased risk of cardiopulmonary complications or mortality after VATS lobectomy, confirming the beneficial effect of this approach in high risk patients and questioning the traditional operability criteria in this subset of patients.[18]

It appears likely that, with the increasing number of patients operated on through VATS, we will be able to verify whether traditional pulmonary thresholds of operability (mostly derived from series of patients operated on through thoracotomy) should be updated.

ANESTHESIA

The anesthetic technique used for VATS lobectomy does not differ from that used for any major thoracic surgical procedure. Induction is performed intravenously and endobronchial intubation takes place following administration of a nondepolarizing neuromuscular blocking drug. Maintenance is with an inhalational agent such as isoflurane.

The patient is then positioned in the lateral decubitus position. It is important to flex the table at the level of the inferior scapular angle to provide maximum spread of intercostal spaces for access. This position facilitates dropping the pelvis away from midline to prevent hindrance of free movement of the camera and other surgical instruments introduced from the inferior port.

One-lung ventilation is necessary to provide an adequate and quiet operating field. There is controversy regarding the use of left-sided tubes. Most believe they should always be used to prevent collapse of the right upper lobe, as it almost always originates close to the carina. Contralateral lung intubation is necessary, however, if major maneuvers are anticipated on the bronchial tree. The successful endobronchial tube position is confirmed with a flexible bronchoscope before the patient is turned to the lateral position.

The choice of double lumen tube or bronchial blocker rests with the team and institutional preference. A double lumen tube is generally preferred because it provides selective ventilation of the contralateral lung, while allowing more rapid collapse of the ipsilateral lung.

Following completion of the resection the residual lung parenchyma should not be reinflated or tested for air leaks before adequate and thorough suctioning of the bronchial tree has taken place. Providing no further actions are required, the chest is closed and spontaneous ventilation is reestablished in the usual manner. Extubation should be accomplished in the operating room and postoperative care is monitored in a high dependency unit.

OPERATION

General principles

A standard set-up is with one monitor placed on each side of the table in front of the surgeon and the scrub nurse.

I perform VATS lobectomies using a 10 mm, 30-degree-angled HD video thoracoscope. The 30-degree scope allows a superior view within the chest cavity.

The surgeon and the assistant are positioned on the anterior (abdominal) side of the patient. The surgeon can change position and place themselves cranially or caudally with respect to the assistant depending on the different steps of the operation.

The scrub nurse is opposite the assistant and follows the operation on a separate screen while still positioned face to face with the operating surgeon.

Initially, a 3.5–4.0 cm anterior utility incision is made without any soft tissue retractor or rib spreading. The wound is protected by a plastic soft tissue retractor kept in place by a ring in the chest cavity and one outside the skin (Alexis retractor, Applied Medical Resources Corporation, Rancho Santa Margarita, California, United States). This incision is usually placed at the 4th–5th intercostal space, between the tip of the scapula and the breast in the anterior axillary line.

Initial inspection is of paramount importance in order to identify any unexpected pathology and adhesions, as well as to assess the level of the diaphragm. A second 2.0–2.5 cm port is positioned more posteriorly at the level of the 7th intercostal space, just anterior to a straight line down from the tip of the scapula.

Typical placement of right and left biportal incisions is shown in **Figure 15.1**.

The camera is usually placed in the utility incision for the upper lobes, whereas it is usually placed in the inferior port for the middle and lower lobes. The camera position can be changed from one port to another if necessary, particularly during specific steps of the operation (parenchymal division, lymphadenectomy, etc.).

Most of the hilar dissection can be performed bluntly, either with a dissecting instrument (peanut) or a thoracoscopic suction device, which also keeps the field dry during dissection. The dissection can be complemented with monopolar diathermy with a long shielded tip. We recommend use of endoscopic forceps with axial handles to assist during this step. An elastic vascular loop is advised for

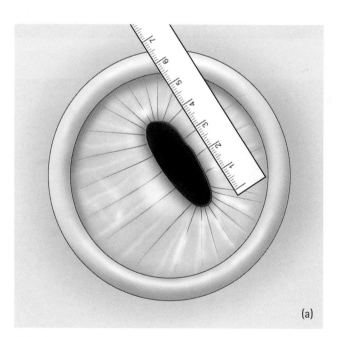

(a)

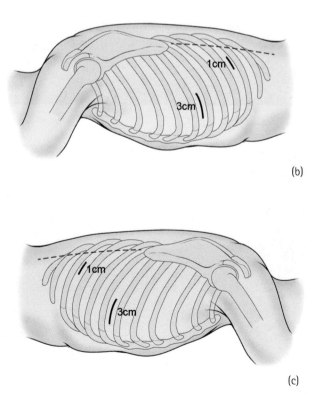

(b)

(c)

15.1a–c

gentle retraction of vessels when the endo-stapler is negotiated around them.

Lobar hilar elements and fissures are divided sequentially, with appropriate endoscopic staplers. For each anatomic lobectomy, the specific pulmonary vein is usually the first structure to be transected.

We use the so-called fissureless or fissure-last approach, in which the fissure is developed at the completion of the procedure after all the hilar elements have been transected. This approach minimizes visceral pleura and parenchymal injury, thus preventing alveolar air leaks. High energy devices can also be used to transect smaller pulmonary artery branches up to the size of 3–4 mm and for lymphadenectomy. At the conclusion of the operation, a single, apical 24 Fr chest tube is placed, generally through the inferior port in a midline position.

Right upper lobectomy

The camera is generally introduced through the utility incision, which facilitates the anterior view of the hilar structures. The lung is reflected posteriorly with endoscopic grasping clamps, usually introduced through the inferior port, and the pulmonary veins are identified. Blunt dissection is performed to identify the superior pulmonary vein and the bifurcation of the upper and middle lobe veins. Once the upper lobe veins have been clearly defined, they are dissected free with the use of a thoracoscopic DeBakey clamp, introduced through the inferior port. Division is accomplished with an endovascular stapler introduced through the inferior port, with the anvil positioned behind the superior pulmonary vein, which is then divided (see **Figure 15.2**). This procedure reveals the underlying pulmonary artery. In a similar manner, the pulmonary arteries to the upper lobe are mobilized and divided, beginning with the truncus anterior. The truncus anterior is first dissected using the DeBakey clamp

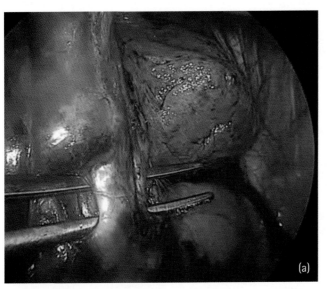
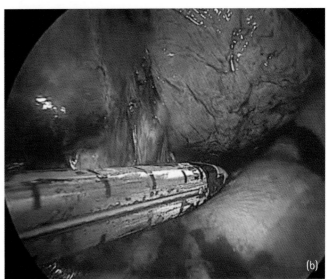

15.2a–b

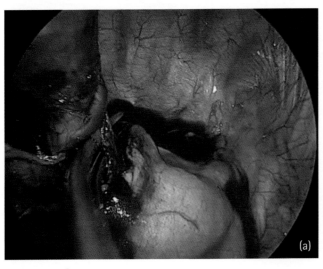
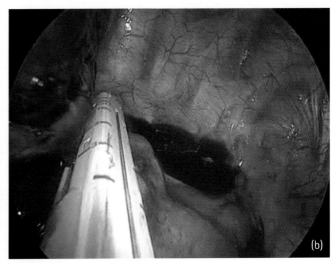

15.3a–b

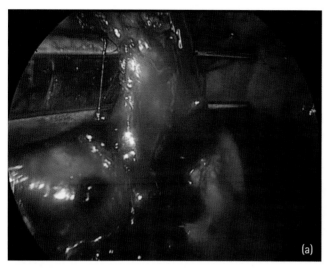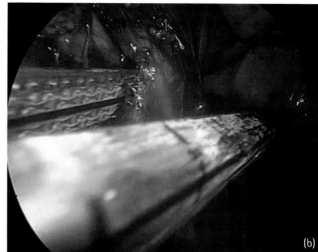

15.4a–b

and subsequently divided using an endoscopic vascular stapler, both introduced through the utility incision (see **Figure 15.3a–b**). The posterior ascending segmental artery may be isolated and divided at this time or after division of the bronchus by using endoscopic vascular clips (Hem-o-lok system), a high energy device or a vascular stapler. The lung is retracted medially and dissection along the posterior pleura is performed at the level of the bronchial bifurcation, which facilitates bronchial dissection later from the anterior approach. Subcarinal lymphadenectomy can be performed at this stage. Changing the position of the camera from the utility incision to the inferior port may facilitate this step by allowing a better view of the posterior mediastinal pleura.

The lung is then reflected posteriorly and the upper lobe bronchus is dissected free from its anterior aspect. The upper lobe bronchus is divided by passing an endoscopic stapler from the utility incision (see **Figure 15.4**). It is generally the last structure to be transected; however, occasionally the bronchus is divided before the dissection of the posterior ascending segmental artery. After division of the bronchus, the fissures are completed using stapling devices (see **Figure 15.5**). This step can be accomplished by alternating the camera from the utility incision to the inferior port. This will depend on the angle of exposure and the most convenient point of entry for the endoscopic stapler. The specimen is finally extracted from the chest in a protective bag (this can be achieved with or without prior removal of the wound protector).

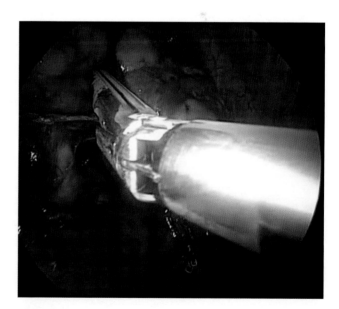

15.5

Right middle lobectomy

The camera is introduced through the inferior port. The pleura overlying the superior pulmonary vein is dissected by blunt and sharp dissection to expose and allow division of the middle lobe vein. The middle lobe vein is encircled by using a thoracoscopic DeBakey clamp, introduced through the utility incision, and subsequently transected by an endoscopic vascular stapler introduced through the same port (see **Figure 15.6a**). Following division of the middle lobe vein, the middle lobe bronchus is nicely exposed. An incomplete anterior oblique fissure should be divided at this stage. This can be accomplished by using an endoscopic stapler introduced from the utility incision.

The bronchus is then isolated, encircled and then closed with a stapler introduced through the utility incision. (see **Figure 15.6b**). During all these steps, the camera remains in the inferior port. After the bronchus is divided, the middle lobe artery branches are exposed. They can be encircled with an endoscopic DeBakey clamp, usually introduced from the utility incision, and transected with an endoscopic vascular stapler also introduced through the utility incision (see **Figure 15.6c**). Endoscopic vascular clips (Hem-o-lok system) can also be used for their division. The horizontal fissure is finally completed with a stapling line drawn in a posterior to anterior fashion via the inferior port.

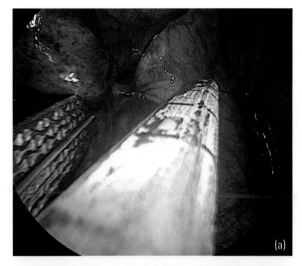

(a)

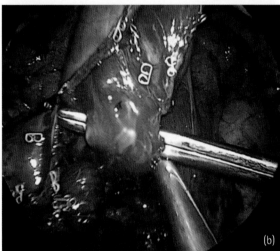

(b)

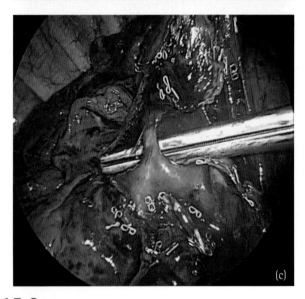

(c)

15.6a–c

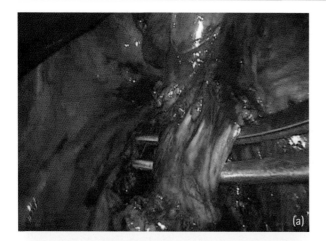

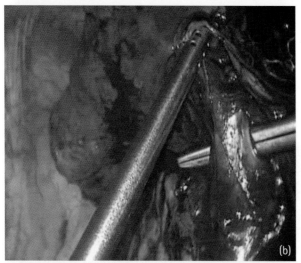

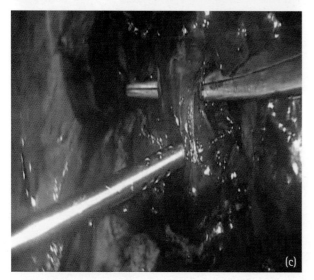

15.7a–c

Left upper lobectomy

The camera is introduced through the utility incision. The lung is reflected posteriorly by using endoscopic grasping clamps introduced from the inferior port. Blunt and sharp dissection is performed to identify both upper and lower lobe venous tributaries. The importance of this step cannot be emphasized enough, as a common venous trunk is a well-known anatomic variation. The superior pulmonary vein is encircled with an endoscopic DeBakey clamp introduced through the inferior port. The vein is then divided with an endoscopic vascular stapler introduced through the same port (see **Figure 15.7a**) and the bronchus is exposed. To facilitate dissection of the bronchus and prevent injury to the pulmonary artery branches, dissection of the lymph nodes between the cephalad aspect of the bronchus and the arterial anterior and apical segments is performed. The anterior and possibly superior branches of the arterial trunk can now be individually exposed and divided by passing an endoscopic DeBakey clamp and, subsequently, a vascular endoscopic stapler through the utility incision (see **Figure 15.7b**). Bronchial dissection and division are now easily accomplished by introducing the endoscopic DeBakey dissector clamp through the inferior port followed by an endoscopic stapler through the same port (see **Figure 15.7c**). Division of the anterior part of the fissure is sometimes recommended to facilitate this step. Care is taken to identify the secondary carina between the upper and lower lobe bronchus at the level of the fissure to prevent the left main bronchus from being erroneously encircled and divided. After the upper lobe bronchus is divided, the apical and posterior branches of the pulmonary artery and the lingular artery are isolated and divided by a single endoscopic vascular stapler or multiple staplers passed through the inferior port. Endoscopic vascular clips (Hem-o-lok system) or high energy devices may be used for smaller caliber vessels. During all these steps, the camera remains in the utility incision. The major fissure is finally divided, with the stapling device generally introduced through the inferior port. The staple line follows a retrograde course of the pulmonary artery, without disturbing the envelope of the visceral pleura.

Lower lobectomy

The camera is introduced through the inferior port. The lung is retracted cranially and the inferior pulmonary ligament is divided by using a long diathermy with a shielded blade. The inferior pulmonary vein is dissected, isolated, and divided in usual fashion, with the endoscopic vascular stapler introduced through the utility incision (see **Figure 15.8a–b**).

The bronchus is exposed by retracting the lobe cranially. The bronchus is dissected from the artery using sharp and blunt dissection and then passing an endoscopic DeBakey clamp through the utility incision. At this time, care is taken

to identify the origin of the middle lobe bronchus on the right, which must be spared. The dissection is followed by division of the lower lobe bronchus by an endoscopic stapler passed through the utility incision and placed just distal to the middle lobe bronchus on the right (see **Figure 15.9a–b**).

The lower lobe artery is then exposed. The arterial trunk is dissected by passing around it a DeBekey clamp introduced by the utility incision and then an endoscopic vascular stapler (see **Figure 15.10a–b**). It is sometimes easier to divide the basilar and superior segmental arteries separately.

Ultimately, the fissure is divided, and the specimen removed.

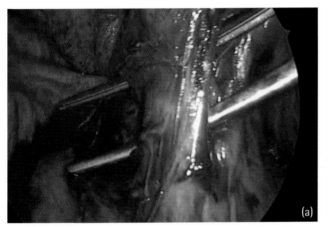
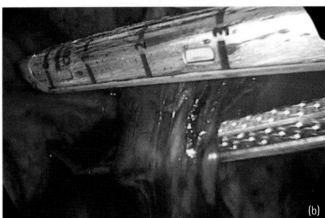

15.8a–b

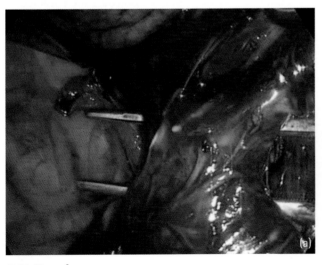
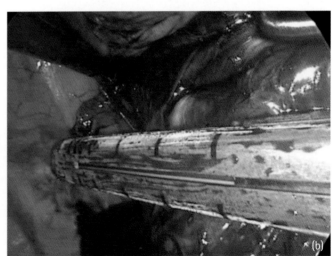

15.9a–b

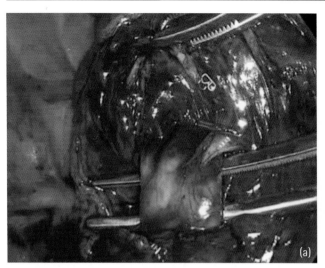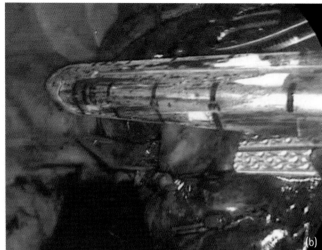

15.10a–b

Lymph node dissection

A systematic lymph node dissection is performed as part of the operation on either the right or the left side. A combination of blunt and sharp dissection is employed by using an endoscopic suction, high energy devices, or diathermy. Long curved thoracoscopic grasping forceps are used to facilitate exposure of the lymph node station by grasping the lymph node packet.

Right paratracheal lymphadenectomy (stations 2R and 4R) is performed by incising the mediastinal pleura above and below the azygos vein. The dissection begins at the tracheobronchial angle and progresses upward. The entire fat pad containing nodes is removed *en bloc* in the area defined by the azygous vein inferiorly, the vena cava medially, the trachea posteriorly, and the subclavian artery superiorly. During this procedure, the camera is introduced from the utility incision and the lung is reflected caudally by a lung grasping clamp or a sponge stick introduced from the inferior port. The dissection is performed through the utility incision.

To approach the subcarinal lymph nodes, the lung is retracted anteriorly and the posterior mediastinal pleura is incised to the level of the azygos vein. The camera is placed through the inferior port to improve visualization of the posterior mediastinum. Station 7 is exposed and removed *en bloc* so that the carinal bifurcation and the opposite bronchus are visualized. The dissection is performed from both the utility incision and the inferior port.

On the left side, nodes are removed *en bloc* from stations 5 and 6; station 7 is removed in a similar fashion to that of the right side. In lower lobe resections, nodes from stations 8 and 9 on the affected side are removed as well.

POSTOPERATIVE CARE

The general principles of postoperative management apply in this setting. Pain control differs between centers but most employ a combination of epidural/paravertebral pain management with patient-controlled analgesia.

One of the major advantages of VATS lobectomy that is promoted is postoperative pain reduction and decreased pain medication requirements.

Patients are encouraged to mobilize early after surgery. Physiotherapy and incentive spirometry are basic requirements. Chest tubes can be removed early in the absence of air leaks.

All necessary information is provided at bedside; hence, the routine use of several chest films and blood tests should be discouraged unless specific indications are present.

In case of prolonged air leak, a portable chest drainage system can be attached and the patient discharged home with follow-up visits at a nurse-led clinic.

OUTCOME

Several case-matched analyses have confirmed the superiority of VATS lobectomy to thoracotomy in terms of postoperative morbidity and, occasionally, mortality.[8,11,19–21] In particular, VATS lobectomy is associated with a reduced risk of respiratory complications and arrhythmia, and shortened hospital stay. These findings have been summarized and statistically confirmed by several systematic reviews and meta-analyses.[10,22–24]

There remains controversy regarding the oncological validity of VATS lobectomy. However, recent systematic reviews and meta-analyses have found improved or at least equivalent long-term survival rates after VATS lobectomy compared with thoracotomy.[22,23,25–27] Other studies from large national or institutional registries found that a VATS resection does not compromise radicality and long-term survival compared with thoracotomy in case-matched cohorts of patients.[28–31] Additionally, VATS lobectomy seems to be associated with a higher rate of completion of adjuvant chemotherapy than open lobectomy.[32,33]

REFERENCES

1. Roviaro CG, Varoli F, Rebuffat C, Vergani C, D'Hoore A, Scalambra SM, Maciocco M, Grignani F. Major pulmonary resections: pneumonectomies and lobectomies. *Ann Thorac Surg.* 1993 Sep; 56(3): 779–83.
2. Kirby TJ, Rice TW. Thoracoscopic lobectomy. *Ann Thorac Surg.* 1993 Sep; 56(3): 784–6.
3. Seder CW, Salati M, Kozower BD, Wright CD, Falcoz PE, Brunelli A, Fernandez FG. Variation in pulmonary resection practices between The Society of Thoracic Surgeons and the European Society of Thoracic Surgeons General Thoracic Surgery databases. *Ann Thorac Surg.* 2016 Jun; 101(6): 2077–84.
4. Swanson SJ, Herndon JE 2nd, D'Amico TA, Demmy TL, McKenna RJ Jr, Green MR, Sugarbaker DJ. Video-assisted thoracic surgery lobectomy: report of CALGB 39802: a prospective, multi-institution feasibility study. *J Clin Oncol.* 2007 Nov; 25(31): 4993–7.
5. Yan TD, Cao C, D'Amico TA, Demmy TL, He J, Hansen H, Swanson SJ, Walker WS; International VATS Lobectomy Consensus Group. Video-assisted thoracoscopic surgery lobectomy at 20 years: a consensus statement. *Eur J Cardiothorac Surg.* 2014 Apr; 45(4): 633–9.
6. Decaluwe H, Petersen RH, Hansen H, Piwkowski C, Augustin F, Brunelli A, Schmid T, Papagiannopoulos K, Moons J, Gossot D; ESTS Minimally Invasive Thoracic Surgery Interest Group. Major intraoperative complications during video-assisted thoracoscopic anatomical lung resections: an intention-to-treat analysis. *Eur J Cardiothorac Surg.* 2015 Oct; 48(4): 588–98.
7. Brunelli A, Kim AW, Berger KI, Addrizzo-Harris DJ. Physiologic evaluation of the patient with lung cancer being considered for resectional surgery: diagnosis and management of lung cancer, 3rd ed: American College of Chest Physicians evidence-based clinical practice guidelines. *Chest.* 2013 May; 143(5 Suppl): e166S–90S.
8. Paul S, Altorki NK, Sheng S, Lee PC, Harpole DH, Onaitis MW, Stiles BM, Port JL, D'Amico TA. Thoracoscopic lobectomy is associated with lower morbidity than open lobectomy: a propensity-matched analysis from the STS database. *J Thorac Cardiovasc Surg.* 2010 Feb; 139(2): 366–78.
9. Paul S, Sedrakyan A, Chiu YL, Nasar A, Port JL, Lee PC, Stiles BM, Altorki NK. Outcomes after lobectomy using thoracoscopy vs thoracotomy: a comparative effectiveness analysis utilizing the Nationwide Inpatient Sample database. *Eur J Cardiothorac Surg.* 2013 Apr; 43(4): 813–17.
10. Cao C, Manganas C, Ang SC, Peeceeyen S, Yan TD. Video-assisted thoracic surgery versus open thoracotomy for non-small cell lung cancer: a meta-analysis of propensity score-matched patients. *Interact Cardiovasc Thorac Surg.* 2013 Mar; 16(3): 244–9.
11. Villamizar NR, Darrabie MD, Burfeind WR, Petersen RP, Onaitis MW, Toloza E, Harpole DH, D'Amico TA. Thoracoscopic lobectomy is associated with lower morbidity compared with thoracotomy. *J Thorac Cardiovasc Surg.* 2009 Aug; 138(2): 419–25.
12. Berry MF, Villamizar-Ortiz NR, Tong BC, Burfeind WR Jr, Harpole DH, D'Amico TA, Onaitis MW. Pulmonary function tests do not predict pulmonary complications after thoracoscopic lobectomy. *Ann Thorac Surg.* 2010 Apr; 89(4): 1044–51.
13. Ceppa DP, Kosinski AS, Berry MF, Tong BC, Harpole DH, Mitchell JD, D'Amico TA, Onaitis MW. Thoracoscopic lobectomy has increasing benefit in patients with poor pulmonary function: a Society of Thoracic Surgeons Database analysis. *Ann Surg.* 2012 Sep; 256(3): 487–93.
14. Jeon JH, Kang CH, Kim HS, Seong YW, Park IK, Kim YT, Kim JH. Video-assisted thoracoscopic lobectomy in non-small-cell lung cancer patients with chronic obstructive pulmonary disease is associated with lower pulmonary complications than open lobectomy: a propensity score-matched analysis. *Eur J Cardiothorac Surg.* 2014 Apr; 45(4): 640–5.

15. Burt BM, Kosinski AS, Shrager JB, Onaitis MW, Weigel T. Thoracoscopic lobectomy is associated with acceptable morbidity and mortality in patients with predicted postoperative forced expiratory volume in 1 second or diffusing capacity for carbon monoxide less than 40% of normal. *J Thorac Cardiovasc Surg.* 2014 Jul; 148(1): 19–28.

16. Kaseda S, Aoki T, Hangai N, Shimizu K. Better pulmonary function and prognosis with video-assisted thoracic surgery than with thoracotomy. *Ann Thorac Surg.* 2000 Nov; 70(5): 1644–6.

17. Nagahiro I, Andou A, Aoe M, Sano Y, Date H, Shimizu N. Pulmonary function, postoperative pain, and serum cytokine level after lobectomy: a comparison of VATS and conventional procedure. *Ann Thorac Surg.* 2001 Aug; 72(2): 362–5.

18. Begum SS, Papagiannopoulos K, Falcoz PE, Decaluwe H, Salati M, Brunelli A. Outcome after video-assisted thoracoscopic surgery and open pulmonary lobectomy in patients with low VO$_2$ max: a case-matched analysis from the ESTS database. *Eur J Cardiothorac Surg.* 2016 Apr; 49(4): 1054–8.

19. Ilonen IK, Räsänen JV, Knuuttila A, Salo JA, Sihvo EI. Anatomic thoracoscopic lung resection for non-small cell lung cancer in stage I is associated with less morbidity and shorter hospitalization than thoracotomy. *Acta Oncol.* 2011 Oct; 50(7): 1126–32.

20. Stephens N, Rice D, Correa A, Hoffstetter W, Mehran R, Roth J, Walsh G, Vaporciyan A, Swisher S. Thoracoscopic lobectomy is associated with improved short-term and equivalent oncological outcomes compared with open lobectomy for clinical Stage I non-small-cell lung cancer: a propensity-matched analysis of 963 cases. *Eur J Cardiothorac Surg.* 2014 Oct; 46(4): 607–13.

21. Falcoz PE, Puyraveau M, Thomas PA, Decaluwe H, Hürtgen M, Petersen RH, Hansen H, Brunelli A; ESTS Database Committee and ESTS Minimally Invasive Interest Group. Video-assisted thoracoscopic surgery versus open lobectomy for primary non-small-cell lung cancer: a propensity-matched analysis of outcome from the European Society of Thoracic Surgeon database. *Eur J Cardiothorac Surg.* 2016 Feb; 49(2): 602–9.

22. Whitson BA, Groth SS, Duval SJ, Swanson SJ, Maddaus MA. Surgery for early-stage non-small cell lung cancer: a systematic review of the video-assisted thoracoscopic surgery versus thoracotomy approaches to lobectomy. *Ann Thorac Surg.* 2008 Dec; 86(6): 2008–16.

23. Chen FF, Zhang D, Wang YL, Xiong B. Video-assisted thoracoscopic surgery lobectomy versus open lobectomy in patients with clinical stage non-small cell lung cancer: a meta-analysis. *Eur J Surg Oncol.* 2013 Sep; 39(9): 957–63.

24. Cai YX, Fu XN, Xu QZ, Sun W, Zhang N. Thoracoscopic lobectomy versus open lobectomy in stage I non-small cell lung cancer: a meta-analysis. *PLoS One.* 2013 Dec; 8(12): e82366.

25. Yan TD, Black D, Bannon PG, McCaughan BC. Systematic review and meta-analysis of randomized and nonrandomized trials on safety and efficacy of video-assisted thoracic surgery lobectomy for early-stage non-small-cell lung cancer. *J Clin Oncol.* 2009 May; 27(15): 2553–62.

26. Zhang Z, Zhang Y, Feng H, Yao Z, Teng J, Wei D, Liu D. Is video-assisted thoracic surgery lobectomy better than thoracotomy for early-stage non-small-cell lung cancer? A systematic review and meta-analysis. *Eur J Cardiothorac Surg.* 2013 Sep; 44(3): 407–14.

27. Taioli E, Lee DS, Lesser M, Flores R. Long-term survival in video-assisted thoracoscopic lobectomy vs open lobectomy in lung-cancer patients: a meta-analysis. *Eur J Cardiothorac Surg.* 2013 Oct; 44(4): 591–7.

28. Berry MF, D'Amico TA, Onaitis MW, Kelsey CR. Thoracoscopic approach to lobectomy for lung cancer does not compromise oncologic efficacy. *Ann Thorac Surg.* 2014 Jul; 98(1): 197–202.

29. Cao C, Zhu ZH, Yan TD, Wang Q, Jiang G, Liu L et al. Video-assisted thoracic surgery versus open thoracotomy for non-small-cell lung cancer: a propensity score analysis based on a multi-institutional registry. *Eur J Cardiothorac Surg.* 2013 Nov; 44(5): 849–54.

30. Lee PC, Nasar A, Port JL, Paul S, Stiles B, Chiu YL, Andrews WG, Altorki NK. Long-term survival after lobectomy for non-small cell lung cancer by video-assisted thoracic surgery versus thoracotomy. *Ann Thorac Surg.* 2013 Sep; 96(3): 951–60.

31. Hanna WC, de Valence M, Atenafu EG, Cypel M, Waddell TK, Yasufuku K, Pierre A, De Perrot M, Keshavjee S, Darling GE. Is video-assisted lobectomy for non-small-cell lung cancer oncologically equivalent to open lobectomy? *Eur J Cardiothorac Surg.* 2013 Jun; 43(6): 1121–5.

32. Petersen RP, Pham D, Burfeind WR, Hanish SI, Toloza EM, Harpole DH Jr, D'Amico TA. Thoracoscopic lobectomy facilitates the delivery of chemotherapy after resection for lung cancer. *Ann Thorac Surg.* 2007 Apr; 83(4): 1245–9.

33. Zhi X, Gao W, Han B, Yang Y, Li H, Liu D, Wang C et al; China Clinical Trials Consortium. VATS lobectomy facilitates the delivery of adjuvant docetaxel-carboplatin chemotherapy in patients with non-small cell lung cancer. *J Thorac Dis.* 2013 Oct; 5(5): 578–84.

16

Robotic approach to lobectomy

BENJAMIN WEI AND ROBERT JAMES CERFOLIO

INDICATIONS/CONTRAINDICATIONS

Robotic-assisted pulmonary lobectomy may be considered for any patient undergoing lobectomy that does not involve complex vascular or airway reconstruction, or chest wall resection. The advantage of minimally invasive chest wall resection, which avoids rib spreading but still resects ribs, is controversial. In our opinion and based on our considerable experience, we favor thoracotomy when chest wall resection is required. Tumors larger than 7 cm (T3), tumors crossing fissures, and centrally located tumors may all be considered for robotic lobectomy with proper patient selection and increasing surgeon experience, but, in general, these factors are relative contraindications to a robotic approach. However, radiologic evidence of N1 nodes, induction chemotherapy and/or radiation, calcified lymph nodes, and prior thoracic surgery are *not* contraindications to robotic lobectomy but a robotic approach should not be selected early in one's learning curve.

The typical contraindications for lobectomy that apply to patients undergoing resection via thoracotomy would also apply to patients undergoing robotic lobectomy. These include, but are not limited to, borderline lung function or medical comorbidities, multistation N2, gross N2 disease, or evidence of N3 disease. Patients with apical lung tumors invading chest wall (Pancoast), tumors with extensive invasion into the mediastinum or esophagus, and contraindications to general anesthesia or single-lung ventilation are also less than ideal for robotic lobectomy. In addition, small indeterminate nodules that require lung palpation for wedge resection are considered by some as a contraindication for robotic lobectomy when a completely portal technique is used, but lung palpation is possible when a robotic-assisted technique is used. However, we have used navigational bronchoscopy with methylene blue tattooing of the nodules to help guide wedge resection when using a robotic approach.

PREOPERATIVE PLANNING

Preoperative evaluation including pulmonary function testing should be obtained. We routinely obtain stress testing to assess for myocardial ischemia, especially in patients who have had a significant smoking history. Complete patient-specific staging should also be performed prior to lung resection. This includes positron emission tomography–computed tomography scan in most patients and the selective use of: brain magnetic resonance imaging or computed tomography (for those who are symptomatic or who have large central adenocarcinomas), endobronchial ultrasound-guided fine needle aspiration, esophageal endoscopic ultrasound-guided fine needle aspiration for biopsy of the posterior inferior lymph nodes and adrenals, and/or mediastinoscopy depending on the tumor size and institutional experience.

When robotic techniques are used, special considerations for robotic proficiency are needed, as we have previously described.[1] These include documented scores of 70% or higher on simulator exercises; certificate of robotic safety training and cockpit awareness; weekly access to the robot; training of the entire personnel, including the bedside assistant; and familiarity with the robotic console and the instruments, and a mandatory mastery of the pulmonary artery from both an anterior and posterior approach.[2]

SURGERY

As with any operation, planning each stage of the procedure is crucial to ensure success. This begins with operating room set-up when a robot is used. The robot adds anxiety to inexperienced robotic surgeons and anesthesiologists. Thus, planning of the room layout prior to the operation is critical and includes the positioning of the bedside cart, the robot, the nurses' table, the monitors, and the patient relative to the anesthesia equipment. Careful planning and communication are mandatory because of the fact that the robot is driven in over the patient's head during lobectomy, the need for two monitors, and the distance between the operating surgeon at the console and the scrub nurse and surgical assistant(s) who stand at the patient's bedside.

Certain concepts specific to operating with robotic assistance should be mentioned here:

- The insertion of robotic instruments deserves special attention, as does the passing of vascular staplers around fragile structures such as the pulmonary artery and/or vein. Carefully orchestrated moves and clear communication is needed between the bedside assistant and the surgeon. We have developed our own communication system between the bedside assistant and the surgeon to prevent iatrogenic injuries. This uses the anvil of the stapler as the hour hand of a clock and the degree of articulation is also quantified and communicated.

- Robotic instruments should initially be inserted under *direct vision* during thoracic surgery. Once safely positioned, instruments then can then be quickly and safely inserted or exchanged for other instruments by properly using the memory feature of the robot that automatically inserts any new instruments to a position that is exactly 1 cm proximal to its latest position. However, if this feature is used, it is incumbent on the surgeon to ensure that no vital structures have moved into the path of that newly placed instrument. The most common structure to do so would be the lung.

Operating room configuration

One possible universal room set-up employed for all types of robotic surgery, including pulmonary resection, is shown in **Figure 16.1**.

CONSOLES

The surgeon console should be positioned so that good communication with the team at the operating table can be established. The da Vinci Surgical System console (Intuitive

Surgical Inc., Sunnyvale, California, United States) contains a microphone that amplifies the voice of the surgeon to the rest of the team. The presence of a second console permits easy exchange of control between surgeon, medical student, resident, or fellow for training purposes; this second console, if used, should be located fairly close to the primary console.

ROBOT/BED

The approach of the robot to the patient's side should be clear of any obstacles. The robot is driven over the patient's head on a 15-degree angle to open up robotic arm 3 over their head and shoulder, as shown in **Figure 16.2**.

In addition, monitors are positioned for a clear view by both the bedside assistants and the scrub nurse.

Depending on the size of the room and the arrangement of immobile structures within it, the table may need to be turned such that the patient's head is located well away from the anesthesia console. A long extension for the endotracheal tubing should be used if this is necessary.

As the robot is set up prior to driving it in over the patient's head, robotic arm 3 should be placed on the robot side opposite to the side of the lobectomy thus if performing a right-sided lobectomy, robot arm 3 should be located on the robot's left when facing it (**Figure 16.2b**).

ASSISTANT

The assistant will be positioned on the patient's ventral side (i.e., in front of the patient's abdomen/chest), with a monitor opposite them.

SCRUB NURSE

The scrub nurse will be positioned with the Mayo stand near or over the patient's feet, as in conventional thoracotomy or video-assisted thoracoscopic surgery (VATS).

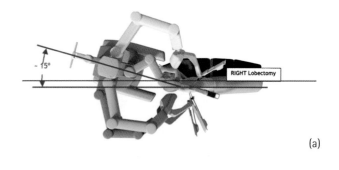

(a)

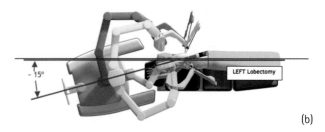

(b)

16.2a–b Angle of approach of robot docking for (A) right side lobectomy and (B) left side lobectomy.

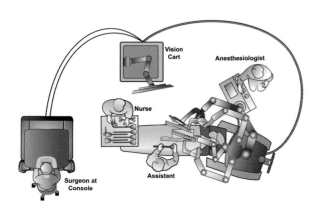

16.1 Operating room configuration for robotic lobectomy.

Patient positioning

General anesthesia is induced and the patient is intubated with a left-sided double-lumen endotracheal tube while supine. Proper placement of the double-lumen tube is facilitated greatly by the use of a flexible pediatric bronchoscope, and is critical to a smooth operation because access to the patient's head and endotracheal tube will be limited by their positioning and the presence of the robot after docking.

After the double-lumen tube is secured, the patient is positioned in lateral decubitus with the operative side up. Images of patient positioning are shown in **Figure 16.3**. An axillary roll is placed. We do not use an arm board but, rather, place the patient with their back at the edge of the table, leaving space in front of their face to fold their arms, taking care to expose the axilla for port placement. We have used this positioning for over 17 years for our thoracotomies, but it is critical when using a four-arm robotic approach, because it allows robotic arm 3 to move on a plane that is below the bed and avoid conflicts with that arm and the operative bed itself. Padding should be used around the arms and head to prevent nerve damage during the case—we use large foam pads.

This technique is easy and quick, requires no special equipment, and is reproducible. We position patients in under 10 minutes. A foam pad also helps protect the back of the patient's head from link two of robotic arm 3. Tape should be used to secure the patient's hips and upper body above the shoulder. The patient should be located with their flank (i.e., space between subcostal margin and iliac crest) directly over the break point of the bed, and the table should be flexed to increase the space between the ribs. A body warmer is applied to the lower body.

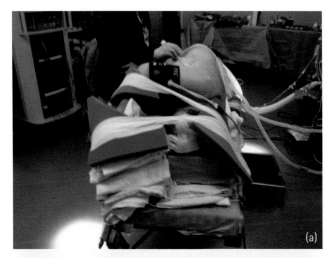
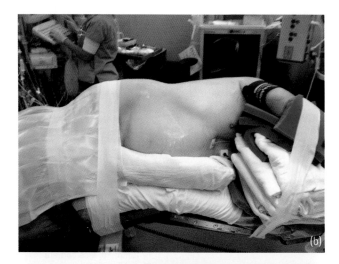
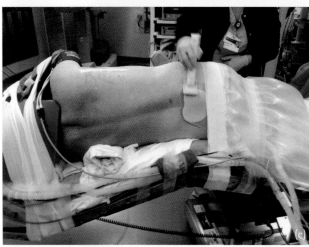
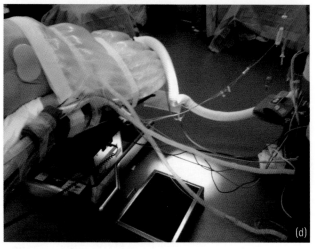

16.3a–d (a) Patient positioning for robotic lobectomy, viewed from the patient's head. Foam pads for protection of pressure points of the head and arms are also shown. (b) Patient positioning for robotic lobectomy, viewed from anterior to the patient. The axilla is exposed widely and the space between the patient's iliac crest and costal margin is located above the break in the bed. (c) Patient positioning for robotic lobectomy, viewed from posterior to the patient. The position of the axillary roll is shown. (d) Patient positioning for robotic lobectomy, showing the distance between the anesthesia ventilator and the patient. Long flexible tubing, used to facilitate this, is taped along the bed with the other monitoring lines to provide easier access to the posterior aspect of the patient if a thoracotomy becomes necessary.

Port placement/Docking

The ports are all inserted in the 7th intercostal space, over the top of the 8th rib, for upper/middle lobectomy, and in the 8th intercostal space, over top of the 9th rib for lower lobectomy.

The ports are marked as follows: robotic arm 3 (5 mm port) is located 1–2 cm lateral from the spinous process of the vertebral body, robotic arm 2 (8 mm) is 10 cm medial to robotic arm 3, the camera port (we prefer the 12 mm camera) is 9 cm medial to robotic arm 2, and robotic arm 1 (12 mm) is placed right above the diaphragm anteriorly. The assistant port (12 mm) is placed as low as possible in the chest, triangulated exactly halfway in between the most anterior robotic port (which is robotic arm 1 in the right chest and robotic arm 2 in the left chest) and the camera port and then as low as possible to remain just above the diaphragm which is being pushed downward by the insufflating humidified carbon dioxide (CO_2) gas (see **Figure 16.4**).

Sequence of port placement

A 5 mm port is placed first in the camera port position and CO_2 insufflation initiated with a pressure of 10 mmHg. We use humidified warm CO_2. An intercostal nerve block with 0.25% bupivacaine with epinephrine is then performed from ribs three to eight by injecting subpleural under direct vision. Then the 5 mm thoracoscope is used to help assist the placement of all of the other ports, which are all placed under direct position. The camera port is placed first, robotic arm 3 is placed second, then robotic arm 2 in the right chest and robotic arm 1 in the left.

The 5 mm VATS camera is then moved to the port for robotic arm 2 and the two most anterior ports (robotic arm 1 in the right chest and 2 in the left) and the access port are placed under direct vision using an exploring needle. Our technique completely avoids all of the diaphragmatic fibers. The 5 mm camera port is then upsized to the 12 mm camera port. We use a 0-degree endoscope for the entire case to help prevent torqueing on the intercostal nerve.

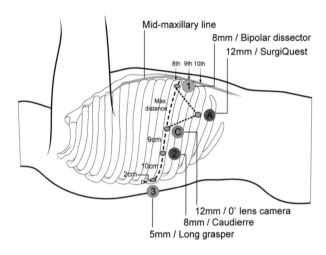

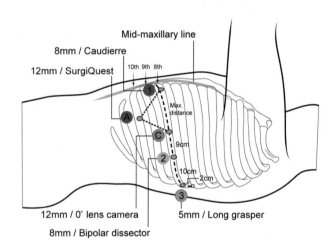

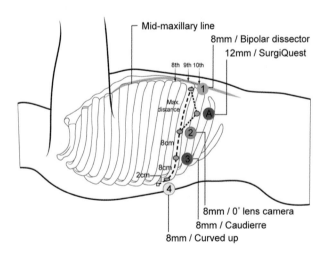

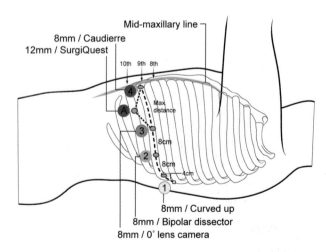

16.4 Port placement for right robotic lobectomy.

Notes: C, camera port; 1, robotic arm 1; 2, robotic arm 2; 3, robotic arm 3; A, assistant port.

16.5 Port placement for left robotic lobectomy.

Notes: C, camera port; 1, robotic arm 1; 2, robotic arm 2; 3, robotic arm 3; A, assistant port.

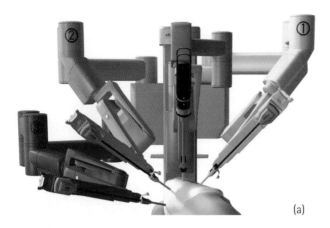

16.6a View of robot docked to patient for right lobectomy.

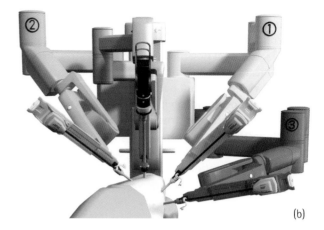

16.6b View of robot docked to patient for left lobectomy.

The port placement for left-sided lobectomy is a mirror image to that just outlined (see **Figure 16.5**). The difference is that robotic arm 3 is next to robotic arm 1, rather than robotic arm 2. The numbering is different, but the locations of the ports are the same.

The robot is brought in at a 15-degree angle toward the patient's face, off the long axis of the bed (see **Figure 16.6**). The robotic arms are docked to the ports, maximizing the amount of space between the arms to avoid collisions. Once the system is docked, the operating room table cannot be moved.

The three instruments used to initiate the operation are as follows: (1) left robotic arm—an 8 mm Cadiere grasper; (2) right robotic arm—an 8 mm bipolar curved thoracic dissector, and (3) robotic arm 3—a 5 mm thoracic grasper.

Mediastinal lymph node dissection

The pleural surface is inspected prior to initiating node dissection and lobectomy to confirm that there are no metastatic lesions.

We perform mediastinal lymph node dissection prior to lobectomy to not only evaluate the lymph nodes but also access arterial and venous branches and the bronchus.

RIGHT SIDE
The inferior pulmonary ligament is divided to access lymph node station 9. It is removed along with lymph node station 8. Robotic arm 3 is used to retract the lower lobe medially and anteriorly to remove lymph nodes from station 7, the subcarinal space. Care is taken to control bronchial arteries. Robotic arm 3 is used to retract the upper lobe inferiorly, while robotic arms 1 and 2 are used to dissect out stations 2R and 4R, clearing the space between the superior vena cava anteriorly, the esophagus posteriorly, and the azygos vein inferiorly. Avoiding dissection too far superiorly can prevent injury to the right recurrent laryngeal nerve that courses around the subclavian artery.

LEFT SIDE
The inferior pulmonary ligament is divided to facilitate the removal of lymph node station 9. The nodes in station 8 are then removed. Station 7 is accessed in the space between the inferior pulmonary vein and lower lobe bronchus, lateral to the esophagus. If still in position, the lower lobe is retracted medially/anteriorly with robotic arm 3 during this process. Absence of the lower lobe facilitates dissection of level 7 from the left. One distinct advantage of the robot when compared with VATS is the dissection of the station 7 lymph node from the left chest. Finally, robotic arm 3 is used to wrap around the left upper lobe and reflect it inferiorly to allow dissection of stations 5 and 6. Care should be taken while working in the aortopulmonary window to avoid injury to the left recurrent laryngeal nerve. Station 2L cannot typically be accessed during left-sided mediastinal lymph node dissection due to the presence of the aortic arch but the 4L node is commonly removed.

General concepts

In general, for a right-handed surgeon, a blunt instrument such as Cadiere forceps is placed in robotic arm 2, which is always the left hand, while the right hand, which is always robotic arm 1, uses a thoracic dissector. We preferentially place a vessel loop under a vessel to be stapled to help elevate it while the stapler is passed under it.

The stapler may be placed through one of three ports—the access port, robotic arm 1, or robotic arm 2. The current design of commercially available white or grey vascular staplers requires a 12 mm port and for the green load stapler, commonly used for the bronchus, a 15 mm port is required. We prefer to remove the trocar and leave it docked to the robotic arm and then place the stapler through the skin incision.

We commonly use a prerolled sponge to absorb blood from the operative field, as well as to facilitate blunt dissection to improve visibility.

Removal of lymph nodes from around bronchovascular structures should be done prior to stapling and dividing, in the interests of both ensuring an oncologically sound operation and facilitating isolation and division of structures.

If significant adhesions are encountered, they may be initially lysed via the assistant port using VATS techniques until safe placement of all the robotic instruments is permitted.

The order in which the structures are isolated and divided during lobectomy varies somewhat depending on patient anatomy. What follows is a general outline of the typical conduct of the operation for each lobectomy.

Right upper lobectomy

1. Retraction of the right upper lobe laterally and posteriorly with robot arm 3 to expose the hilum.
2. The bifurcation between the right upper and middle lobe veins is developed by dissecting the superior pulmonary vein away from the underlying pulmonary artery.
3. The 10R lymph node between the anterior-apical segment arterial branch and the superior pulmonary vein should be removed or swept up toward the lung, thus exposing the anterior-apical segmental branch (see **Figure 16.7**).
4. The superior pulmonary vein is encircled with the vessel loop and then divided. The truncus branch of the pulmonary artery is then divided.
5. The right upper lobe is then reflected anteriorly to expose the bifurcation of the right main stem bronchus (see **Figure 16.8**). There is usually a lymph node (level 11R) here that should be dissected out to expose the bifurcation. The right upper lobe bronchus is then encircled and divided (see **Figure 16.9**). Care must be taken to apply only minimal retraction on the specimen to avoid tearing the remaining pulmonary artery branches.
6. Next, the posterior segmental artery to the right upper lobe is exposed, the surrounding N1 nodes removed, and the artery encircled and divided (see **Figure 16.10**).
7. The upper lobe is reflected again posteriorly, and the anterior aspect of the pulmonary artery is inspected to make sure that there are no arterial branches remaining. If not, the fissure between the upper and middle lobes, and the upper and lower lobes, is then divided with the linear stapler. This is typically done from anterior to posterior, but may be done in the reverse direction if the space between the pulmonary artery and right middle lobe is already developed. During completion of the fissure, the right upper lobe should be lifted up to ensure that the specimen bronchus is included in the specimen.

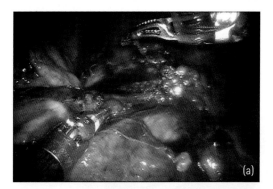

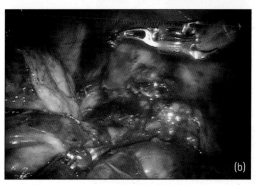

16.7a–b Dissection of lymph node 10R between anterior-apical segment branch and right superior pulmonary vein during robotic right upper lobectomy.

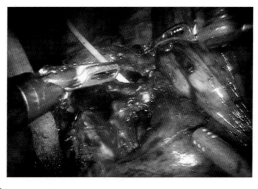

16.8 Anterior retraction of lung to exposure bifurcation of right main stem bronchus.

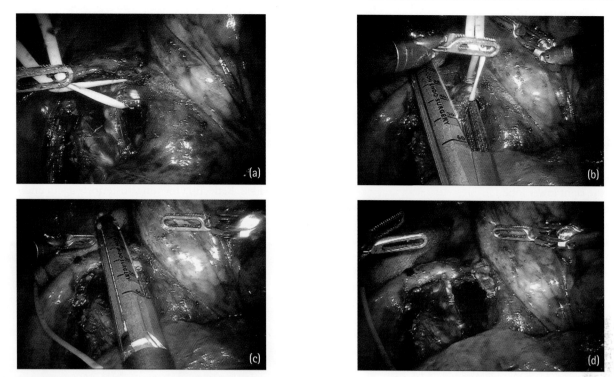

16.9a–d Exposure and division of right upper lobe bronchus. (a) The bronchus is encircled with a vessel loop used to provide traction to allow for better visualization. (b) Applying traction to the vessel loop the endoscopic stapler is passed around the bronchus. (c) The stapler, having been accurately placed to encompass the entire bronchus is closed and fired. (d) The stapler is removed demonstrating the stapled bronchial stump

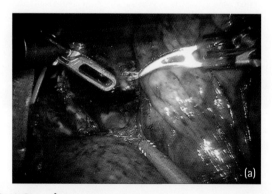
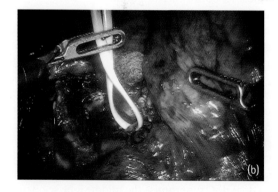

16.10a–b Exposure of right posterior segmental artery.

Right middle lobectomy

1. Retraction of the right middle lobe laterally and posteriorly with robot arm 1 helps expose the hilum.
2. The bifurcation between the right upper and middle lobe veins is developed by dissecting it off the underlying pulmonary artery. The right middle lobe vein is encircled and divided.
3. The fissure between the right middle and lower lobes, if not complete, is divided from anterior to posterior. Care should be taken to avoid transecting segmental arteries to the right lower lobe.
4. The right middle lobe bronchus is then isolated. It will be running from left to right in the fissure. Level 11 lymph nodes are dissected from around it. It is encircled and divided, taking care to avoid injuring the right middle lobar artery that is located directly posterior.
5. Dissection of the fissure should continue posteriorly until the arterial branch to the superior segment of the lower lobe is identified. Then the one or two right middle lobar segmental arteries are isolated and divided.
6. Stapling of middle lobe bronchus and vessels may be facilitated by passing the stapler from posterior to anterior to have a greater working distance.
7. The fissure between right middle and upper lobes is then divided.

Right lower lobectomy

1. The inferior pulmonary ligament should be divided up to the level of the inferior pulmonary vein.
2. The bifurcation between the right superior and inferior pulmonary veins should be dissected. The location of the right middle lobe vein should be positively identified to avoid inadvertent transection.
3. A subadventitial plane on the ongoing pulmonary artery should be established. If the major fissure is not complete, then it should be divided. The superior segmental arterial branch and the right middle lobe arterial branches are identified. The superior segmental artery is isolated and divided. The common trunk to right lower lobe basal segments may be taken as long as this does not compromise the middle lobe segmental artery/arteries; otherwise, dissection may have to extend further distally to ensure safe division.
4. The inferior pulmonary vein is divided.
5. The right lower lobe bronchus is isolated, taking care to visualize the right middle lobe bronchus crossing from left to right. The surrounding lymph nodes, as usual, are dissected, reflected up toward the lung, and the bronchus divided. If there is any question of compromising the right middle lobe bronchus, the surgeon can ask the anesthesiologist to hand-ventilate the right lung to confirm that the middle lobe expands, but the origin of the middle lobe bronchus is usually readily identified.

Left upper lobectomy

1. Retraction of the left upper lobe laterally and posteriorly with robot arm 3 helps expose the hilum.
2. The presence of both superior and inferior pulmonary veins is confirmed, and the bifurcation between the two is dissected.
3. The lung is then reflected anteriorly with robotic arm 3 and interlobar dissection is started, going from posterior to anterior.
4. If the fissure is not complete, then it will need to be divided. Reflecting the lung posteriorly again and establishing a subadventitial plane on the artery will be

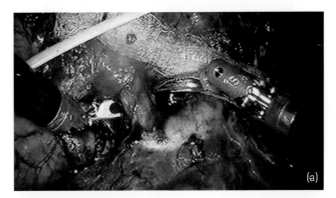

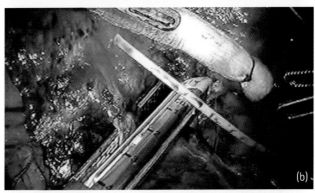

16.11a–b Isolating and dividing a lingular artery during robotic left upper lobectomy.

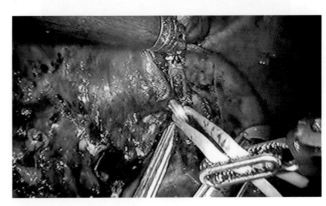

16.12 Isolating and dividing the posterior segmental artery during robotic left upper lobectomy.

helpful. The branches to the lingula are encountered and divided in the fissure during this process (see **Figure 16.11**). The posterior segmental artery is also isolated and divided (see **Figure 16.12**). Division of the lingular artery or arteries can be done before or after division of the posterior segmental artery.

5. The superior pulmonary vein is isolated then divided (see **Figure 16.13**). As the superior pulmonary vein can be fairly wide, it may require that the lingular and upper division branches be transected separately.

6. Often the next structure that can be divided readily will be the left upper lobe bronchus, as opposed to the anterior and apical arterial branches to the left upper lobe. The upper lobe bronchus should be encircled and divided, often passing the stapler from robotic arm 1 to avoid injuring the main pulmonary artery (see **Figure 16.14**).

7. Finally, the remaining arterial branches are encircled and divided.

Left lower lobectomy

1. The inferior pulmonary ligament should be divided to the level of the inferior pulmonary vein. The lower lobe is then reflected posteriorly by robotic arm 3.

2. The bifurcation of the left superior and inferior pulmonary veins should be dissected out.

3. The lung is reflected anteriorly by robotic arm 3. The superior segmental artery is identified. The posterior ascending arteries to the left upper lobe are frequently visible from this view also. The superior segmental artery is isolated and divided. The common trunk to left lower lobe basilar segments may be taken as long as this does not compromise the middle lobar segmental artery/arteries; otherwise, dissection may have to extend further distally to ensure safe division. If the fissure is not complete, this will need to be divided to expose the ongoing pulmonary artery to the lower lobe.

4. After division of the arterial branches, the lung is reflected again posteriorly. The inferior pulmonary vein is divided.

5. The left lower lobe bronchus is isolated. The surrounding lymph nodes, as usual, are dissected and the bronchus divided.

6. For left lower lobectomy, it may be simpler to wait until after resection is performed before dissecting within the subcarinal space for removal of level 7 lymph nodes.

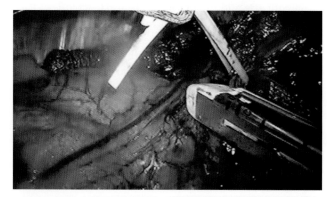

16.13 Isolating and dividing the left superior pulmonary vein during robotic left upper lobectomy.

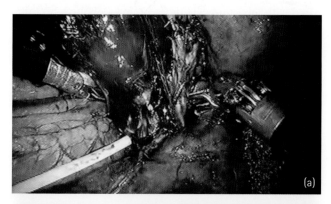

(a)

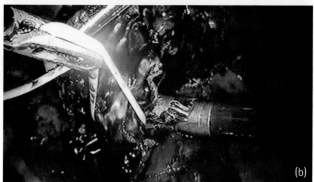

(b)

16.14a–b Isolating and dividing the left upper lobe bronchus during robotic left upper lobectomy.

Specimen removal/Conclusion of operation

1. The "drop zone" for the specimen should be well away from the pulmonary artery, which can be injured during this process if care is not taken. Before the bag is inserted robotic arm 3 is used to hold the specimen. The bag is inserted via the assistant port and robotic arms 1and/ or 2 are used to ensure the bag is deployed under the trocar. This ensures that the bag is opened in the right direction. Robotic arm 3 then drops the specimen in the bag and it then grasps the far lip of the bag to make sure it does not spin, while robotic arms 1 and 2 are used to place the specimen in the bag. Care is taken to make sure the arms are not inside the bag.

2. The chest is irrigated with normal saline, the presence of air leaks checked with insufflation, hemostasis is confirmed, and a 20 Fr chest tube is placed via the most anterior port which is robotic arm 1 in the right chest and robotic arm 2 in the left. The robotic arms are removed under direct vision with insufflation

discontinued to confirm the absence of bleeding. The camera port is removed. The robot is undocked and pushed away from the patient's bed.

3. The bag is removed from the body, usually after enlarging the assistant nonrobotic port posteriorly to avoid injuring the diaphram. Our techniques completely avoid all of the diaphragmatic fibers.

4. The chest tube is secured with a #5 Ethibond suture.

5. The fascial layer in the 12 mm ports is closed with 0 Vicryl suture after the break is removed from the table.

6. The skin is closed in a knotless subcuticular fashion with 3-0 Vicryl suture.

POSTOPERATIVE MANAGEMENT

The management of patients undergoing robotic lobectomy does not differ from that of patients undergoing VATS lobectomy. Our patients go directly to the standard thoracic nursing unit and not the intensive care unit (ICU). Patients generally do well with patient-controlled analgesia or even oral pain medications. Chest tubes are removed when any air leak resolves and at outputs of up to 450 mL/d, depending on the patient. Patients are typically discharged on postoperative day 2 or 3.

COMPLICATIONS

The same complications that can occur after open or VATS lobectomy are possible following robotic lobectomy. We have recently reported the incidence of chylothorax may even be slightly higher in patients undergoing robotic lobectomy, which is probably due to the increased completeness of the mediastinal lymph node dissection.[3] The incidence of atrial fibrillation, pneumonia, blood loss, and pain appears less with robotic-assisted lobectomy than with lobectomy performed via thoracotomy, and similar or favorable when compared with VATS lobectomy.[4]

RESULTS

Reported series of robotic lobectomy to date have been notable for a fairly low conversion rate, low mortality rate, and comparable morbidity to VATS approaches (see **Table 16.1**). With increasing experience, operating times for robotic lobectomy have been shown to decrease; at our institution, robotic lobectomies with complete mediastinal lymph node dissection can routinely be done in 1.5–2.0 hours from incision to skin closure. The single comparison with VATS lobectomy published to date, by Louie et al. (2012), demonstrates similar blood loss, operative time, ICU stay, and length of stay between robotic and VATS lobectomy, but did show benefits for the robotic approach in terms of duration of narcotic use and time to return to usual activities.[4] Park et al. reported 5-year survival rates for 310 patients with stage I non-small-cell lung cancer of ~90% following robotic lobectomy, results comparable to both VATS and open lobectomy.[5,6] Our experience has been that robotic lobectomy facilitates a more thorough and complete mediastinal lymph node dissection, which we believe is associated with a greater accuracy of staging and therefore more optimal adjuvant treatment.[7]

CONCLUSIONS

Robotic pulmonary lobectomy represents an emerging method to achieve an oncologically equivalent, minimally invasive operation that decreases perioperative risk compared with lobectomy via thoracotomy. Robotic lobectomy does seem to offer some special benefits to the surgeon in terms of lymph node dissection, ergonomics, and teachability. The need for highly trained team members who are familiar with both each other and the operation cannot be underestimated for robotic pulmonary lobectomy. A systematic approach to both learning and executing the procedure is highly recommended.

Table 16.1 Results reported by series of robotic-assisted lobectomies

Study	Year	Patients, n	Conversion rate	Morbidity	Perioperative mortality	Median LOS	Other notes
Cerfolio et al.[7]	2011	168	7.7%	27%	0%	2.0 days	Decreased morbidity, improved QOL, shorter LOS than open lobectomy
Park et al.[5,6]	2006	30	12%	26%	0%	4.5 days	
Veronesi et al.[8]	2009	54	13%	20%	0%	4.5 days	Shorter LOS than open lobectomy
Gharagozloo et al.[9]	2009	100	NS	21%	3%	4.0 days	Authors note the steep learning curve

Notes: LOS, length of stay; QOL, quality of life.

REFERENCES

1. Cerfolio RJ, Bryant AS. How to teach robotic pulmonary resection. *Semin Thorac Cardiovasc Surg.* 2013; 25: 76–82.

2. Cerfolio RJ, Bryant AS, Minnich DJ. Starting a robotic program in general thoracic surgery: why, how, and lessons learned. *Ann Thorac Surg.* 2011; 91: 1729–37.

3. Bryant AS, Minnich DJ, Wei B, Cerfolio RJ. The incidence and management of postoperative chylothorax after pulmonary resection and thoracic mediastinal lymph node dissection. *Ann Thorac Surg.* 2014 Jul; 98(1): 232–5.

4. Louie BE, Farivar AS, Aye RW, Vallières E. Early experience with robotic lung resection results in similar operative outcomes and morbidity when compared with matched video-assisted thoracoscopic surgery cases. *Ann Thorac Surg.* 2012; 93: 1598–605.

5. Park BJ, Flores RM, VW Rusch. Robotic assistance for video-assisted thoracic surgical lobectomy: technique and initial results. *J Thorac Cardiovasc Surg.* 2006; 131: 54–9.

6. Park BJ, Melfi F, Mussi A et al. Robotic lobectomy for non-small cell lung cancer (NSCLC): long-term oncologic results. *J Thorac Cardiovasc Surg.* 2012; 143: 383–9.

7. Cerfolio RJ, Bryant AS, Skylizard L, Minnich DJ. Initial consecutive experience of completely portal robotic pulmonary resection with 4 arms. *J Thorac Cardiovasc Surg.* 2011; 142: 740–6.

8. Veronesi G, Galetta D, Maisonneuve P et al. Four-arm robotic lobectomy for the treatment of early-stage lung cancer. *J Thorac Cardiovasc Surg.* 2010; 140: 19–25.

9. Gharagozloo F, Margolis M, Tempesta B et al. Robot-assisted lobectomy for early-stage lung cancer: report of 100 consecutive cases. *Ann Thorac Surg.* 2009; 88: 380–4.

17

Uniportal video-assisted thoracoscopic surgery (VATS)

GAETANO ROCCO

INTRODUCTION

Single-port (uniportal) video-assisted thoracoscopic surgery (VATS) represents an evolution of traditional VATS principles and, at the same time, a formidable return to the geometric configuration of classic open thoracotomies.[1–3] In a way, the uniportal concept is the center of a star system whose satellites exchange technical aspects with the other known thoracic surgical approaches (see **Figure 17.1**). The main feature of the uniportal VATS approach consists of targeting, through a caudocranial (sagittal) plane, any area of surgical interest inside the chest (see **Figure 17.2**). Two advantages result from such a perspective: (1) the procedure allows for a similar approach as is used for open surgery and (2) the reacquisition of the depth of visualization lost with conventional three-port VATS.[3] The latter is based on the

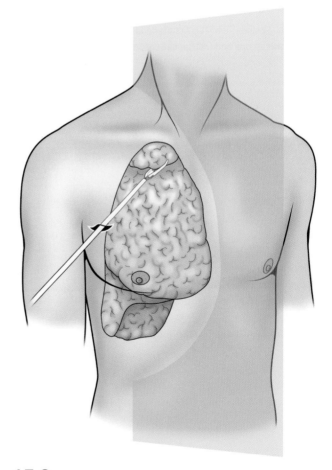

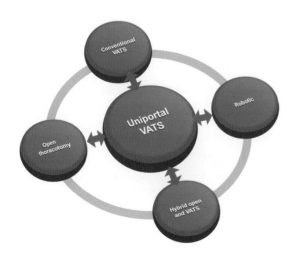

17.1 Uniportal VATS seen as the fulcrum of the armamentarium of the modern thoracic surgeon.

17.2 Caudocranial approach (i.e., sagittal plane) for uniportal VATS.

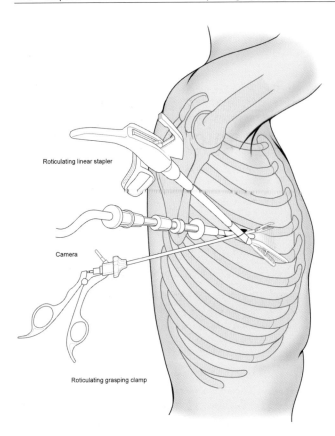

Roticulating linear stapler

Camera

Roticulating grasping clamp

17.3 Schematic of the simultaneous insertion of the videothoracoscope and instrument ensemble during uniportal VATS.

development of a transversal latero-lateral (or anteroposterior) plane, along which the operative instruments are deployed to address the target area.[3] With the current 2-D technology, the surgical maneuvers impede in-depth visualization through a centrally located videothoracoscope because of the torsion angle created by the operative instruments (see **Figure 17.3**).[3,4] As a result, traditional three-port VATS demands an extent of hand–eye coordination to overcome the geometrical obstacle originating from this torsion angle (see **Figure 17.4a**).[4] This hand–eye coordination represents an added difficulty, especially during hilar dissection during VATS lobectomy, and this has possibly undermined the more universal acceptance of the procedure, which is otherwise appealing. Conversely, in the uniportal approach, the eye "accompanies" in depth the stems of the instruments, which are deployed parallel to each other along the sagittal plane, and effectively represents an extension of the surgeon's hands (see **Figure 17.4b**).[4] At present, the similarity between open and uniportal VATS is as close as it can get. In addition, the articulated jaws or graspers can be positioned so as to avoid bite closure on the target area, which could, in turn, obstruct the in-depth view. Furthermore, the fulcrum of the operative instruments is inside the chest—at a short distance from the actual lesion. This characteristic assimilates uniportal VATS to robotic surgery; indeed, robotic surgery is considered to be the minimally invasive surgical approach that most closely duplicates the technical features of open thoracotomy (see **Figure 17.1**).

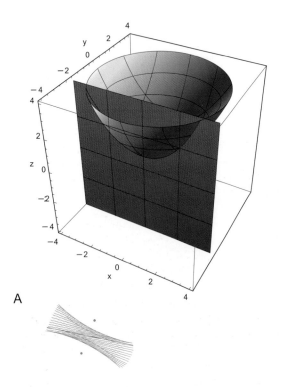

A

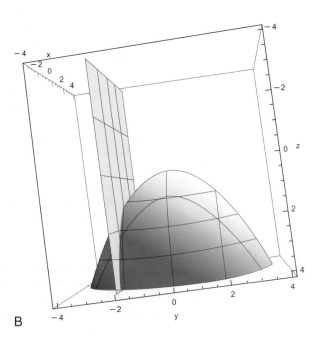

B

17.4a–b (a) The torsion angle resulting from instrument interaction along a transversal plane obstructing in-depth visualization through 2-D imaged conventional three-port VATS; (b) 2-D imaged uniportal VATS enabling improved in-depth visualization of the surgical field.

The concept of using a thoracoscope and instrumentation through the same small incision dates back to a report by Singer in 1924.[5] Uniportal VATS has since been described for sympathectomy and the diagnosis of pleural conditions.[6,7] The general consensus is that the main advantage of uniportal VATS is to provide a minimally invasive approach that can be used in conjunction with loco-regional anesthesia to fast track surgical candidates to diagnostic or therapeutic procedures.[1] In this setting, the triad one port–one intercostal–less pain seems justified, albeit that definitive evidence (i.e., a prospective, randomized trial) has yet to be published.[8,9]

PREOPERATIVE PLANNING

The technical feasibility of uniportal VATS is heavily dependent on preoperative planning of the surgical coordinates necessary to identify the location of the single incision. In this setting, the scapular angle line—that is, *longitude*—defines the distinction between anteriorly and posteriorly located incisions. The *latitude* is defined by the intercostal space at a level that must warrant sufficient distance between the single port and target lesion to avoid videothoracoscope-instrument interference.[2] Longitudinal and latitudinal coordinates usually allow for placing the incision so as to "face" the target area inside the chest. Accordingly, lesions located in the middle lobe are best approached through incisions located posterior to the scapular angle line; conversely, lesions located in the apical segment of the lower lobe are best addressed

from incisions located anterior to the scapular angle line. The intercostal space selected depends on the caudocranial level where the lesion is found in the lung. As an example, if the lesion is in the apex of the right upper lobe, an incision should be placed at the fourth or fifth intercostal space. Once the incision is made (see **Figure 17.5a**), the distribution of the surgical personnel varies so that the first surgeon and his/her assistant work from the same side, looking at the same monitor (see **Figure 17.5b**).

UNIPORTAL VATS FOR DIAGNOSTIC PURPOSES

Recurrent pleural or pericardial effusions, early empyemas, interstitial lung disease, peripheral pulmonary nodules, or ground glass opacities, as well as pleural or mediastinal masses and lymph node biopsy, are all amenable to uniportal VATS, yielding precise histological diagnosis and short hospitalizations.[2,6,10,11] Interestingly, selected awake patients can be operated on under a combination of loco-regional anesthesia and sedation.[12] Typically, an epidural catheter is positioned at the T5-6 level and a single shot of 1% Ropivacain solution (10 mg/mL diluted to 5 mg/mL, for a total dose of 15 mL = 75 mg) is administered.[12,13] In addition, the patient is given intravenous (IV) midazolam (4 mg), fentanyl (100 mcg) and propofol (0.5 mg/kg/h up to a total of 30 mg in 1 hour), along with supplemental oxygen by nasal prongs in order to maintain arterial oxygen saturation above 90%.[12,13]

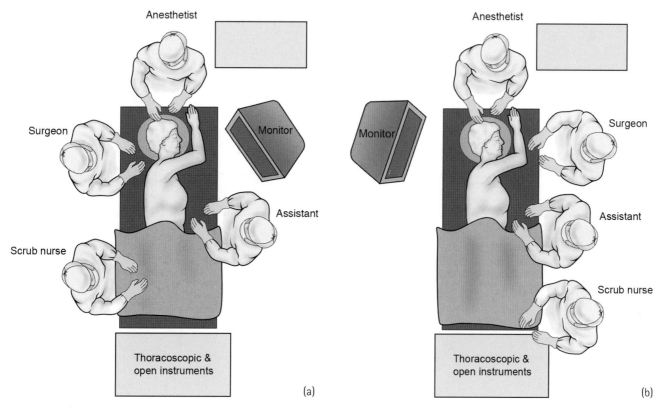

17.5a–b   Distribution of the theater personnel before the incision (a) and after the incision (b) for a uniportal VATS procedure.

SURGICAL TECHNIQUE FOR UNIPORTAL VATS FOR PLEURAL CONDITIONS

As a rule, diagnostic uniportal VATS is performed through a single 1.0–1.5 cm incision located along a virtual thoracotomy line in the fifth intercostal space, usually anterior to the scapular line if the pleural effusion occupies two-thirds or more of the chest cavity.[14] When the pleural effusion is less significant, needle probing is used to identify the most recumbent site compatible with safe performance of the procedure and convenient chest drain placement. A 24 Fr chest drain is passed through a 10 mm trocar inserted through the single incision and the pleural fluid aspirated and routinely sent for cytology. As a rule, a 5 mm trocar is then used to introduce a 5 mm 0-degree videothoracoscope to explore the posterior chest wall and the diaphragm. The trocar is removed along the stem of the videothoracoscope to gain more operative space at the incision level. Later, the videothoracoscope is tilted toward the assistant's side, and the anterior chest wall, pericardium, and diaphragm are visualized. At this point, biopsy forceps are introduced parallel to the videothoracoscope. If talc pleurodesis is needed, the insufflator is inserted parallel to the thoracoscope, which is slightly retracted to visualize the tip of the insufflators in order to better direct talc aspersion. Talc poudrage is completed by rotating the thoracoscope and insufflator ensemble to cover all areas of the chest cavity.

SURGICAL TECHNIQUE FOR UNIPORTAL VATS WEDGE RESECTION

The perfect size for single-port VATS—in line with the extreme minimally invasive philosophy behind this technique—is one fingerbreadth measured at the knuckle—that is, 2.5 cm (see **Figures 17.6 and 17.7**).[3] The intercostal space is opened flush to the superior border of the underlying rib

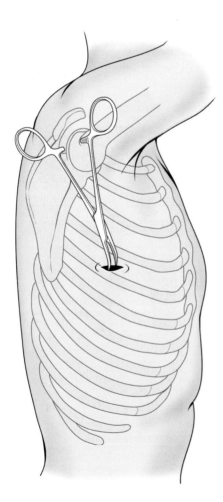

17.6   Length of the incision for uniportal VATS wedge resection.

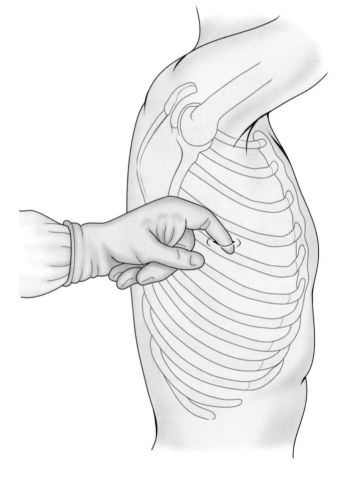

17.7   The standard length of incision has to accommodate one surgeon's fingerbreadth.

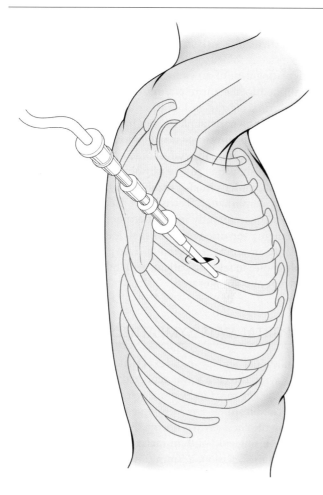

17.8 The endostapler is articulated outside the chest and inserted in the same fashion as one would insert a mediastinoscope under the pre-cervical fascia.

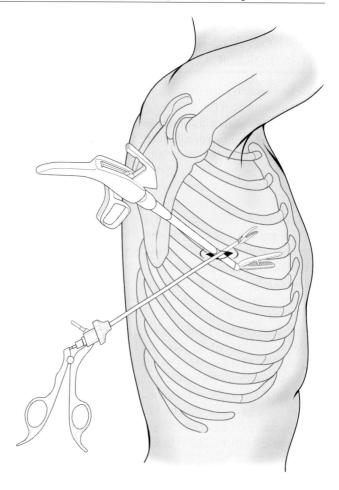

17.9 Intraoperative view of the simultaneous insertion of the videothoracoscope and instrument ensemble.

so as to allow for 1 cm lateral movements on each side. The following step is the introduction of a 0- or 30-degree 5 mm videothoracoscope without trocar, which is retracted along the thoracoscope stem.[3] Next, articulating endograspers and an endostapler are inserted to suspend and resect the pulmonary target area along a craniocaudal (sagittal) plane (see **Figures 17.8 and 17.9**). The reciprocal position of the instruments and the thoracoscope can vary during the procedure to facilitate surgical maneuvers.[3] The placement of soft tissue retractors is discouraged, to avoid subtracting room for the instruments and thoracoscope. Once the nodule is visualized or identified with an ultrasound probe,[15] the area of parenchyma containing the nodule is marked and resected (see **Figure 17.10**).

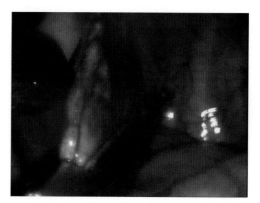

17.10 Uniportal VATS wedge resection of the lung; the endograsper is suspending the parenchyma to be resected while the endostapler is positioned at the base of the parenchyma to complete the resection.

RESULTS OF UNIPORTAL VATS FOR DIAGNOSIS AND TREATMENT OF INTRATHORACIC CONDITIONS

A 10-year study reported that uniportal VATS for the diagnosis and treatment of intrathoracic conditions was performed in up to 28% of thoracic surgical candidates.[2] Of the 644 uniportal VATS procedures, over 50% were used to diagnose pleuropericardial conditions, while 29% were needed for wedge resections. The remaining 21% of surgeries were performed for pre-thoracotomy exploration of the chest cavity, diagnosis of mediastinal masses, sympathectomy, and debridement of early stage empyemas or hemothoraces. The median operative time was 18 and 22 minutes for diagnostic uniportal VATS and wedge resection, respectively. In addition, median postprocedure chest tube duration was 4 days (range, 2–20) and 2 days (range, 0–6) for pleural effusions and wedge resections, respectively, inclusive of the day of chest drain insertion. Furthermore, the median postoperative hospitalizations were 5 and 4 days, respectively, for pleural effusions and wedge resections; these figures included the operative day. Overall, 146 pulmonary nodules were resected by uniportal VATS; the median size was 1.6 cm (range, 0.4–3.2) and the median margin from the nodule was 1.2 cm (range, 0.5–2.1). Of the 146 nodules, 69 were proven to be primary lung cancers, 77 secondary deposits from an extrathoracic cancer, and 33 benign lesions.[2]

UNIPORTAL VATS FOR PNEUMOTHORAX

One of the most appropriate indications for uniportal VATS seems to be represented by the management of pneumothorax.[3,16] The presence of a chest drain, often placed in an emergency setting, and of a usually visible target lesion (i.e., a bleb or bulla) make the single-port approach immediately feasible both under general or loco-regional anesthesia.[13] Wedge resection of the apex and apical pleurectomy or talc pleurodesis are easily accomplished through uniportal VATS using articulating instruments.[3] In particular, a scratch pad appropriately folded and cut to size can be mounted on the articulating arm of an endograsper.[16] The scratch pad can be applied to the entire circumference of the inner chest wall by rotating the endograsper arm.[3,16] The initial tear induced in the parietal pleura can be used as starting point for an apical pleurectomy using endo Kitners to elevate the parietal pleura from the endothoracic fascia.[16] Alternatively, a thorough abrasion can be easily obtained by extending the procedure, under visual control, onto the remaining chest wall and diaphragm. Likewise, any blebs or bullae can be resected concomitantly in any peripheral area of the lung by changing the orientation of the videothoracoscope and operative instrument ensemble. Talc pleurodesis is also a viable choice in selected patients with bilateral symptomatic recurrent pneumothoraces.

UNIPORTAL VATS SYMPATHECTOMY

My colleagues' and my initial experience with bilateral single access sympathectomy was reported in 2004 and updated in 2007.[17] The main indications were palmar hyperhidrosis and facial blushing. The technique consists of sequentially entering the chest cavities during the same operative session through a single 0.5–1.0 cm incision located in the axilla.[17] Through this incision, a 5 mm 0-degree videothoracoscope is inserted along with an endograsper. In our experience, the use of an articulating endograsper is preferred to be able to mobilize the lung apex as necessary. As a rule, the sympathetic chain, with its T2 and T3 ganglia, was identified and divided by means of a diathermy hook.[17] The diathermy hook is pressed against the rib; by applying low voltage electricity, the surgeon makes sure to separate the nerve endings and to laterally extend the sympathectomy for 3–5 cm to include the so-called Kuntz fibers.[17]

UNIPORTAL VATS MAJOR LUNG RESECTIONS

Gonzalez-Rivas and his colleagues from Coruña University Hospital deserve the credit for having recently expanded the indications of uniportal VATS to include major lung resections.[18,19] The authors have described the evolution of the single-port technique from multiple-port down to only two-port lobectomy.[18] Of the original uniportal VATS technique,[3] Gonzalez-Rivas and colleagues have maintained the caudocranial approach to the target structure in the lung hilum and the introduction of multiple instruments through the same incision along with the videothoracoscope, which is usually located at one edge of the incision; the full use of laterality for the surgical maneuvers; and, the insertion of the chest drain through the same incision at the end of the procedure.[18] However, the typical approach to uniportal VATS major pulmonary resection is an anterior one for all possible lobar resections and pneumonectomy,[20] with a length for the utility and operative incision, which is larger (up to 5 cm) than the one used for the classic uniportal VATS wedge resection to accommodate the extracted specimen (see **Figure 17.11**).[18] The anterior single-port incision was sufficient to ensure safe lobar resection and adequate nodal dissection, as later demonstrated in the work of other groups.[21,22] Standard open instrumentation can be used, although articulated or specifically devised instruments have also been recommended to facilitate hilar dissection. After uniportal VATS lobectomy, while the mean operative time was 154 minutes, the median duration of chest drain insertion was 2 days (range, 1–16) whereas the median length of stay in the hospital was 3 days (range, 1–14) with neither operative nor 30-day mortality.[18]

CONCLUSIONS

By 2014, virtually all routine thoracic surgical procedures could be done by uniportal VATS.[9] While the issues of feasibility and safety seem to have been solved, the jury is still out as to the results of the uniportal technique compared with those of conventional three-port VATS. It appears intuitive that conditions like pleural effusions, pneumothoraces, and hyperidrosis need to be managed through a single-port incision to fast track patients by reducing morbidity. When it comes to major resections, postoperative pain, and long-term oncologic outcomes will provide the crucial benchmark for comparison between uniportal and other surgical approaches.

REFERENCES

1. Rocco G. One-port (uniportal) video-assisted thoracic surgical resections: a clear advance. *Journal of Thoracic and Cardiovascular Surgery*. 2012; 144(3): S27–31.
2. Rocco G, Martucci N, La Manna C, Jones DR, De Luca G, La Rocca A et al. Ten-year experience on 644 patients undergoing single-port (uniportal) video-assisted thoracoscopic surgery. *Annals of Thoracic Surgery*. 2013; 96(2): 434–8.
3. Rocco G, Martin-Ucar A, Passera E. Uniportal VATS wedge pulmonary resections. *Annals of Thoracic Surgery*. 2004; 77(2): 726–8.
4. Bertolaccini L, Rocco G, Viti A, Terzi A. Geometrical characteristics of uniportal VATS. *Journal of Thoracic Disease*. 2013; 5(Suppl. 3): S214–16.
5. Moisiuc FV, Colt HG. Thoracoscopy: origins revisited. *Respiration*. 2007; 74(3): 344–55.
6. Rocco G. History and indications of uniportal pulmonary wedge resections. *Journal of Thoracic Disease*. 2013; 5(Suppl. 3): S212–13.

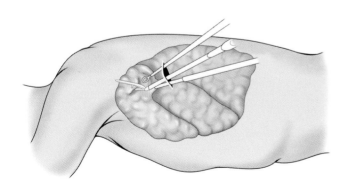

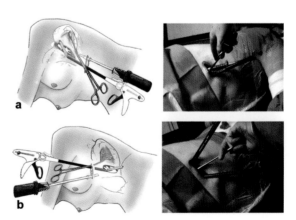

17.11 Instrument disposition for uniportal VATS lobectomy; the videothoracoscope is routinely kept at one side of the incision to facilitate surgical maneuvers.

7. Rocco G. VATS and uniportal VATS: a glimpse into the future. *Journal of Thoracic Disease.* 2013; 5(Suppl. 3): S174.

8. Atkinson JL, Fode-Thomas NC, Fealey RD, Eisenach JH, Goerss SJ. Endoscopic transthoracic limited sympathotomy for palmar-plantar hyperhidrosis: outcomes and complications during a 10-year period. *Mayo Clinic Proceedings.* 2011; 86(8): 721–9.

9. Roubelakis A, Modi A, Holman M, Casali G, Khan AZ. Uniportal video-assisted thoracic surgery: the lesser invasive thoracic surgery. *Asian Cardiovascular and Thoracic Annals.* 2014; 22(1): 72–6.

10. Rocco G, Brunelli A, Jutley R, Salati M, Scognamiglio F, La Manna C et al. Uniportal VATS for mediastinal nodal diagnosis and staging. *Interactive Cardiovascular and Thoracic Surgery.* 2006; 5(4): 430–2.

11. Rocco G, La Rocca A, La Manna C, Scognamiglio F, D'Aiuto M, Jutley R et al. Uniportal video-assisted thoracoscopic surgery pericardial window. *Journal of Thoracic and Cardiovascular Surgery.* 2006; 131(4): 921–2.

12. Rocco G, Romano V, Accardo R, Tempesta A, La Manna C, La Rocca A et al. Awake single-access (uniportal) video-assisted thoracoscopic surgery for peripheral pulmonary nodules in a complete ambulatory setting. *Annals of Thoracic Surgery.* 2010; 89(5): 1625–7.

13. Rocco G, La Rocca A, Martucci N, Accardo R. Awake single-access (uniportal) video-assisted thoracoscopic surgery for spontaneous pneumothorax. *Journal of Thoracic and Cardiovascular Surgery.* 2011; 142(4): 944–5.

14. Salati M, Brunelli A, Rocco G. Uniportal video-assisted thoracic surgery for diagnosis and treatment of intrathoracic conditions. *Thoracic Surgery Clinics.* 2008; 18(3): 305–10, vii.

15. Rocco G, Cicalese M, La Manna C, La Rocca A, Martucci N, Salvi R. Ultrasonographic identification of peripheral pulmonary nodules through uniportal video-assisted thoracic surgery. *Annals of Thoracic Surgery.* 2011; 92(3): 1099–101.

16. Jutley RS, Khalil MW, Rocco G. Uniportal vs standard three-port VATS technique for spontaneous pneumothorax: comparison of post-operative pain and residual paraesthesia. *European Journal of Cardio-thoracic Surgery.* 2005; 28(1): 43–6.

17. Rocco G. Endoscopic VATS sympathectomy: the uniportal technique. *Multimedia Manual of Cardiothoracic Surgery.* 2007; 2007(507): MMCTS.2004.000323.

18. Gonzalez-Rivas D, Paradela M, Fernandez R, Delgado M, Fieira E, Mendez L et al. Uniportal video-assisted thoracoscopic lobectomy: two years of experience. *Annals of Thoracic Surgery.* 2013; 95(2): 426–32.

19. Gonzalez-Rivas D, Fieira E, Mendez L, Garcia J. Single-port video-assisted thoracoscopic anatomic segmentectomy and right upper lobectomy. *European Journal of Cardio-thoracic Surgery.* 2012; 42(6): e169–71.

20. Gonzalez-Rivas D, Delgado M, Fieira E, Mendez L, Fernandez R, de la Torre M. Uniportal video-assisted thoracoscopic pneumonectomy. *Journal of Thoracic Disease.* 2013; 5(Suppl. 3): S246–52.

21. Tam JK, Lim KS. Total muscle-sparing uniportal video-assisted thoracoscopic surgery lobectomy. *Annals of Thoracic Surgery.* 2013; 96(6): 1982–6.

22. Wang BY, Tu CC, Liu CY, Shih CS, Liu CC. Single-incision thoracoscopic lobectomy and segmentectomy with radical lymph node dissection. *Annals of Thoracic Surgery.* 2013; 96(3): 977–82.

18

Segmentectomy

WENTAO FANG, CHENXI ZHONG, AND ZHIGANG LI

RATIONALE FOR SEGMENTECTOMY

Segmentectomy was first performed in 1939 for the treatment of benign pulmonary diseases such as bronchiectasis and tuberculosis. Shortly thereafter, anatomic pulmonary segmentectomy was also employed for primary lung cancers. The study by Jensik et al. in 1979 showed that segmentectomy was safe and feasible for selected patients with non-small-cell lung cancer (NSCLC).[1] Since then, whether segmentectomy is comparable to lobectomy has been an area of controversy.

In 1995, the Lung Cancer Study Group reported a randomized trial in stage IA (T1N0M0) NSCLC, comparing limited resection in 122 patients (82 segmentectomies and 40 wedge resections) with lobectomy in 125 patients.[2] The results showed that, compared with lobectomy, limited resection was associated with 75% increase in recurrence ($p = .02$), tripling of local recurrence ($p = .008$), 30% increase in overall death ($p = .08$), and 50% increase in cancer death ($p = .09$). The inclusion of nonanatomic wedge resections in the limited resection group tends to bias the results in favor of lobectomy and subsequent studies have not confirmed the results found in the Lung Cancer Study Group report. Thereafter, lobectomy has been considered the standard procedure for early stage NSCLC, while sublobar resection is reserved only for those who could not tolerate lobectomy due to marginal lung function and/or significant comorbidities. However, the size of the lesion to be resected should be taken into consideration, given that, in the seventh edition of the Union for International Cancer Control staging system for NSCLC, T1 disease is now subdivided into T1A (≤2 cm) and T1B (>2 cm).[3] The Lung Cancer Study Group trial included all T1N0M0 tumors of size up to 3 cm, and it did not stratify the results between T1A and T1B.[2] In a more detailed retrospective study involving 1272 stage I NSCLC patients, the 5-year cancer-specific survivals were similar after lobectomy (92.4%) or segmentectomy (96.7%) when the tumor size was ≤20 mm.[4]

It should also be noted that the Lung Cancer Study Group trial came from the time when only TNM (tumor node metastasis) staging was considered for surgical strategy. With the increased use of computed tomography (CT) screening, small peripheral ground glass opacity (GGO) lesions, which would have been difficult or even impossible to detect on routine chest X-ray, have been encountered more frequently in daily practice. These lesions often correspond to rather indolent early stage adenocarcinomas. Emerging data have shown that these GGO lesions seldom have lymphatic involvement. Compared with standard lobectomy, sublobar resection may offer equivalent local control and disease-free survival for these patients. The International Association for the Study of Lung Cancer, together with the American Thoracic Society and European Respiratory Society, recently proposed a new histologic classification system for lung adenocarcinomas, highlighted by the introduction of adenocarcinoma in situ (AIS; small adenocarcinomas <3 cm in diameter with pure lepidic growth) and minimally invasive adenocarcinoma (MIA; small solitary adenocarcinomas showing predominant lepidic growth with ≤5 mm invasion).[5] It is appropriate at this time to reevaluate the indication and selection of surgical approach and specifically, the extent of resection, incorporating both anatomical (TNM) and biological behavior (histologic subtyping) of the tumor.

Meanwhile, segmentectomy should be distinguished from nonanatomic wedge resection, as the latter was applied to up to one-third of the patients in the limited resection arm of the Lung Cancer Study Group trial.[2] The advantages of segmentectomy over nonanatomic wedge resection are at least twofold: first, by dissecting the segmental vessels and bronchus, hilar and segmental lymph nodes can be harvested systematically; second, anatomic segmentectomy also enables a deeper parenchymal resection and a safer margin for relatively centrally located lesions.

Moreover, surgical management of early stage lung cancer has changed greatly with the introduction of minimally invasive video-assisted thoracoscopic surgery (VATS).[6] In the case of lobectomy, there is a large body of evidence demonstrating that VATS is associated with decreased morbidity and mortality, shorter hospital stay, less postoperative pain, earlier return to normal life, better quality of life, and superior compliance with adjuvant therapy. VATS even has potentially better oncologic results, making it now the preferred approach over open lobectomy. When segmentectomy is performed via VATS, it is not simply to revive a procedure that previously was used infrequently but to add new meaning to "minimally invasive" lung cancer surgery to include parenchymal sparing, in addition to the other advantages of VATS noted above. For small early stage lung cancers, VATS segmentectomy may be expected to achieve excellent oncologic results with very low morbidity and mortality. A retrospective study conducted at our hospital compared clinical outcomes between VATS segmentectomy and lobectomy in patients with small-sized (≤2 cm) stage IA tumors.[7] There were no in-hospital deaths in either group. Local recurrence rates were similar after VATS segmentectomy (5.1%) and lobectomy (4.9%), and no significant difference was observed in 5-year overall or disease-free survivals following both procedures.

INDICATIONS FOR SEGMENTECTOMY

Pulmonary segmentectomy is often indicated for benign lesions such as those caused by infectious diseases, and may also be used selectively in patients with NSCLC. For small GGO lesions, segmentectomy is sometimes used to establish a histologic diagnosis, as fine needle biopsy has been shown to be quite unsatisfactory in such situations. The overall diagnostic yield from fine needle aspiration is merely 51% for GGO dominant lesions (GGO ratio >50%) and only 35% for GGO dominant lesions smaller than 10 mm. In addition, these lesions are sometimes extremely difficult to locate when using a VATS approach, making a wedge resection very challenging.

As mentioned earlier, segmentectomy has been accepted and used as an alternative for those high-risk lung cancer patients who are deemed unable to tolerate lobectomy. The potential benefits of segmentectomy compared with lobectomy are less surgical risk and better preservation of pulmonary function, while its advantage over nonanatomic wedge resection is superior oncologic outcome. Until recently, the indication for segmentectomy in good-risk patients who have no contraindication to lobectomy was not only unclear but questionable on oncologic grounds. Both tumor size and biology should be considered in determining the feasibility and efficacy of segmentectomy. Retrospective data from single or multiple institutions demonstrate that segmentectomy provides acceptable local control for tumors sized 2 cm or smaller, provided that at least a 2 cm resection margin can be achieved.[8] GGO-type tumors represent an excellent indication for segmentectomy. For pure GGO lesions corresponding to AIS or MIA, even tumors up to 3 cm

can be considered for segmentectomy. A near 100% disease-free survival rate can be expected after complete resection.[9]

Several studies have shown that width of resection margin is an important factor in maintaining local control following segmentectomy.[7] A safe margin of greater than 2 cm might be reasonable, as resection margins less than 2 cm have been shown to be associated with an increased incidence of local recurrence. Based on this concern, if a tumor is located on the edge of diseased segment or a safe resection margin cannot be guaranteed intraoperatively, multiple segmental resections or lobectomy should be performed.

For lung cancer patients, preoperative staging should be completed to confirm the absence of nodal (mediastinal or hilar) disease. Small tumors, especially those appearing on CT to be air-containing lesions, are associated with a lower likelihood for lymphatic spread, which is another reason why they are excellent candidates for segmental resection. Still, careful intraoperative exploration of hilar and mediastinal lymph nodes should be performed to exclude occult metastases and ensure the appropriateness of segmentectomy. Conversion to standard lobectomy is indicated when a frozen section of a mediastinal or hilar lymph node demonstrates the presence of metastatic disease. Segmentectomy should be oncologically more effective than nonanatomic wedge resection, since it includes dissection of intersegmental, intralobar, and interlobar lymph nodes.

While anatomically less lung parenchyma is resected by segmentectomy than lobectomy, it does not necessarily result in a similar amount of pulmonary function preserved. This is affected by multiple factors, including the number, location, and quality of the segment resected. Resecting more than three segments has been shown to leave only 0.1 L of forced expiratory volume in 1 second in the remaining lobe. Recognizing this, basal segmentectomy of the lower lobes with preservation only of the superior segment, though technically feasible, is seldom indicated.

GENERAL STRATEGY FOR SEGMENTECTOMY

Technically, all segments can be approached surgically. The superior segments of the lower lobes, the lingular segment and the upper division of the left upper lobe, and posterior segment of the right upper lobe, in decreasing order of frequency, are the most common segmentectomies performed. Other individual segmental resections, such as upper lobe superior or anterior segmentectomy, are feasible but less commonly performed. Basal segmentectomy is seldom indicated, as it saves very little pulmonary function of the remaining lower lobe.

Segmentectomy can be performed thorough standard lateral thoracotomy or via a VATS approach. Compared with thoracoscopic lobectomy, VATS has been applied to anatomic segmentectomy only recently. Technically, thoracoscopic segmentectomy is considered to be more difficult than thoracoscopic lobectomy. Thoracic surgeons should be familiar with the three-dimensional anatomical relationship of pulmonary segments to accomplish a segmentectomy successfully. Still, it has been proven to be safe and oncologically effective. No matter whether via an open or minimally invasive approach, it is imperative to make certain that standard dissection and oncologic principles are not compromised.

Open segmentectomies are often approached through a lateral thoracotomy via the fifth intercostal space. In performing a minimally invasive thoracoscopic segmentectomy, a standard three- or four-hole approach, with the major utility port in the fourth or fifth intercostal space, is the usual technique. The entire chest cavity should first be inspected to rule out signs of unexpected advanced disease, such as pleural dissemination or concomitant additional pulmonary nodules. Except for high-risk patients who cannot tolerate lobectomy, mediastinal or hilar nodal involvement should always lead to conversion to standard lobectomy, so as to ensure lymphatic clearance. Usually, the tumor should be palpated to confirm that segmentectomy is the correct procedure to ensure an adequate resection margin; otherwise, a bi-segmentectomy or lobectomy would be a better choice.

During segmentectomy, the segmental pulmonary veins, arteries, and bronchus are dissected and stapled separately. Thoracoscopic segmentectomy usually begins with identification and dissection of the segmental vein. Subsequently, the bronchus or the artery is divided, depending on the segment to be resected. Alternatively, the arterial branches can be identified and mobilized before the segmental veins are divided, but the more logical approach takes the segmental vein first. Some authors stated that this might minimize engorgement of the segment and facilitate further maneuvering, but in our experience, this has not been the case. Mobilizing arterial branches to the posterior segment of the upper lobes or the apical segment of the lower lobes often requires dissection of the major fissure. In the major fissure, the main pulmonary artery can be exposed, demonstrating its continuation into the lower lobe. On the right side, the lower lobe superior segmental branch can be identified at the posterior part of the major fissure. The posterior ascending and the middle lobe branches originate opposite each other, and go, respectively, to the posterior segment of the upper lobe and the middle lobe.

On the left side, the pulmonary artery crosses superiorly above the left main bronchus to become the most posterior structure in the hilum. The apicoposterior and anterior segmental branches are located anteriorly and superiorly. A separate posterior segmental branch is often found posteriorly on the main pulmonary artery, just at or above the major fissure. In the major fissure, the lingular branches, directed anteriorly, and the superior segment branch, posteriorly, are located across from each other on the continuation of the pulmonary artery. The surgeon must be mindful of the high variability in pulmonary artery branching, and carefully identify and confirm each branch before ligation.

In performing VATS segmentectomy, the pulmonary vessels are usually divided using endostaplers or endo-clips, with or without the help of energetic devices such as a Harmonic scalpel. After vascular division, the segmental

bronchus is then identified and divided with an endostapler, or divided sharply and closed with interrupted absorbable sutures. The segmental bronchus is first clamped and the lung inflated before stapling for further confirmation of the correct anatomic location. Alternatively, a bronchoscopy can be helpful to confirm the correct segmental bronchus has been identified.

Division of the intersegmental plane is sometimes the most challenging part of a segmentectomy. Selected jet ventilation in the diseased segmental bronchus may help delineate the correct plane.[10] In our experience, identification of the intersegmental plane can be achieved by repeated ventilation of the ipsilateral lung after the segmental bronchus is clamped. The first several puffs will probably serve to delineate the parenchyma aerated by that bronchus. Due to the large degree of intersegmental cross-ventilation through collateral pores of Kohn, it may be helpful to inflate the entire lung, clamp the segmental bronchus, and then collapse the lung while observing the delineation between residually inflated and actively deflating lung. In addition, the divided vascular and bronchial structures can be used as landmarks to guide this process. There are two ways to divide the segmental parenchyma: via the so-called open division or with the use of a stapling device. The advantage of open division with electrocautery or simply by "stripping" the intersegmental plane using the venous supply as a guide, is greater preservation of lung volume. However, this technique is associated with increased risk of air leak and oozing from the raw surface of the lung, which could be problematic after operation, though both the air leak and bleeding usually stop spontaneously in a short period if the correct plane has been entered. Staple division results in a pneumostatic separation of the intersegmental plane, minimizing the troublesome issue of air leak, but this comes at the expense of more volume loss, as the visceral pleural layers are drawn together during the act of stapling. The intersegmental plane is stapled according to the inflation–deflation line and at least a 2 cm parenchymal resection margin should be guaranteed in segmentectomy for malignant diseases. When using staplers to divide the intersegmental plane, care should be taken to ensure they are placed exactly in the right position so as to avoid inadvertently stapling the adjacent segmental vein or bronchus. This may result in engorgement or atelectasis and repeated infection of the remaining lobe. Inflation of the remaining lung after the stapler is approximated but not yet fired is often helpful in avoiding inadvertent injury of the adjacent segmental bronchus.

SPECIFIC SEGMENTAL RESECTIONS

Upper division segmentectomy of the left upper lobe

This segmentectomy begins with the dissection of the anterior hilum. After the upper division branches of the left superior pulmonary vein are divided (see **Figure 18.1**), the upper division bronchus, located directly behind the pulmonary vein, is readily exposed (see **Figure 18.2**). Under thoracoscopy, this can easily be visualized. It is then divided with an endostapler, after the location of the lingular segment bronchus is confirmed. Alternatively, the anterior and apical pulmonary artery branches can be exposed and dissected first. This may also facilitate passing of endostapler through the bronchus during VATS segmentectomy (see **Figure 18.3**). As described earlier, there is usually a posterior arterial branch located just at or above the major fissure. This can be dissected either anteriorly after the segmental bronchus is divided, or posteriorly from the major fissure (see **Figure 18.4**). Segmentectomy is then completed with division of the intersegmental plane, as previously described. In case of a fully developed major fissure, fixation of the remaining lingular segment to the left lower lobe is advisable to prevent torsion of this segment.

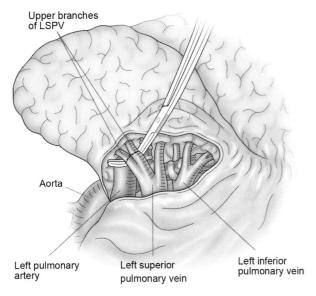

18.1 The upper division branches of the left superior pulmonary vein are divided.

Notes: LSPV, left superior pulmonary vein.

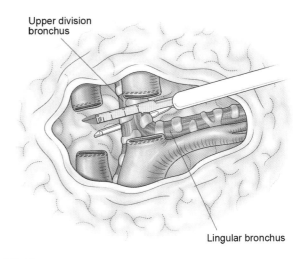

18.2 The upper division bronchus of the left upper lobe is exposed and stapled, sparing the lingular bronchus.

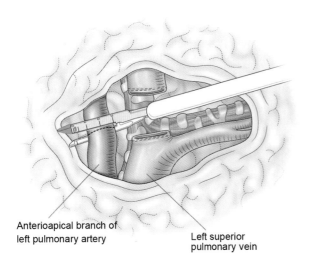

18.3 The anterior and apical pulmonary artery branches are divided and stapled.

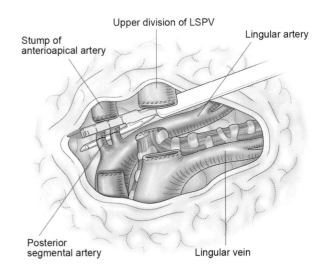

18.4 The posterior segmental artery is exposed and stapled.

Notes: LSPV, left superior pulmonary vein.

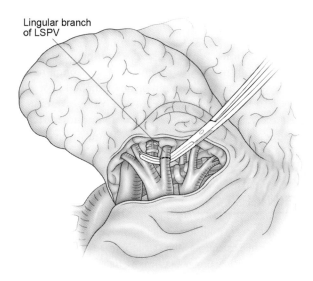

18.5 The lingular branch of the left superior pulmonary vein is exposed.

Notes: LSPV, left superior pulmonary vein.

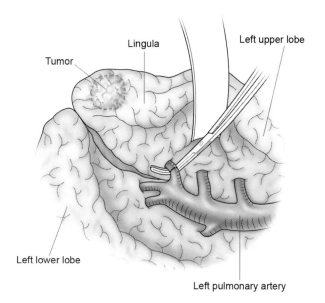

18.6 The lingular branches of the left pulmonary artery are exposed after the major fissure is opened.

Left upper lobe lingular segmentectomy

Resection of the left lingular segment is somewhat similar to right middle lobectomy. The lung is retracted posteriorly, and the hilar pleura is incised to expose the lingular branch of the superior pulmonary vein (see **Figure 18.5**). After the lingular vein is divided, dissection of the lingular bronchus can be undertaken at its bifurcation from the left upper lobe bronchus. The major fissure is then opened, beginning anteriorly, to expose the lingular branches of the pulmonary artery (see **Figure 18.6**). There are usually two branches that supply this segment that originate either separately side by side or from one single stem at the anterior end of the pulmonary artery before it continues on to the left lower lobe. Division of the intersegmental plane starts from the hilum anteriorly to the midline of the major fissure posteriorly, with stapling devices, after this plane is identified and confirmed.

Superior segmentectomy of the lower lobes

Removal of the lower lobe superior segment is often initiated with dissection of the pulmonary artery in the major fissure. The superior segment branch can be approached directly if the major fissure is well developed. Otherwise, the posterior portion of the major fissure can be opened and divided with a stapler. Once this is done, the segmental artery can be isolated and divided (see **Figure 18.7**). This will provide excellent exposure to the superior segment bronchus, which runs deep to the artery. The superior segment vein can be identified as the uppermost separate tributary running into the inferior pulmonary vein, and can be approached after opening the hilar pleura posteriorly (see **Figure 18.8**).

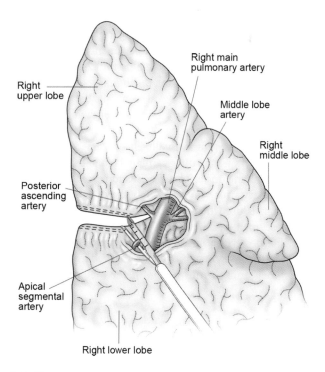

18.7 The apical segment artery of the right lower lobe is divided and stapled after the posterior portion of the major fissure is developed.

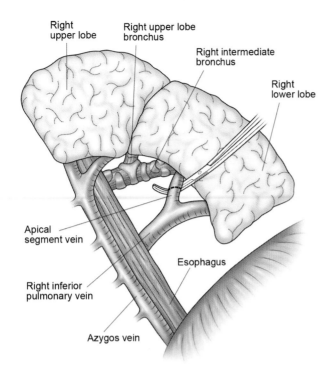

Right upper lobe
Right upper lobe bronchus
Right intermediate bronchus
Right lower lobe
Apical segment vein
Esophagus
Right inferior pulmonary vein
Azygos vein

18.8 The apical segmental vein of the right lower lobe is identified as the upper most separate tributary running into the inferior pulmonary vein.

Right upper lobe segmentectomies

Individual segmental resections of the right upper lobe are technically more demanding. Apical segment resection begins by opening the hilar pleura adjacent to the azygous vein. The apical branch of the anterior pulmonary artery trunk is identified and divided. The apical segmental bronchus is then approached posteriorly and dissected after dividing the right posterior bronchial artery branch. The apical segment branch of the pulmonary vein is usually encompassed in the staple line when dividing the intersegmental plane using staplers.

In performing posterior segmentectomy, related branches of pulmonary artery and vein can be exposed and divided in the major fissure when opened. Alternatively, the bronchus to this segment can be tracked along the right upper lobe bronchus posteriorly and distally, dissected first, and divided.

The anterior segment is often approached from the medial aspect, beginning with incision of the mediastinal pleura along the hilum. The anterior segmental vein is then exposed, ligated, and divided. Care must be taken not to compromise other branches of the superior pulmonary vein. The anterior segmental pulmonary artery, likewise, can be identified as it branches from the anterior trunk. The horizontal fissure is then opened to expose the anterior segmental bronchus posterior to the pulmonary vein. When the bronchus is divided and its distal stump retracted up and forward, the intersegmental plane can be stapled without injury to the remaining hilar structures.

REFERENCES

1. Jensik RJ, Faber LP, Kittle CF. Segmental resection for bronchogenic carcinoma. *Ann Thorac Surg.* 1979; 28: 475–83.
2. Lung Cancer Study Group, Ginsberg RJ, Rubinstein LV. Randomized trial of lobectomy versus limited resection for T1N0 non-small cell lung cancer. *Ann Thorac Surg.* 1995; 60: 615–22.
3. Sobin LH, Gospadarowicz MK, Wittekind C (eds). (2009) *TNM Classification of Malignant Tumours*, 7th edition. Oxford, UK. Wiley-Blackwell. pp. 138–47.
4. Okada M, Nishio W, Sakamoto T et al. Effect of tumor size on prognosis in patients with non-small cell lung cancer: the role of segmentectomy as a type of lesser resection. *J Thorac Cardiovasc Surg.* 2011; 129: 87–93.
5. Travis WD, Brambilla E, Noguchi M et al. International Association for the Study of Lung Cancer/American Thoracic Society/European Respiratory Society international multidisciplinary classification of lung adenocarcinoma. *J Thorac Oncol.* 2011; 6: 244–85.
6. Onaitis MW, Petersen RP, Balderson SS et al. Thoracoscopic lobectomy is a safe and versatile procedure: experience with 500 consecutive patients. *Ann Surg.* 2006; 244: 420–5.
7. Zhong C, Fang W, Mao T et al. Comparison of thoracoscopic segmentectomy and thoracoscopic lobectomy for small-sized stage IA lung cancer. *Ann Thorac Surg.* 2012; 94: 362–7.
8. Swanson SJ. Video-assisted thoracic surgery segmentectomy: the future of surgery for lung cancer? *Ann Thorac Surg.* 2010; 89: S2096–7.
9. Smith CB, Swanson SJ, Mhango G et al. Survival after segmentectomy and wedge resection in stage I non-small-cell lung cancer. *J Thorac Oncol.* 2013; 8: 73–8.
10. Okada M, Mimura T, Ikegaki J et al. A novel video-assisted anatomic segmentectomy technique: selective segmental inflation via bronchofiberoptic jet followed by cautery cutting. *J Thorac Cardiovasc Surg.* 2007; 133: 753–8.

19

Combined bronchial and pulmonary artery sleeve resections

ABEL GÓMEZ-CARO AND LAUREANO MOLINS

INTRODUCTION

In centrally located lung cancer, resection is frequently associated with massive parenchyma extirpation and high rates of morbidity and mortality. Pneumonectomy (PN) has a significantly greater incidence of mortality compared with lesser pulmonary resections and results in substantial declines in lung function and quality of life, precluding adjuvant treatments or further lung resection. In the search for alternative strategies, sleeve lobectomy (SL) has become the gold standard for centrally located lung tumors that otherwise would not be resectable by simple lobectomy. Sparing lung function may allow patients with very limited lung function and those treated with chemoradiotherapy to overcome prohibitive surgical risk and be candidates for intervention. About 10%–14% of all lung tumors and nearly 60% of central tumors may be amenable to sleeve resection with combined pulmonary artery (PA) and bronchial reconstruction techniques. Several thoracic surgery teams have developed an aggressive parenchyma-sparing policy, with a reported PN:SL ratio of at least 1:3, decreasing the PN rate to 5%.

Management of centrally located non-small-cell lung cancer may combine various surgical techniques to avoid PN without compromising the long-term oncological results. Surgical options include PA reconstruction or replacement, alleviation of bronchial mismatch, and in some cases, resection of more than one lobe and airway anastomoses in segmental bronchi.

PREOPERATIVE EVALUATION

Preoperative assessment of potential surgical candidates includes taking the clinical history; performing a physical examination; standard blood tests; chest radiographic analysis; bronchoscopy; and thoracic, abdominal, and cerebral computed tomography scan, as well as 18F-fluoro-D-glucose positron emission tomography. Suggestion of ipsilateral mediastinal lymph node metastases (N2 disease) requires histologic confirmation using the most appropriate invasive methods; if confirmed, neoadjuvant treatment is needed before the candidate can be considered for resection, based on response to therapy. Functional tolerance of PN must be established before SL can be attempted. In very carefully selected cases with high probability of complete resection without neoadjuvant therapy, the SL strategy could be considered even with poor lung function that precludes PN. The predicted postoperative forced expiratory volume in 1 second is estimated either with the 19-segment method, which multiplies baseline function by the percentage of lung segments that remain after resection, or with isotopic scanning where needed.

ANESTHESIA

Systematic bronchoscopy is done before surgery and repeated in theater by the operating surgeon to assess intraluminal tumor extension from segmental or main bronchi in order to macroscopically anticipate the potential site of anastomoses. If laser or mechanical resection is needed, rigid bronchoscopy should be performed. Double-lumen tube intubation is preferred over a bronchial blocker in these operations. If extended SL (lobe plus one or two segments) is carried out, jet ventilation may be employed if desaturation occurs during the procedure and is useful to identify the segmental plane if extended SL is needed. Epidural catheterization is routinely used, if not contraindicated, to improve postoperative care and physiotherapy. Antibiotics may be started if there is evidence of ongoing infection; if not, regular prophylactic protocol is followed.

SURGICAL TECHNIQUE

Posterolateral thoracotomy with or without serratus dorsi muscle sparing is the preferred approach. Comfortable and excellent exposure is essential for technically demanding procedures such as bronchial and PA reconstruction. If vascular reconstruction is required positioning the clamps also requires adequate exposure and precise surgical technique, following accepted vascular principles in order to avoid postoperative anastomotic complications.

1. During thoracotomy, if bronchovascular reconstruction is planned, an intercostal flap including the parietal pleural is harvested and preserved before any rib spreading, to be used to cover the anastomosis and to separate the PA and bronchial sutures. An exploration

of the thoracic cavity is completed before performing any irreversible steps in the procedure. Technical and oncological feasibility of the parenchymal-sparing technique is evaluated preoperatively in the outpatient clinic, with the final decision made by the surgeon during the procedure.

Left-side double-sleeve resection

PA reconstruction—lateral resection, end-to-end anastomoses, patch reconstruction, or replacement—is most frequent on the left side (60%–70% of cases), mainly because of the short left main PA and its relation to the mainstem bronchus. Lateral PA resection, patches, or end-to-end anastomoses may be performed on the right side, but replacement by

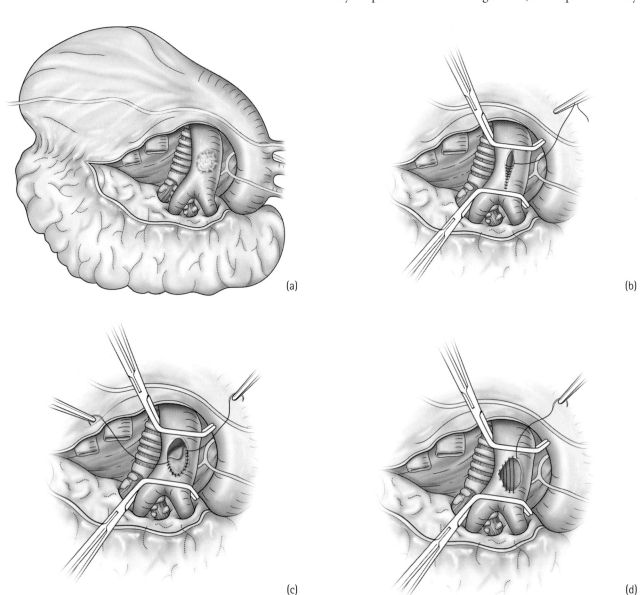

(a)

(b)

(c)

(d)

19.1a–d (a) Tumor involving the PA branch at take-off; (b) Tangential suture (with clamps); (c) tangential inverted suture (with clamps); (d) patch for PA reconstruction (with clamps).

conduit is rarely required. In general, lateral resection is performed when the branch take-off or less than 25% of the PA caliber is tumor involved. Although lateral clamping is the simplest procedure, systemic heparin and central clamping are safer and more easily achieve an adequate artery caliber and healthy anastomosis. When more than about a third of the artery is involved, reconstruction should be performed using either a patch (autologous or bovine pericardium, autologous vein, etc.) or end-to-end anastomosis, depending on the surgeon's experience or preferences. In our experience, end-to-end anastomosis tends to be preferred because it is simple, quick, and easily performed along with the bronchial sleeve resection. A long artery segment invaded by the tumor may require PA replacement with biological conduit (see **Figure 19.1**).

2. On either side, when the PA is involved, intrapericardial control of the main PA should be achieved. Lymph nodes of the aortopulmonary window may complicate the main artery and bronchus dissection. The superior pulmonary vein is encircled intra- or extrapericardially and divided, allowing full exposure of the proximal PA and better exposing the artery to permit optimal clamp placement for proximal control. The left main PA is clamped as far proximally as possible, with distal control achieved by clamping the artery within the fissure.

   Fused fissures and inflamed tissues are frequent in these cases, and may result in persistent postoperative air leak that can cause concern regarding anastomotic failure. Careful surgical technique is required to avoid this problem, allowing the surgeon to sleep better at night. These central tumors usually extend throughout the fissure and may involve the superior segment of the lower lobe. When an extended SL (lobe plus one or two segments) is required, the intersegmental plane must be identified, with or without the use of jet ventilation in order to complete the anatomic segmentectomy.

The segments involved are removed *en bloc* with the lobe by developing the intersegmental plane, usually with electrocautery and scissors. We avoid the use of mechanical staplers in order to optimize reexpansion of remnant lung in an attempt to fill the entire thoracic cavity. Once the specimen is removed, the raw surface of the lung parenchyma is checked for bleeding and air leaks and may be reinforced with pulmonary sealant (see **Figure 19.2**).

3. When the PA segment is involved by the tumor (<25% of all sleeve reconstructions), it must be resected *en bloc* with the specimen. Systemic heparin sodium (5000 units/h) is intravenously administered before any PA clamping and not reversed during operation. Soft atraumatic vascular clamps are used on the proximal PA (Satinsky curve clamp) and distal (bulldog or femoral clamp) disease-free segments of the PA. Proximal clamp placement must provide sufficient space to allow for construction of the anastomosis. If an extensive PA reconstruction is planned, division of the ligamentum arteriosum prior to placing the proximal clamp greatly facilitates mobilization of the proximal portion of the PA, leaving enough space for the anastomosis. The phrenic and vagus nerves and, specifically, the left recurrent laryngeal nerve should be identified and preserved, if possible, but there should be no hesitation in sacrificing these structures if doing so will permit a complete resection. Ideally, one should avoid taking both the phrenic and the vagus nerves. If resection of the vagus nerve is necessary, one should try to take it distal to the take-off of the left recurrent laryngeal nerve. To avoid injuries after both anastomoses are complete, systematic mediastinal dissection with *en bloc* lymph node resection of station 7 is performed before the reconstruction and clamping (see **Figure 19.3**).

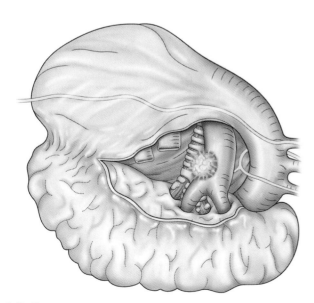

19.2 Before clamping.

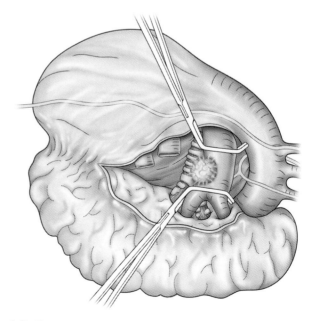

19.3 Clamping of left PA.

4. Once the fissure is opened, the PA and bronchus are circumferentially divided using a scalpel. The distal bronchial opening is always close to the origin of segmental bronchi (if not oncologically precluded); a trapezium-like section, involving less of the distal bronchus wall, is recommended to minimize the tension of the anastomoses (see **Figure 19.4a**). Bronchial and arterial margins are assessed routinely by frozen section to ensure R0 resection. The bronchial anastomosis should be performed prior to the vascular reconstruction. *En bloc* resection of the tumor, lung parenchyma, and PA is performed. The PA section should be placed at least 5 mm distal to the proximal clamp to allow for construction of the anastomosis (see **Figure 19.4b**).

5. Avoidance of excessive tension on both the bronchial and vascular anastomoses is essential and should not be a problem. Bronchial tension can be decreased with several maneuvers, including the routine use of division of the inferior pulmonary ligament. A U-shaped pericardial release incision around the inferior pulmonary vein allows for an extra 1–2 cm and causes no additional morbidity. If necessary for better exposure, rolled packing can be placed at the bottom of the thoracic cavity to lift the lower lobe and facilitate anastomosis. If tension tears the tissues (damaged by inflammation, previous chemoradiotherapy, fissure

dissection, etc.) during PA anastomoses, a PN or PA replacement should be considered at this stage. Completion PN in a reoperation has a high incidence of complications and mortality. Bronchus manipulation must be very gentle to protect the tissues and bronchial blood supply. Use of the electrocautery of surrounding tissues should be avoided and bronchial arteries must be spared during dissection and lymphadenectomy.

The bronchial anastomosis is begun on the membranous aspect using an absorbable monofilament 4-0 suture with a double needle. The initial stitch is placed in the middle of the membranous portion of the distal bronchial segment and main bronchus to avoid torsion of the bronchial axis, with running suture leading away from the surgeon until the cartilaginous junction. The other needle is used at this point and membranous portion is completed. Corner stitches are placed and tension of the running suture is checked and tied with the knots outside. The first stitch (again, double needle and absorbable monofilament 4-0) is placed at the middle of the cartilaginous portion and the anastomosis is completed by interrupted stitches every 2–3 mm, alternating sides to avoid telescoping. The cartilage sutures should encompass the entire bronchial wall and involve approximately a 3–4 mm length of bronchus to ensure a solid anastomosis (see **Figure 19.5**). Extremely large caliber discrepancies

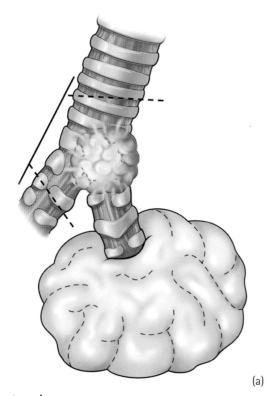

(a)

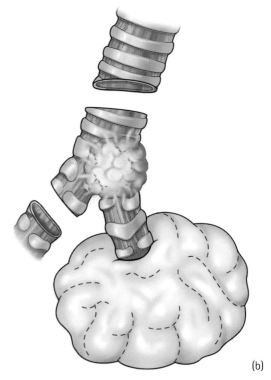

(b)

19.4a–b Trapezoid bronchial cut. (a) Lines show the cuts to be made in the mainstem bronchus. The proximal cut is made first to assure complete resection. The cut is made between cartilage rings to assure a clean edge to facilitate the anastomosis. The distal cut is made beyond the lesion but as close as possible so as to preserve distal length. (b) The sleeve of bronchus has been resected. Note the clean bronchial edges that allow for an accurate anastomosis with the best chance of healing.

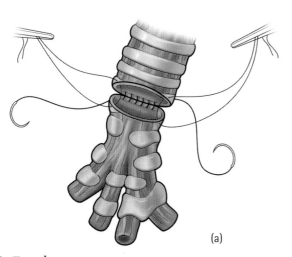
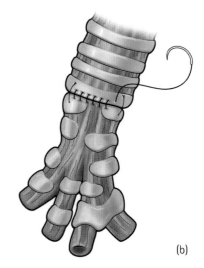

19.5a–b Detail of the suture technique used for the anastomosis. (a) membranous face; (b) cartilaginous face.

between the proximal and distal bronchial segments are uncommon in routine SL, but are a frequent finding in extended SL. These can be reconciled by narrowing the proximal stump by passing 4-0 absorbable monofilament sutures through the membranous portion and adjacent ends of the stump's cartilaginous ring to achieve plication and substantial narrowing. We prefer this small variation over telescopic suture, which could result in healing problems during the postoperative course. In general, we consider this hybrid anastomosis (running and interrupted suture) quicker, safe, and equivalent to using all interrupted sutures to adjust the caliber discrepancies. *After* filling the thoracic cavity with saline, we routinely check the suture line for air leaks using a peak airway pressure of 30 mmHg, and we perform bronchoscopy prior to leaving theater. Any air leak on the bronchial suture should be reinforced using interrupted sutures, ignoring the needle hole leaks. If the bronchial anastomosis is not perfect, this is the moment to redo or correct. A few hours or days later, correction will be more difficult for both the surgeon and the patient (see **Figure 19.5a and b**).

6. PA anastomoses are performed using systemic and local heparin to avoid in situ thrombosis. If distal clamping is very tight after bronchial anastomosis, the clamp can be removed and the inferior pulmonary vein can be clamped discontinuously to avoid intralobar venous thrombosis. After 20 minutes, when the bulldog clamp is removed, there is very little backflow due to the surgical atelectasis, and distal anastomosis can be carried out without further maneuvers.

   End-to-end anastomosis is started using a nonabsorbable monofilament 5-0 to 6-0 running suture, beginning in front of the principal surgeon and at the bottom of the anastomosis. The PA is then refilled by local heparin-saline and the proximal clamp is partially opened to allow 25%–50% flow reperfusion,

while a gentle ventilation of the spared lobe quickly enhances lung perfusion. The anastomosic suture is tied after air purge during the low-flow reperfusion, and the clamp is totally removed after 10–15 minutes. A pedicled intercostal flap is used to wrap the bronchial anastomoses and split vascular anastomoses, especially in the case of a double sleeve, large caliber discrepancies, and neoadjuvant chemoradiotherapy. Close surveillance of the spared lobe is needed during closing to detect thrombosis or any other technical complications. As the PA is a low-pressure system, a small arterial leak may go unnoticed in the operating room. In our experience, postoperative anticoagulation or antiplatelet therapy is not needed for PA reconstruction when using biological materials; we start it only when indicated because of associated diseases (see **Figure 19.6**).

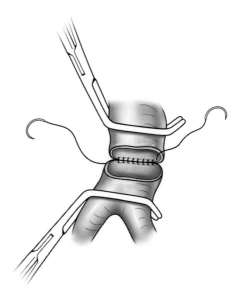

19.6 Arterial anastomosis.

Right-side double-sleeve resection

The basic and most frequent location for this resection is tumor at the origin of the right upper lobe bronchus. If an associated PA reconstruction is required, usually a lateral resection suffices and only very rarely is an end-to-end anastomosis necessary. On the right side, dissection of the mainstem should be performed from the posterior aspect, and subcarinal lymphadenectomy is performed prior to division of the bronchus. The bronchus intermedius dissection is performed from behind and the bronchus encircles just proximal to the take-off of the bronchus to the superior segment of the lower lobe. Once the artery to the superior segment is identified, the posterior fissure is dissected and the adequacy of resection is confirmed. In general, the superior pulmonary vein control is less challenging because the central tumors are more distant.

Dissection and division of the superior pulmonary vein, preserving the middle lobe vein, allows excellent exposure of the artery for clamping. Azygos vein division can facilitate access to paratracheal and hilar lymph nodes and facilitate exposure of the right main PA and main bronchus. On the right side, intrapericardial control of the PA is recommended to allow adequate room for clamping if the central tumor is close to the right PA origin. Essentially, PA reconstruction is performed as described for the left side, using systemic and local heparin (see **Figures 19.7 through 19.9**).

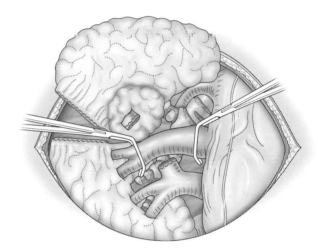

19.7 Right-side arterial control.

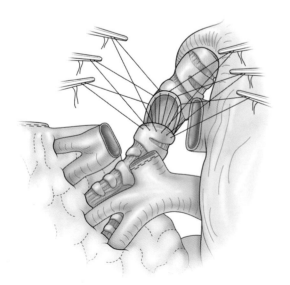

19.8 Bronchial anastomosis right side.

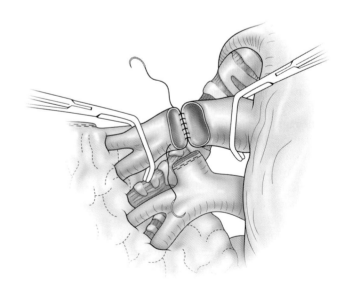

19.9 PA anastomosis right side.

Lower sleeve resection

This type of resection is performed when the upper lobe is spared of a central tumor involving the bronchial division. On the right side, the tumor usually involves the bronchus intermedius and extends proximal to upper lobe bronchus take-off. If the upper lobe bronchus or membranous portion close to the main bronchus is involved, the upper lobe bronchus can be anastomosed in the right main bronchus after middle and lower lobe resection. On the left side, lower lobe tumors involving the mainstem bronchus proximal to the upper lobe take-off but sparing the upper lobe are candidates for sparing the upper lobe and anastomosing it to the left mainstem bronchus. These procedures, at times, may be more complex than regular SL, due to caliber discrepancies and frequently associated vascular resection.

Caliber discrepancies between proximal and distal bronchial stumps can be corrected by reducing the proximal stump, inserting 5-0 absorbable monofilament stitches through the membranous portion and adjacent ends of the stump's cartilaginous ring to achieve plication and substantial narrowing. Correcting the size discrepancy allows the anastomosis to be carried out as previously described. A continuous running 4-0 or 5-0 absorbable monofilament suture is placed from the cartilaginous membranous juncture to the middle of the cartilaginous wall. The rest of the anastomosis is performed using interrupted sutures. Each suture is inserted through the full thickness of the bronchial wall, and all knots are tied outside. During these anastomoses, torsion should be carefully prevented due to the weakness of the lobar bronchus and the direction change of the bronchial axis (see **Figures 19.10 through 19.12**).

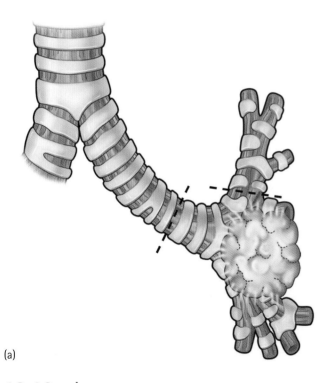

(a)

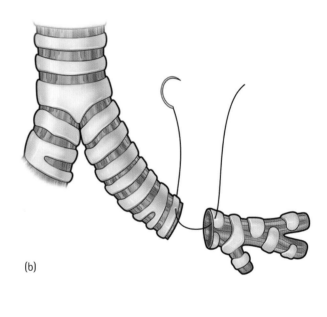

(b)

19.10a–b Lower SL in right side.

Note: Right lower lobe

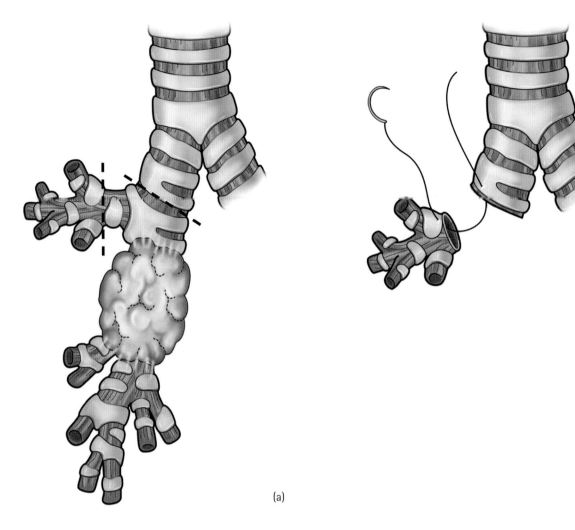

(a)

(b)

19.11a–b Lower resection left side.

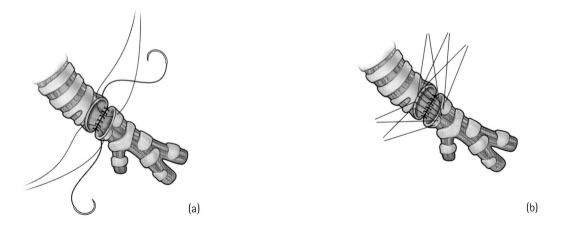

(a)

(b)

19.12a–b (a) The anastomosis is begun by approximating the membranous portion of the bronchus using a continuous suture.
(b) Following completion of the membranous portion interrupted sutures are used to complete the cartilaginous portion of the anastomosis.

Pulmonary artery reconstruction by patch

Patches are a widely accepted option for PA reconstruction when tumor involvement is lateral and exceeds 50% of the caliber, or when a direct suture is either impossible or may result in a very narrow artery. All cases amenable to patch reconstruction can be easily performed using an end-to-end anastomosis with an excellent result. Following resection of the bronchus and the PA, the arterial reconstruction, whether patch or end to end, should be done prior to bronchial reconstruction to avoid prolonged clamp time. Biological patch (autologous or heterologous pericardium or pulmonary vein) can be used and results in a very low rate of thrombosis and excellent performance. Autologous patch material from the pericardium should be harvested anterior to phrenic nerve. Bovine pericardial tissue is another available option that requires no extra preparation time. The patch should be oval shaped and as small as possible to maintain artery tension, and suturing should be done with double-armed, monofilament 6-0 running suture. Double landmarks at the superior and inferior edges are sutured first to maintain the tension during suturing. A small needle minimizes tissue injury and needle hole bleeding, and is essential if a pericardial patch is used. The suture starts from the top of the artery and is tied using the landmark stitches. This technique is not always easy, for several reasons; poor malleability of the pericardial patch is probably the most important of these, because oozing may result during the first hours after surgery and a small leak may go unnoticed, with serious consequences (see **Figure 19.13**).

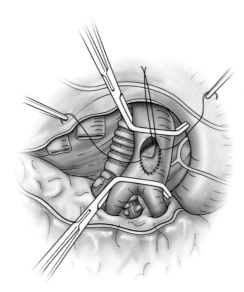

19.13 Following resection of a portion of the circumference of the PA a pericardial patch is placed to close the defect so as to prevent any narrowing of the artery.

Pulmonary artery reconstruction by conduit

The last option to avoid PN is PA replacement using biological material. In our opinion, the use of other foreign materials should be avoided due to the high incidence of thrombosis and infection and the need for lifelong anticoagulation. Options such as autologous or cryopreserved allograft arteries or bovine pericardium have been suggested to replace the artery and avoid PN.

In general, anastomoses are performed using systemic and local heparinization to avoid in situ thrombosis, as described earlier. The selected conduit should be constructed to the right caliber and size. Similar caliber to the proximal stump artery should be achieved, with a smooth decrease in caliber to match the distal stump. The conduit length must be as short as possible to prevent kinking but avoid tension. Traction sutures inserted in stumps should be gently pulled to reduce tension when tying anastomotic sutures, and can also be used as landmarks to prevent artery twist. Running nonabsorbable 6-0 monofilament suture is used for the end-to-end distal anastomosis. Usually, this reconstruction is the more technically demanding due to the proximity to the origin of the superior segment arterial branch and should be performed first. The distal clamp should be removed for this anastomosis, and the corresponding pulmonary vein can be intermittently clamped if there is a major backflow. Most often the backflow after 15–25 minutes is very low because of the surgical atelectasis of the lobe, and the vascular anastomosis can be carried out without any distal clamp. After completion, the anastomosis is checked for any leak with heparin-saline before starting the proximal anastomosis. Sometimes the superior segment branch is very close to the anastomosis and should be divided to avoid unexpected thrombosis starting at that point. After division, the proximal anastomosis is performed checking for correct size, length, and absence of twisting in the conduit.

Once the anastomoses are completed, backflow is allowed before the distal anastomosis is tied, allowing air drainage from the circuit. The proximal clamp is then removed and a close surveillance of the spared lobe is carried out during the preclosure protocol to detect thrombosis, color change, or any other technical complications such as small arterial leaks.

Once the lobe is reinflated, the arterial conduit should be carefully assessed. If the conduit is too large, unexpected kinking can occur at the anastomosis of the implanted conduit and lead to thrombotic or ischemic complications.

After both anastomoses are complete, we routinely cover the bronchial anastomosis, especially when the patient has undergone induction chemoradiotherapy, or if there was a large caliber discrepancy between the proximal and distal bronchial segments.

The use of biological conduits and autologous or bovine pericardium is an intriguing option, primarily because of some presumed resistance to infection and avoidance of the need for anticoagulation or antiplatelet therapy beyond the first month—and it may be the only option when an unexpected PA replacement is needed. Cryopreserved allografts

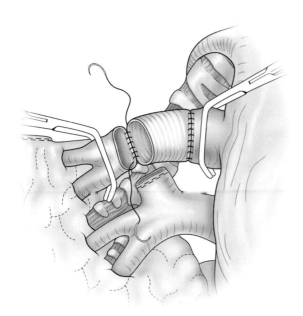

19.14 Right-side conduit.

have the added advantage of better malleability and adaptability to any kind of intrathoracic vessel, particularly in intrapulmonary PA replacement. The thrombosis risk with a nonbiological prosthesis mandates lifelong anticoagulation, and the grafts are not completely resistant to infection. In addition, these conduits lack malleability and adaptability compared with biological grafts, especially cryopreserved allografts, and are therefore less appropriate for most intrapulmonary PA replacement.

Overall, PA reconstruction has proven to be a reliable and useful operation for parenchymal sparing in central tumors and, compared with PN, offers better immediate and long-term results in terms of complications, survival, quality of life, and substantially better respiratory function (see **Figure 19.14**).

POSTOPERATIVE CARE

All patients should spend at least the first 24 hours in the intensive care unit. Postoperative care starts in theater, with a bronchoscopy to check the anastomoses, clean the airway, and take samples. In some cases, surgical revision will be mandatory to avoid short- and long-term healing problems that will be impossible to resolve later. Bronchoscopy should be repeated in the event of sputum retention during the first postoperative days. Some patients may require a mini- or regular tracheotomy for airway cleaning. Pain relief and physiotherapy to avoid lung infection and cleaning of airways to prevent anastomosis failure are essential. A routine bronchoscopy is recommended on the seventh postoperative day, or before discharge, whichever comes first. In general, clear dehiscence should be surgically treated by completion PN,

especially if a vascular reconstruction also has been done. Early dehiscence within 5 days is frequently related to technical issues and reanastomosis can be attempted, although the reported success rate is low.

PA reconstructions (lateral resection, end-to-end anastomoses, and patch or conduit replacement) usually do not require anticoagulation or antiplatelet agents if biological patch material or conduits are used. Postoperative low-molecular weight heparin is routinely used, as in other pulmonary resections. Low steroid doses are recommended to reduce secretion retention and atelectasis, facilitate parenchymal reexpansion, and minimize the risk of dehiscence and granuloma formation.

Daily chest X-ray is performed, even in absence of clinical symptoms. Any clinical or radiological change should be taken seriously, and angio-CT scan may reveal any patency problems. Partial artery thrombosis can be treated with heparinization if there is no associated pulmonary infarction and the pulmonary vein is unobstructed. In our experience artery thrombosis after reconstruction typically leads to completion PN.

Finally, any residual pleural space following extended SL can be managed by adjusting the duration of drainage (depending on clinical and radiological follow-up) and level of suction (gentle during mechanical ventilation and interrupted as soon as possible).

OUTCOMES

Sleeve lobectomies can be performed safely and should be considered in all central tumors in lieu of PN. Induction chemoradiotherapy does not preclude these parenchymal-sparing techniques; indeed, it may even minimize postoperative complications. There is valuable information in the literature concerning the safety of SL after chemoradiotherapy showing no increased incidence of anastomosic complications, morbidity, and mortality.

Sleeve resection to spare well-functioning pulmonary parenchyma is an excellent strategy to reduce postoperative complications and respiratory impairment and improve quality of life and length of survival. In addition, there is reliable information about higher rates of adjuvant therapy completion with sleeve resection patients compared with PN patients.

PA reconstruction for lung-sparing surgery is an infrequent procedure. Among the experienced centers, SL represents less than 14% of all pulmonary resections for lung cancer and only 25% of these require pulmonary reconstruction. Most vascular reconstructions are tangential patches, followed by end-to-end anastomoses, and, finally, very few PA replacements by various types of conduits. Prosthetic and biological substitutes have been used for this purpose. Prosthetic materials, including polytetrafluoroethylene and Gore-Tex, are readily available, easy to use, and can be adjusted perfectly to the PA diameter. The main issues related to their use are the high frequency of early thrombosis, potential infectious complications (especially in the case of double-sleeve resection), and the need for long-term anticoagulation therapy. Biological substitutes—arterial or venous allografts or autologous pericardium conduits—have been used with satisfactory results, and homologous saphenous or pulmonary veins are possible alternatives. However, the latter require time-consuming intraoperative procedures, produce variable outcomes related to graft shrinkage or twisting, and are not always available. Cryopreserved arterial allografts offer substantial advantages: availability in tissue banks, bacteriologic safety, and no need for anticoagulation therapy. Their ability to resist infection has been demonstrated by vascular surgeons in the routine use of cryopreserved allografts to address aortic prosthesis infection.

The most-feared complications after SL are bronchial fistulae (<3%). Most often, if the anastomosis is still viable, these should be conservatively managed with antibiotics, thoracic drain, etc. Flap cover may offer an excellent solution without extra morbidity during the first surgery, if performed well. Any air leakage should be monitored for cessation or increase, and bronchoscopy will reveal whether the healing process is satisfactory or PN completion is needed. Mortality after failed spared lobe resection is very high, with technical issues that can be impossible to resolve.

When PA reconstruction is associated with SL, any bleeding (drain or hemoptysis) should be taken seriously to rule out PA fistulae. Reoperation to assess the anastomosis and flap health is recommended over waiting for massive hemoptysis.

Early PA thrombosis is rare and usually linked to technical pitfalls. An angio-CT scan allows for the identification of PA flow and will inform the surgical decision. Conservative treatment with heparin should not be attempted and PN completion is mandatory in these cases.

Our experience suggests that PA reconstruction after extended resection of centrally located lung tumors is feasible with acceptable morbidity. These procedures could avoid PN in selected patients. Long-term follow-up seems to make clear the beneficial effects of avoiding PNs with similar local recurrence rates and extended long-term survival. Therefore, increased use of these techniques may be desirable and, despite their complexity, promote better surgical results.

FURTHER READING

Berthet JP, Boada M, Paradela M, Molins L, Matecki S, Marty-Ané CH, Gómez-Caro A. Pulmonary sleeve resection in locally advanced lung cancer using cryopreserved allograft for pulmonary artery replacement. *Journal of Thoracic and Cardiovascular Surgery*. 2013; 146(5): 1191–7.

Berthet JP, Paradela M, Jimenez MJ, Molins L, Gómez-Caro A. Extended sleeve lobectomy: one more step toward avoiding pneumonectomy in centrally located lung cancer. *Annals of Thoracic Surgery*. 2013; 96(6): 1988–97.

Fadel E, Yildizeli B, Chapelier AR, Dicenta I, Mussot S, Dartevelle PG. Sleeve lobectomy for bronchogenic cancers: factors affecting survival. *Annals of Thoracic Surgery*. 2002; 74(3): 851–8; discussion 858–9.

Gómez-Caro A, Boada M, Reguart N, Viñolas N, Casas F, Molins L. Sleeve lobectomy after induction chemoradiotherapy. *European Journal of Cardio-thoracic Surgery*. 2012; 41(5): 1052–8.

Gómez-Caro A, Garcia S, Reguart N, Cladellas E, Arguis P, Sanchez M, Gimferrer JM. Determining the appropriate sleeve lobectomy versus pneumonectomy ratio in central non-small cell lung cancer patients: an audit of an aggressive policy of pneumonectomy avoidance. *European Journal of Cardio-thoracic Surgery*. 2011; 39(3): 352–9.

Gómez-Caro A, Martinez E, Rodríguez A, Sanchez D, Martorell J, Gimferrer JM, Haverich A, Harringer W, Pomar JL, Macchiarini P. Cryopreserved arterial allograft reconstruction after excision of thoracic malignancies. *Annals of Thoracic Surgery*. 2008; 86(6): 1753–61; discussion 61.

Venuta F, Ciccone AM, Anile M, Ibrahim M, De Giacomo T, Coloni GF et al. Reconstruction of the pulmonary artery for lung cancer: long-term results. *Journal of Thoracic and Cardiovascular Surgery*. 2009; 138(5): 1185–91.

20

Superior sulcus tumors

VALERIE W. RUSCH

INTRODUCTION

Pancoast tumors, properly known as "superior sulcus non-small-cell lung carcinomas," are particularly challenging to manage because they invade vital structures at the thoracic inlet, including the brachial plexus, subclavian vessels, and spine. Originally described in 1924 by Henry K. Pancoast,[1] a radiologist at the University of Pennsylvania, this subset of non-small-cell lung carcinomas (NSCLCs) was considered inoperable and thus fatal, until the late 1950s. In 1956, Chardack and MacCallum described treatment of a Pancoast tumor by *en bloc* resection of the right upper lobe, chest wall, and nerve roots, followed by adjuvant radiotherapy leading to a 5-year survival. In 1961, Shaw and colleagues reported a patient who became symptom free after 30 Gy of radiotherapy and went on to a successful resection.[2] This treatment strategy was then applied to 18 more patients with good local control and long-term survival. Based on this experience, the standard approach to these challenging tumors involved induction radiotherapy, and *en bloc* resection and this became the standard of care for Pancoast tumors over the next 40 years. In 1994 and 2000, the largest published retrospective studies from Memorial Sloan Kettering Cancer Center defined negative prognostic factors including mediastinal lymph node metastases, vertebral and subclavian vessel involvement, and incomplete resection.[3,4] Complete (R0) resection was achieved in only 64% of patients with T3N0 disease and 39% of patients with T4N0 disease, and locoregional relapse was the most common site of tumor recurrence. Anatomic lobectomy was associated with a better outcome than sublobar resection and intraoperative brachytherapy did not enhance overall survival. This retrospective study documented the results of "standard" treatment for resectable Pancoast tumors and emphasized the need for novel therapeutic approaches.

As combined modality therapy was increasingly being used for other locally advanced NSCLC subsets (e.g., Stage IIIA [N2] disease), induction chemoradiotherapy followed by surgical resection was studied in a large North American prospective multi-institutional Phase II trial (T3, T4 N0-1, M0 Pancoast tumors.[5] A total of 110 eligible patients received induction therapy using two cycles of cisplatin and etoposide chemotherapy along with 45 Gy of concurrent radiotherapy. Patients with stable or responding disease then underwent thoracotomy and resection followed by two more cycles of chemotherapy. Induction therapy was well tolerated, allowing 75% of enrolled patients to go on to thoracotomy. R0 resection was achieved in 91% of T3 and 87% of T4 tumors. Approximately one-third of patients had no residual viable disease, one-third had minimal residual microscopic disease, and one-third had gross residual tumor on final pathology. Patients who had a R0 resection experienced 53% survival at 5 years and the most common sites of relapse were distant rather than locoregional. Additional studies, including a

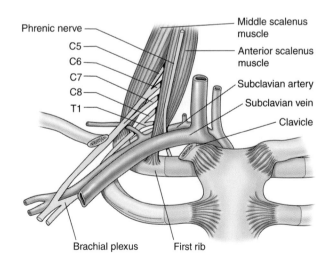

20.1 The key anatomical landmarks that affect resection of Pancoast tumors.

multicenter prospective clinical trial from Japan, confirm these results and establish induction chemoradiotherapy and surgery as standard care for resectable Pancoast tumors.[6]

ANATOMY OF PANCOAST TUMORS

The pulmonary sulcus is defined as the posterior costovertebral gutter, and extends from the first rib to the diaphragm. The superior pulmonary sulcus encompasses the most apical aspect of the gutter. Surgical resection of superior sulcus tumors requires an understanding of the complex anatomy of this area and of the thoracic inlet, the superior aperture of the thoracic cavity bounded by the first thoracic vertebra (T1) posteriorly, the first ribs laterally, and the superior border of the manubrium anteriorly.

The thoracic inlet can be separated into three compartments based on the insertion of the anterior and middle scalene muscles on the first rib and the posterior scalene muscle on the second rib (see **Figure 20.1**). The anterior compartment is located in front of the anterior scalene muscle and contains the sternocleidomastoid and omohyoid muscles, and the subclavian and internal jugular veins and their branches. Tumors in this location invade the first intercostal nerve and first rib, resulting in pain in the upper and anterior chest wall. The middle compartment, located between the anterior and middle scalene muscles, includes the subclavian artery, the trunks of the brachial plexus, and the phrenic nerve that lies on the anterior surface of the anterior scalene muscle. Tumors found in the middle compartment invade the anterior scalene muscle, the phrenic nerve, the subclavian artery, and the trunks of the brachial plexus and middle scalene muscle and present with signs and symptoms related to direct compression or infiltration of the brachial plexus, such as pain and paresthesias in the ulnar distribution. The posterior compartment contains the nerve roots of the brachial plexus, the stellate ganglion and the vertebral column, the posterior aspect of the subclavian artery, the paravertebral sympathetic chain, and the prevertebral musculature. Tumors in this area invade the transverse processes and vertebral bodies, as well as the spinal foramina, and are associated with Horner's syndrome (ptosis, miosis, and anhydrosis); brachial plexopathy (weakness of the intrinsic muscles of the hand); paralysis of the flexors of the digits resembling a "claw hand"; and diminished sensation over the medial side of the arm, forearm, and hand (related to C8 and T1 destruction).

INITIAL ASSESSMENT

Superior sulcus masses associated with chest and arm pain may be due to other pathologic processes, including infectious conditions like tuberculosis or malignant disorders such as lymphoma, primary chest wall tumors, or metastatic disease from other neoplasms. A diagnosis of NSCLC must be confirmed before starting treatment and is best obtained by transthoracic fine needle aspiration.

The extent of disease should be evaluated before surgical resection is considered. Computed tomography (CT) of the chest and upper abdomen, including the adrenals, with intravenous contrast, whole body fluorodeoxyglucose positron emission tomography (FDG-PET), and brain magnetic resonance imaging (MRI) should be done to exclude metastatic disease in extrathoracic sites and the mediastinum. Pancoast tumors are, by definition, at least Stage IIB lung cancers, with a significant risk of mediastinal nodal involvement. Further staging by endobronchial ultrasound and/ or mediastinoscopy should be considered if CT or positron emission tomography suggest N2 or N3 disease.

Due to the anatomical location, MRI is essential to defining tumor extent and resectability.[7] The brachial plexus, subclavian vessels, vertebrae, and neural foramina are best visualized by MRI. T1 nerve root resection is well tolerated, but resection of the C8 nerve root and lower trunk of the brachial plexus generally leads to permanent loss of intrinsic hand and lower arm function. Radiographic evidence of spine involvement, or neurologic symptoms and signs suggestive of nerve root or brachial plexus pathology, necessitates joint evaluation of these patients by a thoracic surgeon and a spine surgeon. At Memorial Sloan Kettering, the resection of Pancoast tumors is planned jointly by the thoracic surgeon and spine neurosurgeon.[8]

SURGICAL APPROACHES TO RESECTION

The goal of any cancer operation is complete resection of the tumor with pathologically negative margins (R0 resection). Due to their unique location, R0 resection of Pancoast tumors is technically challenging, and includes upper lobectomy, involved chest wall with or without the subclavian vessels, portions of the vertebral column and T1 nerve root, and dorsal sympathetic chain. Pancoast tumors may be approached through an extended high posterolateral thoracotomy incision (Paulson's incision) or through an anterior approach popularized by Dartevelle.

Posterior approach

The patient is positioned in the lateral decubitus position but rotated slightly anteriorly, to provide exposure to the paravertebral region (see **Figure 20.2**). A standard posterolateral thoracotomy is performed in the fifth intercostal space and the chest explored to make sure that there is no evidence of metastatic disease. If the tumor appears resectable, the incision is extended superiorly to the base of the neck following a line midway between the spinous process and the edge of the scapula. Extension of the incision anteriorly around the anterior border of the scapula up toward the axilla, as originally popularized by Masaoka and colleagues in Japan, facilitates elevation of the scapula and enhances exposure.[9] The scapula is elevated away from the chest wall with either a rib-spreading retractor (see **Figure 20.3**) or internal mammary retractor with good visualization of the apex of the chest (see **Figure 20.4**). The scalene muscles are detached from the first and second ribs and the first rib exposed. Involved ribs

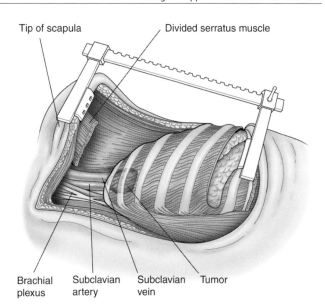

20.3   The fifth intercostal space is entered for exploration. If the initial exploration indicates that the lesion is resectable, the incision is extended up to the C7 prominence, and the trapezius muscle and the rhomboids are divided. The Finochietto retractor is positioned with the inferior blade resting on the sixth rib and the superior blade under the tip of the scapula. The retractor is cranked open, elevating the scapula off of the chest wall. The maneuver exposes the apex of the chest. The posterior scalene is divided with cautery.

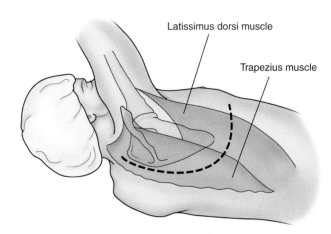

20.2   The posterior approach that is used for the resection of most Pancoast tumors. The patient is placed in the lateral decubitus position, rotated slightly anteriorly. The posterolateral thoracotomy incision is extended to the base of the neck. Anteriorly, the incision can contour the anterior aspect of the scapula up to the midaxillary line to facilitate elevation of the scapula.

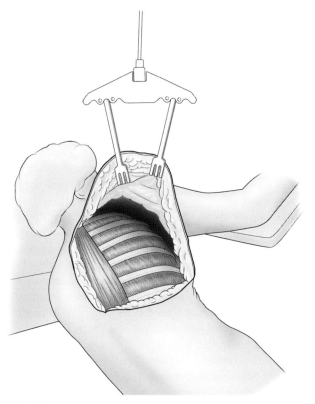

20.4   An alternate approach to gain exposure to the first rib and superior sulcus is to use an internal mammary retractor to elevate the tip of the scapula.

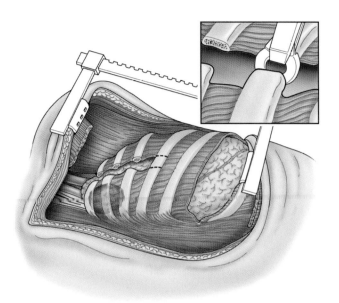

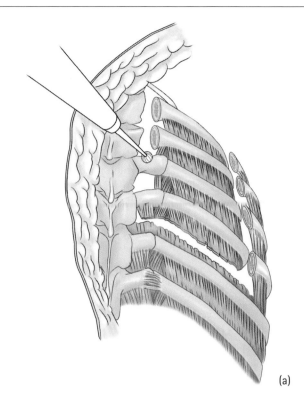

(a)

20.5 The middle and anterior scalenes are dissected off the first rib in the subperiosteal plane, recognizing that the brachial plexus and subclavian vessels lie superior to the first rib. Dividing the scalene muscles is made easier by placing the first rib on downward traction. The anterior scalene muscle inserts on the first rib between the subclavian vein and artery. Initially, the first rib is dissected in the subperiosteal plane. This step frees the rib of the medial and anterior scalenes without risking injury to the brachial plexus or phrenic nerve. The exact location to begin the chest wall resection is determined by observing the extent of tumor from within the chest. Usually, a 4 cm margin is necessary. The dissection begins at the inferior margin and progresses superiorly. It is easiest to divide the rib to be taken at the anterior aspect first and then divide posteriorly. The inferior ribs are taken working up toward the first rib.

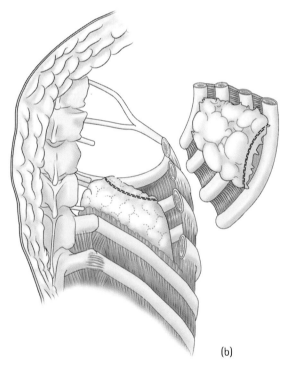

(b)

are divided anteriorly to allow for a 4 cm margin away from the tumor (see **Figure 20.5**). Care is taken to visualize and control the intercostal neurovascular bundle. To facilitate the posterior dissection, the erector spinae muscles are retracted off the thoracic spine, allowing for visualization of the costovertebral gutter. To provide an adequate posterior margin, the transverse processes and rib heads are usually resected *en bloc* (see **Figure 20.6a and b**). This approach ensures a better posterior margin of resection than does disarticulation of the rib heads from the transverse processes. Intercostal nerves are meticulously ligated before division to prevent leak of cerebrospinal fluid. Bleeding near the neural foramina is carefully controlled with bipolar electrocautery. The T1 nerve root is examined for tumor involvement and ligated if necessary. Frozen sections are used liberally during the operation to determine the necessary extent of resection. After the chest wall resection is completed, the detached chest wall is allowed to fall into the chest cavity and an upper lobectomy and mediastinal lymph node dissection is completed in the

20.6a–b Completion of posterior component of chest wall resection. The paraspinal muscles are dissected to expose the junction of the laminae and transverse processes. The drill is used to resect the transverse processes distal to the pedicle to expose the neural foramen (a). For a Type C resection, the laminae, facet joints, and pedicles are resected to expose the lateral dura. The chest wall is then pushed forward, and the nerve roots are ligated at the distal neural foramen. *En bloc* chest wall and tumor resection are accomplished (b).

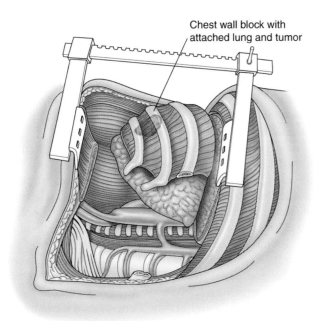

Chest wall block with attached lung and tumor

20.7 Once the chest wall has been divided and freed, it is left in continuity with the lung, and a formal lobectomy with lymph node dissection is performed.

standard fashion (see **Figure 20.7**). Reconstruction of the chest wall is not necessary unless the defect created is larger than the first three ribs, in which case the angle of the scapula can herniate into the chest cavity, causing pain and impaired shoulder motion. If a chest wall reconstruction is needed, a 2 mm thick PTFE patch is sutured to the margins of resection.

Tumors involving the vertebral bodies and epidural region

Vertebral body invasion by Pancoast tumors is not a con-traindication to surgical resection. The development of better instrumentation for spine stabilization now permits a more aggressive approach to these tumors. Currently, with multimodality therapy, T4 lesions with vertebral body or epidural extension can be considered for resection with cura-tive intent.[10] At Memorial Sloan Kettering, spine MRI images are used to divide tumors into four classes, A–D, based on the degree of spinal column and neural tube involvement. Class A and B tumors are T3 lesions that are amenable to complete R0 resection. Class A tumors involve only the periosteum of the vertebral bodies and Class B tumors are limited to the rib heads and distal neural foramina. Class C and D tumors are T4 lesions that are not amenable to *en bloc* resection but can still be completely resected. Class C tumors extend into the neural foramina, have limited or no vertebral body involvement but do have unilateral epidural compression. Class D tumors involve the vertebral column, either the vertebral body and/or lamina with or without epidural compression. Class A, B, and some Class C tumors

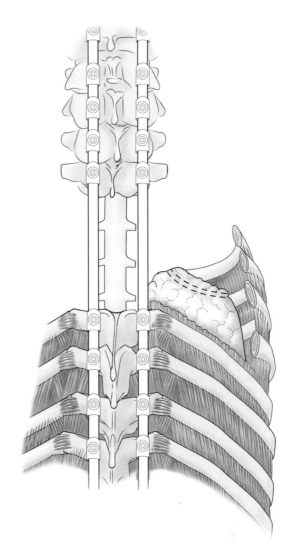

20.8 Illustration depicting a posterolateral transpedicular approach for a Class D tumor with bilateral posterior segmental fixation.

can be approached through a posterolateral thoracotomy. A high-speed drill is used to remove involved vertebral bodies. The posterior longitudinal ligament is removed and provides a margin on the anterior dura. The disc spaces adjacent to the tumor are exenterated to aid in spinal fixation. Anterior reconstruction alone is sufficient for resections of one to two vertebral bodies. Autologous bone from the iliac crest or nondiseased rib, allograft fibula, or methyl methacrylate with Steinman pins can all be used for reconstruction.

Class D tumors that involve the posterior elements (spinous process, laminae, and pedicles) are resected through a combined anterior/posterior approach. Patients are posi-tioned prone and a posterior midline incision made. The involved areas of the spinous process, laminae, and pedicles are resected. Epidural tumor is dissected off the dura and a multilevel resection of affected nerve roots done. Posterior fixation is accomplished in order to maintain coronal and sagittal stability (see **Figure 20.8**). If soft tissue over the reconstruction is inadequate, muscle flap rotation by a plastic surgeon can be done to reduce the risk of skin breakdown and infection of the spine hardware. Once the posterior resection and reconstruction is complete, the incision is closed, the patient turned to the lateral decubitus position, a posterolateral thoracotomy performed, and the lung and chest wall resection completed.

Anterior approaches

Pancoast tumors that involve the subclavian vessels are best approached anteriorly. Although several different approaches have been described, the anterior transcervical approach, originally described by Dartevelle and modified by others, is considered the standard approach for this subset of Pancoast tumors.[11,12,13]

The patient is positioned supine with the neck hyperextended and the head turned to the opposite side of the lesion. An inverted L-shaped incision is carried down the anterior border of the sternocleidomastoid muscle and extended below the clavicle to the level of the second intercostal space, then turned horizontally following a parallel line below the clavicle to the deltopectoral groove (see **Figure 20.9**). The sternal attachment of the sternocleidomastoid is divided,

along with the insertion of the pectoralis major. A myocutaneous flap is then folded laterally, exposing the thoracic inlet. The scalene fat pad is excised and sent for frozen section to determine lymph node involvement. If the tumor is deemed resectable, the upper part of the manubrium is divided and the incision carried into the second intercostal space via an L-shaped incision. The involved section of the subclavian vein is resected but not reconstructed (collateral venous flow around this area being sufficient).

Next, the anterior scalene muscle is divided at its insertion into the first rib. The phrenic nerve is identified and preserved. The subclavian artery is resected and reconstructed with an 8 or 10 mm PTFE graft (see **Figure 20.10**). The middle scalene muscle is detached above its insertion on the first rib to expose the C8 and T1 nerve roots. These are dissected in a lateral-to-medial direction up to the confluence of the lower trunk and brachial plexus. The ipsilateral prevertebral muscles and paravertebral sympathetic chain and stellate ganglion are then resected off the anterior aspect of the vertebral bodies of C7 and T1. The T1 nerve root is commonly divided just lateral to the T1 intervertebral foramen.

Attention is now given to the chest wall resection. The anterolateral arch of the first rib is divided at the costochondral junction and the second rib is divided at its midpoint. The third rib is dissected on its superior border, in a posterior

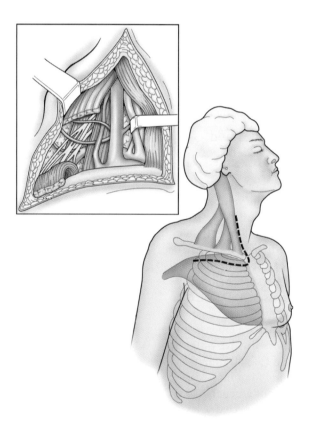

20.9 An L-shaped incision is made along the medial border of the sternocleidomastoid down to the sternal notch and then out along the inferior border of the clavicle to the deltopectoral groove. The subcutaneous tissues are divided, exposing the clavicle, manubrium, and first and second ribs. The manubrium is divided using an L-shaped incision and is elevated along with the attached clavicle to expose the subclavian vessels and brachial plexus.

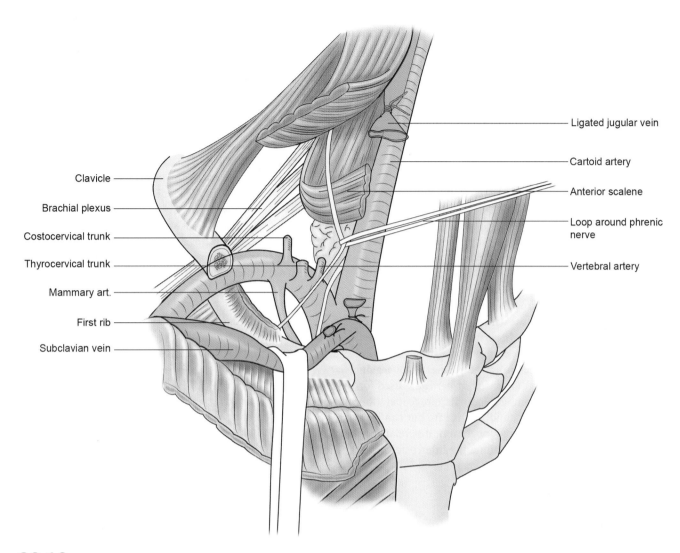

20.10   The phrenic nerve and subclavian vein are retracted. The anterior scalene muscle is divided to expose the subclavian artery.

Labels on figure: Ligated jugular vein; Cartoid artery; Anterior scalene; Loop around phrenic nerve; Vertebral artery; Clavicle; Brachial plexus; Costocervical trunk; Thyrocervical trunk; Mammary art.; First rib; Subclavian vein

direction, toward the costovertebral angle and the first two through three ribs are disarticulated from the transverse processes. From this cavity, an upper lobectomy is completed. If exposure for the lobectomy and chest wall resection is inadequate, the anterior incision is closed and the patient turned to the lateral decubitus position. The remainder of the resection can then be performed via a posterolateral thoracotomy incision.

ANESTHETIC CONSIDERATIONS

Lung isolation with a left-sided double-lumen tube or right-sided bronchial blocker can be used depending on surgeon and anesthesiologist experience and preference. Intra-arterial blood pressure monitoring and large bore intravenous (IV) access should be placed on the side opposite the tumor. If

there is potential for superior vena cava or innominate vein resection, venous access via the femoral region or lower extremity is advisable. Central venous catheterization on the nonoperative side may be considered if adequate IV access is unavailable or if the patient's cardiovascular reserve is limited and perioperative use of vasoactive agents is anticipated. If spine stabilization is required, it is our practice at Memorial Sloan Kettering to employ somatosensory and motor evoked potential monitoring intraoperatively. The cause of reversible changes during surgery is often compression of segmental spinal arteries or spinal cord hypoperfusion, and can lead to spinal cord infarction unless corrected, usually by pharmacologically elevating the patient's blood pressure. During neurophysiologic monitoring, it is customary to employ minimal inhalation anesthesia balanced by total intravenous anesthetic regimens with Bispectral brain monitoring when feasible. Since lobectomy or pneumonectomy is needed in some cases, judicious fluid administration is recommended due to the risk of postoperative pulmonary edema and respiratory distress in these patients. Initiating good pain control intraoperatively, usually via an epidural catheter, aids postoperative mobilization and pulmonary toilet. Patients with preoperative pain will have taken opioid analgesics prior to surgery, will have opioid tolerance, and require a multi-modal approach by a pain specialist, including drugs against neuropathic pain, nonsteroidal anti-inflammatory agents, and continuous nerve block in extreme cases.

POSTOPERATIVE CONSIDERATIONS

The most common postoperative complications are respiratory (atelectasis, pneumonia) related to postoperative pain. Good pain management and respiratory care are key. The patient should be mobilized the first postoperative day and given vigorous chest physiotherapy. Awake bronchoscopic suctioning may be required to clear retained secretions. Other complications are those usually seen after pulmonary resection, including supraventricular cardiac dysrhythmias, bleeding, wound infection, or empyema. Chylothoraces can occur after extensive dissection in the paravertebral region (either right- or left-sided). Infection of hardware used for spine stabilization is uncommon but can require reoperation and drainage. Cerebrospinal fluid leak is rare but can be a serious complication requiring reoperation; it is related to inadequate closure of the dura along the intercostal nerve roots at the level of the spinal foramina.

REFERENCES

1. Pancoast HK. Superior pulmonary sulcus tumor. *J Am Med Assoc* 1932; 99: 1391–6.
2. Shaw RR, Paulson DL, Kee JL, Jr. Treatment of the superior sulcus tumor by irradiation followed by resection. *Ann Surg.* 1961; 154: 29–40.
3. Ginsberg RJ, Martini N, Armstrong JG et al. The influence of surgical resection and brachytherapy in superior sulcus tumor. *Ann Thorac Surg.* 1994; 57: 1440-5.
4. Rusch VW, Parekh KR, Leon L et al. Factors determining outcome after surgical resection of T3 and T4 lung cancers of the superior sulcus. *J Thorac Cardiovasc Surg.* 2000; 119: 1147–53.
5. Rusch VW, Giroux DJ, Kraut MJ et al. Induction chemoradiation and surgical resection for superior sulcus non-small cell lung carcinomas: Long-term results of Southwest Oncology Group Trial 9416 (Intergroup Trial 0160). *J Clin Oncol.* 2007; 25: 313–18.
6. Kunitoh H, Kato H, Tsuboi M et al. Phase II trial of preoperative chemoradiotherapy followed by surgical resection in patients with superior sulcus non-small cell lung cancers: Report of Japan Clinical Oncology Group trial 9806. *J Clin Oncol.* 2008; 26: 644–9.
7. Freundlich IM, Chasen MH, Varma DG. Magnetic resonance imaging of pulmonary apical tumors. *J Thorac Imaging.* 1996; 11: 210–22.
8. Rusch VW, Bilsky MH. En bloc resection of thoracic tumors involving the spine. *Oper Tech Thorac Cardiovasc Surg.* 2007; 12: 266–78.
9. Niwa H, Masaoka A, Yamakawa Y, Fukai I, Kiriyama M. Surgical therapy for apical invasive lung cancer: Different approaches according to tumor location. *Lung Cancer.* 1993; 10: 63–71.
10. Bolton WD, Rice DC, Goodyear A et al. Superior sulcus tumors with vertebral body involvement: A multimodality approach. *J Thorac Cardiovasc Surg.* 2009; 137: 1379–87.
11. Dartevelle PG, Chapelier AR, Macchiarini P et al. Anterior transcervical-thoracic approach for radical resection of lung tumors invading the thoracic inlet. *J Thorac Cardiovasc Surg.* 1993; 105: 1025–34.
12. Masaoka A, Ito Y, Yasumitsu T. Anterior approach for tumor of the superior sulcus. *J Thorac Cardiovasc Surg.* 1979; 78: 413–15.
13. Grunenwald D, Spaggiari L, Girard P, Baldeyrou P. Transmanubrial approach to the thoracic inlet. *J Thorac Cardiovasc Surg.* 1997; 113: 958–9.

21

Lung volume reduction surgery

CLAUDIO CAVIEZEL AND WALTER WEDER

HISTORY

Chronic obstructive pulmonary disease is a major and well-known health problem. It was first described as large air spaces in human lung specimens by Ruysch in 1691[1] and by Floyer in 1698.[2] A few decades later, the first comprehensive clinical and pathological report of a case was published by Watson in 1764.[3] Despite optimal medical therapy and pulmonary rehabilitation, many patients remain disabled and even now lung transplantation is still an option only for a few.

By 1924, Reich had already described the use of pneumoperitoneum in the treatment of pulmonary emphysema due to its effect on the diaphragm.[4] His work was followed by Piaggio-Blanco et al. and Carter et al. in 1937[5] and 1950,[6] respectively. By restoring the normal diaphragmatic arch with the pneumoperitoneum, they made contraction downward of the flattened muscle possible again. They also could describe a decrease in residual volume (RV) and an increase in vital capacity.

Lung volume reduction surgery (LVRS) was then first described by Brantigan and Mueller in 1957[7] and reintroduced by Cooper et al. in 1995.[8]

With many observational studies during the 1990s and a large randomized study in 2003 (National Emphysema Treatment Trial [NETT][9]), LVRS has now been shown to improve lung function, exercise capacity, health status, and even survival in patients with emphysema, and therefore has become an internationally established procedure.

PRINCIPLES AND JUSTIFICATION

LVRS downsizes the hyperinflated lung to a more physiologic size. This makes the diaphragmatic dome move upward and increases the area of muscle apposed to the rib cage.[10] This effect improves maximal ventilator and exercise capacity by optimizing the match between the size of the lungs and the rib cage.[11] LVRS improves global inspiratory muscle strength and the contribution of the diaphragm to inspiratory pressure generation and tidal volume.[12,13] The major effects consist of a reduction in static lung volumes (functional residual capacity and RV), with an associated increase in lung elastic recoil. The latter leads to a reduction in the degree of airflow obstruction and hyperinflation.[14]

These effects are independent from emphysema morphology, and therefore patients with heterogeneous emphysema can benefit from LVRS as well as patients with homogeneous morphology.[15]

Although LVRS has been introduced as a minimal-invasive procedure[16] and its principles have internationally been established, patient selection is still a key issue and should be performed with a multidisciplinary emphysema board at specialized centers.

PREOPERATIVE ASSESSMENT AND PREPARATION

Despite nicotine abstention and completed pulmonary rehabilitation, there are defined indications for LVRS, with evidence-based probability for benefit.

The NETT showed significant benefit for patients with upper-lobe-predominant heterogeneous emphysema with low exercise capacity.[9]

As already mentioned, homogeneous emphysema morphology is no contraindication to LVRS, as long as the disadvantage of resected parenchyma contributing to gas exchange is compensated by the beneficiary effect of downsizing the hyperinflated lung.[15] Symptomatic and large bronchiectasis, recurrent infectious exacerbations, and a daily prednisone intake of more than 20 mg are contraindications for LVRS.

Lung function

LVRS is offered to selected patients with severe obstruction, as defined by forced expiratory volume in 1 second (FEV1) between 20% and 45% of the predicted value, hyperinflation greater than 150%, and residual volume to total lung capacity ratio (RV/TLC) of more than 60%.

The achieved 6-minute walking distance should be between 150 and 450 m.

A diffusing capacity lower than 20% is not a contraindication if FEV1% is greater than 20% in heterogeneous emphysema.

Imaging

The most reliable method of obtaining information on the degree and distribution of emphysema is chest computed tomography (CT) scanning. Lung perfusion scintigraphy has a limited role in prediction of outcome, but it may help to identify target areas for resection in LVRS candidates with homogeneous CT morphology.[17]

Cardiac risk

The left ventricle ejection fraction should be greater than 30%, whereas a mean pulmonary arterial pressure above 35 mmHg, significant arrhythmias, exercise-induced syncope, and myocardial infarction within the last 6 months are contraindications to LVRS.[18] If peak systolic pulmonary artery pressure is above 45 mmHg on echocardiogram, right-sided heart catheterization is required.

ANESTHESIA

LVRS is typically performed under general anesthesia, with one-lung ventilation established with a double-lumen endotracheal tube. Especially when performed bilaterally, additional epidural analgesia is recommended for a smoother, less eventful postoperative course, due to better ventilation performance (ambulation, coughing, and use of incentive spirometer). Inspiratory pressures must be monitored and minimized in the ventilated lung, especially after the first side has been operated, to prevent rupture of the staple lines.

OPERATION

The operation can be performed as an open or thoracoscopic (video-assisted thoracoscopic surgery [VATS]) procedure and may be done unilaterally or bilaterally or staged bilaterally. The authors prefer one-staged bilateral VATS LVRS in bilateral emphysema.

VATS approach

PATIENT POSITIONING (see Figure 21.1)

When a bilateral procedure is planned for upper-lobe-predominant emphysema, the patient is situated in a supine position with both arms raised, allowing access to both sides without changing the patient's position.

Unilateral or bilateral procedures, in cases of lower-lobe-predominant emphysema, are performed in the lateral decubitus position. Unless there is a massive air leak after the first side is completed, the patient has to be turned to complete the procedure on the opposite side.

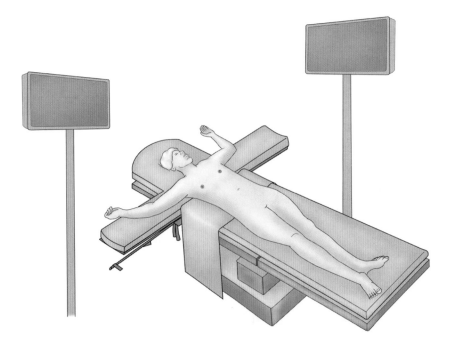

21.1

INCISIONS (see **Figure 21.2**)

The incisions for bilateral LVRS in upper-lobe-predominant emphysema are situated just below the inframammary crease in the 4th or 5th intercostal space in the midclavicular, anterior axillary, and median axillary lines. The incisions are preferably placed in the same intercostal space to minimize postoperative pain. For the left side, we often choose to place the incisions in the 5th intercostal space and more laterally due to the position of the heart. We use three 11.5 mm trocars, with a 10 mm endoscope, 10 mm grasps, and 10 mm stapling devices.

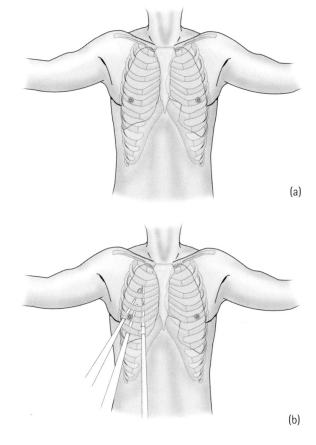

(a)

(b)

21.2a–b

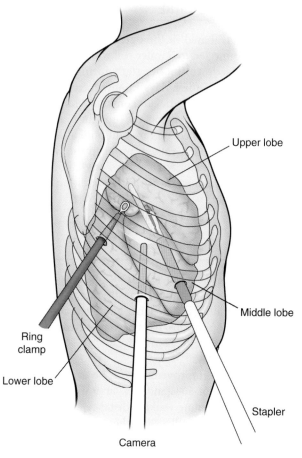

Upper lobe

Middle lobe

Ring clamp

Lower lobe

Stapler

Camera

21.3

When the procedure is performed in the lateral decubitus position, the incision placement might be slightly more dorsal or lower, but depends on the emphysema type as well (see **Figure 21.3**).

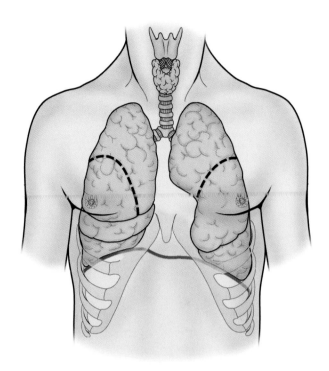

21.4

DEFINING THE TARGET-VOLUME (see Figure 21.4)

The target areas and the extent of resection differ between various types of emphysema. The lung is resected in areas that show the most severe emphysematous destruction on imaging studies (CT scan) corresponding to the intraoperative macroscopic appearance. In patients with upper-lobe-predominant emphysema, approximately 30%–50% of the upper lobe is resected. The target-volume can be approximated from the difference between the predicted and the desired value of TLC. In patients with homogeneous emphysema, it is more difficult to define the amount and site of resection, since clearly defined target areas are absent. We preferentially choose the upper lobes and approximately 30%–40% are resected.

STAPLING (see Figures 21.5 through 21.7)

Before resection, the defined target area is prepared by compressing the lung parenchyma along the line of the proposed staple line with a clamp or grasper. Manipulation and contact with the lung should be limited, as the emphysematous lung is very soft and even touching it with the stapler can make a hole. Before introducing the stapler, the lung should be aligned so it can slide easily across the stapler. A reinforced endostapler is then introduced (i.e. through the anterior VATS port) along the precompressed region of the lung. We generally use a 60 mm long endostapler with 4.8 mm staples. This stapling procedure is repeated until the target area is resected. In case of upper-lobe-predominant emphysema, the resection often starts at the level of the azygos vein or the aortic arch. The resected area appears like a hockey stick. The specimen is then removed through one port with or without the use of an endobag.

CHEST CLOSURE

After resection, one chest tube is placed and the reinflation is checked under direct vision. In case of massive air leak, the stapling lines are checked first. The port incisions are closed and the opposite side is approached after establishing one-lung ventilation. In patients in the supine position, the operation table might be tilted from one side to the other.

Open approach

In our experience, adhesions might be the only indication for an open approach. Nevertheless, every LVRS should be attempted as a video-assisted procedure.

If severe adhesions are present and cannot be safely lysed by VATS, an anterolateral thoracotomy in the 4th or 5th intercostal space is performed. Defining target areas and stapling are the same as in thoracoscopic LVRS. Due to the extensive adhesiolysis, we place two chest tubes before closure of the chest. Once LVRS has been done as an open procedure, the operation is limited to the ipsilateral side, and LVRS for the opposite side is postponed for at least 6–12 months.

POSTOPERATIVE CARE

Patients are extubated in the operating room. The chest tube(s) are connected to a water seal with suction of −5 cm H_2O. Prophylactic antibiotics start during the operation and are continued for 5 days in absence of pneumonia. Depending on comorbidities and on unilaterality or bilaterality of the procedure patients are brought to the intensive care unit or an intermediate care unit until at least the first postoperative day. Generally, transfer to the ward is possible on the first postoperative day. Early ambulation and frequent physiotherapy are critical, in addition to optimal pain management.

OUTCOME

Pulmonary complications after LVRS have been reported to be as high as 30%, though mostly these are prolonged air leaks. Respiratory insufficiency and pneumonia are rare. Mortality rates up to 5.5% have been reported,[18] but in our own experience, this rate hardly exceeds 1%. Mean hospitalization time is 12 days.[19]

Lung function improvement can be expected with an increase of FEV1 of 50% and 35% after 6 and 12 months, respectively. Six-minute walking distance increases to 60% after 6 months and is still 58% higher after 12 months.[15,20]

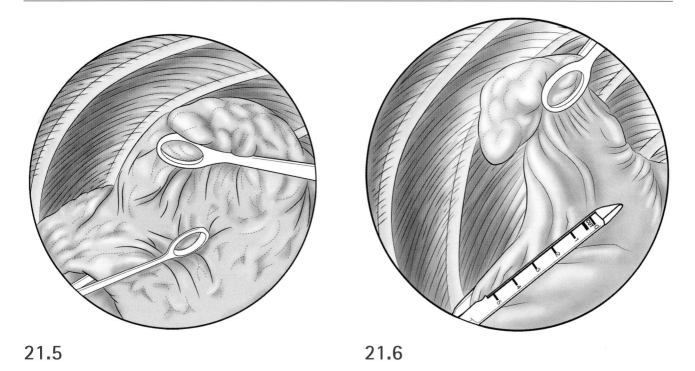

21.5

21.6

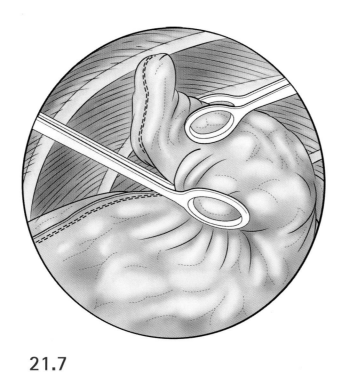

21.7

REFERENCES

1. Ruysch F. *Observationum anatomico-chirurgicarum centuria*. Amsterdam: Boom; 1691: obs. XIX, XX.
2. Floyer J. *A treatise of the asthma*. London: Wilkin; 1698.
3. Watson W. An account of what appeared on opening the body of an asthmatic person. *Philos Trans*. 1746; 54: 239–45.
4. Reich L. Der Einfluss des Pneumoperitoneums auf das Lungenemphysem [The influence of the pneumoperitoneum on the pulmonary emphysema. *Wien Arch Inn Med*. 1924; 8: 245–60. German.
5. Piaggio-Blanco RA, Piaggio-Blanco RO, Caimi RA. Mejorías sintomáticas del enfisema por el neumoperotoneo [Symptomatic improvements in emphysema due to pneumoperotoneum]. *Arch Urug Med Cir Espec*. 1937; 10: 273–83. Spanish.
6. Carter MG, Gaensler EA, Kyllonen A. Pneumoperitoneum in the treatment of pulmonary emphysema. *N Engl J Med*. 1950; 243: 549–58.
7. Brantigan OC, Mueller E. Surgical treatment of pulmonary emphysema. *Am Surg*. 1957; 23: 784–804.
8. Cooper JD, Trulock EP, Triantafillou AN et al. Bilateral pneumectomy (volume reduction) for chronic obstructive pulmonary disease. *J Thorac Cardiovasc Surg*. 1995; 109: 106–16; discussion 116–19.
9. Fishman A, Martinez F, Naunheim K, et al; National Emphysema Treatment Trial Research Group. A randomized trial comparing lung-volume-reduction surgery with medical therapy for severe emphysema. *N Engl J Med*. 2003; 348: 2059–73.
10. Cassart M, Hamacher J, Verbandt Y et al. Effects of lung volume reduction surgery for emphysema on diaphragm dimensions and configuration. *Am J Respir Crit Care Med*. 2001; 163: 1171–5.
11. Fessler HE, Permutt S. Lung volume reduction surgery and airflow limitation. *Am J Respir Crit Care Med*. 1998; 157: 715–22.
12. Bloch KE, Li Y, Zhang J et al. Effect of surgical lung volume reduction on breathing patterns in severe pulmonary emphysema. *Am J Respir Crit Care Med*. 1997; 156: 553–60.
13. Benditt J, Wood DE, McCool FD et al. Changes in breathing and ventilatory muscle recruitment patterns induced by lung volume reduction surgery. *Am J Respir Crit Care Med*. 1997; 155: 279–84.
14. Sciurba FC, Rogers FM, Keenan RJ et al. Improvement in pulmonary function and elastic recoil after lung-reduction surgery for diffuse emphysema. *N Engl J Med*. 1996; 334: 1095–9.
15. Weder W, Tutic M, Lardinois D et al. Persistent benefit from lung volume reduction surgery in patients with homogeneous emphysema. *Ann Thorac Surg*. 2009; 87: 229–36; discussion 236–7.
16. Russi EW, Stammberger U, Weder W. Lung volume reduction surgery for emphysema. *Eur Respir J*. 1997; 10: 208–18.
17. Thurnheer R, Engel H, Weder W et al. Role of lung perfusion scintigraphy in relation to chest computed tomography and pulmonary function in the evaluation of candidates for lung volume reduction surgery. *Am J Respir Crit Care Med*. 1999; 159: 301–10.
18. Naunheim KS, Wood DE, Krasna MJ et al. National Emphysema Treatment Trial Research Group. Predictors of operative mortality and cardiopulmonary morbidity in the National Emphysema Treatment Trial. *J Thorac Cardiovasc Surg*. 2006; 131: 43–53.
19. Meyers BF, Yusen RD, Guthrie TJ et al. Results of lung volume reduction surgery in patients meeting a national emphysema treatment trial high-risk criterion. *J Thorac Cardiovasc Surg*. 2004; 127: 829–35.
20. Bloch KE, Georgescu CL, Russi EW et al. Gain and subsequent loss of lung function after lung volume reduction surgery in cases of severe emphysema with different morphologic patterns. *J Thorac Cardiovasc Surg*. 2002; 123: 845–54.

22

Pleural space problems

KONRAD HOETZENECKER AND WALTER KLEPETKO

PLEURAL EMPYEMA WITHOUT BRONCHOPLEURAL FISTULA

Pleural empyema is, by definition, a collection of pus within the naturally existing anatomical cavity of the pleura. It is, in most cases, a sequela of a pneumonitis that has gained contact to the pleural cavity. According to demographic studies, it accounts for six out of 100 000 hospitalizations in the United States, with a twofold increase within the last 10 years. Although pleural empyema is a rare clinical condition, it has a high mortality of 7.2%.[1]

The pathogens traditionally associated with empyema are *Streptococcus pneumoniae*, *Streptococcus pyogenes*, and *Staphylococcus aureus*. The triphasic nature of the disease is well established. In the early phase (Stage I, exudative phase) the pleural cavity is filled with superinfected pleural effusion, or pus. If these fluid retentions are not evacuated, a fibropurulent state (Stage II) develops, which is finally replaced by a fibrothorax (Stage III, consolidated phase). The lung is trapped by a thick peel of inflammatory tissue causing a contraction of the hemithorax, the mediastinum to shift, the diaphragm to elevate, and the spaces between the ribs to narrow (see **Figure 22.1**).

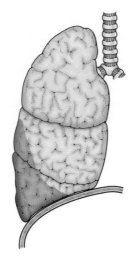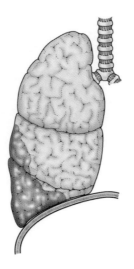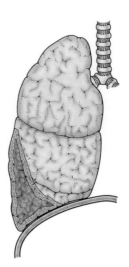

22.1

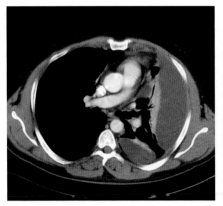
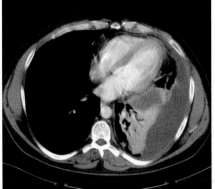
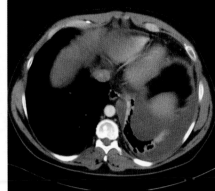

22.2 Typical CT scan of a pleural empyema.

Preoperative evaluation includes a thoracic computed tomography (CT) scan with contrast agent. It provides information on the location and extent of the empyema, degree of loculation, and the integrity of the underlying lung parenchyma. A contrast-enhanced pleura and a multiloculated pleural collection are a typical picture found in most cases (see **Figure 22.2**).

The management of pleural empyema is based on a stage-wise approach.

Conservative management/Chest tube

In the early phases, an insertion of a chest tube might be sufficient. To completely evacuate all effusion, a chest tube of sufficient size (at least 28 Fr) should be placed directly in the most dependent location, specifically into the costodiaphragmatic recesses and advanced in a posterior direction.[2] If the lung does not fully expand after chest tube insertion, a decortication is necessary (see **Figure 22.3**).

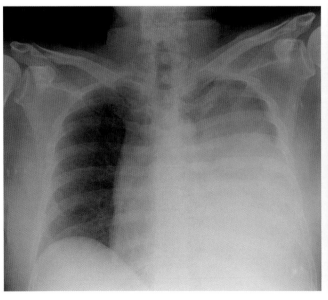
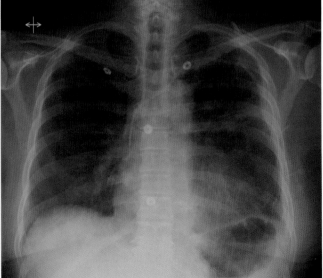

22.3 Chest radiographs of a Stage I empyema successfully managed by chest tube placement.

Thoracoscopic decortication

Thoracoscopic decortication should be the treatment option of choice for Stage II empyema. There is sufficient evidence that thoracoscopic decortication has a superior outcome in terms of postoperative morbidity, complications, and length of hospital stay when compared with open decortication for Stage II empyema. When the history of infected effusion is less than 3 weeks, a thoracoscopic approach is usually successful. If the empyema has been present for a longer time, a minimal-invasive approach is more difficult, due to dense adhesions and the presence of a thick visceral peel.

TECHNIQUE

The procedure is usually done with a three-port technique. (see **Figure 22.4**) The preoperative CT scan helps to place the ports in the right place. One port in the 6th or 7th intercostal space anterior axillary line, one port in the 7th or 8th intercostal space posterior axillary line, and a small working port (3 cm incision) in the 5th intercostal space midaxillary line provide a good exposure of the lower pleural cavity. Care should be taken not to injure the lung when placing the ports. It is advisable to bluntly create a working space in the pleural cavity with a finger before inserting any instruments. First, the pleural space has to be completely visualized by breaking up loculations and by clearing any gelatinous fibrinous deposits. In a next step, the visceral pleura is freed from the beginning cortex with the use of ring forceps, curettes, and peanut dissectors. Special care should be taken not to injure the surface of the lung. Intermittent ventilation helps to visualize the right plane for decortication and to detect any residual trapping of the lung. A complete mobilization is the goal for a good postoperative result, since a residual space is a setup for recurrent infection. Complete reexpansion of the lung to completely obliterate the space is the goal. To accomplish this, it is especially critical to mobilize the lower lobe away from the diaphragm and the anterior aspect of the lung from the mediastinum. Care must be taken to protect the phrenic nerve during this preparation step. If adequate progress is not being made because of too dense adhesions and a complete decortication is impossible with an inadequate expansion of the lung, a conversion to open decortication should be performed. At the end of the operation, complete hemostasis should be achieved and the pleural cavity irrigated with warm water or an antibiotic solution. Two chest tubes are placed and the ports are closed.

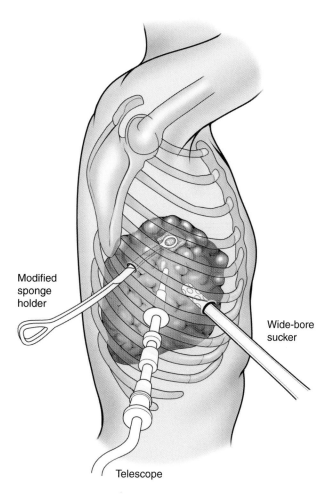

Modified sponge holder

Wide-bore sucker

Telescope

22.4

Open decortication

Open decortication should be reserved for Stage III or complicated Stage II empyema. The incision is placed in the 5th or 6th intercostal space. Care should be taken to avoid opening an intercostal space that is too low, since the diaphragm is always elevated due to the shrinkage of the pleural cavity. Although a posterolateral approach has traditionally been preferred and facilitates perfect vision, muscle-sparing thoracotomies can be used without impairment of visualization. After the intercostal muscles are dissected a blunt—if necessary, extrapleural—development of the pleural space next to the thoracotomy is advisable before inserting the chest retractor. This releases tension on the ribs in order to avoid fractures during spreading. A resection of ribs, as suggested by some authors, is not necessary in most cases. The thickened parietal pleura and peel are incised with a scalpel until the visceral pleura is identified. Then the thick peel is meticulously removed in a blunt way, taking care to maintain the appropriate plane between the visceral pleura and the peel. (see **Figure 22.5**) A mild inflation of the lung usually eases this maneuver, since it provides some needed countertraction necessary in maintaining the appropriate plane. A complete mobilization is important, and small superficial injuries of the lung are often unavoidable but usually seal within the first hours after the operation. Deep tears of the lung should be closed with absorbable suture material. At the end of the procedure, hemostasis is obtained, the pleural cavity is irrigated with warm saline or an antibiotic solution, and two chest tubes are placed. In severely compromised patients, a sufficient hemostasis is sometimes impossible to achieve. In these selected cases, packing of the pleural cavity using towels is advisable.

Small abscess formations found during the decortication should be closed by capitonnage with reinforced sutures. Necrotizing pneumonia, extensive pulmonary abscess formations, and lung gangrene are rare situations. They always require resection of all devitalized pulmonary structures. In most cases, an anatomical resection (septic lobectomy, pneumonectomy) is necessary. In these cases, it is of utmost importance to reinforce the bronchial stump with well-vascularized muscle or a pericardial flap.

Open treatment

For multimorbid patients who are considered not fit enough for an open decortication, an open window thoracostomy (Eloesser flap) in combination with a vacuum-assisted closure (VAC) device can be considered. VAC therapy allows an acceptable reexpansion of remaining lung and a sterilization of the pleural cavity in most cases.

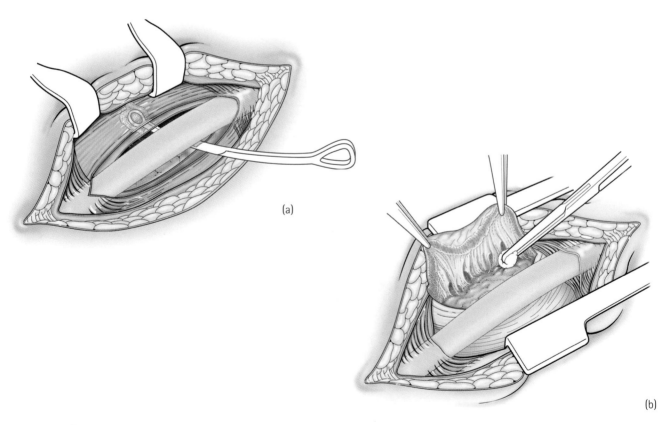

(a)

(b)

22.5a–b

Postresectional pleural empyema

Postresectional pleural empyema may occur after anatomical as well as wedge resections. The incidence for postlobectomy empyema is 2%. For wedge resections, it is considerably lower. Infections of the pleural space after lung resections are nearly always associated with prolonged air leaks. In contrast to the pleural space, which is a highly sterile region, the lung itself is often colonized by pathogens. During a prolonged air leak, the pleural space can be contaminated with pathogens resident in the lung breaking the natural antimicrobial barrier of the pleural space. In early stages, a chest tube placement and intravenous antibiotics provide sufficient treatment. In advanced stages, an open window thoracostomy with/without intrathoracic VAC treatment, followed by a muscle transposition, might be necessary.

POSTPNEUMONECTOMY EMPYEMA

Postpneumonectomy empyema (PPE) is a serious complication in thoracic surgery, which carries a high mortality. The reported incidence ranges from 2% up to 7%; however, these numbers may be underestimated because of delayed presentation and occurrence of the disease.[3] In general, PPE can be classified as PPE with a bronchopleural fistula (BPF) or PPE without a BPF, the latter being rather rare (comprising only 15%).

Risk factors for the development of PPE include local (long bronchial stump, disrupted blood supply, preexistent empyema, postoperative mechanical ventilation, right pneumonectomy, neoadjuvant radiotherapy) and systemic factors (poor nutritional status, diabetes). A proper surgical technique is a prerequisite to reduce the risk of a PPE. When performing the lymphadenectomy at the time of resection, special care should be taken to avoid devascularization of the main bronchus and carinal region. The bronchial stump should be stapled at the level of the carina to avoid a long bronchial stump. Right bronchial stumps are at higher risk for the development of a BPF. This is due to minimal mediastinal coverage compared with the left side, where the stump will usually retract in the mediastinum beneath the aorta. The bronchial stump should always be covered with vascularized tissue after a pneumonectomy. This includes, according to local availability, a pedicled pericardial fat pad, a diaphragmatic or an intercostal muscle flap, an azygos flap, or a combination thereof.

PPE can present days to years after the initial surgery. Diagnosis is difficult, since the clinical presentation can be quite subtle, especially in late occurring fistulas. The most reliable diagnostic tool has been shown to be a constantly high C-reactive protein, with a sensitivity of 100% and a specificity of almost 92%. Radiological imaging should always include a chest X-ray and if in doubt a CT scan. Air in the pleural cavity, a convex expansion of the pneumonectomy space, and a reversal of the physiological ipsilateral mediastinal shift are signs highly suspicious of PPE. A bronchoscopy should always be performed to exclude a bronchial stump fistula. It is of note that a small stump dehiscence may be missed easily during bronchoscopy. An injection of methylene blue and monitoring of the drained pleural fluid help to identify a small BPF.

Treatment

DRAINING THE PLEURAL SPACE

As many patients with PPE present with a fulminant course and a preseptic or septic condition, stabilization of the patient is the primary goal. Draining of the pleural space is the most important initial measure. This controls the septic process and prevents aspiration of pleural fluid through the BPF to the remaining lung. The chest tube should be placed above the old thoracotomy to avoid a subphrenic malposition due to the chronic shrinkage of the pneumonectomy cavity. Broad intravenous antibiotic coverage should be started immediately and adapted according to the culture results of obtained pleural fluid specimens. This can be supported by insertion of an irrigation catheter applying topical antibiosis into the thoracic cavity. The most common organisms cultured from PPE specimens are *Staphylococcus aureus* and *Pseudomonas aeruginosa*.

The further treatment algorithm is dependent on the following factors: early versus late fistula, large versus small bronchial defects, the patient's overall condition, and the extent of intrapleural infection. In general, surgical management of PPE includes three different steps.

1. Closure of the BPF

The surgical approach to reach the hilum can be difficult, especially for late fistula, when the hilar structures are covered by a dense cortex. For right-sided problems, a redo thoracotomy is the best option. The old skin incision can be used; however, the chest cavity should be entered one intercostal space higher. This maneuver facilitates the use of an undamaged intercostal muscle flap (if needed) for the buttressing of the reclosed bronchus. For left-sided stump problems, access through a left-sided repeat thoracotomy is not advisable. The stump is usually deeply positioned in the mediastinum below the aorta and very hard to dissect. An alternative approach through a right-sided thoracotomy or a transsternal approach eases the preparation of the stump through a formerly untouched area.[4]

After exposing the hilum, the bronchial stump is carefully dissected, leaving the blood supply intact. Small fistulas can be visualized by positive airway ventilation under water seal. There are several ways to manage the fistula. If the stump is long enough, a more central reclose with a commercial stapling device can be done. If there is too little space to insert a stapler, the bronchus should be reclosed with interrupted reinforced monofilament sutures. The neostump should be buttressed with either an intercostal muscle flap or a pedicled pericardial flap. For patients with older fistulas, a direct closure without tension is sometimes not possible. In these cases, the bronchial opening is closed by directly suturing a muscle flap or omentum onto the fistula.

2. Debridement and sterilization of the pleural cavity

Sterilization of the pleural cavity is an essential step in the successful treatment of PPE. The postpneumonectomy cavity is a noncollapsible space, which is filled by bradytrophic, contaminated tissue. Due to the advanced scarring, systemic antibiotics only reach the cavity insufficiently and a thorough debridement of all necrotic or infected tissue in the pleural cavity is a prerequisite to reach sterility.

According to the grade of infection, singular or repeated debridements are necessary. Mild infections of the thoracic cavity can be treated by a singular removal of infected material, and a subsequent sealing with viable tissue (myoplasty, omental flap). Omental flaps are—in our opinion—the best option. Although a median laparotomy is required for their preparation, they are able to effectively contain residual minor infection.

In most cases, however, sterility cannot be reached in a single stage, and multiple procedures will be required. The old concept of creating a thoracic window, initially developed for the treatment of tuberculosis, is still the approach of choice in many centers. This procedure combines repeated debridements through a thoracic window (Eloesser flap, open window thoracostomy) with later closure after sterilization is completed. The technique results in a high rate of success, although treatment requires a prolonged hospital stay and the thoracostomy procedure is disfiguring and related to high morbidity. Therefore, alternative procedures have been proposed recently. An accelerated treatment omitting the thoracic window by performing repeated debridements in the operating room and packing with iodine dressings was proposed by Schneiter and colleagues (2008).[5] This technique resulted in a definite closure of the chest within 8 days and a success rate of 100%. Alternatively, in cases with only moderate infectious changes of the thoracic cavity, a single thoracic debridement procedure followed by prolonged antibiotic irrigation can be successful. Another novel approach is vacuum-assisted management of the infected pleural cavity. The negative-pressure wound therapy stimulates an accelerated sterilization of the cavity, avoiding prolonged hospitalization and facilitating an early closure of the thoracic window.

3. Sealing of the cavity

Successful sterilization of the pleural space is a prerequisite before the postpneumonectomy cavity can be closed. The cavity should be completely sealed with vascularized vital tissue (muscle flap, omental flap). If the remaining space is too large, this can be combined with a limited thoracoplasty, removing the first three ribs. A complete thoracoplasty is associated with high morbidity and disfiguration and should rarely be performed. Alternatively, if no vital flaps are available, the cavity can be obliterated with antibiotic solution.

ENDOBRONCHIAL PROCEDURES

Endoscopic treatment options to close small BPF have been anecdotally described in the literature.[6] The bronchial defects can either be bridged by coated stents or directly closed by glues, coils, balloon catheter occlusion, or by repeated application of silver nitrate. These techniques can be successful for defects less than 3 mm but are not advisable for a larger bronchial stump dehiscence. One must remember that infection in the pleural space is the major issue; closure of the bronchial fistula must be considered strictly as an adjunct to ultimately sterilizing and obliterating the space.

MUSCLE FLAPS AND OMENTAL FLAP

Muscles are an ideal material for filling the pleural space and for covering bronchial stump fistulas. They are well vascularized and can be rotated to nearly any region of the thoracic cavity. The survival of the muscle depends on the preservation of its blood supply during preparation. The following muscles can be used for intrathoracic transposition.

Intrathoracic muscle flaps

DIAPHRAGMATIC MUSCLE FLAP

This flap can be easily used to cover a BPF. Its vascular pedicle is the phrenic artery, which runs below the phrenic nerve on the inferior aspect of the muscle. The flap is prepared in a U-shaped fashion and is rotated to the lung hilum. Care should be taken to avoid a torsion or extensive tension on the pedicle. The remaining rent in the diaphragm is closed with interrupted sutures (see **Figure 22.6**).

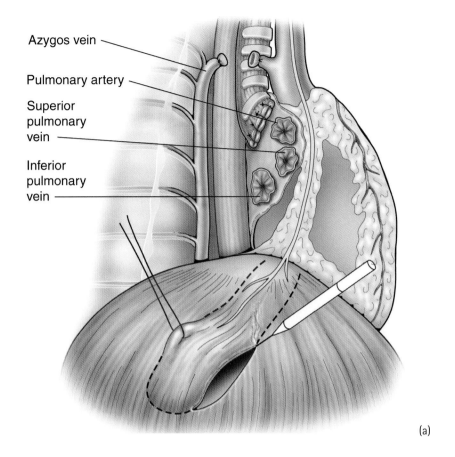

Azygos vein

Pulmonary artery

Superior
pulmonary
vein

Inferior
pulmonary
vein

(a)

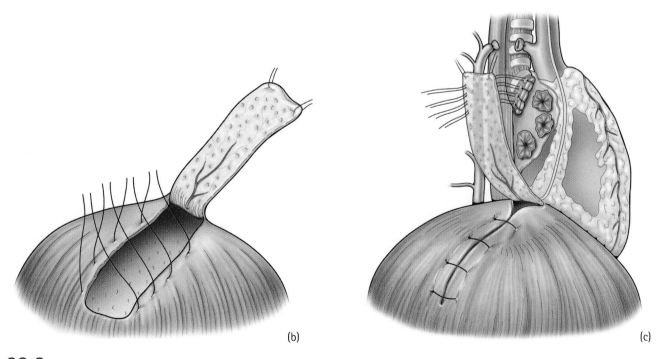

(b)

(c)

22.6a–c

INTERCOSTAL MUSCLE FLAP

Intercostal muscle flaps are very helpful in covering a BPF. They can be completely mobilized and nearly every part of the thoracic cavity can be reached with these muscle flaps. The technique of harvesting is easy. The flap should be prepared before inserting a rib spreader to avoid damage to the neuromuscular pedicle by extensive crushing. The muscle is prepared by an incision of the periosteum of two neighboring ribs and by blunt dissection along both edges. Alternatively, one rib can be resected to obtain better exposure to the flap. The neuromuscular bundle is divided at the ventral aspect, thus enabling a rotation of the muscle flap toward the hilar region (see **Figure 22.7**).

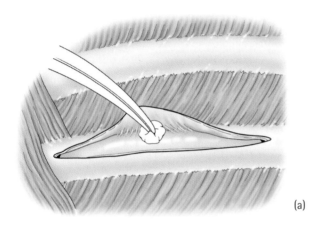

(a)

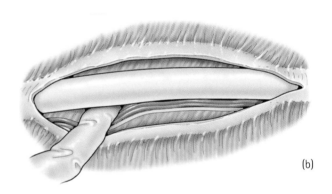

(b)

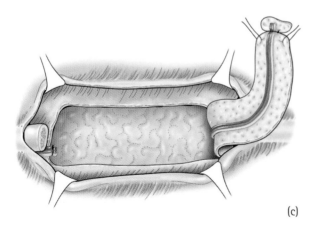

(c)

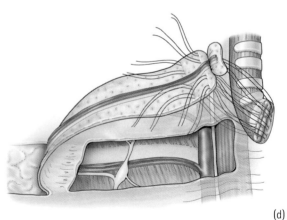

(d)

22.7a–d

Extrathoracic muscle flaps

PECTORALIS MAJOR

The pectoralis major receives its blood supply from branches of the internal mammary artery and the thoracoacromial artery, the latter serving as the vascular pedicle of the flap. It is most commonly used to cover sternal defects but can be rotated intrathoracically to cover a BPF originating from an upper lobe bronchus. The use of this muscle results in the loss of the anterior axillary fold, limiting the cosmetic results. In addition, the functionality of the shoulder and upper limb is impaired.

The muscle is completely dissected free from its origins and insertions in order to advance it through a small window created by a partial resection of the second or third rib (see **Figure 22.8**).

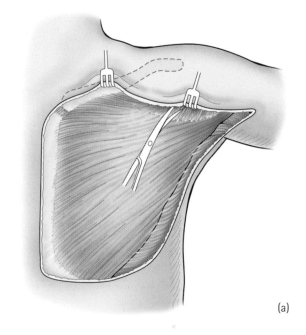

(a)

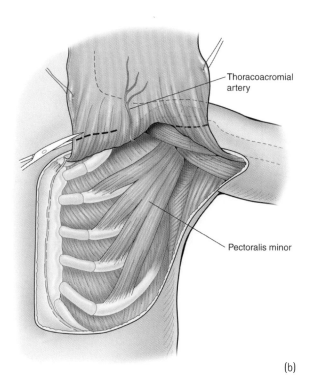

Thoracoacromial artery

Pectoralis minor

(b)

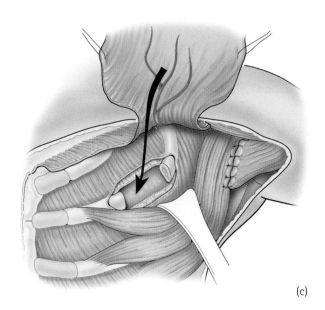

(c)

22.8a–c

LATISSIMUS DORSI

The latissimus dorsi is the largest muscle of the chest wall and is an optimal muscle to fill up a PPE cavity. It receives its blood supply from the thoracodorsal artery, which serves as the vascular pedicle. However, a previously transected latissimus dorsi after full posterolateral thoracotomy cannot be used as a flap, as the distal portion of the muscle beyond the previous transection line will become necrotic. The muscle is divided from its posterior and inferior attachments and is raised based on the thoracodorsal vessels. Vascular branches to the serratus anterior can be divided and the muscle is transposed in the thoracic cavity through a small window created by a partial resection of the second or third rib (see **Figure 22.9**).

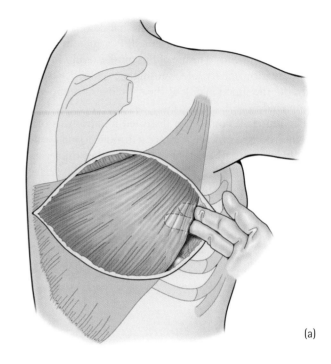

(a)

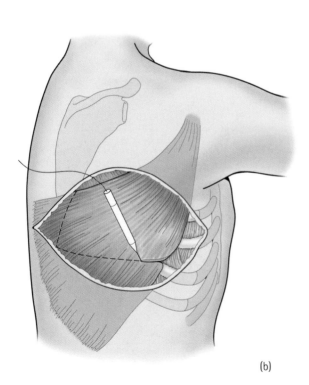

(b)

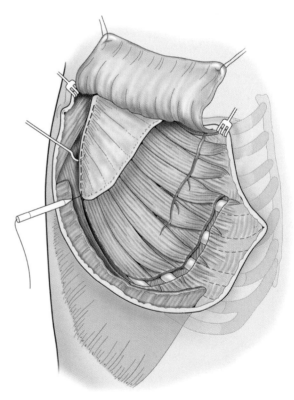

(c)

22.9a–c

SERRATUS ANTERIOR

If the latissimus dorsi cannot be used as a flap due to prior posterolateral incision, the serratus anterior serves as an alternative. The muscle receives its blood supply from the lateral thoracic artery, which serves as the pedicle. All muscular insertions from the ribs and the scapula are detached. Again, the muscle is rotated into the thoracic cavity by creating a small window by a partial resection of the third rib. The use of this flap will result in a scapula alata in most cases (see **Figure 22.10**).

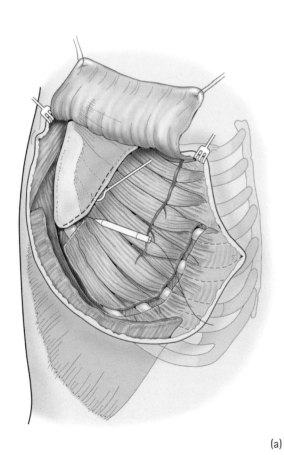

(a)

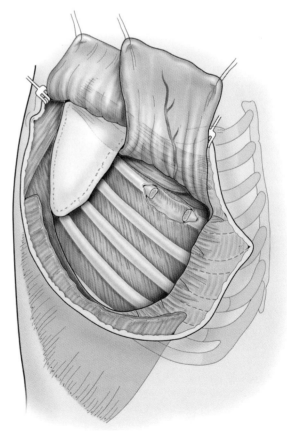

(b)

22.10a–b

OMENTUM FLAP

The omentum flap is an ideal flap to control residual infection. It is well vascularized by the epiploic vessels and can be completely mobilized, reaching all portions of the pleural cavity. A pedicled flap can be created using either the right or the left gastroepiploic artery. The omentum is divided from the greater curvature of the stomach, and the posterior fold of the omentum has to be released from the transverse colon. The flap is then transposed into the thoracic cavity by a small incision in the diaphragm.

A drawback to using an omentum flap is the need for an additional upper midline laparotomy for its preparation (see **Figure 22.11**).

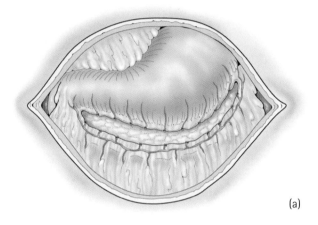

(a)

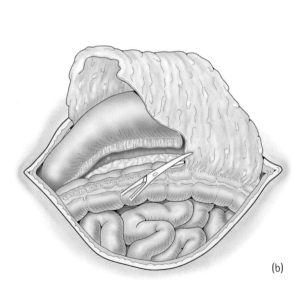

(b)

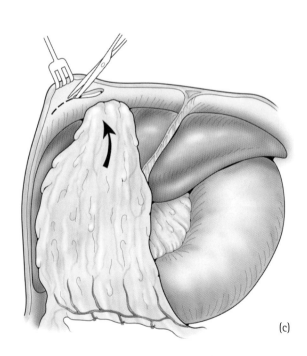

(c)

22.11a–c

MANAGEMENT OF POSTOPERATIVE AIR LEAKS AFTER LUNG RESECTIONS

The incidence of air leaks after lung resections is high. Up to 60% of all patients will show some grade of air leakage during the water submersion test after parenchymal resections. The majority of small air leaks stop within the first few hours after surgery. However, when air leakage extends to postoperative day 5, a prolonged postoperative air leak (PAL) is established by definition. PAL is the most prevalent postoperative complication, with an incidence of around 20%. The prolonged need for chest tube drainage is not only associated with increased morbidity (pain, immobility, restricted ventilation) but also leads to considerably increased health costs. In addition, a heightened mortality rate is associated with PAL, mainly due to the higher likelihood of developing empyema and pneumonia caused by the prolonged pleuroparenchymal communication. Several risk factors have been found predisposing for the development of PAL: a low predicted forced expiratory volume in 1 second, upper lobe resection, incomplete fissures, emphysema, pleural adhesions, and previous thoracic operations.

Prevention of PAL

Major air leakage found during the water submersion test should be repaired immediately during the operation. Besides placing stiches to reclose the lung surface, there are several intraoperative techniques to prevent the development of PAL.[7]

SEALING OF THE LUNG

There are several sealing products on the market, including liquid fibrin sealants, synthetic hydrogels, glutaraldehyde-bovine-albumin-based bioadhesives and collagen fleece-bound sealants. Small diffuse parenchymal defects can be easily closed by these sealing devices, especially if the lung parenchyma is fragile and placing sutures results in aggravation by tearing of the parenchyma. According to the literature, lung sealants are effective in reducing PAL, and their application results in shorter time to chest tube removal.[8]

REDUCING PLEURAL SPACE: PLEURAL TENTING, PNEUMOPERITONEUM, PHRENIC CRUSHING

Pleural tenting is a rather old technique, first proposed in 1956 by Miscall et al., that has been rediscovered lately. The technique is rather easy to apply. The apical aspect of the parietal pleura is completely dissected from the endothoracic fascia and the free lateral margin is sutured to the muscle fibers of the 4th intercostal space in order to form a tent. A pneumoperitoneum is produced by puncturing the diaphragm with a Veress needle and injecting air into the abdomen. This results in a temporary elevation of the diaphragm, reducing the postoperative pleural space and sustaining the symphysis of the two pleural surfaces. Both techniques result in a higher likelihood of sealing small parenchymal defects. Alternatively, the phrenic nerve can be crushed, leading to a temporary paralysis of 3–6 months, but this technique rarely is used.

BUTTRESSING OF STAPLE LINES

The development of varied height staples has minimized the mechanical stress placed on the staple line, and therefore air leakage originating from staple lines is mostly limited to severely emphysematous lung tissue. Reinforced staple lines have been successfully applied to overcome this problem. Synthetic materials (e.g., polytetrafluoroethylene) as well as biological tissues (e.g., bovine pericardium) can be used for this purpose.

SUCTION VERSUS NO SUCTION

The application of suction to chest tubes after pulmonary resection is common practice in thoracic surgery. The idea behind this practice is that negative pressure might enhance the approximation of the lung to the chest wall, resulting in earlier sealing of small parenchymal leaks. This is opposed by evidence from patients undergoing lung volume reduction surgery, where the application of $-20\,cm\ H_2O$ led to prolonged air leaks due to increased air flow preventing a closure of small parenchymal defects. Several randomized controlled trials found that suction with water seal was not superior in terms of duration of postoperative air leak and the development of PAL when compared with water seal alone.[9]

Treatment of PAL

The treatment algorithm for PAL first presumes differentiation into parenchymal air leakage and early BPFs. In most cases, a leak from the alveoli will be the underlying mechanism of PAL; however, if there is clinical suspicion of BPF, a bronchoscopy should be performed. Early BPF requires immediate operative revision and reclosure of the bronchial stump.

PAL due to parenchymal leakage can be treated in the following ways:

- The vast majority of PALs will eventually close in the course of time. Chest tubes should be reduced to one drainage tube and a mobile drainage system or a chest drain valve can be installed. Patients can be fully mobilized and discharged from hospital with these devices. Prolonged antibiotic coverage is necessary and patients should be regularly checked up on, on an outpatient basis. When air leakage subsides and chest radiography is inconspicuous, the chest tube can be removed.
- There is limited evidence that installation of autologous blood in the pleural space might be successful in treating PAL. As the exact volume of blood is not clear and the risk of infections and empyema is increased, this is not routinely used.

- Another novel approach is the temporary implantation of an endobronchial one-way valve into the affected segmental or subsegmental bronchus.

If conservative treatment fails and a considerable air leakage remains, rethoracotomy and surgical closure of the parenchymal defect are recommended. Electronic chest tube systems allow a quantitative assessment of the air leak and can show a long-term trend over certain period. These devices considerably facilitate the decision-making process relative to the need to return to the operating room for repeat thoractomy and surgical closure of the air leak.

REFERENCES

1. Grijalva CG, Zhu Y, Nuorti JP, Griffin MR. Emergence of parapneumonic empyema in the USA. *Thorax*. 2011 Aug; 66(8): 663–8.
2. Davies HE, Davies RJ, Davies CW; BTS Pleural Disease Guideline Group. Management of pleural infection in adults: British Thoracic Society Pleural Disease Guideline 2010. *Thorax*. 2010 Aug; 65(Suppl 2): ii41–53.
3. Abbas AES, Deschamps C. Postpneumonectomy empyema. *Curr Opin Pulm Med*. 2002 Jul; 8(4): 327–33.
4. Moreno P, Lang G, Taghavi S, Aigner C, Marta G, De Palma A, Klepetko W. Right-sided approach for management of left-main-bronchial stump problems. *Eur J Cardiothorac Surg*. 2011 Oct; 40(4): 926–30.
5. Schneiter D, Grodzki T, Lardinois D, Kestenholz PB, Wojcik J, Kubisa B, Pierog J, Weder W. Accelerated treatment of postpneumonectomy empyema: a binational long-term study. *J Thorac Cardiovasc Surg*. 2008 Jul; 136(1): 179–85.
6. Lois M, Noppen M. Bronchopleural fistulas: an overview of the problem with special focus on endoscopic management. *Chest* 2005 Dec; 128(6): 3955–65.
7. Venuta F, Rendina EA, De Giacomo T, Coloni GF. Postoperative strategies to treat permanent air leaks. *Thorac Surg Clin*. 2010 Aug; 20(3): 391–7.
8. Malapert G, Hanna HA, Pages PB, Bernard A. Surgical sealant for the prevention of prolonged air leak after lung resection: meta-analysis. *Ann Thorac Surg*. 2010 Dec; 90(6): 1779–85.
9. Deng B, Tan QY, Zhao YP, Wang RW, Jiang YG. Suction or non-suction to the underwater seal drains following pulmonary operation: meta-analysis of randomised controlled trials. *Eur J Cardiothorac Surg*. 2010 Aug; 38(2): 210–15.

23

Video-assisted thoracoscopic surgery (VATS) sympathectomy

YOUNG K. HONG AND M. BLAIR MARSHALL

HISTORY

Dorsal sympathectomies have been performed since the beginning of the twentieth century, with the earliest reported by Alexander in 1889.[1] Initially, they were used to treat a variety of ailments unrelated to the sympathetic nervous system, such as epilepsy, angina pectoris, and glaucoma. Before the invention of endotracheal intubation, upper thoracic sympathectomies were performed via a posterior or supraclavicular approach. The initial video-assisted thoracoscopic surgery (VATS) sympathectomy, performed in 1978, demonstrated a less invasive and effective method to operate safely within the thoracic cavity.[2] Since then, the thoracoscopic approach has been the most widely used and accepted standard approach for sympathectomy.[3] The majority of these procedures are performed for primary palmar hyperhidrosis, with a smaller fraction of patients having a VATS sympathectomy for upper extremity ischemia. Currently, we use a bilateral video-assisted technique, with a 2 mm, 0-degree rigid thoracoscope, which allows it to be performed as an outpatient procedure.

PRINCIPLES AND JUSTIFICATION

Hyperhidrosis is a condition characterized by excess secretion from eccrine sweat glands that are stimulated by acetylcholine released from postganglionic neurons. Although not life threatening, hyperhidrosis can be psychologically traumatic and socially disabling for the individual. Topical creams and lotions are usually ineffective and are accompanied by side effects that are intolerable for most. Iontophoresis—electrical water bath—can be effective; however, it requires frequent use to maintain its efficacy, with infrequent, though troublesome, side effects of paresthesias, scaling, and fissure of the skin. Patients may be placed on beta-blockers or antidepressants by some physicians, but these therapies are generally ineffective. The only oral preparation found to be effective is Robinul (glycopyrrolate), a synthetic anticholinergic, but this also causes blurred vision, dry mouth, and urinary retention as side effects. We routinely give oral sympatholytic agents to all hyperhidrosis patients. Approximately 65% of patients are well controlled on this regimen, and we reserve sympathectomy for those who fail. While botulinum toxin has been demonstrated to be an effective alternative therapy, the effects are temporary, with a median duration of 3–6 months, and thus repetitive treatments are required, which can be expensive.

In addition to their use for palmar and axillary hyperhidrosis, thoracic sympathectomies may be performed to treat severe facial blushing and ischemic distal upper extremities due to small vessel disease of varying etiology.

TERMINOLOGY AND NOMENCLATURE

Historically, sympathectomy was performed without a uniform standard nomenclature to describe the various techniques used, the anatomic levels of blockade, and descriptions of symptoms, making comparison of outcome data between various institutions difficult. There was no consensus on the optimal level of sympathectomy for blockade of craniofacial, axillary, or palmar hyperhidrosis. As a result, the Society of Thoracic Surgeons released its "Expert consensus for the surgical treatment of hyperhidrosis" in 2011.[4] A new international nomenclature was recommended for describing the level of sympathectomy by referring to the rib level (R) rather than the vertebral level. In addition, the nomenclature includes terms for describing the techniques used in the procedure; specifically, "cauterized," "clipped," "cut," and "removal" of a segment of the sympathetic chain.

PREOPERATIVE ASSESSMENT AND PREPARATION

As the majority of patients presenting for a sympathetomy are young and healthy, we do not routinely perform any preoperative testing other than a complete history and physical examination. Any history of endocrine disorders should be completely evaluated prior to performing the operation. For those patients with comorbidities, the standard preoperative guidelines for general endotracheal anesthesia should be observed. Patients should be counseled preoperatively about the risks of sympathectomy, which include, but are not limited to, compensatory sweating, bradycardia, gustatory sweating, and Horner's syndrome. While Horner's syndrome or bradycardia are rarely seen (0.7%–3.0% incidence), compensatory sweating is common, with an incidence range of 30%–98%, and patients should be made well aware of this possibility prior to agreeing to the procedure. In our experience, the majority of patients experience some degree of compensatory sweating; it is the rare patient who does not. The lower incidence noted in the range described was probably reported in series where the authors either didn't look for compensatory sweating or simply ignored it. *We tell all patients to expect compensatory sweating.* The mechanism for sweating will be interrupted for the dermatome affected by the level of the sympathectomy. Thus, for thermoregulation, other parts of the body must secrete more sweat to maintain body temperature during periods of exercise or warm weather. It is important to set patients' expectations in advance, as this affects their satisfaction with the procedure overall.

ANESTHESIA

1. Our current technique uses a 2 mm thoracoscope, a Veress needle, and a 5 mm port. The procedure is performed under general anesthesia with a single-lumen endotracheal tube. The patient is positioned supine, with arms abducted to 90 degrees at the shoulder and the elbows flexed. One needs to pay special attention to positioning of the arms to avoid an inadvertent brachial plexus injury. (See **Figure 23.1**).

2. After draping, the table is flexed to bring the torso up to approximately 45 degrees. This maneuver allows gravity to assist in dropping the lungs away from the apex to allow for optimal visualization. Bilateral upper extremity temperature probes are placed and baseline temperatures are recorded for each hand. However, we have found increased digital temperature less reliable when the nerve is clipped as opposed to being divided. (See **Figure 23.2**.)

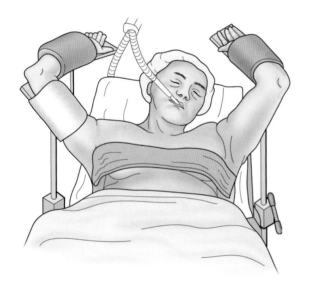

23.1

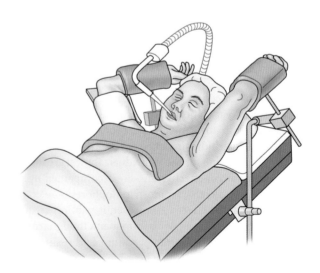

23.2

SURGICAL PROCEDURE

3. The table is rotated away from the operative side. Two intercostal spaces along the anterior axillary line are marked for placement of trocars. The superior one is located in the inferior margin of the axillary hair line, in approximately the second or third intercostal space, just posterior to the border of the pectoralis. (See **Figure 23.3**).

4. The second trocar is placed in the fifth intercostal space in the midaxillary line. The first trocar is placed through the inferior site while ventilation is being held. Carbon dioxide (CO_2) insufflation is used to reflect the lung away from the chest wall. One must ensure that the pressure limit on CO_2 insufflation is set below 10 mmHg to avoid hemodynamic compromise. (See **Figure 23.4**).

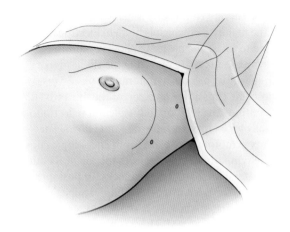

23.3

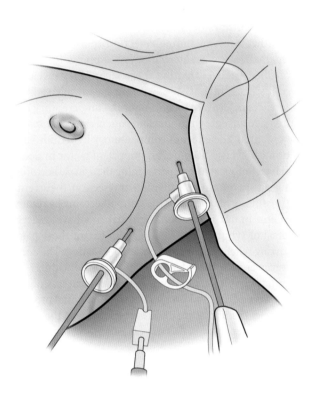

23.4

5. Once the apex of the lung is sufficiently reflected away from the apical chest wall, the second trocar is placed under direct vision. The sympathetic chain is identified, and the ribs are counted by initially identifying the first rib, the majority of which is hidden. Electrocautery is used to incise the pleura to allow visualization of the sympathetic chain overlying the rib head. For craniofacial or palmar symptoms, we place 5 mm endoscopic clips at the level top of the third rib (R3). We continue the incision in the pleural reflection laterally for 3 cm to include the Kuntz fibers. For axillary symptoms, we place 5 mm endoscopic clips on the sympathetic chain at both the top of R4 and of R5. Bilateral intercostal nerve blocks for postoperative analgesia are placed using 0.5% bupivacaine. Next, the CO_2 is evacuated, the lung is allowed to reexpand, and the trocars are removed. There is no need for routine placement of pleural drainage for these procedures, since there is no ongoing air leak as the parenchyma has not been violated. The identical procedure is performed on the opposite side. No skin sutures are needed. Dressings are placed. (See **Figure 23.5a through c**.)

Different authors have reported different techniques for sympathectomy, including resection of a portion of the sympathetic chain, cauterization, or clipping. Randomized controlled trials evaluating these techniques revealed an overall success rate of 95%, with no statistically significant differences in terms of pneumothorax, compensatory hyperhidrosis, recurrent symptoms, and patient satisfaction.[5] Given the potential side effect of compensatory hyperhidrosis, the option of reversal becomes an important factor in deciding which technique to use in performing the sympathectomy. By using clips, as opposed to division or resection, there remains the possibility of reversal of the sympathectomy by removing the clips. In our institution, eight patients have undergone reversal of sympathetic clipping, with five of those patients reporting relief of their compensatory sweating. The successful reversal patients all had the clips removed within 75 days of initial clip placement, while the three unsuccessful procedures were performed over a year after the initial procedure. We expect them to ultimately reverse, but given the slow rate of nerve regeneration, this will take additional time.

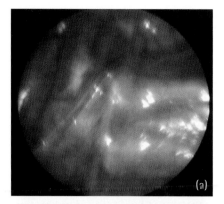

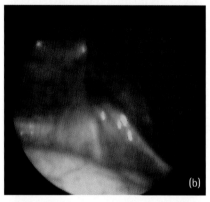

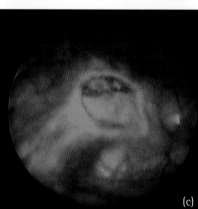

23.5a–c

POSTOPERATIVE CARE

Immediately following the procedure, a chest X-ray is routinely performed to evaluate for pneumothorax. It is not uncommon to have one or even bilateral small apical pneumothoraces from residual CO_2 left in the pleural space. If a small residual pneumothorax is noted, we place the patients on nasal cannula oxygen to expedite reabsorption. If any question of a parenchymal injury exists, we repeat a chest X-ray within 2 hours of the initial one. For those with an increasing pneumothorax, a small 6 or 7 Fr pleural catheter is placed rather than a chest tube. The leak usually seals in less than 24 hours.

Postoperative pain control is superior with intercostal nerve blocks and minimizes the requirement for either oral or intravenous opioid analgesia. The majority of patients are discharged home on the same day.

OUTCOME

For those patients undergoing sympathectomy for hyperhidrosis, most are very satisfied with their immediate results. The reported success of the procedure ranges from 85% to 98% for palmar hyperhidrosis but is only about 70% for axillary hyperhidrosis.[6,7] Although the sympathetic innervation of the feet should not be affected with this approach, 50% of patients report improvement in pedal symptoms. For those patients who fail to note improvement of their symptoms or develop a recurrence, we have performed repeat sympathectomies. For these individuals, we usually cut the pleura and underlying tissue laterally along the rib head to ensure division of any aberrant nerves.

The majority of the morbidity associated with this procedure is compensatory hyperhidrosis. As noted earlier, this is a common problem and occurs in approximately 30%–98% of patients. For most, the issue of compensatory sweating proves to be insignificant, and the patient will gladly trade this for what they had previously suffered. However, in a small fraction of patients, the compensatory sweating is actually reported to be worse than their original problem. Meta-analysis of single-ganglia and multiple ganglia sympathectomy suggests a lower risk of moderate/severe compensatory hyperhidrosis in single-ganglia blockade versus multiple ganglia blockade.[5] Additional complications include gustatory sweating (35%), with other rare (1%) complications such as Horner's syndrome, parenchymal injury, bleeding, and prolonged pain.

SUMMARY

VATS sympathectomy is a definitive, safe, and effective treatment for patients who suffer from craniofacial, palmar, or axillary hyperhidrosis, with the highest success rate reserved for those suffering from hand sweating. Various techniques such as electrocautery lesions, resection, and clip placement have been used for blockade of the sympathetic chain at the appropriate level corresponding to a patient's symptoms. Compensatory hyperhidrosis is a known and common side effect and should be discussed in detail with the patient preoperatively. By using minimally invasive methods and bilateral intercostal nerve blocks, and there being a lack of intrapleural drainage, the procedure may be performed in an ambulatory setting with patients being discharged home on the same day and experiencing immediate relief of their embarrassing social problem.

REFERENCES

1. Alexander W (1889). *The treatment of epilepsy.* Y.J. Pentland, Edinburgh, p. 228.
2. Kux M. Thoracic endoscopic sympathectomy in palmar and axillary hyperhidrosis. Arch Surg 1978; 113: 264–6.
3. Inan K, Goksel OS, Uçcak A, Temizkan V, Karaca K, Ugur M, Arslan G, Us M, Yilmaz AT. Thoracic endoscopic surgery for hyperhidrosis: comparison of different techniques. *Thoracic Cardiovascular Surgery.* 2008; 56: 4: 210–13.
4. Cerfolio RJ, De Campos JRM, Bryant AS, Connery CP, Miller DL, DeCamp MM, McKenna RJ, Krasna MJ. The Society of Thoracic Surgeons expert consensus for the surgical treatment of hyperhidrosis. *Annals of Thoracic Surgery.* 2011; 91: 1642–85.
5. Deng B, Tan QY, Jiang YG, Zhao YP, Zhou JH, Ma Z, Wang RW. Optimization of sympathectomy to treat palmar hyperhidrosis: the systemic review and meta-analysis of studies published during the past decade. *Surgical Endoscopy.* 2011; 25: 1893–1901.
6. Lee DY, Yoon YH, Shin HK, Kim HK, Hong YJ. Needle thoracic sympathectomy for essential hyperhidrosis: intermediate-term follow-up. *Annals of Thoracic Surgery.* 2000; 69: 251–3.
7. Goh PM, Cheah WK, De Costa M, Sim EK. Needlescopic thoracic sympathectomy: treatment for palmar hyperhidrosis. *Annals of Thoracic Surgery.* 2000; 70: 240–2.

24

Lung transplantation

PAULA MORENO

HISTORY

James Hardy performed the first lung transplantation (LT) in a human in 1963. The patient, a 58-year-old prisoner diagnosed with a squamous cell carcinoma in his left main bronchus, underwent single left LT.[1] Despite the initial success, the patient developed renal failure and died on postoperative day 18. Nearly 40 additional procedures were done worldwide in the following 15 years, all of them unsuccessful as a result of primary graft failure, airway complications, and multiorgan failure. The advent of cyclosporine and the refinement in surgical technique heralded clinical success. In 1981, the Stanford Group led by Norman Shumway performed the first human heart-lung transplantation (HLT).[2] The first successful single lung transplantation (SLT) was performed in 1983 by Joel Cooper and colleagues from Toronto.[3] Three years later, the same group reported the first *en bloc* double lung transplantation (DLT) through a median sternotomy using full cardiopulmonary bypass (CPB).[4] The introduction of the clamshell incision allowed for superb exposure of the pleural cavity, while providing adequate access for performing the left atrial anastomosis.[5]

PRINCIPLES

Indications for LT include any chronic end-stage pulmonary disease, refractory to maximal medical therapy or for which no medical therapy exists. Currently, chronic obstructive pulmonary disease (COPD) is the leading indication for LT, followed by idiopathic pulmonary fibrosis (IPF), cystic fibrosis (CF), emphysema due to alpha-1 antitrypsin deficiency, and idiopathic pulmonary arterial hypertension (IPAH). For septic lung diseases and certain pulmonary hypertensive disorders, the extent of disease mandates the removal of both lungs. During the early years of LT, this was achieved with combined heart-DLT. This technique was first replaced by *en bloc* DLT using CPB and a tracheal anastomosis, and finally by bilateral sequential LT through a clamshell incision.[4,5] The procedure involves three major anastomoses: (1) bronchus, (2) pulmonary artery (PA), and (3) left atrium (LA). Bronchial artery revascularization is not routinely performed. Brain-dead donors remain the main source of lung grafts for transplantation. However, only 20% of potential donors, even those whose other organs are perfectly suitable, provide lungs that are usable for transplantation.

DONOR LUNG PROCUREMENT

Donor selection criteria

The lung is especially vulnerable to being damaged as a result of trauma, aspiration, ventilator-related pneumonia, or fluid overload. Moreover, brainstem death itself may cause lung injury, which may be worsened in the posttransplant period as a result of primary graft dysfunction (PGD). The standard criteria for choosing an ideal donor lung are shown in Table 24.1.[6] However, many of these clinical criteria were chosen arbitrarily in the early years of LT. Indeed, the use of less than optimal or marginal donor lungs has not been associated with poorer outcomes and the use of such lungs has allowed for expansion of the donor pool.

Operation

DONOR LUNG PROCUREMENT

The donor chest is opened by median sternotomy, extending the incision inferiorly to the pubis, to permit extraction of the abdominal organs. Thymic remnants are dissected until the innominate vein is identified. The pericardium is widely opened in an inverted T fashion and the heart is exposed and examined. Both pleurae are incised along the reflection and the lungs are examined, looking for areas of atelectasis, edema, or contusion. A compliance test is performed by disconnecting the ventilator at end inspiration, and should result in a prompt deflation of the lungs.

1. The intrapericardial superior vena cava (SVC) is isolated and encircled with two No. 2 silk ligatures, and the inferior vena cava (IVC) is encircled with a single No. 2 silk ligature. The SVC is retracted to the left to allow the right main PA to be dissected away from the SVC and the ascending aorta (AA). The AA and main PA are dissected free from one another and each encircled with an umbilical tape. A 4-0 polypropylene suture is placed in the distal main PA in purse-string fashion for the pulmoplegia cannula and a 2-0 purse-string suture is placed in the AA for the cardioplegia cannula. The posterior pericardium between the aorta and the SVC is incised and the distal trachea is exposed. Once the

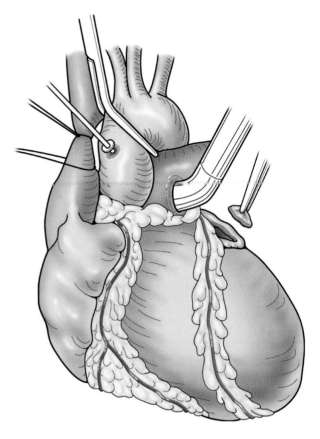

24.1 Donor lung procurement.

thoracic dissection is completed, the donor is given a systemic dose of heparin (300 units/kg). The AA is cannulated for cardiac preservation and the proximal main PA is cannulated with a 14 mm bullet-tipped perfusion cannula. A 500 mcg bolus of prostaglandin E1 (PGE1) is injected directly into the PA. Close attention should be paid to the systemic blood pressure, as this bolus may result in systemic hypotension. Shortly after, the SVC is doubly ligated and the IVC is divided above the clamp to decompress the right heart. After three or four heartbeats, the heart empties of blood, the AA is cross-clamped, and cardioplegia is initiated. The tip of the left atrial appendage is generously incised to

Table 24.1 Traditional lung transplant donor selection criteria

Age <55 years
ABO compatibility
Smoking history ≤20 pack-year
Clear chest X-ray
PaO_2 ≥300 mmHg (FiO_2 1.0, PEEP = 5 cm H_2O; 5 min)
Fiber-optic bronchoscopy with no evidence of aspiration or purulent secretions
Absence of significant chest trauma

Notes: FiO_2, Fraction of inspired oxygen; PaO_2, Partial pressure of oxygen at sea level; PEEP, positive end-expiratory pressure.

decompress the left heart, and the lung flush is initiated. Perfadex, 60 mL/kg at 4°C, is used as preservation solution. The pericardial sac and both pleural spaces are topically cooled with ice slush saline, while gentle ventilation of both lungs is continued. Toward the end of lung perfusion, the effluent should run almost clear. After completion of the cardioplegia and the pulmoplegia, the aortic and pulmonary cannulae are removed and the heart is then extracted. The SVC is divided between the ligatures, the aorta is transected proximal to the cross-clamp and dissected off the right PA, and the distal main PA is transected, starting at the cannulation site (**Figure 24.1**).

2. Cooperation of the heart and lung teams is of paramount importance, especially regarding the site of division of the left atrial cuff and the site of cannulation and division of the main PA. The heart is retracted to the right and an incision is made in the LA, midway between the coronary sinus and the left pulmonary veins (PVs). The incision is extended superiorly over the roof of the LA, and inferiorly, parallel to the coronary sinus. An adequate cuff of LA should have a small rim of atrial muscle around each of the PV orifices (**Figure 24.2**).

3. Once the heart is removed, the trachea is encircled and doubly stapled using a TA stapling device, keeping the lungs at end-tidal inflation. The trachea is then divided between the staple lines, and all superior mediastinal tissue is incised. The pericardium is incised from one side to the other, the pulmonary ligaments are divided, and the donor lung block is removed after dividing the descending aorta (**Figure 24.3**).

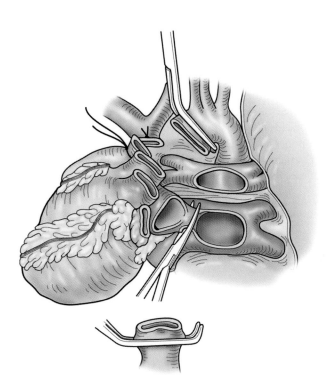

24.2 Donor cardiectomy.

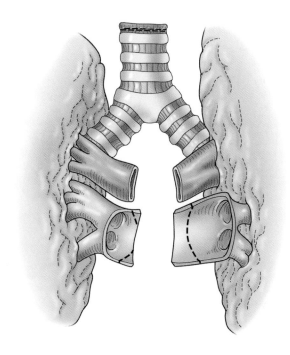

24.3 Donor lung block.

SPLITTING THE DONOR LUNG BLOCK

Once on the back table, an additional retrograde flush is made. With the same PA cannula inserted into the PVs, the perfusate is vented through the main PA and continued until the effluent runs clear, with no clots. For DLT, the lung block is triple-bagged and placed on ice in the transport box. On occasion, the lung block must be split at the donor hospital, when two single lung recipients are going to be transplanted at different institutions (twinning procedures). In this case, the PA is divided at the level of its bifurcation, the LA is divided at midline, and the posterior pericardium is divided from below upward. Any residual mediastinal tissue is dissected free, and the proximal left main bronchus is doubly stapled and divided between the staple lines, which separates the two lungs. Then, the grafts are triple-bagged and transported as described.

Donation after circulatory death and the use of *ex vivo* lung perfusion

Recently, new strategies have been developed to potentially increase the lung donor pool, such as the use of lungs from donors after circulatory death—donation after circulatory death (DCD)—and the use of *ex vivo* lung perfusion (EVLP).[7] Controlled DCD is the most accepted and used DCD type for donation.[8] A warm ischemic time is added to the cold ischemic period. The process of DCD donor lung evaluation and procedure is as follows: life-sustaining therapies are withdrawn from the DCD donor at a planned time, which subsequently leads to patient death and then, organ retrieval can proceed; five minutes after the declaration of

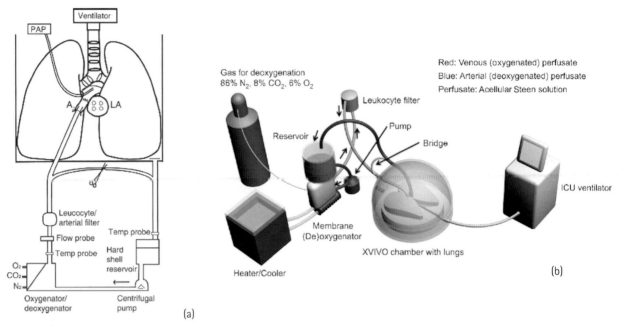

24.4a–b (a) Scheme of EVLP protocol, Lund. (b) Scheme of EVLP protocol, Toronto.

cardiac death, the donor is reintubated and reventilated; finally, the lungs are procured and preserved in the standard way, with in situ antegrade flush and retrograde flush on the back table.

Another novel strategy to overcome the shortage of donor lungs is EVLP, which is used to optimize and recover organs initially deemed unsuitable for transplantation.[9] Contrary to standard cold static preservation, EVLP provides physiologic normothermic lung perfusion and allows for functional reassessment prior to implantation.

4. The lungs are perfused with a specifically designed solution (Steen solution) through the PA, and ventilated mechanically following a protective strategy. Clinically, the two most practiced EVLP methodologies are the Lund and the Toronto protocols[8,9] (**Figure 24.4a and b**).

SINGLE LUNG TRANSPLANTATION

Preoperative assessment and preparation

RECIPIENT SELECTION

Candidates must be free of significant comorbidities and sufficiently fit to tolerate the procedure. The most frequent conditions to be considered for SLT are COPD and interstitial lung diseases. Also, SLT may be the procedure of choice for older patients or those who would not tolerate the longer anesthetic time of DLT. Absolute contraindications are listed in **Table 24.2**. The side to be transplanted depends on several factors. Ideally, one should choose the lung that demonstrates the poorest function on lung perfusion scanning. However, for patients with previous thoracic operations like talc pleurodesis, the "virgin" side is preferable.

Table 24.2 Absolute contraindications to LT

Malignancy in the last 2 years (other than nonmelanoma skin cancer)
Noncurable extrapulmonary infection (chronic active viral hepatitis B, hepatitis C, HIV)
Significant dysfunction of other vital organs (especially heart, liver, and kidney)
Significant chest wall/spinal deformity
Active or recent cigarette smoking, drug or alcohol dependency (last 6 months)
Severe psychiatric illness
Documented noncompliance with medical therapy
Absence of a consistent or reliable social support system

Anesthesia

Sedation outside of the operating room is not recommended as it may precipitate a cardiorespiratory arrest due to hypoxemia, hypercapnia or increased pulmonary vascular resistance resulting in acute right ventricular failure. A thoracic epidural catheter is usually placed once the patient arrives at the operating room. Standard monitoring is shown in Table 24.3. Transesophageal echocardiography (TEE) is also recommended to evaluate right ventricular function, distention, tricuspid regurgitation, left- and right-sided preload, the adequacy of left heart filling and volume status, assessment of air emboli after de-airing maneuvers, and to estimate right ventricular cardiac output, especially during and after PA clamping and unclamping. One-lung ventilation (OLV) is achieved with a double lumen endotracheal tube. In IPF patients, oxygenation can be maintained at the expense of increasing inflation pressures, which may result in hypercapnia or increased end-tidal partial pressure of carbon dioxide (PCO_2). In addition, hypotension during trial PA clamping anticipates the need for CPB. Monitoring of the patient undergoing DLT is as for SLT. However, bronchial toilet is of paramount importance for patients with septic lung disease. These patients are initially intubated with a single lumen endotracheal tube and fiber-optic bronchoscopy is performed to allow vigorous suctioning of purulent secretions. This maneuver reduces the need for CPB due to respiratory insufficiency while on OLV. Due to the risk of development of noncardiogenic pulmonary edema in the reimplanted lung, it is extremely important to avoid excessive fluid administration.

OPERATION

The patient is positioned in a lateral decubitus position, with a roll under the chest. Proper padding to the elbows and knees will avoid postoperative complications, such as venous thrombosis or nerve compression. In addition, a prophylactic venous compression system is placed on the lower extremities in every patient. A posterolateral thoracotomy is made, entering the chest through the 5th intercostal space. In patients with a small thorax, it is recommended to enter the pleural space through the 4th rather than the 5th intercostal space. A Finochietto retractor is placed and slowly opened to spread the ribs. Optionally, a Tuffier rib retractor can be placed in a perpendicular direction to retract the skin and the serratus anterior muscle. Double lung ventilation is continued whenever possible, to minimize the aggravation of hypoxia secondary to intrapulmonary shunt. Adhesions, if any, and the inferior pulmonary ligament are divided. Due to the small chest cavities of fibrotic patients, it is helpful to place a heavy traction suture (0 silk) into the fibrous dome of diaphragm, which is brought out of the chest and secured after pulling down the diaphragm with the suture. The pleura is incised anteriorly at the hilum, and special care should be taken to avoid injury to the phrenic nerve. Even if the patient is hemodynamically stable, the PA should be clamped for a trial period of 10–15 minutes to ensure that both ventilation and perfusion of the dependent lung only can be tolerated. If the patient does not tolerate OLV, in case of ventilatory compromise (acidosis, hypoxemia, hypercapnia), or hemodynamic instability (hypotension, dysrhythmias, right ventricular dysfunction, increased PA pressures) during this maneuver, they should be placed on extracorporeal lung support (ELS).

Table 24.3 Standard monitoring of the lung transplant recipient

1. Vascular

    Radial artery line

    Large peripheral venous line

    Multi-lumen central venous access

    Swan-Ganz catheter (continuous PA monitoring)

2. Heart

    Five-lead electrocardiography

    Pulse oximetry

    Transesophageal echocardiography

3. Kidney

    Urinary output (Foley catheter)

4. Temperature monitoring

5. Active warming

6. Capnography

PNEUMONECTOMY

5. Recipient pneumonectomy is performed only after the donor lung arrives in the operating room. The PA branches are ligated and divided, and the main trunk of the PA is divided beyond this level. The superior and inferior PVs are dissected to their first branches and divided. An Endo GIA stapler can help in the division of the PA and both PVs and should be placed as far distally on the vessel as possible, to leave a long cuff. The last structure to be divided is the main bronchus, which is transected two cartilaginous rings proximal to the upper lobe bronchus orifice. A No. 15-blade scalpel is used to open the bronchus, which is transected at right angles to its axis, and between rather than through cartilaginous rings. Excessive dissection around the peribronchial tissues is to be avoided, to ensure adequate blood supply to the bronchial anastomosis (see **Figure 24.5**).

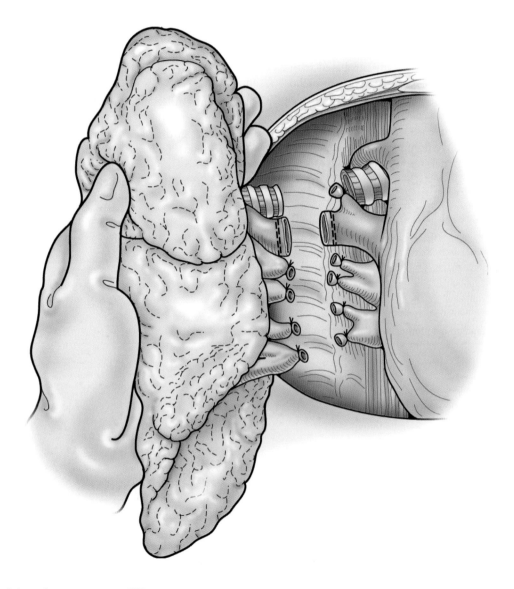

24.5 Recipient of pneumonectomy SLT.

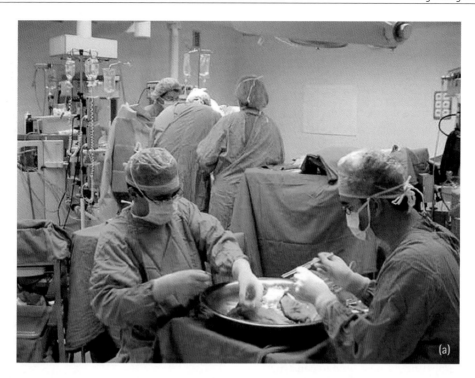

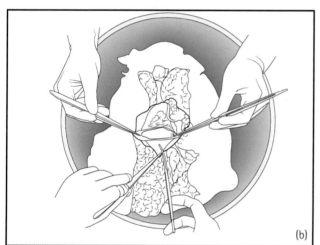

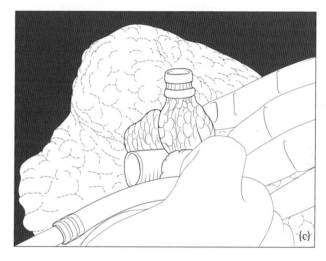

24.6 Bench dissection: (a) surgeons at the back table; (b) allograft separation; (c) allograft ready for implantation.

PREPARATION OF THE HILUM

Once the native lung is removed from the operative field, secretions in the open proximal bronchus are suctioned. Before implanting the lung graft, the pulmonary hilum has to be prepared for the anastomoses. The PA is dissected as central as possible and mobilized off adjacent structures to permit the placement of a vascular clamp for proximal control. Next, the PV stumps are grasped and retracted anteriorly, laterally and posteriorly to permit circumferential opening of the pericardium. For right LT, the interatrial groove (Sondergaard's groove) must be dissected to safely place a Satinsky vascular clamp. Meticulous hemostasis in the posterior mediastinum is achieved at this point of the operation, because this area is difficult to reach once the graft has been implanted.

BENCH DISSECTION

6. An additional allograft dissection is performed to prepare the bronchus, the PA, and the atrial cuff for the anastomoses. The donor PA is identified and cut appropriately short to avoid kinking once the anastomosis is complete. The atrial cuff is identified and freed from the pericardium. Then, the stapled end of the bronchus is transected and cultures of secretions are sent. Secretions are suctioned and lavaged with a few milliliters of saline and the donor bronchus is trimmed within two cartilaginous rings of the upper lobe bronchus takeoff (see **Figure 24.6a through c**).

IMPLANTATION

The donor lung, wrapped in cold gauze, is placed in the posterior portion of the chest cavity. Continued recooling of the graft can be achieved by regularly placing ice slush on the lung surface.

7. The anastomoses start from the most posterior and proceed to the most anterior hilar structure (bronchus → PA → LA). The membranous portion of the bronchial anastomosis is performed first, with a running 4-0 PDS (polydioxanone) suture. The cartilaginous wall can usually be sutured in a running fashion. In case of size mismatch, a telescoping anastomosis with the donor bronchus outside might be unavoidable. When the bronchial anastomosis is completed, the chest cavity is flooded with cold saline and the suture is checked for air leaks (see **Figure 24.7**).

8. The second anastomosis to be performed is the PA. A PA clamp is applied, taking care to not apply the clamp to the Swan-Ganz catheter. The clamp is secured to the skin with a silk suture to immobilize it and prevent it from sliding out or springing open prematurely. A running 5-0 polypropylene suture is used to construct the anastomosis. Before tying both sutures in the middle, the PA is filled with heparinized saline to check the suture line for leaks and identify any leaking point needing additional stitches (see **Figure 24.8a and b**).

9. The last anastomosis to be performed is the LA. Judd-Allis clamps are applied to the superior and inferior PVs stumps, a Satinsky vascular clamp is placed on the recipient atrial cuff and secured to the skin with a No. 2 silk. The staple lines of the superior and inferior vein stumps are incised, and both venous openings are joined into a single orifice. An end-to-end running anastomosis is performed, using a 4-0 polypropylene suture. The

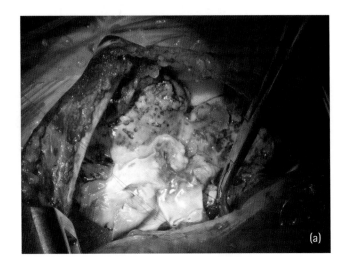

(a)

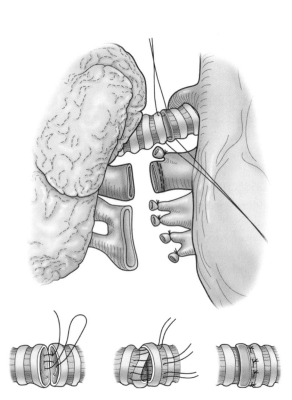

24.7 Implantation. Bronchial anastomosis.

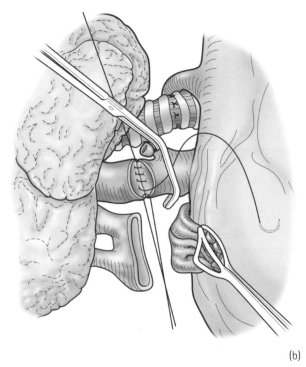

(b)

24.8 Implantation. PA anastomosis. (a) The pulmonary arterial anastomosis is completed with a running suture of 5-0 polypropylene. (b) Note the division of the ligamentum arteriosum and the placement of the clamp on the recipient pulmonary artery.

back wall is sutured from the bottom corner to the top corner, using an everting mattress suture to prevent any atrial muscle from remaining inside the anastomosis. The two suture ends are left untied for flushing and deairing of the graft after reperfusion. The anesthetist should suction all the secretions from the implanted lung. My routine practice before reperfusion consists of the administration of 1 g of methylprednisolone intravenously together with the antioxidants acetylcysteine (2 g intravenous [IV]) and vitamin C (1 g IV) as free radical scavengers, to minimize the development of reperfusion edema. The patient is then placed in Trendelenburg position and ventilation is started. The silk ties securing the PA clamp and the Satinsky vascular clamp are both cut. The PA clamp is gradually opened to fill the PA, and this makes the lung turn its appearance progressively from pale to pink, as the warm blood perfuses it. The Satinsky vascular clamp is gradually opened too, and the perfusion solution first, followed by blood thereafter and some air bubbles, will appear at the atrial suture line. When blood comes from the atrial suture line without any air bubble, the two suture ends are tied and the Satinsky vascular clamp removed from the field. It is of paramount importance to avoid initial volume overload to the implanted lung. For this, the PA clamp is reapplied and maintained half-open for 10–15 minutes (the so-called controlled pressure reperfusion). Alternatively, partial manual compression of the artery can be performed. At the end of this period, the PA clamp is completely removed. Both vascular anastomoses are checked for hemostasis, and additional polypropylene sutures are placed as needed. Two 28 Fr chest tubes are positioned: one is placed superiorly toward the apex, and the other is placed inferiorly, at the costodiaphragmatic sinus. Finally, the thoracotomy is closed in layers and the double lumen endotracheal tube is changed to a single lumen one. Fiber-optic bronchoscopy is performed to check the bronchial anastomosis and to vigorously suction secretions and blood clots from the airway.

10. Extracorporeal lung support (ELS is required in approximately one-third of cases. It can be used either electively (in the case of pretransplant pulmonary hypertension, lobar transplantation, reduced pulmonary vascular bed, concomitant cardiac repair), during the implantation of the graft (if the native lung is not able to maintain ventilation), or during the implantation of the second graft in the case of a DLT. During the procedure, the need for ELS is anticipated by the development of hypoxia, hypercapnia, or hemodynamic instability, usually indicating right ventricle failure. Right ventricle dysfunction is managed with milrinone, while reperfusion edema may improve with the use of inhaled nitric oxide and PGE1 infusion. Systemic hypotension is a relatively frequent event during LT, usually secondary to mediastinal manipulation and vasodilation. Thus,

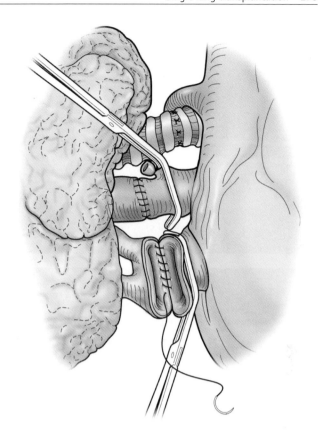

24.9   Implantation. LA anastomosis.

treatment with norepinephrine, vasopressin, and phenylephrine may improve gas exchange. However, these are only supportive measures. The question is whether to choose standard CPB or extracorporeal membrane oxygenation (ECMO), which is determined by the indications, and availability in and expertise of each individual transplant center. Recently, many lung transplant groups have taken to using ECMO instead of CPB.[10] Ideally, one should choose to use standard CPB for those cases in which extremely high blood turnover is expected due to previous operations and significant adhesions, or when concomitant cardiac surgery is needed. In all other cases, venoarterial ECMO support is preferable (see **Figure 24.9**).

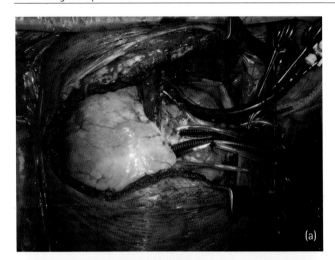

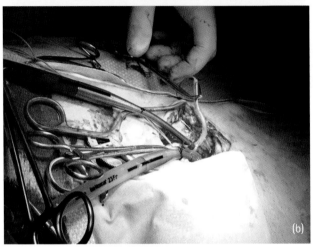

24.10a–b ELS cannulation: (a) central cannulation; (b) peripheral cannulation (right groin).

11. The mode of cannulation can be central or peripheral. In right thoracotomies or clamshell incisions, the right atrium and the AA are cannulated. In left thoracotomies, the cannulas are placed in the main PA and the descending aorta. The right groin via the common femoral vein (21F to 28F) and common femoral artery (15F to21F) is the preferred site for peripheral ECMO cannulation. At the end of the procedure, the patient is progressively weaned from ECMO if hemodynamically stable, as long as there is no evidence of significant reperfusion edema or right ventricular failure. On the contrary, ECMO support, if required, is continued into the postoperative period by switching from central to peripheral cannulation (see **Figure 24.10a and b**).

DOUBLE LUNG TRANSPLANTATION

Preoperative preparation and assessment

Patients with septic lung disease require a DLT to remove the entire focus of sepsis. A single lung graft is doomed to fail if a septic lung remains in place. Pleural spaces of these patients are often severely distorted by recurrent bacterial infection, and adhesions are usually dense and very vascular. Furthermore, enlarged lymph nodes are frequently found at the hilum, obscuring the dissection of the PA and main bronchus. LT candidates with obstructive lung disease will do well with either SLT or DLT. Patients younger than 55 years who are fit enough to tolerate the bilateral procedure and those with larger chest cavities are usually candidates for DLT. Slightly superior actuarial survival is observed for COPD patients undergoing DLT compared with those undergoing SLT, probably due to avoidance of the risks of severe hyperinflation and occult sepsis of the remaining native lung. DLT in emphysema patients is technically straightforward, sternal splitting can be avoided, and CPB is usually not required. Also, marginal donor lungs can be used in these patients, as some degree of reversible donor lung dysfunction is usually tolerable. The advent of disease-specific medical therapies for IPAH has significantly reduced patient referral for LT programs. However, transplantation remains the gold standard for patients who fail medical therapy. As a rule, patients with IPAH do not require HLT unless there is a significant anatomic heart defect. Furthermore, results with SLT or DLT for primary pulmonary hypertension are comparable to or better than HLT, with a trend toward a survival benefit with DLT over SLT. In addition, severe right heart dysfunction is reversible after SLT or DLT, due to the rapid reduction in pulmonary vascular resistance that results following placement of the lung allograft. It is likely that DLT results in better unloading of the right heart, leading to a more benign postoperative course. However, the threshold for unrecoverable right ventricular dysfunction is unknown but experience has shown reversibility of right ventricular dysfunction in the majority of cases. The approach to DLT has changed significantly since its inception. The original procedure was performed through a median sternotomy and the donor lungs were implanted *en bloc* with a single tracheal anastomosis, with the patient on full CPB. The bilateral sequential operation was introduced in 1989 and has become the standard approach. The sternal-sparing approach was introduced in 1996 and may be used in selected patients with emphysema, but it might be inappropriate for patients with small pleural cavities where exposure would prove difficult. The lung with the least perfusion, as judged by preoperative quantitative ventilation and perfusion scans, is resected and replaced first, as this strategy decreases the likelihood of needing intraoperative CPB.

POSITION

12. The patient is positioned supine with the chest elevated by a roll under the back and the arms tucked at their side. Alternatively, the arms can be abducted or lifted upward and fixed to the ether screen. The entire chest is exposed from the neck to the umbilicus, and laterally to each posterior axillary line (see **Figure 24.11**).

INCISION

13. Our incision of choice is the bilateral transsternal anterolateral thoracotomy (clamshell incision). The curvilinear skin incision runs along the inframammary crease and crosses the sternum at the level of the fourth intercostal space. The lower edge of the pectoralis major muscle is divided and lifted up with its overlying skin and soft tissues. In patients with substantial breast tissue, a heavy silk suture is used to retract both breasts cephalad. The chest is entered laterally at the fourth intercostal space. The internal mammary vessels are ligated or clipped and divided, and a Gigli saw is used to divide the sternum transversally. Two twin Finochietto chest retractors are placed and smoothly opened to gradually spread the ribs vertically. The retrosternal space is exposed and sternomediastinal ligaments are progressively freed by blunt dissection. Both pleural spaces are examined and adhesions, if any, divided. The dissection continues on the side where the lung is to be replaced first. The mediastinal pleura is opened, exposing the hilum. It is important to perform bilateral pleural adhesiolysis and complete mobilization of pulmonary hila before explantation of

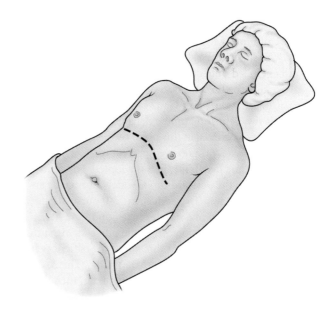

24.11 Patient's position for DLT.

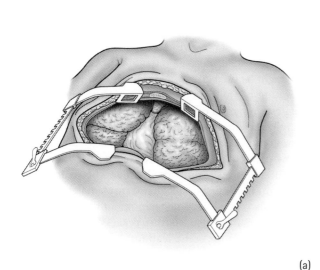

(a)

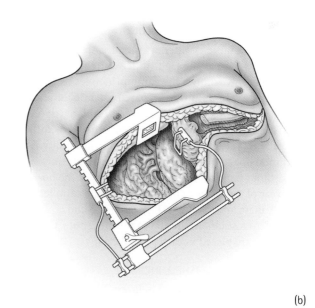

(b)

24.12a–b Clamshell incision. (a) The bilateral thoracosternotomy (clamshell) incision is placed in an inframammary location. The sternum is divided in a transverse fashion and the chest is entered through bilateral fourth intercostal spaces. Two Finochietto retractors are placed for maximum exposure. (b) Alternatively instead of dividing the sternum bilateral anterior thoracotomies may be performed. This eliminates the problem with sternal healing but limits somewhat the exposure as compared to that available when the sternum is divided. The Finochietto retractor is used to spread the ribs while the Balfour retractor spreads the soft tissue.

the first lung, as this minimizes the time that the newly implanted lung is exposed to the entire cardiac output. The pulmonary ligament is incised toward the inferior PV. The superior PV, PA, and inferior PV are dissected and encircled outside the pericardium. A clamp is used to occlude the PA for a trial period of 10–15 minutes, ensuring that the Swan-Ganz catheter is not grasped. By this time, the lung can be deflated. Monitoring of the patient is crucial at this point of the procedure. In case of hypoxia, progressive hypercapnia, low pH, or hemodynamic instability, ELS is adopted. For central cannulation, the pericardium is widely opened in an inverted T fashion. Two concentric 2-0 purse-string sutures are placed in a standard fashion in the AA, followed by one 4-0 polypropylene purse-string suture in the right appendage. At this point, the patient is fully heparinized intravenously with 300 IU/kg. The AA and the right appendage are then cannulated in turn, and ELS is begun. The pneumonectomy is then completed. The superior PV, PA, and inferior PV are transected; the bronchus is sectioned; and the specimen is removed from the field (see **Figure 24.12a and b**).

IMPLANTATION OF THE FIRST LUNG

The recipient's pulmonary hilum is prepared for the three anastomoses as described for SLT. The lungs to be implanted have been previously separated and dissected on a back table, to prepare the bronchus, the PA, and the atrial cuff for the anastomoses (bench dissection). The donor lung, wrapped in cold gauze, is brought to the operative field and placed in the posterior portion of the mediastinum. The anastomoses are completed in the standard fashion of bronchus, PA, and LA.

IMPLANTATION OF THE SECOND LUNG

The operating table is tilted as much as possible to the opposite side (i.e., to the right in left lung implantation). Pneumonectomy follows the same principles as the contralateral side. The hilum is prepared for implantation of the graft analogous to the right-sided implantation. The LA anastomosis on the left side is often the most difficult technically to perform, and hemodynamic instability is not uncommon due to mediastinal retraction. Gentle traction by the assistant's hand and intermittent release of the heart aid in recovery of the systemic blood pressure. On completion of the three anastomoses, the graft is ventilated and reperfused in a standard fashion. At the end of the procedure, two 28 Fr chest drains are placed in each pleural cavity.

CLOSURE OF THE CLAMSHELL INCISION

14. The thoracotomy is closed in layers. My colleagues and I have replaced classic sternal wire fixation with semirigid fixation using two nitinol (nickel-titanium) thermo-reactive clips, placed at each side of the sternum. Electrocautery is used to create a tunnel through the intercostal space, just adjacent to the sternum, to set the clip. Great care should be taken to avoid injury to the internal thoracic vessels. Thereafter, four pericostal sutures are placed on each hemithorax and tied. This aids in keeping the sternum closed. When the proximal and distal parts of the sternum are put together, the distance between intercostal spaces is measured to choose the clip size. The clip is then cooled with ice and set on special forceps. Cooling makes the clip malleable and easy to fit into the intercostal space. Once placed, the clip is heated using a gauze embedded in hot saline. The pectoralis major muscle, subcutaneous tissue, and skin are closed in layers with absorbable sutures. At the conclusion of the procedure, the double lumen endotracheal tube is switched to a single lumen endotracheal one, and fiber-optic bronchoscopy is then performed to check the anastomosis (see **Figure 24.13a through e**).

POSTOPERATIVE CARE

The patient is transported intubated to the intensive care unit (ICU) and mechanical ventilation is continued until the patient is stable. Protective ventilation is used to minimize barotrauma in the newly implanted lungs. Most patients can be extubated in the first 48 hours posttransplantation. However, for those recipients who will probably require prolonged mechanical ventilation, early tracheostomy should be performed to aid in ventilatory weaning. Adequate negative fluid balance should be maintained, keeping the patient "dry" through aggressive diuresis. Ventilation–perfusion mismatches are minimized in DLT, so the postoperative course of an uncomplicated DLT recipient is generally smoother than that of a SLT recipient. In SLT, due to size and compliance discrepancy between the transplanted lung and the native one, air trapping, mediastinal shift due to hyperinflation of the native lung, or even tension pneumothorax may occur. For instance, peak airway pressure must be managed accordingly and the use of positive end-expiratory pressure (PEEP) is generally avoided, especially after SLT for COPD. Low-level PEEP might be used after SLT or DLT for other indications. Positioning of the patient with the transplanted side up facilitates ventilation of the graft. Fiber-optic bronchoscopy is liberally used to clear secretions from the airway and check the anastomosis.

Many patients require vasopressors during the surgical procedure. However, most of them can be weaned from these agents in the first hours after transplantation if aggressive diuresis is used. Hypotension may then be secondary to hypovolemia but also to other processes, such as sepsis, vascular anastomotic complications, left or right ventricular failure, pulmonary thromboembolism, or native lung hyperinflation. Some degree of pulmonary edema in the newly implanted lung is almost universal, due to increased vascular permeability and impairment of lymphatic drainage. Therefore, optimal fluid for volume replacement is of paramount importance.

The immunosuppression regimen is begun just before or immediately after surgery. A standard triple-drug regimen,

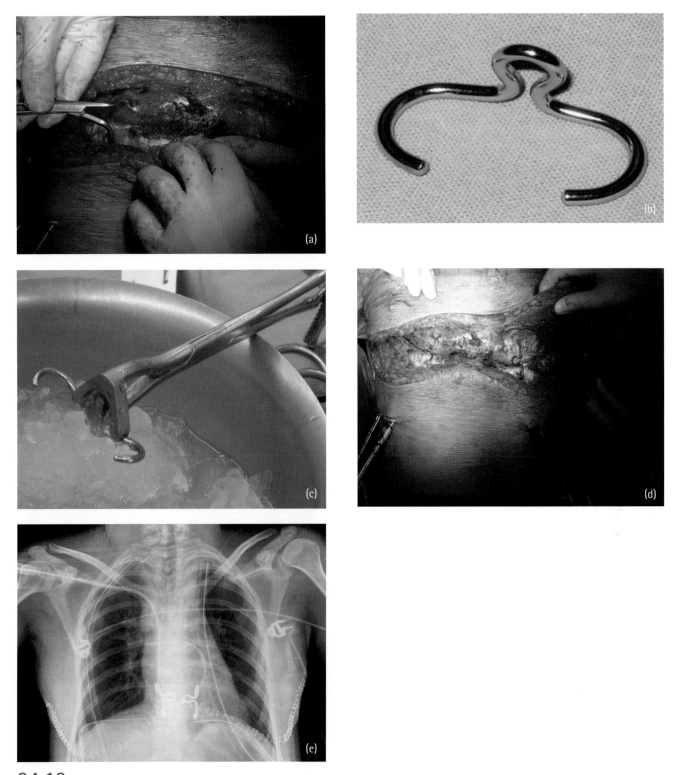

24.13a–e Clamshell closure: (a) measurement clip size; (b) nitinol clip; (c) nitinol clip placed on ice; (d) chest closed with pleural drains in situ; (e) postoperative chest X-ray showing nitinol clips.

including a calcineurin inhibitor (cyclosporin/tacrolimus), an antimetabolite agent (mycophenolate/azathioprine), and steroids, is used for maintenance therapy. Induction immunosuppression with cytolytic agents is also used in many centers to reduce doses of standard immunosuppressants. Acute rejection episodes occur in more than 50% of recipients within the first year following LT, regardless of the immunosuppressive regimen used. Treatment consists of a 3-day course of 10–15 mg/kg/day of IV methylprednisolone.

Primary graft failure may occur in up to 20% of patients in the early posttransplantation period, and manifests within the first 72 hours as hypoxemia; copious and proteinaceous secretions; leukocytosis, low-grade fever; elevated pulmonary arterial pressures; pulmonary infiltrates on chest X-ray, typically most extensive in perihilar regions; and difficulty in ventilating the patient secondary to decreased lung compliance. Differential diagnoses are acute rejection, infection, venous anastomosis complications, and cardiogenic pulmonary edema. Inhaled nitric oxide (10–40 ppm) may improve hemodynamics and ventilation–perfusion matching in some patients. Alternatively, nebulized epoprostenol can be used. Recently, ECMO has been added to the armamentarium of PGD management.

Infections are common among LT recipients, due to the continued exposure of the graft to the external environment. Thus, antimicrobial therapy is administered to every patient, starting intraoperatively with broad-spectrum antibiotics. In case of LT for a CF recipient colonized by multiresistant *Pseudomonas aeruginosa*, inhaled colistin or tobramycin is added to the antimicrobial regimen. *Pneumocystis jirovecii* pneumonia prophylaxis is started immediately after transplantation, with trimethoprim-sulfamethoxazole. Prophylactic viral medication is given on the basis of the recipient/donor CMV and EBV status.

Appropriate analgesia in the early postoperative phase is crucial. IV fentanyl is used in the first hours/days in the ICU. Furthermore, an epidural catheter aids in achieving pain control, combined with IV nonsteroidal anti-inflammatory drugs for the first days.

Chest tube drainage is monitored carefully for hemorrhage or significant air leak. Bleeding is more frequent following CPB or in those patients who required takedown of extensive pleural adhesions and may require surgical reexploration. There should be no hesitation in taking a patient back to the operating room in the presence of hemorrhage. Following extubation, the apical chest tubes are removed in the absence of air leaks, usually in the first 48 hours posttransplant. On the contrary, the basal chest tubes are usually maintained until the fifth to seventh posttransplant day, because of the frequent occurrence of pleural effusions, especially following DLT.

REFERENCES

1. Hardy JD, Webb WR, Dalton ML Jr, Walker GR Jr. Lung homotransplantation in man. *JAMA*. 1963 Dec 21; 186: 1065–74.
2. Reitz BA. The first successful combined heart-lung transplantation. *J Thorac Cardiovasc Surg*. 2011 Apr; 141(4): 867–9.
3. Grossman RF, Frost A, Zamel N et al. Results of single-lung transplantation for bilateral pulmonary fibrosis. The Toronto Lung Transplant Group. *N Engl J Med*. 1990 Mar 15; 322(11): 727–33.
4. Patterson GA, Cooper JD, Goldman B et al. Technique of successful clinical double-lung transplantation. *Ann Thorac Surg*. 1988 Jun; 45(6): 626–33.
5. Kaiser LR, Pasque MK, Trulock EP, et. al. Bilateral sequential lung transplantation: the procedure of choice for double-lung replacement. *Ann Thorac Surg*. 1991 Sep; 52(3): 438–45; discussion 445–6.
6. Botha P, Rostron AJ, Fisher AJ, and Dark JH. Current strategies in donor selection and management. *Seminars in Thoracic and Cardiovascular Surgery*. 2008; 20(2): 143–51.
7. Cypel M, Yeung Y, Machuca T et al. Experience with the first 50 ex vivo lung perfusions in clinical transplantation. *Journal of Thoracic and Cardiovascular Surgery*. 2012; 144(5): 1200–7.
8. de Antonio DG, Marcos R, Laporta R et al. Results of clinical lung transplant from uncontrolled non-heart-beating donors. *Journal of Heart and Lung Transplantation*. 2007; 26(5): 529–34.
9. Ingemansson R, Eyjolfsson A, Mared L et al. Clinical transplantation of initially rejected donor lungs after reconditioning ex vivo. *Annals of Thoracic Surgery*. 2009; 87(1): 255–60.
10. Aigner C, Wisser W, Taghavi S, Lang G, Jaksch P, Czyzewski D, and Klepetko W. Institutional experience with extracorporeal membrane oxygenation in lung transplantation. *European Journal of Cardio-thoracic Surgery*. 2007; 31(3): 468–74.

25

Management of postoperative chylothorax

MAXIM ITKIN AND JOHN C. KUCHARCZUK

INTRODUCTION

Traumatic chylothorax is a result of the direct or indirect trauma to the thoracic duct (TD) or its branches and the type most frequently encountered by surgeons. These injuries complicate thoracic, cardiac, and head/neck surgical procedures involving the anatomical areas where the TD or its branches reside. The incidence of chylothorax complicating pulmonary resections can be as high as 4%, and a recent report suggests the incidence may be rising given the increased frequency of extensive resections and lymph node dissection.[1] Postesophagectomy TD leaks result in a statistically significant increase in 30-day major morbidity (85% vs. 46%; $p < .001$) and mortality (17.7% vs. 3.9%, $p < .001$)

compared with no TD leak.[2] The development of a postoperative TD leak has a significant impact on the patient's course.

Anatomically, the TD is a 2–5 mm vessel that originates at the cisterna chyli in the retrocrural area of the abdomen and then travels in the posterior mediastinum, finally draining into the left subclavian vein. It serves as a main drainage conduit of the lymphatic system. Unfortunately, the TD anatomy is highly variable; less than 40% of patients have "classic" anatomy, described as a solitary duct entering the chest on the right side between the esophagus and azygous vein (see **Figure 25.1**). The variable anatomy, in addition to the difficulty in visualizing the TD, increases the risk of intraoperative injury.[3]

The TD collects lymphatic fluid from most of the parts of

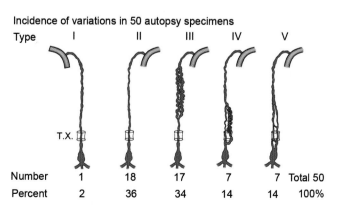

Incidence of variations in 50 autopsy specimens

Type	I	II	III	IV	V	
Number	1	18	17	7	7	Total 50
Percent	2	36	34	14	14	100%

T.X.

25.1 TD variability by autopsy study.

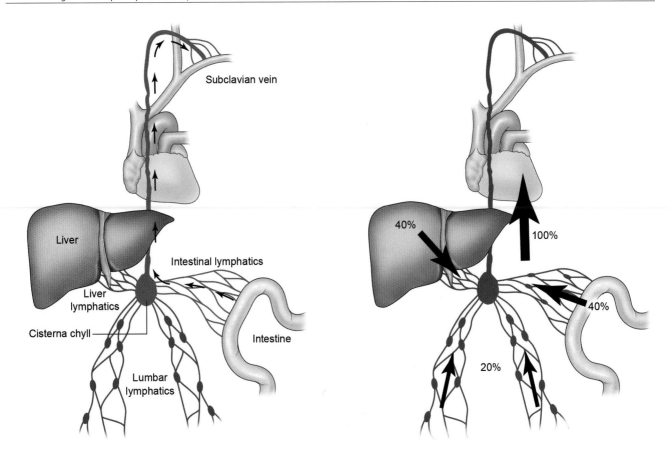

25.2a–b   (A) Schematic representation of the chyle path from the intestine through cisterna chyli and TD. (B) Percentage of the contribution of the lymphatic flow from intestine (chyle), liver, and soft tissue to the flow in the TD.

the body. "Chyle," the lymph that originates in the intestine, contains a high concentration of chylomicrons absorbed from the gastrointestinal (GI) tract (see **Figure 25.2**) and constitutes approximately 40%–60% of the flow in the TD. The liver lymph, which is rich with proteins, contributes an additional 40% of the lymphatic fluid in the TD. Prolonged drainage of TD contents leads to depletion of circulating T-lymphocytes and significant nutritional depletion due to protein loss. It is the loss of the protein component from the TD fluid that decreases the intravascular oncotic pressure, resulting in fluid leakage and anasarca.

The traditional management of traumatic TD leaks includes pleural drainage, low fat diets to decrease the gut lymphatic flow, nutritional support, and time, hoping for spontaneous closure of the leak.[4,5] Electing to manage a TD leak conservatively depends greatly on the volume of the output. High volume leaks will rarely close with conservative management, since the volume is correlated with the size of the rent in the vessel. A low volume leak resulting from the avulsion of a small branch of the duct will often close with the management described. Assuming watchful waiting with pleural drainage, minimal fat intake, and nutritional support are attempted, the waiting time to declare conservative management a failure traditionally has been 2–3 weeks, which has often resulted in an immune- and nutritionally depleted

patient. The advent of thoracic duct embolization (TDE) and improved lymphangiogram techniques have allowed us to reengineer our management pathway for traumatic TD leaks. At present, in our institution, patients with postoperative TD leak are started immediately on intravenous nutritional support. They are kept without oral intake for 72 hours and given an enteral fat challenge. If the TD leak has not resolved spontaneously, they are taken for lymphangiogram and TDE. If TDE fails, the lymphangiogram is used to accurately define the patient's precise TD anatomy and, ideally, the site of leakage to aid in the plan for operative TD ligation. This early intervention approach allows us to minimize the nutritional and immunologic imbalances that accompany an ongoing TD leak, especially ones where the volume output is large.

DIAGNOSIS OF CHYLOTHORAX

In cases of the postsurgical chylothorax, the leakage of "milky" fluid from the chest tubes following the administration of enteral fat may or may not be diagnostic, and confirmation of the presence of chyle should be determined. An elevated triglyceride level relative to the serum triglyceride level, in addition to a high percentage of lymphocytes in the fluid, is used to biochemically confirm the diagnosis. Triglyceride levels are in 200–300 mg/mL and higher in patients on a regular diet but are significantly lower in patients on a fat-free diet, in which case TD is confirmed by a high lymphocyte count. In cases of uncertainty, we repeat an enteral fat challenge test by giving the patient cream.

TD VISUALIZATION AND TD EMBOLIZATION

The concept of TDE was initially described and tested by Dr. C. Cope at the University of Pennsylvania.[6,7] Cope found that visualization of the lymphatic system and TD following a lymphangiogram could increase the treatment success and use of a minimally invasive, percutaneous, transabdominal approach for TDE. The need for a traditional pedal lymphangiogram represented the main hindrance to the widespread use of TDE, as few interventional radiologists are experienced with this technique, since it is rarely used. Recently, a new technique of ultrasound-guided intranodal lymphangiogram has allowed most operators to easily acquire the experience to successfully perform a meaningful lymphangiogram.[8]

Access to the inguinal lymph node is obtained using a 25-gauge spinal needle under ultrasound guidance. The needle tip is positioned in the hilum of the node. Using fluoroscopy, confirmation of the position of the needle tip is determined by injecting an oil-based contrast agent (Ethiodol; Savage Laboratories, Melville, New York, United States) by hand or using a balloon inflator filled with contrast. If the needle is in the optimal position, immediate opacification of the lymphatic vessels is observed. A volume of approximately 6 mL of oil-based iodinated contrast injected in each groin is usually enough to opacify the abdominal and pelvic lymphatics (see **Figure 25.3**). A "saline push," an injection of saline following the infusion of contrast, is used to further advance the contrast toward the central lymphatic system.

Using this new and innovative technique has simplified and improved the procedure and decreased procedural time. In a recent publication using these improvements, the TD was visualized, successfully catheterized, and embolized in all patients.[9]

Following opacification of the target lymphatic vessels in the abdomen (lumbar lymphatics, cisterna chyli), a 21- to 22-gauge needle is used transabdominally to access the lymphatic system. A stiff 0.046 cm wire is advanced into the central lymphatic system, followed by a 3 Fr microcatheter.

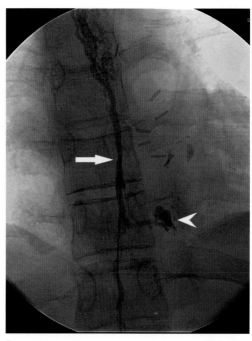

25.4 Fluoroscopic image showing injection with the contrast of the distal part of the TD through the microcatheter (arrow) demonstrating the leak (arrowhead) in patient with chylous microcatheter leak after resection of a left posterior mediastinal mass.

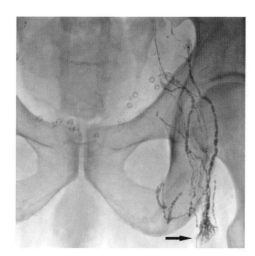

25.3 Fluoroscopic image of the pelvis demonstrating contrast material in the lymphatic vessels after injection in the groin lymph node (arrow).

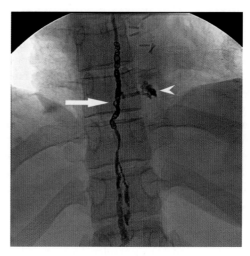

25.5 Spot image of the glue and coil cast (arrow) in the TD post successful embolization of the leak (white arrowhead).

Water-soluble iodinated contrast is injected through the catheter to define the TD anatomy and the cause of the chylous leak (see **Figure 25.4**). Once the location of the leak is identified, embolization is carried out through the catheter using a combination of endovascular coils and N-butyl cyanoacrylate glue (Trufill; Cordis Corporation, Fremont, California, United States) (see **Figure 25.5**). Embolization with glue only is reserved for those patients with leakage from multiple small branches.[10–12]

SURGICAL LIGATION

Ligation of the TD has been described using both video-assisted thoracoscopic surgery and traditional open techniques.[13] In general, we prefer to proceed through a small low thoracotomy to try to ligate the TD as low as possible within the chest in an attempt to ligate the duct prior to any branching (see **Figure 25.6**). We do not make any attempt to find or ligate the actual site of the leak; rather, we perform an *en masse* ligation to include all tissue between the aorta, the esophagus, and the spine. We avoid the use of clips, which can shear the duct, making a difficult situation worse. Instead, we incise the pleura overlaying the spine and gently place a blunt right-angled clamp around the entire tissue bundle, which is then ligated with two heavy silk ligatures (see **Figure 25.7**). An enteral fat challenge is given at the start of the procedure, either via a nasogastric or an enteric feeding tube, to allow us to see whether the ligation has completely occluded the TD. Often, it will take 30–45 minutes following the administration of fat to ensure that no leak is present following ligation.

RESULTS

The success rate of the TD ligation exceeds 70%.[2] Although this result is promising, the operative risk and potential morbidity that accompany open ligation, and our observed improved outcomes with the nonoperative approach, make TDE our preferred initial approach.[9–12,14,15] When we cannot accomplish successful TDE, we proceed to surgical ligation using the lymphangiogram as a road map or guide.

The largest series of TDEs in treating traumatic TD leaks included 109 patients, with an overall success rate of 71% using "intent to treat."[9] In patients in whom the duct was able to be successfully catheterized, embolization resulted in resolution of the leak in 64 of 71 patients (90%). In 18 of the 33 unsuccessful catheterization cases, needle interruption of the TD was performed and resulted in resolution of the chylothorax in 72% of patients. In 20 patients who had failed previous surgical ligation, embolization, or interruption, we attempted 17 TDEs and were successful in 15 (88%). We also examined the patients who had failed TD ligation and then came to TDE. The most common causes of the TD ligation failure were missed TD, incomplete ligation of the TD, and leakage from the stump of the ligated duct.

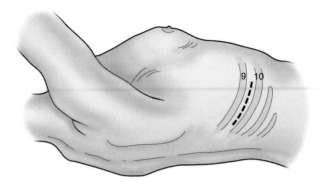

25.6 Patient position and incision for surgical ligation of the TD.

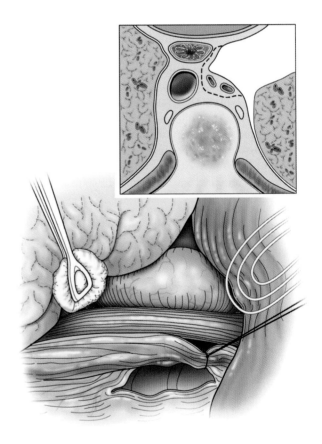

25.7 The thoracic duct is located on the spine and the tissue between the aorta and esophagus is encircled and ligated. No attempt is made to specifically isolate the thoracic duct but it is encompassed by this mass ligation.

CONCLUSION

In recent years, our group and others have developed an innovative and thoughtful algorithm for the evaluation and treatment of postoperative TD leaks. Through refinement of techniques, including intranodal lymphangiogram and transabdominal TDE we have been able to successfully manage the majority of these patients nonoperatively. As a result of this experience, our institution has become a referral center for patients with TD leaks, allowing us to further study the TD and continue to improve our outcomes for control of postoperative TD leaks.

REFERENCES

1. Misthos P, Kanakis MA, Lioulias AG. Chylothorax complicating thoracic surgery: conservative or early surgical management? *Updates Surg.* 2012; 64(1): 5–11.
2. Shah RD, Luketich JD, Schuchert MJ, Christie NA, Pennathur A, Landreneau RJ, Nason KS. Postesophagectomy chylothorax: incidence, risk factors, and outcomes. *Ann Thorac Surg.* 2012; 93(3): 897–903; discussion 903–4.
3. Kausel H. W., Reeve T. S., Stein A. A., Alley R. D., Stranahan A., Anatomic and pathologic studies of the thoracic duct. *J Thoracic Surg.* 1957; 34: 631.
4. Hashim SA, Roholt HB, Babayan VK, Vanitallie TB. Treatment of chyluria and chylothorax with medium-chain triglyceride. *N Engl J Med.* 1964; 270: 756–61.
5. Ramos W, Faintuch J. Nutritional management of thoracic duct fistulas: a comparative study of parenteral versus enteral nutrition. *JPEN J Parenter Enteral Nutr.* 1986; 10(5): 519–21.
6. Cope C. Percutaneous thoracic duct cannulation: feasibility study in swine. *J Vasc Interv Radiol.* 1995; 6(4): 559–64.
7. Cope C. Diagnosis and treatment of postoperative chyle leakage via percutaneous transabdominal catheterization of the cisterna chyli: a preliminary study. *J Vasc Interv Radiol.* 1998; 9(5): 727–34.
8. Nadolski GJ, Itkin M. Feasibility of ultrasound-guided intranodal lymphangiogram for thoracic duct embolization. *J Vasc Interv Radiol.* 2012; 23(5): 613–16.
9. Itkin M, Kucharczuk JC, Kwak A, Trerotola SO, Kaiser LR. Nonoperative thoracic duct embolization for traumatic thoracic duct leak: experience in 109 patients. *J Thorac Cardiovasc Surg.* 2010; 139(3): 584–9; discussion 589–90.
10. Cope C, Kaiser LR. Management of unremitting chylothorax by percutaneous embolization and blockage of retroperitoneal lymphatic vessels in 42 patients. *J Vasc Interv Radiol.* 2002; 13(11): 1139–48.
11. Litherland B, Given M, Lyon S. Percutaneous radiological management of high-output chylothorax with CT-guided needle disruption. *J Med Imaging Radiation Oncol.* 2008; 52(2): 164–7.
12. Binkert C, Yucel E, Davison B, Sugarbaker D, Baum R. Percutaneous treatment of high-output chylothorax with embolization or needle disruption technique. *J Vasc Interv Radiol.* 2005; 16(9): 1257–62.
13. Bryant AS, Minnich DJ, Wei B, Cerfolio RJ. The incidence and management of postoperative chylothorax after pulmonary resection and thoracic mediastinal lymph node dissection. *Ann Thorac Surg.* 2014 Jul; 98(1): 232–5; discussion 235–7.
14. Cope C. Management of chylothorax via percutaneous embolization. *Curr Opin Pulm Med.* 2004; 10(4): 311–14.
15. Chen E, Itkin M. Thoracic duct embolization for chylous leaks. *Semin Intervent Radiol.* 2011; 28(1): 63–74.

26

Outpatient thoracic surgery

LAUREANO MOLINS, JUAN J. FIBLA, AND JORGE HERNÁNDEZ

INTRODUCTION

The term "ambulatory surgery" was coined by J. E. Davis in 1986. Outpatient surgery, also called "major ambulatory surgery" or "day surgery," can be defined as a surgical or diagnostic procedure performed under general, locoregional, or local anesthesia with or without sedation, requiring postoperative care and returning home the same day of surgery. It must be distinguished from "short-stay surgery" in which a major surgical procedure stay lasts between 1 and 3 days. Other terms such as "early discharge surgery" have been discarded for being inaccurate or confusing terms.

The classification of levels of surgery, according to Davis, are:

- Level I: procedures performed on an outpatient basis under local anesthesia requiring no special postoperative care (minor surgery)
- Level II: major surgical procedures requiring specific postoperative care without hospitalizing (outpatient/ambulatory surgery)
- Level III: surgery that requires hospitalization
- Level IV: surgery that requires highly specialized or critical care

"Major surgery" is a variety of surgery with a complexity that requires special or intensive postoperative care. However, thanks to advances in surgical and anesthetic techniques, some of these procedures can now be performed on an outpatient basis without an overnight stay in the hospital. According to the International Association for Ambulatory Surgery, such procedures should not be urgent; be performed within a normal working day; and not exceed a duration of 12 hours, including postoperative recovery.

Several potential advantages of these procedures arise: decreased costs through more efficient resource use; increased hospital bed availability; lower risk of resistant bacterial strain transmission; and quicker return to family, social, and working life. Outpatient surgery must meet all these goals, offering the same guarantees and quality of care as conventional surgery for the same type of surgical procedure.

Outpatient surgery was born in the United Kingdom in the mid-twentieth century under the auspices of the public health system. Its original purpose was to reduce surgical waiting times. One of the first experiences was reported in 1909 by James H. Nicoll who, at the Glasgow Royal Hospital for Sick Children, performed 8988 operations on children without hospitalization.

This system of surgical activity was quickly built on and developed in the United States, powered by a health care system based on private hospitals and insurance companies. Before long, it proved not only to be a cost-effective and safe therapeutic modality but also improved patient care by simplifying the administration of diagnostic and therapeutic processes.

OUTPATIENT THORACIC SURGERY

Ambulatory surgery has gained wide popularity and satisfaction among patients. As an alternative to conventional hospitalization, outpatient surgery has grown internationally over the past 20 years. However, there has been little on outpatient thoracic surgery in the international medical literature since the first publication by Vallieres et al. in 1991 detailing outpatient mediastinoscopy.

Thoracic surgery as a specialty has been slow to get into the dynamics of outpatient surgery. This low use of outpatient surgery programs appears to be due to several causes. The anatomical complexity of the chest, the requirement for prolonged postoperative recovery, significant postoperative pain, the possibility of serious complications, and the frequent need to leave a postoperative chest drain, in addition to other factors, has limited the number of thoracic procedures that may safely be done in an outpatient setting. The pressure of waiting lists, the concern regarding legal liability and low demand by patients are other nonmedical reasons causing this phenomenon.

The last 25–30 years has seen significant technological advances. First, the appearance of videothoracoscopic approaches has led to the realization of many surgical procedures replacing more aggressive and traumatic approaches with minimally invasive techniques. Second, minimally invasive surgery often causes less postoperative pain, which results in better postoperative rehabilitation and earlier return of the patient to their daily activities. Third, advances in the anesthetic field, such as improved selective endobronchial intubation devices as well as the optimization of anesthetic drugs used during surgery, can greatly facilitate the work of the surgeon. Today, we can objectively quantify postoperative pulmonary air leak with new drainage systems available on the market, and the use of postoperative chest X-rays may be replaced by other imaging techniques. Specifically, the use of the portable chest ultrasound technique allows for the examination of the patient at the bedside, in the operating room, or in the recovery room, with the ability to safely repeat the examination as often as necessary without relying on the radiology department and without additional exposure to x-irradiation.

With all these innovations, there has been a gradual reduction in the length of stay following surgical procedures for which, years ago, prolonged postoperative care that increased hospital stay was required. Short-stay units and outpatient surgery, previously found exclusively in other surgical specialties, have allowed the inclusion of programs in outpatient thoracic surgery, adding different surgical procedures progressively.

REGULATION

Ambulatory surgery programs aim to meet the demand of patients suffering from various pathologies quickly and efficiently, reducing cost without decreasing the benefit of the treatment given to the patient, yet allowing for maximum safety and satisfaction.

These programs require specific, strict, and rigorous regulation. In the United Kingdom, certification of ambulatory surgical programs is controlled through various regulations within the National Health Service. European countries such as Spain also have established regional or national standards for regulation. A consequence of this regulation requires specific valid indicators documenting the optimization and quality management of the offered day surgery:

- The substitution index (SI) is defined as the ratio of the number of outpatients to the total number of procedures, expressed as a percentage.
- The admission rate (AR) is defined as the ratio of the number of unplanned admissions (any reason) to the total number of outpatient procedures, expressed as percentage.
- The readmission rate (RR) is defined as the ratio of the number of unplanned admissions after discharge from the total number of outpatient procedures, expressed as percentage.

Patient and procedure selection are the most important determinants to a safe and effective outpatient thoracic surgical program. Proper selection decreases the number of unplanned hospitalizations. Therefore, strict procedure selection criteria should be established in relation to the pathology present while also taking into account the experience of each thoracic unit.

SURGICAL PROCEDURES

Currently, potential cases amenable to outpatient surgery include:

- Video-mediastinoscopy and anterior mediastinotomy for surgical staging of lung cancer and/or biopsy of a mediastinal mass/lymphadenopathy
- Video-assisted thoracoscopic surgery (VATS) bilateral sympathectomy/clipping to treat palmar/axillary hyperhidrosis and facial blushing
- Video-assisted thoracoscopic surgery lung biopsy (VATS-LB) for interstitial lung disease
- VATS resection/biopsy of lung nodules (with/without previous hookwire localization)
- VATS staging of lung cancer (lymph node biopsy of lymph node stations 5, 6, 7, 8, 9; VATS exploration of the pleural cavity in pleural effusions; biopsy/excision of pleural masses
- VATS biopsy/resection of mediastinal tumors
- Limited chest wall procedures: rib resection/extraction of Nuss bar
- Other: diagnostic-therapeutic bronchoscopy; supraclavicular lymph node biopsy; computed-tomography (CT)-guided fine needle aspiration (FNA) of lung, mediastinal, chest wall and pleural nodules /masses

All these procedures are included within the level II classification of Davis. With the exception of supraclavicular lymph node biopsy, pleural biopsy, and endobronchial explorations that can be accomplished with local anesthesia and sedation, all other procedures are performed under general anesthesia. Thoracoscopic techniques require selective bronchial intubation and lung collapse and, in most cases, a chest tube postoperatively that will be withdrawn in the recovery room.

SELECTION CRITERIA

Each thoracic surgical unit should establish the criteria for the selection of patients in its ambulatory surgery program. Most of the previously named surgical procedures may be included in a program of ambulatory thoracic surgery, but in order to accomplish it, first, one has to keep this possibility in mind, and, second, the team must have the necessary motivation and involvement.

Medical criteria

The program should maintain quality of care. Patients classified according to the American Society of Anesthesiology (ASA) physical status classification system as ASA I and II should be included regardless of age. Patients who are judged ASA III should be selected only after taking into account the extent and type of comorbidity.

Personal criteria

The patient must understand and accept the conditions and be motivated to be included in a program of outpatient surgery. It is vital to have their complete involvement in the process, actively collaborating in the operation, reflected by signing the surgical consent following a thorough discussion informing them of the proposed procedure and the implications of doing it in an outpatient setting.

Socio-familiar criteria

The patient should have the support of a family member or friend, who is capable and responsible, to assist them during the first 24–48 hours postoperation. The patient should be provided with a phone number to communicate with the unit if necessary. Usually, outpatient programs include exclusion criteria, limiting the distance between home and hospital or the time taken to cover that distance (1–2 hours).

It is of vital importance to evaluate these general rules in each particular case before deciding if the patient should participate in the outpatient program.

OUR OUTPATIENT THORACIC SURGERY PROGRAM

Our outpatient thoracic surgery program (OTSP) at Sagrat Cor University Hospital, Barcelona, began in April 2001 and, as of December 2013, 814 patients have participated. The program is composed of a multidisciplinary team of surgeons; anesthesiologists; nurses; administrative staff; and, of course, most important, patients. In our view, preoperative, intraoperative, and immediate postoperative anesthetic management is a fundamental part of the process of outpatient surgery. The aim is the early awakening of the patient in the surgical theater in order to facilitate a quick recovery and discharge within a few hours of the surgical procedure with less pain and anxiety. This requires preoperative sedation (diazepam 5–10 mg) and a combination of anesthetic agents, including short-acting relaxants (atracurium, succinylcholine), inhalation agents (sevoflurane, nitrous oxide), intravenous anesthetic drugs (propofol), short-acting opioids (alfentanil, remifentanil), and intercostal nerve blocks. Postoperative analgesia is administered in the recovery room, avoiding derivatives of morphine and meperidine, which delay the recovery process. The patient remains at the recovery room for 20–40 minutes prior to being transferred back to the major ambulatory unit (see **Figure 26.1a and b**) where they remain for 4–6 hours, until they meet the criteria required to be discharged home—specifically, normal values of blood pressure, heart rate, and oxygen saturation; full recovery of consciousness; tolerance to oral liquids; ambulation without assistance; spontaneous voiding; absence of, or moderate pain; and no signs of decompensation of associated comorbidities. The patient is provided with a phone number so they can call the anesthesiologist on call to ask any questions. Our nurses contact the patient the morning after, and the patient is visited by a member of the surgical team within 1 week.

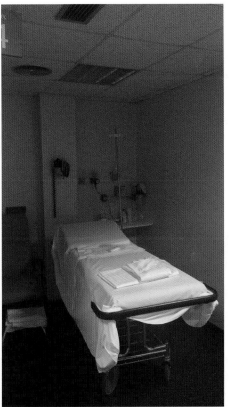

(a)

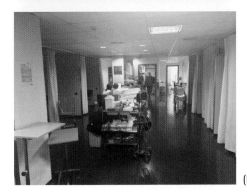

(b)

26.1a–b (a) Major ambulatory surgery unit box. (b) Major ambulatory surgery unit, nursing control.

There are several reasons why patients originally scheduled for an outpatient procedure may need to be admitted, and these include conversion to thoracotomy; bleeding; an air leak; arrhythmia; nausea/vomiting; pain; urinary retention; pneumothorax; and, sometimes, social reasons. Causes for admission following discharge from the outpatient unit include pneumothorax, hemothorax, pain, and pneumonia.

Outpatient mediastinoscopy

The first published indication for ambulatory thoracic surgery was cervical mediastinoscopy for lung cancer staging. Currently in our unit, mediastinoscopy represents the most commonly performed major ambulatory procedure, probably due to the fact that postoperative drainage is not needed.

In our Department of Thoracic Surgery, by December 2013, 392 mediastinoscopies had been done as outpatient surgeries. The results have been very satisfactory, showing an SI of 82.9% (392 of 473 patients, AR of 1.78% (seven patients), and admission rate following discharge of 0.7% (three patients). According to series published to date by various authors (see **Table 26.1**), outpatient mediastinoscopy has proven to be a safe and effective procedure.

At present, the indications for mediastinoscopy are decreasing because of alternative less invasive procedures with excellent diagnostic accuracy, such as endobronchial ultrasound–transbronchial needle aspiration, or endoscopic ultrasound–transbronchial needle aspiration (EBUS-TBNA or EUS-TBNA, respectively).

Outpatient lung biopsy

Thoracoscopic lung biopsy (VATS-LB) is the definitive procedure for diagnosis in patients with diffuse interstitial lung disease or pulmonary nodules, although only a few articles have been published to date relating to performing this as an outpatient procedure. The need to leave a postoperative chest drain is the main reason that mandates the patient's inpatient hospitalization. Several authors, such as Russo and colleagues in 1998, showed that it is safe to remove the chest drain within the first 90 minutes following VATS-LB. Other

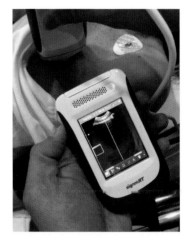

26.2 Chest ultrasound study.

authors have confirmed that it is safe to completely avoid the use of a chest drain following lung biopsy for the diagnosis of interstitial lung disease.

Our OTSP excluded patients with a forced expiratory volume in 1 second (FEV1) or diffusion capacity of the lung for carbon dioxide (D_{LCO}) of less than 30%. The procedure is performed using a double-lumen endotracheal tube or by selective bronchial intubation using a single lumen tube. With the patient in the lateral decubitus position, two or three ports are used and one or two stapled wedge resections are performed. In the recovery room, we use portable chest ultrasound (see **Figure 26.2**) to assess lung reexpansion in the operated hemithorax. Using this technique, we have been able to successfully document lung reexpansion with high sensitivity (92.86%), specificity (87.50%), positive predictive value (PPV; 98.11%) and negative predictive value (NPV; 63.64%) when compared with chest radiograph. The chest drain is removed in the recovery room if there is no air leak or evidence of ongoing bleeding. Using digital drainage systems that objectively quantify an air leak if present, in addition to the amount of fluid, has been an important determinant in our decision-making. After 30–40 minutes, the patient is transferred back to the short-stay facility and if they meet the discharge criteria as described, are discharged home within 4–6 hours of surgery.

Table 26.1 Outpatient mediastinoscopy

Study	N	SI	AR	RR
Valleries et al.	158	21.0%		
Bonadies et al	65	54.0%	1.50%	4.0%
Cybulsky and Bennett	1015	96.0%	9.80%	0.9%
Souilamas et al.	20	40.0%	0.00%	2.5%
Molins et al.	297	83.4%	1.30%	0.0%
Molins et al. (present study)	392	82.9%	1.78%	0.7%

Notes: N, number of patients; SI, substitution index; AR, admission rate; RR, readmission rate.

Table 26.2 Outpatient lung biopsy

Study	N	SI	AR	RR
Blewett et al.	32	NA	0.00%	
Chang et al.	62	NA	27.50%	1.60%
Molins et al.	66	57.9%	3.00%	3.00%
Molins et al. (present study)	115	62.8%	3.47%	2.60%

Notes: N, number of patients; SI, substitution index; AR, admission rate; RR, readmission rate.

Up to December 2013, outpatient VATS-LB was performed in 115 patients, with an SI of 62.8% (115 of 183 patients, AR of 3.47% (four patients), and RR of 2.60% (three patients). Note that the SI decreases because these patients have poor lung function that often precludes them from being considered for outpatient surgery. There has been no mortality in our OTSP. Our results are comparable to those reported by others performing outpatient lung biopsy (see **Table 26.2**).

At present, indications for lung biopsy in diffuse interstitial lung disease may be decreasing with the emergence of less invasive procedures that have good diagnostic accuracy, such as endoscopic cryobiopsy.

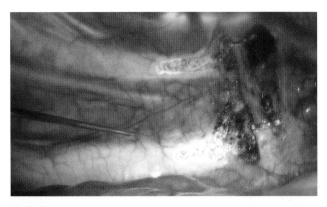

26.3 Systematic infiltration of the intercostal spaces after sympathetic clipping.

Outpatient thoracic sympathectomy/clipping

In recent years, there has been a significant increase in the use of thoracoscopic sympathectomy for the treatment of primary palmar/axillary hyperhidrosis and facial blushing. Patients are usually young people who are prone to nausea, vomiting, and have a lower tolerance for postoperative pain. The key to successfully incorporating these patients in an outpatient program is the anesthetic technique and premedication with anti-emetic agents and analgesia.

Thoracic sympathectomy has been part of our outpatient program since 2003, and up until 2007, the technique employed was sectioning a portion of the sympathetic chain. Starting in 2007, we changed from sectioning the nerve to using a clipping technique that would allow for the potential to possibly reverse the procedure. The operation is performed with selective bronchial intubation using a single lumen tube. With the patient in semi-Fowler's position, two ports are used and, systematically, intercostal spaces are infiltrated (see **Figure 26.3**) with local anesthetic (0.5% bupivacaine with adrenaline or 0.2% ropivacaine). Small-bore chest tubes are used and removed while the patient is in the theater or shortly after arrival in the recovery room, where we monitor with portable chest ultrasound to ensure the complete reexpansion of both lungs and compare scans with the chest X-rays. After 30–40 minutes, the patient is transferred back to the short-stay facility and, once they meet the discharge criteria previously described, they are discharged to home within 4–6 hours of surgery.

From 2003 to 2013, 307 sympathectomies were performed in our program of outpatient surgery, with an SI of 83% (307 of 370 patients AR of 3.90% (ten patients), and RR of 1.95%

Table 26.3 Outpatient thoracic sympathectomy

Study	N	SI	AR	RR
Grabham et al.	20	–	10.0%	–
Hsia et al.	47	–	0.0%	–
Baumgartner and Toh	309	–	0.3%	1.2%
Hsia et al.	262	–	0.0%	–
Doolabh et al.	180	–	1.7%	–
Miller et al.	205	–	–	–
Molins et al.	117	71.3%	0.85%	1.7%
Molins et al. (present study)	307	83.0%	3.9%	1.95%

Notes: N, number of patients; SI, substitution index; AR, admission rate; RR, readmission rate.

(six patients). Based on our experience and that of other series published to date by various authors (see **Table 26.3**), outpatient thoracic sympathectomy has proved to be a safe and effective procedure.

Solitary or multiple pulmonary nodules: outpatient VATS resection

Patients with solitary or multiple pulmonary nodules may also be selectively included in a program of outpatient surgery. Resection of pulmonary nodules by VATS, with either diagnostic or curative intention, does not differ technically from performing VATS-LB. If the procedure is being performed strictly for diagnostic purposes, inclusion in the outpatient program is fairly clear cut. However, in the patient with a solitary pulmonary nodule being resected with curative intent, other factors must be taken into account before scheduling the patient for outpatient surgery. If the nodule is highly suspected of being benign, outpatient surgery may be appropriate, but if the nodule is of unknown etiology and suspected of being a primary lung carcinoma, the likelihood of performing an anatomic pulmonary resection is significant, thus mandating a longer period of chest drainage and precluding doing the procedure on an outpatient basis. We believe that for thoracoscopic localization of small peripheral lung nodules, it is helpful to use a CT-guided harpoon (see **Figure 26.4**), prior to resection by minimally invasive surgery. Our team has successful outpatient experience, with 76 cases performed since 2004, resulting in a fast and safe surgical procedure.

Other outpatient thoracic procedures

We and others also have used the outpatient setting to perform other procedures, including VATS staging of lung cancer (biopsy of lymph node stations, 5, 6, 7, 8 and 9); VATS exploration of the pleural cavity for pleural effusions and biopsy/excision of pleural masses; VATS biopsy/resection of mediastinal tumors; chest wall procedures, including rib resection/extraction of Nuss bar; diagnostic-therapeutic bronchoscopy; supraclavicular lymph node biopsy; and CT-guided FNA of lung, mediastinal, chest wall, and pleural nodules/masses.

These procedures have been included in our program on a case by case basis with the same fundamentals of the other more standardized procedures, demonstrating that the outpatient thoracic program can be expanded to other surgical procedures.

ECONOMIC IMPACT

The economic impact is a very important issue in any major ambulatory surgical program. Theoretically, increasing the percentage of operations performed on an outpatient basis should result in reduced healthcare expenditure and allow more patients to be treated using the same amount of resources. Performing more procedures in the outpatient setting will result in less reimbursement to the hospital compared with what is paid for an inpatient stay but provide an overall benefit to society by expending less money on healthcare.

In the 2006 paper from our thoracic surgical service, we presented the economic data based on results obtained from treating 300 patients in our outpatient surgical unit. The average length of stay for patients undergoing lung biopsy, mediastinoscopy, and sympathectomy for hyperhidrosis was only 1 day. The median cost of an outpatient VATS-LB was €1257.78, compared with €1743.88 for a 1-day hospital stay, so the final cost savings (€486.10) was not as great as in hospitals where the baseline hospital stay was somewhat longer. Comparing the average hospital stay for a lung biopsy in Spanish hospitals with similar activity level (2 days), the saving per patient would have been greater (€972.20). This estimate of the economic impact was applied only to variable hospital costs (bed, meals, energy, laundry, and so on), considering the fixed costs similar to conventional hospitalization (personnel and so on), without the real benefit of being able to include the income gained when another patient occupies the bed of the patient treated as an outpatient.

SUMMARY

Although the role of ambulatory thoracic surgery has increased over the past two decades, it has not reached the level of use seen in other surgical specialties. Therefore, there is significant scope for extending its use routinely for selected thoracic surgical procedures.

It is important to continually look to integrate an outpatient surgery within the context of a full service thoracic surgical program. Results should be collected and evaluated using specific validation indicators to ensure the proper functioning of each outpatient program. It is essential to have the commitment of an entire multidisciplinary team, but it is even more important to have patient buy in to be able to take full advantage of the outpatient setting.

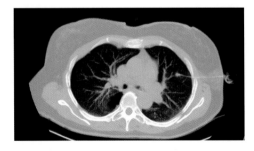

26.4 CT-guided placement of a hookwire in a small pulmonary nodule before VATS resection.

Improvements in anesthetic management have allowed us to extend the range of outpatient surgical procedures, largely due to the excellent postoperative pain management and improved recovery. Recent technological advances, such as endoscopic suturing devices, new digital drainage systems, and the use of lung ultrasound, allow for early and safe chest tube removal. These factors, when used together, have allowed us to increase the number of procedures that potentially can be included in a program of ambulatory thoracic surgery. Therefore, procedures including lung resections, VATS-LB, and even resection of solitary pulmonary nodules can be successfully performed in an outpatient setting.

The overall economic impact of an outpatient surgical program in a given unit and, specifically, the amount of cost savings will depend on the baseline expenditures for the same procedure when done as an inpatient procedure.

In our experience, video-assisted mediastinoscopy, lung biopsy, bilateral sympathectomy, and lung nodule resection can be safely performed in an OTSP. Further experience is needed to increase the SI and expand the OTSP to include additional procedures. Currently, VATS is well established in many thoracic procedures, a fact which suggests an increase in its use in the present and future that can allow new procedures to be included as outpatient surgeries, reserving hospitalization for more complex procedures or for patients who do not meet the established criteria.

FURTHER READING

Baumgartner FJ, Toh Y. Severe hyperhidrosis: clinical features and current thoracoscopic surgical management. *Ann Thorac Surg.* 2003 Dec; 76(6): 1878–83.

Blewett CJ, Bennett WF, Miller JD, Urschel JD. Open lung biopsy as an outpatient procedure. *Ann Thorac Surg.* 2001; 71: 1113–15.

Bonadies J, D'Agostino RS, Ruskis AF, Ponn RB. Outpatient mediastinoscopy. *J Thorac Cardiovasc Surg.* 1993 Oct; 106(4): 686–8.

Chang AC, Yee J, Orringer MB, Iannettoni MD. Diagnostic thoracoscopic lung biopsy: an outpatient experience. *Ann Thorac Surg.* 2002 Dec; 74(6): 1942–6; discussion 1946–7.

Cybulsky IJ, Bennett WF. Mediastinoscopy as a routine outpatient procedure. *Ann Thorac Surg.* 1994 Jul; 58(1): 176–8.

Davis JE, ed. (1986) *Major Ambulatory Surgery.* Baltimore: Williams & Wilkins. 274–82.

Doolabh N, Horswell S, Williams M et al. Thoracoscopic sympathectomy for hyperhidrosis: indications and results. *Ann Thorac Surg.* 2004 Feb; 77(2): 410–4; discussion 414.

Fibla JJ, Molins L, Blanco A et al. Video-assisted thoracoscopic lung biopsy in the diagnosis of interstitial lung disease: a prospective, multi-center study in 224 patients. *Arch Bronconeumol.* 2012; 48: 81–5.

Fibla JJ, Molins L, Simón C, Pérez J, Vidal G. Early removal of chest drainage and outpatient program after videothoracoscopic lung biopsy. *Eur J Cardiothorac Surg.* 2006; 29(4): 639–40.

Grabham JA, Raitt D, Barrie WW. Early experience with day-case transthoracic endoscopic sympathectomy. *Br J Surg.* 1998 Sep; 85(9): 1266.

Hsia JY, Chen CY, Hsu CP et al. Outpatient thoracoscopic sympathicotomy for axillary osmidrosis. *Eur J Cardiothorac Surg.* 2003 Sep; 24(3): 425–7.

Hsia JY, Chen CY, Hsu CP, Shai SE, Yang SS. Outpatient thoracoscopic limited sympathectomy for hyperhidrosis palmaris. *Ann Thorac Surg.* 1999; 67: 258–9.

Luckraz H, Rammohan KS, Phillips M et al. Is an intercostal chest drain necessary after video-assisted thoracoscopic (VATS) lung biopsy? *Ann Thorac Surg.* 2007; 84: 237–9.

Miller DL, Force SD. Outpatient microthoracoscopic sympathectomy for palmar hyperhidrosis. *Ann Thorac Surg.* 2007 May; 83(5): 1850–3; discussion 1853.

Molins L. [Ambulatory chest surgery]. *Arch Bronconeumol.* 2007 Apr; 43(4): 185–7.

Molins L, Fibla JJ, Pérez J et al. Outpatient thoracic surgical programme in 300 patients: clinical results and economic impact. *Eur J Cardiothoracic Surg.* 2006; 29: 271–5.

Molins L, Mauri E, Sánchez M et al. Locating pulmonary nodules with a computed axial tomography-guided harpoon prior to videothoracoscopic resection: experience with 52 cases. *Cir Esp.* 2012; 91: 184–8.

Russo L, Wiechmann RJ, Magovern JA et al. Early chest tube removal after video-assisted thoracoscopic wedge resection of the lung. *Ann Thorac Surg.* 1998 Nov; 66(5): 1751–4.

Souilamas R, D'Attellis N, Nguyen-Roux S, Giomborani R. Outpatient video-mediastinoscopy. *Interact Cardiovasc Thorac Surg.* 2004 Sep; 3(3): 486–8.

Vallieres E, Page A, Verdant A. Ambulatory mediastinoscopy and anterior mediastinotomy. *Ann Thorac Surg.* 1991; 52: 1122–6.

SECTION II

Esophageal surgery

27

Endoscopy

EWEN A. GRIFFITHS AND DEREK ALDERSON

INTRODUCTION

Flexible upper gastrointestinal endoscopy is the principal method for the evaluation and treatment of a wide range of conditions of the esophagus, stomach, and duodenum. With advances in equipment and technology over the last 50 years, complete visualization of the upper gastrointestinal tract mucosa can be achieved, with targeted tissue sampling and therapeutic intervention (dilatation, polypectomy, endoscopic ablation/resection, stent insertion) being performed as necessary. Flexible endoscopy has largely replaced rigid endoscopy and contrast radiology as the first-line investigation of choice. While the basic controls have changed little over the years, digital technology with high resolution imaging and magnification means that the modern endoscope differs markedly from the early flexible fiberscopes of the 1960s. Still images and videos can be captured easily and training is enhanced by all parties viewing the procedure on the same screen.

Surgeons have been influential in the developments of endoscopic assessment of the upper gastrointestinal tract, but in certain countries around the world they have now relinquished this role to their medical gastrointestinal colleagues. However, esophagogastric and thoracic surgeons have an increasing incentive to ensure that endoscopic techniques, both diagnostic and therapeutic, are integral to their surgical practice. Advanced endoscopic treatment for achalasia, gastro-esophageal reflux disease, and obesity are emerging and are beginning to compete with the more traditional surgical methods of treatment. There is also an increasing role of combining endoscopic visualization intraoperatively during certain operations to improve the outcome of surgical therapy. Surgeons need to reengage with this domain to the benefit of their patients.

This chapter summarizes the indications, techniques, and uses of upper gastrointestinal endoscopy. Modern assessment of the esophagus is not carried out as an isolated procedure and is performed in conjunction with assessment of the stomach and duodenum. However, in this chapter, we focus on the esophagus and the gastro-esophageal junction (GEJ) and uses of flexible endoscopy directly relevant to esophageal surgeons.

RIGID ESOPHAGOSCOPY

The need for rigid esophagoscopy is rare. Achieving proficiency with this technique is difficult nowadays. **Figure 27.1** shows rigid esophagoscopy equipment—esophagoscopes (A), biopsy forceps (B), and suctioning devices (C). Its main disadvantages are that general anesthesia is required, it is technically difficult in patients with restricted cervical mobility, and there is a small rate of perforation. By comparison, the risk of perforation with diagnostic flexible esophagoscopy is negligible. When lesions are at or close to the upper esophageal sphincter, visualization and biopsy can be easier with a rigid endoscope, where a combination of general anesthesia to eliminate swallowing and a greater instrument

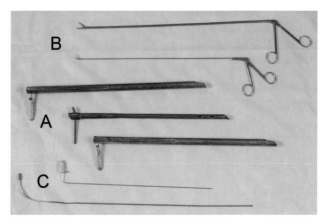

27.1 Rigid esophagoscopy equipment.

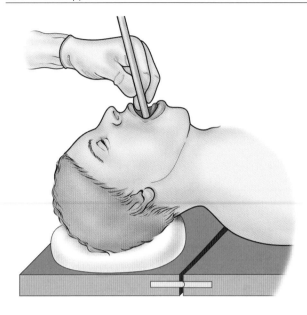

27.2

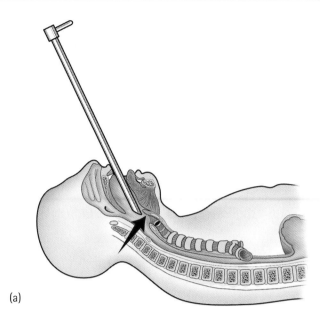

(a)

diameter can be helpful. While some surgeons maintain that the removal of large impacted foreign bodies can be easier with a large bore rigid tube and appropriately sized grasping forceps, the wide range of instrumentation designed for use with flexible endoscopes and a semirigid overtube has largely superseded the rigid procedure.

Under general anesthesia, the patient is placed supine on an operating table where the head end of the table can be adjusted. The esophagoscope should be checked and connected to the light cable. An adequate length suction device and biopsy forceps should be available on a tray beside the surgeon. The upper teeth are protected by a gum guard. The surgeon holds the rigid esophagoscope in the right hand while the left stabilizes the patient's mandible and protects the teeth. During insertion of the scope, the head is initially held forward in the "sniffing" position while the scope is placed to the left side of the oropharynx (see **Figure 27.2**). The epiglottis is visualized and pushed out of view by the beak of the endoscope. Once the cricopharyngeus is passed, the head is extended to eliminate the angle of the mouth and pharynx, and the endoscope gently enters the esophagus (see **Figure 27.3a through c**). The esophagus can then be examined under direct vision.

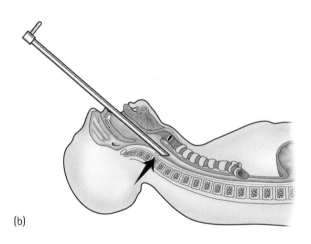

(b)

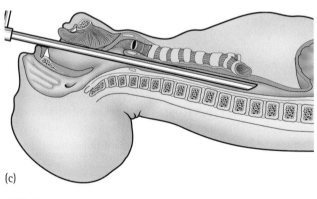

(c)

27.3a–c

FLEXIBLE UPPER GASTROINTESTINAL ENDOSCOPY

Indications

Table 27.1 indicates the common reasons for flexible endoscopic assessment of the esophagus. It is clearly indicated in patients complaining of dysphagia, odynophagia, and persistent heartburn, or those with an abnormal contrast study or computed tomography (CT) scan, or who have other symptoms suspicious of esophagogastric cancer. However, its role has vastly expanded to include uses in the therapeutic, intraoperative, postoperative, and surveillance settings.

Upper gastrointestinal endoscopes

A wide variety of endoscopes of different types, lengths, and diameters are available (see **Figure 27.4**, which shows a thin gastroscope [A], standard gastroscope [B], side-viewing duodenoscope [C], linear endoscopic ultrasound [EUS] scope [D], radial EUS scope [E], and therapeutic double channel gastroscope [F]). The endoscopist should ensure that the type used matches the intended procedure.

Modern standard endoscopes are designed to be placed transorally and have an approximate diameter of 10 mm with a 2.8 mm or greater working channel. The basic features

(channels for insufflation, suction, and biopsy) and controls (up/down, right/left tip deflection) have changed little over the years. With the exception of echoendoscopes and duodenoscopes, all are forward viewing, with the image captured on a chip at the tip of the endoscope, rather than transmission via fiber-optic cables. The most advanced scopes come with high definition, zoom, or narrow band imaging settings. The working channel allows insertion of an array of accessories, including biopsy forceps, snares, injection needles, guide wires, and balloon dilators. Unlike colonoscopes, which have

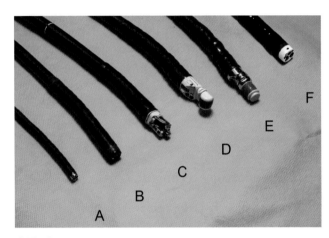

27.4   Range of different endoscopes available.

Table 27.1   The indications for flexible examination of the esophagus

	Scenario
Diagnosis	Dysphagia, odynophagia, reflux symptoms, abnormal contrast study or CT scan
	Other symptoms, such as iron deficiency anemia, weight loss, cervical lymphadenopathy
Advanced diagnosis of Barrett's/ Staging of malignancy	Narrow band imaging
	Chromoendoscopy
	Endoscopic ultrasound $\pm$ FNA
Therapeutic	Dilatation of strictures
	Achalasia dilatation/Botox injection/POEM
	Radiofrequency ablation of Barrett's esophagus
	Endoscopic mucosal resection
	Esophageal stent insertion
	Variceal banding or injection
Intraoperative	Staging laparoscopy
	Minimal invasive esophagectomy
	Heller's cardiomyotomy
	Revisional antireflux surgery
	Hiatus hernia/Gastric volvulus
	Protection of the GEJ during gastro-esophageal surgery
Postoperative	Assessment of anastomotic leaks/strictures
	Assessment of wrap position after fundoplication
Surveillance	Barrett's esophagus
	Varices
	Achalasia
	Malignancy

Notes: FNA, fine needle aspiration; POEM, peroral endoscopic myotomy.

some degree of torque along the shaft so that the instrument can be rotated by twisting, the shorter endoscopes used in the upper gastrointestinal tract are most easily rotated by the operator's body position and hands rather than attempting to twist the endoscope.

Ultrathin endoscopes (less than 6 mm diameter) can be passed in the unsedated patient transnasally. There is some evidence they may be better tolerated in some patients. These narrow diameter scopes are particularly useful to negotiate tight esophageal strictures, avoiding the need for dilatation and allowing precise evaluation of the length and nature of the stricture. The working channel, however, is only about 2 mm in diameter and biopsies are therefore small. Nasendoscopy has limited therapeutic value because of the small channel, but it can be used to negotiate strictures so that a guide wire can be placed safely, prior to a therapeutic maneuver. Endoscopes with two working channels (dual channel endoscopes) are useful for therapeutic work including endoscopic resections and for the control of upper gastrointestinal bleeding.

Flexible endoscopy technique

Most endoscopies are performed as outpatient procedures either with conscious sedation (usually achieved with a short-acting benzodiazepine) or local anesthetic throat spray. Pulse, blood pressure, and oxygen saturation should be monitored throughout the procedure. Patients are prepared for endoscopy by being nil by mouth for 6 hours, although this may need to be extended in patients with chronic obstructive symptoms, such as suspected achalasia or delayed gastric emptying. Examination should include the entire gastrointestinal tract as far as the second part of the duodenum, even when symptoms seem confined to the esophagus.

The most common position for the examination is the left lateral decubitus, with the neck flexed. Under general anesthesia, the patient can be supine and intubation aided by the anesthetist providing a chin lift. A dental guard is used to protect the endoscope, which is passed under direct vision over the tongue to the back of the oropharynx where the epiglottis and larynx are visualized. Slight neck flexion and an instruction to swallow, while maintaining the endoscope in the midline, will allow the endoscope to pass the cricopharyngeus and into the cervical esophagus. Gentle pressure only should be used and particular care taken in elderly patients who potentially have cervical osteophytes or symptoms suspicious of a pharyngeal pouch.

The endoscope is advanced under direct vision with gentle air insufflation to provide an optimal view. Minor indentations into the esophageal wall can occur at the level of the aortic arch and left atrium, but the critical landmark is identification of the GEJ that is usually about 40 cm from the incisor teeth (see **Figure 27.5**). Under normal circumstances, this is also the squamocolumnar junction and is easily identified as a Z-shaped line of demarcation between the pale pink squamous esophageal mucosa and the redder columnar lining of the stomach. This junction can be difficult to identify in the presence of a hiatus hernia or when the lower esophagus is covered by a columnar epithelium (Barrett's esophagus). The most useful visual clue is careful inspection of the mucosal vascular pattern, which, in the lower esophagus, has a characteristic palisaded appearance. The termination of gastric folds is less reliable. Detailed endoscopic examination is best performed as the instrument is withdrawn, and it is therefore preferable to reach the duodenum with insufflation and minimal use of suction unless a large fluid residue is a problem. This avoids mucosal suction artifact, reduces the risk of the endoscope looping in a very dilated stomach, minimizes patient discomfort, and facilitates maneuverability.

The duodenal bulb (which has no circular folds) is inspected. The scope is angled right and upward and rotated 90 degrees clockwise to enter the second part of the duodenum. While views of the distal duodenum can be obtained, it is only necessary if there is a clinical reason to do so. The papilla of Vater is not easily viewed using an end-viewing gastroscope. The scope is withdrawn through the pylorus. The stomach is inflated so that the rugal folds are flattened out and full mucosal views can be obtained. The antrum and body are examined withdrawing the scope in a spiral fashion on careful withdrawal. Identification of the incisura angularis is a useful landmark. Retroflexion of the scope allows visualization of the fundus and cardia. Lesions are mapped, biopsied as necessary, and conventionally both anatomic location and a measurement from the incisor teeth,

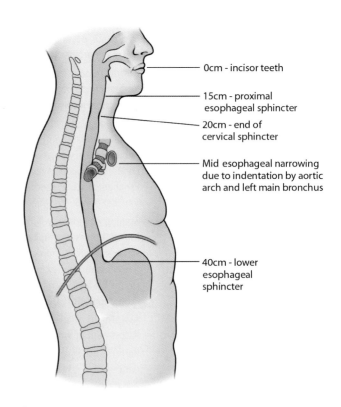

0 cm - incisor teeth

15 cm - proximal esophageal sphincter

20 cm - end of cervical sphincter

Mid esophageal narrowing due to indentation by aortic arch and left main bronchus

40 cm - lower esophageal sphincter

27.5 Landmarks of the esophagus at endoscopy.

as indicated by markings on the shaft of the endoscope, are described. Care should be taken with the measurements to ensure that the endoscope is straight and most of the stomach is deflated before complete withdrawal from the stomach (residual air should be removed to ensure the patient is comfortable after the procedure). The esophagus is then also assessed during withdrawal.

BIOPSY TECHNIQUE AND RECOMMENDED NUMBER OF SAMPLES

The "turn and suction" technique of endoscopic biopsies allows better acquisition of larger mucosal samples to aid in histological diagnosis. The biopsy forceps are advanced into the lumen, opened, and then withdrawn backward to be close to the tip of the endoscope. The endoscope tip is then turned gently into the wall of the esophagus and the suction button is depressed to suck the mucosa into the biopsy forceps, which are then closed. After the endoscope is straightened and air introduced to the lumen, the biopsy can be taken by pulling the forceps and avulsing the mucosal sample. This technique is especially useful for Barrett's surveillance biopsies. The recommended number of biopsy samples obtained for different esophageal conditions are shown in **Table 27.2**. It is particularly important in malignancy to ensure adequate numbers of biopsies are taken so that an accurate histological diagnosis is made on the first endoscopy. Increasingly, immunohistochemical tests may be required both for diagnostic purposes (gastrointestinal stromal tumors [GIST]) and to guide therapy (human epidermal growth factor receptor 2 [HER-2]).

BLIND AREAS

The area immediately below the cricopharyngeus is a potential blind spot during flexible upper gastrointestinal endoscopy. This area needs careful evaluation just prior to withdrawal through the upper esophageal sphincter. The fundus of the stomach can only be viewed in its entirety by retroflexion and then rotation of the endoscope.

Table 27.2 Recommended biopsy schedule for esophageal pathology

Disease	Tissue sampling
Esophageal malignancy	>8 samples (ideally 10–12)
Gastro-esophageal reflux disease	Targeted biopsies of any irregular mucosa Grade C/D esophagitis should be biopsied as there is a risk of underlying Barrett's esophagus or malignancy
Nondysplastic Barrett's esophagus	Four-quadrant biopsies every 2 cm, with additional biopsies of any irregular or nodular mucosa
Dysplastic Barrett's esophagus	Four-quadrant biopsies every 1 cm, with additional biopsies of any irregular or nodular mucosa
Eosinophilic esophagitis	2–4 biopsies from the proximal and distal esophagus
Candida esophagitis	Biopsies of the affected area (usually proximal esophagus) ± brush cytology

Specific scenarios and features

MALIGNANCY

The proximal, distal, and circumferential extent of the tumor should be accurately measured from the incisor teeth and its morphology (polypoid, nodular, ulcerated, stricturing) noted. The distance from the GEJ should be assessed to help plan further operative resection if indicated. Associated lesions such as Barrett's esophagus should also be measured and documented. The appropriate number of diagnostic biopsies should be obtained.

ESOPHAGITIS

Esophagitis can be caused by a variety of factors. The most common is gastro-esophageal reflux, but it can be also caused by bile reflux, infection, medication, alcohol, stasis, and caustic ingestion. A number of autoimmune conditions can be complicated by esophagitis and chronic inflammation, such as Crohn's disease, which, while rare, can affect the esophagus. For most of these disorders, a careful history may raise suspicion about the likely diagnosis, such as odynophagia and immunosuppression in patients with infective causes. Reflux esophagitis is usefully graded using the Los Angeles (LA) system, which describes the severity of inflammation from A to D (see **Table 27.3**). A carefully detailed description and photographs should be standard practice, as this classification is based on the worst grade seen at any point. Biopsy at the index endoscopy should be undertaken, and, in patients with ulcerative esophagitis, follow-up endoscopy after appropriate treatment is recommended to ensure an underlying malignancy is not missed. Signs of an incompetent antireflux mechanism are often also present with free esophagogastric reflux during the procedure. The presence of any associated hiatus hernia should be carefully sought.

HIATUS HERNIA

Hiatal herniation, where some part of the stomach comes to lie above the diaphragmatic crura, is classified as shown in **Figure 27.6**. Sliding hiatus hernia (Type I; see **Figure 27.6a**) is usually recognized endoscopically by a double narrowing as the endoscope is advanced down the esophagus. The proximal narrowing corresponds to the lower sphincter and is close to the visible GEJ. A second area of narrowing is then identified at the level of the diaphragmatic crura. On retroflexion, the cardia does not close snugly around the endoscope. Para-esophageal (rolling) hernias can prove difficult to negotiate, especially when large and not known to be present. There is always a degree of gastric volvulus that accompanies a large para-esophageal hernia. The GEJ may be in its normal position (Type II; see **Figure 27.6b**) or dislocated into the mediastinum when there are sliding and rolling components (Type III; see **Figure 27.6c**). These very large mixed hernias result in an upside-down stomach that is difficult to fully examine endoscopically. To pass into the distal stomach, it is best to use minimal air insufflation and avoid over distending the stomach, as this blocks passage of the scope into the antrum. If the whole stomach and duodenum cannot be viewed, a contrast study is the best technique to define the anatomy. A CT scan may be needed to identify other viscera contained within the hernia sac (Type IV; see **Figure 27.6d**). Further information on hiatus hernia, including laparoscopic repair, can be found in Chapter 39, "Laparoscopic large hiatus hernia repair."

Table 27.3 The LA classification of reflux esophagitis

Severity	Definition
Grade A	One or more mucosal breaks no longer than 5 mm, none of which extends between the tops of the mucosal folds
Grade B	One or more mucosal breaks more than 5 mm long, none of which extends between the tops of two mucosal folds
Grade C	Mucosal breaks that extend between the tops of two or more mucosal folds, but which involve less than 75% of the esophageal circumference
Grade D	Mucosal break that involves at least 75% of the esophageal circumference

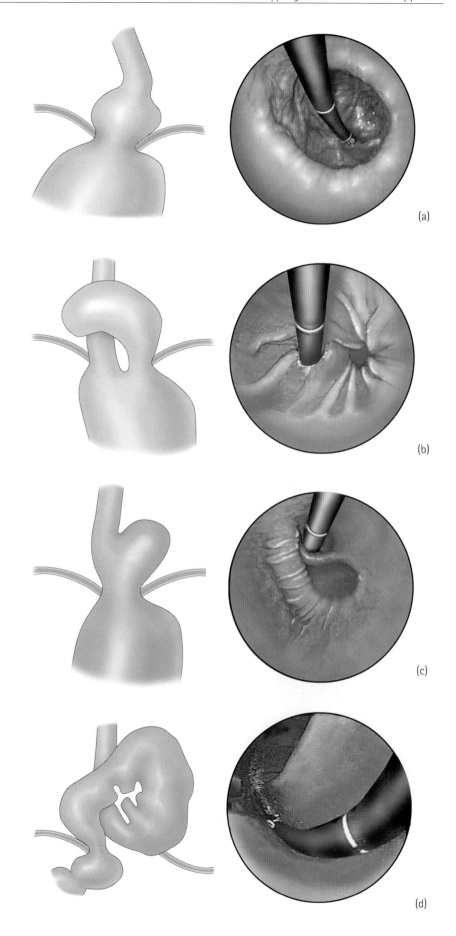

(a)

(b)

(c)

(d)

27.6a–d Types of hiatal hernia.

BARRETT'S ESOPHAGUS

In this condition, the esophagus is lined with columnar epithelium within which intestinalization occurs, with goblet cells producing mucus. Barrett's esophagus should be graded using the Prague C and M (C—circumferential extent, M—maximum extent) criteria to allow standardization. **Figure 27.7** shows an illustration of a Prague C3M7 Barrett's esophagus. It is important to assess any degree of associated hiatal herniation by locating the GEJ. The upper extent of the gastric folds, sphincter "pinch," cylindrical shape, and the point of crural narrowing have to be used rather than the squamocolumnar junction.

Chromoendoscopy using dye is occasionally a useful adjunct. A wide variety of dyes have been used. Iodine stains squamous mucosa and may be helpful to identify the upper end of a Barrett's segment. Dyes that preferentially stain columnar epithelia, such as methylene blue, can be used similarly. Magnification endoscopy, autofluorescence, and narrow band imaging are all useful techniques to enhance the detail of the Barrett's mucosa, particularly in the context of identifying suspicious areas that can then be targeted for biopsy.

PREVIOUS ANTIREFLUX SURGERY

Management of patients who have had antireflux surgery and develop recurrent or new symptoms can be challenging. Together with contrast radiology and 24-hour pH studies, careful endoscopic assessment is valuable. Endoscopic views of failed antireflux surgery are usually quite characteristic. Normal appearances of a properly constructed and functioning fundoplication include an intra-abdominal wrap measuring 2–3 cm in length with no gastric mucosa above it, absence of any gap between the shaft of the endoscope and the wrap, and no evidence of twisting (the markings on the scope are in the same orientation as the wrap). Location of the GEJ should therefore be assessed in relation to the crura, the amount of gastric tissue above and below the fundoplication noted, and the anatomy of the fundoplication characterized. An associated para-esophageal hernia should be sought.

The typical features of an intrathoracic fundoplication, partially disrupted wrap, and twisted wrap are illustrated in **Figure 27.8a through d**: A shows the normal endoscopic appearance, B demonstrates intrathoracic migration of fundoplication, C shows a partial disruption, and D shows a twisted total fundoplication.

Please see Chapter 40, "Revisional antireflux surgery," for further information on this topic.

ACHALASIA

In early achalasia, the esophagus may appear normal. A lack of peristalsis, and a nonrelaxing lower esophageal sphincter may be subtle findings. Typically, however, the esophagus is dilated and contains food and debris. The lower esophageal sphincter is closed and opens with slight resistance. It is important to assess the gastric cardia for malignancy and exclude pseudoachalasia. Refer to Chapter 41, "Laparoscopic cardiomyotomy for achalasia," and Chapter 42, "Per oral endoscopic myotomy (POEM) for achalasia," for more on this topic.

ESOPHAGEAL PERFORATION

Endoscopic assessment of patients with spontaneous and iatrogenic esophageal perforation is important. If iatrogenic, the nature of the injury (caused by a guide wire, graduated dilator, or balloon) should be evaluated. The size and location of the perforation influences management, and while many endoscopic perforations can be managed nonoperatively, careful monitoring of the patient, antibiotics, and proper nutritional support are essential. With spontaneous perforation, the mucosal injury is usually longer than the muscular defect and endoscopic assessment can help in deciding what operative approach is best. Endoscopy can also identify underlying pathology and guide radiological intervention as appropriate. Refer to Chapter 37, "Perforation of the esophagus."

THE EARLY POSTESOPHAGECTOMY PATIENT

Flexible endoscopy accurately identifies anastomotic leaks or gastric conduit ischemia in patients who have recently had esophagectomy with appropriate symptoms or signs. The anastomosis can be inspected in detail for integrity and the size of any defect noted. The viability of the gastric conduit can be assessed. Endoscopy is particularly important when there are concerns about a cause for deteriorating respiratory performance. Portability of the equipment means that the

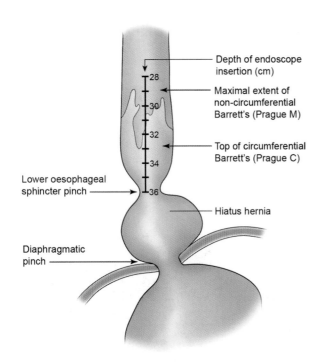

27.7 Prague C and M criteria for standardized measurement of Barrett's esophagus.

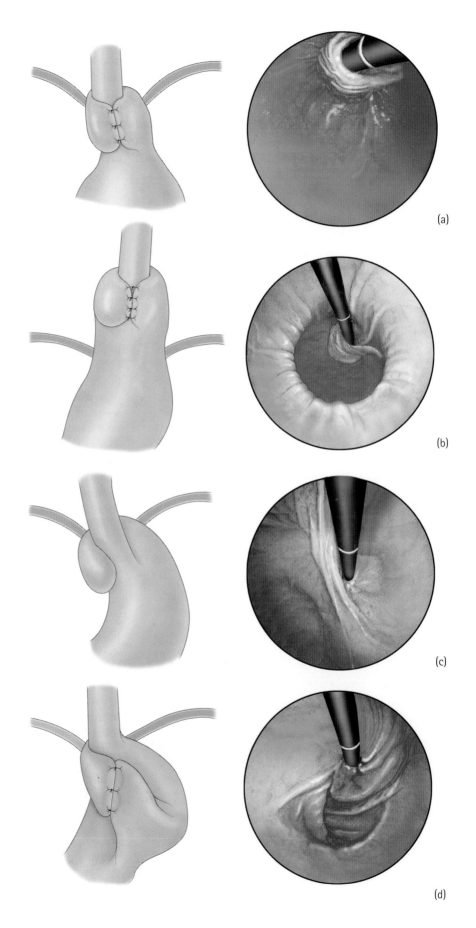

27.8a−d Endoscopic views after antireflux surgery.

(a)

(b)

(c)

(d)

procedure can take place within a critical care environment. Endoscopic visualization will nearly always determine the need for intervention. More on this topic can be found in Chapter 28, "Esophageal stents," and Chapter 37, "Perforation of the esophagus."

CAUSTIC INJURIES

Strong alkalis and acids can be ingested either accidentally or in attempted suicide. The type of agent, its concentration, and the volume ingested determine the amount of damage. Acids tend to cause more gastric damage than alkalis, due to the induction of intense pylorospasm and pooling in the antrum. Early endoscopy is essential, with inspection of the entire esophagus and stomach. A gray/black eschar carries the greatest risk of perforation. Local hemorrhage from the damaged segment is common as the endoscope is passed. With minor injuries, there may only be mucosal edema and these patients can be safely fed. Endoscopy is therefore used to determine the need for nutritional support, as well as the level of care required. Significant stricturing occurs in about half of the patients who have had a severe mucosal injury. The role and timing of repeated endoscopies with or without dilatation are controversial. It is preferable in the early phase of the condition, as the fibrotic phase of healing takes at least 3 months to become established. This assumes that emergency surgery for extensive necrosis or perforation is not required.

Therapeutic upper gastrointestinal endoscopy

ESOPHAGEAL DILATATION

Patients with dysphagia due to gastro-esophageal reflux disease, anastomotic strictures, and those with short radiotherapy-induced or caustic strictures are good candidates for esophageal dilatation. Dilatation of malignant strictures should be avoided, especially in patients who have potentially resectable tumors, where perforation may result in tumor dissemination within the chest or an inability to deliver curative treatment as a result of sepsis. Dilatation of malignant strictures should only be used as a preliminary to stent

placement. With the development of narrow stent delivery systems, this has largely become unnecessary.

Balloon and mechanical dilators are equally effective in dilating esophageal strictures and there are no obvious clinical differences between the two techniques. **Figure 27.9** shows the variety of endoscopic dilators: standard controlled radial expansion (CRE) balloon dilator (A), achalasia balloon dilator (B), inflation devices for the balloon dilators (C), and a range of Savary-Gillard dilators (D). Mechanical dilators exert an additional shearing force, whereas balloon dilators exert a uniform radial force throughout the stricture, and in theory this may be beneficial and reduce the perforation risk. Complex strictures, which are long, tortuous, or associated with diverticula are best dilated with guide-wire-based systems under fluoroscopic guidance.

Dilatation technique

Placement of a guide wire through the stricture is the vital first step. With difficult strictures, it may be necessary to confirm position of the guide wire within the gastrointestinal tract. Passage of a catheter over the guide wire, contrast injection, and radiologic confirmation may be required. Balloon dilators can be passed through the biopsy channel of the endoscope or the endoscope can be removed, the dilator passed over the guide wire and the endoscope then passed separately to visualize the procedure. CRE balloons placed under endoscopic visualization are usually between 13 and 15 mm in diameter but narrower balloons should be used with very tight strictures at the initial procedure. The balloon is placed across the stricture and inflated under endoscopic control using the manufacturer's instructions. The balloon is kept inflated for between 1 and 2 minutes. After deflation, the stricture should be examined and, if successful, the endoscope should pass.

Graduated dilators (e.g., Savary-Gillard bougies) are made of polyvinyl and come in a range of diameters between 5 and 20 mm. They have a tapered tip with a radiologically visible band. They are passed over a flexible-tipped guide wire. Prior to dilatation, the soft tip of the guide wire should be placed at least into the proximal stomach (we prefer proximal duodenum) and the same constraints apply here as outlined for balloon dilatation previously. Placement of the bougie into a warm bath makes the plastic flexible and allows for a smoother insertion. Serial dilatations using the "rule of three" is an accepted method of using these types of dilators. The initial dilator should be slightly larger than the estimated stricture diameter, and no more than three consecutive dilators in increments of 1 mm should be passed in a single session. Any resistance should be noted and excessive force avoided. Many strictures require more than one session for the patient's symptoms to be adequately treated.

Achalasia dilatation should be carried out under fluoroscopic visualization after a 4-day period on a liquid diet to ensure the esophagus is clear of solid food debris. Endoscopy is performed, under sedation with opiate analgesia or general anesthetic. A guide wire is placed into the stomach and the endoscope removed. Achalasia balloons are between 30 and

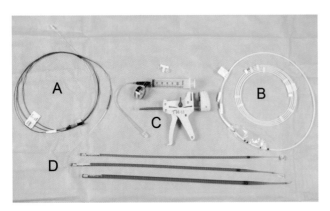

27.9 Range of endoscopic dilators.

40 mm in diameter when fully inflated. Most endoscopists use smaller balloons for the initial procedure, but there is little evidence that there are major differences in outcomes regarding success or complication rates. The chosen balloon is lubricated, passed over a guide wire, followed by the endoscope, and inflated under radiologic control. Radio-opaque markers aid accurate placement. The aim is to forcibly disrupt the lower esophageal sphincter. The balloon is inflated, using a pressure gauge, to 7 psi for 2 minutes. The waist of the balloon, which corresponds to the lower esophageal sphincter, should be obliterated on the fluoroscopic image. The esophagus and GEJ are then inspected endoscopically to exclude iatrogenic perforation. After the procedure, the patient should be observed closely before discharge, but day-case dilatation is feasible in fit patients. Any signs or symptoms of esophageal perforation should be investigated promptly (see Chapter 37, "Perforation of the esophagus"). Patients who fail to be relieved of their symptoms can be dilated again with a wider diameter balloon.

REMOVAL OF FOREIGN BODIES

A variety of techniques can be used to remove foreign bodies endoscopically, including the use of forceps, nets, snares, and tripod-type graspers. Patients who present with food bolus obstruction and no obvious cause should have esophageal biopsies taken either at the time of index endoscopy or at a later date to exclude eosinophilic esophagitis. Food boluses can be removed piecemeal with the use of nets and gentle pushing pressure of smaller pieces into the stomach. After removal of any foreign body, the esophagus should be inspected for underlying disease, perforation, or ischemic injury.

Occasionally, it is advisable to move a sharp foreign body into the stomach, allowing a change its position so that the sharp edge trails on removal. During removal of sharp foreign bodies such as razor blades or needles, the esophagus can be protected by the use of an overtube (see **Figure 27.10**). The short esophageal overtube (see **Figure 27.10a**) is used to protect the proximal esophagus when retrieving foreign bodies in the distal esophagus, while the long esophageal overtube (see **Figure 27.10b**) protects the GEJ and whole of the esophagus while retrieving foreign bodies from the stomach or duodenum. The lubricated overtube is positioned over the most proximal part of the endoscope, which is placed so

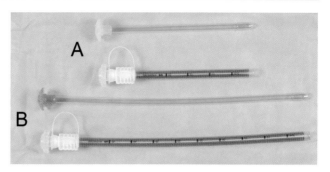

27.10 Long and short esophageal overtube.

that the overtube can be railroaded over the endoscope and into the esophagus. The endoscope is removed, the overtube capped to create a seal for insufflation, and the endoscope reinserted, allowing the object to be drawn into the overtube protecting the esophagus.

ENDOSCOPIC ULTRASOUND

The use of EUS has allowed the endoscopist to look beyond the mucosa of the esophagus and accurately stage esophageal cancer. EUS can also assess nodal disease beyond the surgical field and allow targeted fine needle aspiration (FNA) of suspicious lymph nodes. It is especially useful for assessing local resectability and excluding invasion to structures such as the aorta, tracheo-bronchial tree, diaphragmatic crura and pericardium. The accuracy of EUS in staging local invasion (T stage) is 80%–90%, compared with only 50%–60% with CT imaging. Echoendoscopes come in radial and linear types (see **Figure 27.4d and e**). Radial echoendoscopes provide cross-sectional views of the layers of the gastrointestinal tract, and are used to characterize these wall layers to determine the depth of tumor invasion, appearance of lymph nodes, presence of free fluid, and limited views of other organs such as the left lobe of the liver. Linear probes provide a sector scan in the line of the shaft of the instrument and are therefore ideally suited to interventional procedures and biopsy of structures deep to the mucosa or beyond the esophageal wall, as a needle will be seen completely in the ultrasound plane. The linear instrument is also equipped with Doppler capability to allow vessels to be identified and avoided.

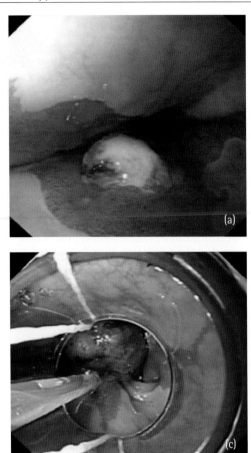

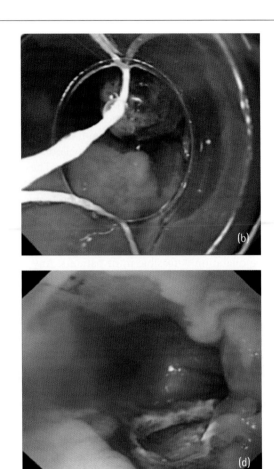

27.11a–d EMR in Barrett's esophagus.

ENDOSCOPIC MUCOSAL RESECTION

Although a detailed account of endoscopic mucosal resection (EMR), especially indications, is beyond the scope of this chapter, the esophageal surgeon needs to have a good working knowledge of this procedure. Different techniques have been described including saline lift EMR, "suck and cut" EMR, and "suck and ligate" EMR. In the esophagus, it can be used to excise areas of high-grade dysplasia and early malignancy. The resected lesion should be orientated accurately and pinned out for the pathologist to careful examine. **Figure 27.11** shows the standard suck and ligate EMR technique: A shows an early malignant lesion in Barrett's esophagus; B shows saline injection into the submucosal layer, suction of the lesion into the endoscopic banding device, and deployment of the ligation band; C shows removal of the lesion with an endoscopic snare and diathermy; and D demonstrates the final endoscopic view.

LAPAROENDOSCOPIC SURGERY

The combination of an endoscopic procedure during a laparoscopic operation is described as laparoendoscopic surgery. It is an important part of the esophageal surgeon's armamentarium. Endoscopic visualization of the adequacy of cardiomyotomy during surgery for achalasia is widely used. The GEJ can be precisely defined; assessment can be made whether the myotomy extends far enough proximally and distally; mucosal perforations can be excluded. Intraoperative endoscopy is important with localized gastric surgery such as GIST excision, to ensure completeness of resection and where protection of the GEJ is required. Endoscopy can be helpful during revisional antireflux operations where a luminal view can provide extra information before and after hiatal dissection, as well as disclosing mucosal injuries. Resection margin assessment that might alter the extent and nature of the surgery during esophagectomy can be difficult when there is a Barrett's segment that extends close to the thoracic inlet, with early tumors that are not easily felt or during minimal access surgery, where the loss of tactile sensation means that visual clues about the proximal extent of a tumor might be important. Intraoperative endoscopy helps in all of these situations. It is important that laparoscopic ports are placed *before* endoscopy during these combined procedures because overzealous gas insufflation can make intra-abdominal visualization difficult as the stomach and proximal small bowel distend with gas. Surgeon and endoscopist should carefully coordinate maneuvers to avoid inadvertent injury and to gain the best from both laparoscopic and endoscopic views.

COMPLICATIONS

Complications are uncommon after diagnostic flexible endoscopy, but include sedation-related complications, aspiration, bleeding, and perforation. Sedation-related complications are largely avoidable by carefully titrating the dose of benzodiazepines and adhering to guidelines on the use of conscious sedation. Reversal agents, if required, should be immediately available. Chest pain, breathlessness, subcutaneous emphysema, fever, and tachycardia are all potential features of perforation. Its risk increases in patients with an obstructing lesion or when intervention is added. With diagnostic endoscopy, this is probably the case in 1 in 4000 procedures, and intervention is thought to increase risk at least tenfold. Bleeding is usually minor and self-limiting. Therapeutic endoscopists who perform EMR or polypectomy should be well trained in endoscopic techniques of hemostasis, including adrenaline injection, heater probe application, clip application, and Hemospray.

FURTHER READING

American Society for Gastrointestinal Endoscopy (ASGE) Standards of Practice Committee, Sharaf RN, Shergill AK, Odze RD, Krinsky ML, Fukami N, Jain R et al. Endoscopic mucosal tissue sampling. *Gastrointest Endosc.* 2013 Aug; 78(2): 216–24.

Dent J. Endoscopic grading of reflux oesophagitis: the past, present and future. *Best Pract Res Clin Gastroenterol.* 2008; 22(4): 585–99.

Gustafson LM, Tami TA. MD. Flexible versus rigid esophagoscopy: a practical comparison for otolaryngologists. *Curr Opin Otolaryngol Head Neck Surg.* 2000 Jun; 8(3): 227–31.

Kuppusamy MK, Felisky C, Kozarek RA, Schembre D, Ross A, Gan I, Irani S, Low DE. Impact of endoscopic assessment and treatment on operative and non-operative management of acute oesophageal perforation. *Br J Surg.* 2011 Jun; 98(6): 818–24.

Levine DS, Reid BJ. Endoscopic biopsy technique for acquiring larger mucosal samples. *Gastrointest Endosc.* 1991 May–Jun; 37(3): 332–7.

Mittal SK, Juhasz A, Ramanan B, Hoshino M, Lee TH, Filipi CJ. A proposed classification for uniform endoscopic description of surgical fundoplication. *Surg Endosc.* 2013 Apr; 28(4): 1103–9.

Riley SA, Attwood SE. Guidelines on the use of oesophageal dilatation in clinical practice. *Gut.* 2004 Feb; 53(Suppl. 1): i1–6.

Sharma P, Dent J, Armstrong D, Bergman JJ, Gossner L, Hoshihara Y, Jankowski JA et al. The development and validation of an endoscopic grading system for Barrett's esophagus: the Prague C and M criteria. *Gastroenterology.* 2006 Nov; 131(5): 1392–9.

Standards of Practice Committee, Egan JV, Baron TH, Adler DG, Davila R, Faigel DO, Gan SL et al. Esophageal dilation. *Gastrointest Endosc.* 2006 May; 63(6): 755–60.

28

Esophageal stents

NABIL P. RIZK AND SARAH K. THOMPSON

A recent American College of Gastroenterology study reviewed the available evidence regarding the various uses of esophageal stents and provided an assessment of the quality of the evidence and the strength of the recommendations for a range of indications. The researchers found that the most common indications for the use of esophageal stents were malignant obstruction, extrinsic compression, refractory strictures, and esophageal perforations and leaks. The incidence of these indications has increased significantly during the last two decades, as has as the number of patients undergoing stent placement, as stent technology has evolved and the safety and ease of stent placement have improved. In this chapter, we will briefly review the evolution of stent technology, including the current standard of care, the technique for stent placement, and the various indications for placement of an esophageal stent.

STENT TECHNOLOGY

Esophageal stent technology has evolved significantly during the past two decades, replacing rigid prosthetic stents such as the Celestin tube and Atkinson's tube—which were difficult to deploy and were associated with high complication (perforation, migration, occlusion, airway compression) and mortality rates—with self-expandable metallic stents (SEMS). The advantage of SEMS over rigid stents was initially confirmed in a prospective trial published in 1993, and SEMS have since become the standard of care. SEMS are primarily composed of a metallic mesh of nickel-titanium metal alloy (nitinol), which allows the stent to retain its shape and to conform to a variety of shapes while maintaining adequate radial pressures. Initially, stents were fully uncovered (fully exposed metallic mesh component), but because of the occurrence of tumor and granulation tissue ingrowth between the wire mesh, partially covered stents that primarily used polytetrafluoroethylene as the covering material were developed. An advantage of partially covered stents is that the covered component minimizes ingrowth while leaving the metal ends exposed, which allows the stent to attach to the underlying mucosa and lessens the risk of stent migration. Currently, the various brands of partially covered SEMS differ with regard to design, including the presence or absence of braiding (braiding shortens the length of the stent during deployment by 30% on each end), length, diameter, radial strength, and deployment mechanism. However, numerous studies have found there is no meaningful advantage of any of the currently available brands of partially covered SEMS.

INDICATIONS FOR STENT INSERTION

Esophageal stents in unresectable disease

An increasing incidence of esophageal cancer in the Western hemisphere is occurring without a concomitant increase in the rate of early detection. Consequently, the number of patients presenting with advanced stage disease (not appropriate for surgery or irradiation) is increasing at an alarming rate, and the need to provide these patients with

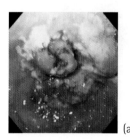 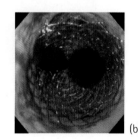

28.1 Esophageal lumen obscured by a malignant obstruction (a). A self-expandable metallic stent (SEMS) has been inserted to open up the lumen of the esophagus before initiation of chemoradiotherapy (b).

palliative treatment options to maintain their quality of life is increasingly relevant. Among the most debilitating symptoms in patients with advanced stage esophageal cancer is dysphagia. Advancements in stent technology during the past two decades have dramatically improved the management of this condition, by far the most common indication for the placement of an esophageal stent. Unlike for other indications, the goal of treatment of malignant strictures and obstruction from tumor encroachment is to durably improve dysphagia while minimizing the risks of the intervention and the need for reinterventions. Overall, when SEMS are used to palliate malignant esophageal obstruction, they are cost-effective, efficient, and successful at palliating patients (see **Figure 28.1**).

Esophageal stents for trachea-esophageal fistula

Malignant trachea-esophageal fistula (TEF) occurs in 5%–15% of patients with esophageal cancer. TEFs can occur as a direct consequence of tumor invasion, or they can be iatrogenic in patients who have received chemoradiation, which were probably invading the airway wall. A bronchoscopic examination should be performed to exclude airway invasion before contemplating radiation treatment in any patient with a bulky proximal or mid-esophageal tumor. Once a fistula occurs, the life expectancy of the patient is 1–3 months. The most common site of invasion and fistula formation is the trachea, followed by the left mainstem bronchus. Given the typically poor prognosis and physical condition of patients

with TEFs, surgical management is rarely indicated (diversion or bypass), and so a durable yet minimally invasive treatment is the most appropriate. Most often, these patients are managed with partially covered SEMS with a high success rate; alternatively, airway stents are a possible choice. Occasionally, parallel airway and esophageal stents are required to occlude the fistula in these patients (**Figure 28.2a and b**).

Esophageal stents before chemoradiation in surgically resectable disease

The need for stent placement in patients with a locally advanced tumor has diminished significantly as treatment algorithms have become more standardized, effective, and better tolerated. In most of these patients, dysphagia rapidly improves with induction doses of chemo-/radiotherapy, such that stents are no longer necessary. Most patients can be managed with enteral feeding access (i.e., nasoenteric tube). However, there are occasions when stents are necessary, either because of complete obstruction or because of an inadequate initial treatment response, in which case a temporary stent may help to relieve dysphagia. In these patients, the stent will need to be removed during the course of treatment; therefore, a fully covered SEMS is typically placed, since these are the easiest to retrieve. The risk of stent migration in these patients is relatively low, because of the narrowness of the lumen, but it becomes more problematic over time if treatment response causes significant tumor regression.

Esophageal stents for postesophagectomy complications

One relatively common complication following an esophagectomy for cancer is anastomotic leak at the gastroesophageal anastomosis. An effective treatment for leak is the placement of a stent to cover the site of dehiscence, which stops contamination of the mediastinum and allows for earlier oral intake. Typically, fully covered SEMS are used for this indication and are kept in place for approximately 4–6 weeks. Reported success rates at sealing the leak range from 80% to 90% (for more on this indication, refer to Chapter 37, "Perforation of the esophagus").

A less common but more dreaded postoperative complication is iatrogenic fistula between the airway and the conduit/esophagus. This complication is uncommon (<1%) but is associated with high morbidity and mortality. It most likely results from a combination of anastomotic leak and an unrecognized intraoperative airway injury. Most patients with this complication are acutely ill and present with a respiratory infection, and the accepted management has been to reoperate; take down the anastomosis; divert the esophagus; and, if the patient is sufficiently stable, remove the gastric conduit. Some have reported repairing the site of the fistula and placing an interposed muscle flap, although this is frequently not technically feasible. In the few patients

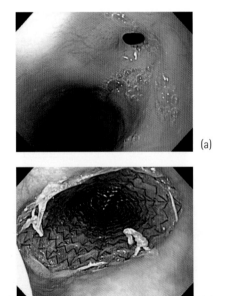

(a)

(b)

28.2 An iatrogenic post-chemoradiation fistula between the proximal esophagus and the trachea (a). A fully covered self-expandable esophageal stent (SEMS) has been inserted to occlude the fistula (b).

with this complication who are not acutely ill and for who ongoing lung contamination is a lesser concern, there is the option of placing a stent in the esophagus. This approach has been reported by some to successfully seal the fistula and allow the fistula to heal. In such cases, fully covered SEMS should be used.

TECHNIQUE OF ESOPHAGEAL STENTING

A preoperative contrast swallow and/or computed tomography scans of the neck, chest, and abdomen are obtained. We prefer to insert the stent in the operating theater with the patient under general anesthesia. Generally, patients are intubated with a single lumen endotracheal tube. Both fluoroscopic and endoscopic equipment is required.

The stent can be placed in either the supine or lateral position. In our institution, either approach is used depending on surgeon preference. Endoscopy is performed first to evaluate the location of the stricture/leak/fistula. If a narrow stricture, a skinny endoscope may be necessary to evaluate the distal extent. If a complete or near-complete obstruction is present, a guidewire is placed carefully under fluoroscopic guidance into the stomach. Gentle dilatation using a Savary-Gilliard technique is used up to a diameter of 7 mm, so the skinny

endoscope can then be inserted through the stricture. Under fluoroscopic guidance, radio-opaque markers are placed at the proximal and distal aspects of the stricture/leak/fistula. If the patient is in the supine position, this can be done with paperclips on the patient's chest (see **Figure 28.3**). If in the lateral position, a radio-opaque solution is generally injected endoscopically (either iopromide or ethiodized oil) at the proximal and distal aspects.

A guidewire is then placed into the first part of the duodenum. The appropriate stent is passed over the guidewire and deployed into position using fluoroscopy (see **Figure 28.4**). For a malignant stricture, we prefer to use an 18 mm diameter partially covered stent rather than a 24 mm diameter stent, as no difference has been noted postoperatively with respect to diet, but considerably less pain is experienced with the smaller diameter stent. For a perforation/leak, a fully covered stent is advisable with a large enough diameter to exert sufficient radial force to seal the perforation and prevent stent migration.

Once deployed, the stent can be maneuvered proximally if needed, using endoscopic graspers. Ideally, the stent should be placed with at least 3 cm of extension beyond both the proximal and distal extent of the stricture/perforation/fistula. In the upper esophagus, a 2 cm proximal margin is acceptable provided the top of the stent does not encroach on the upper esophageal sphincter. It is of course preferable to position the stent accurately from the outset, and err toward more proximal placement, as the stent may migrate distally (see **Figure 28.5**).

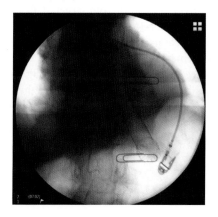

28.3

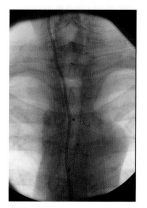

28.4

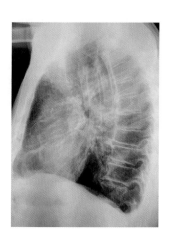

28.5

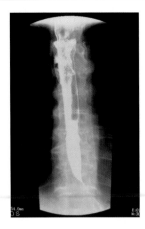

28.6

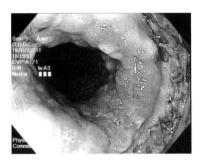

28.7

Following placement of the stent, the endoscope is reinserted to confirm accurate proximal position. We advise against inserting the endoscope through the stent for fear of injuring the endoscope and/or causing distal migration. A contrast swallow is not routinely performed poststent insertion, unless the patient reports ongoing dysphagia/vomiting/pain (**Figure 28.6**). Very occasionally, the stent does not expand completely. In this scenario, it is useful to perform pneumatic balloon dilation, but we advise waiting at least 24–48 hours for maximal stent expansion to occur. All patients are seen by our dietician and remain on a minced/soft diet indefinitely.

COMPLICATIONS FROM STENTS AND STENT PLACEMENT

Although common (approximately 30%–50%), procedural and stent-related complications with the current stent technologies are rarely lethal. Aspiration, bleeding, airway compromise, perforation, and malpositioning are all possible complications at the time of stent placement. Depending on the scenario, some iatrogenic stent-related perforations might require operative intervention, either for repair, resection and reconstruction, or diversion; however, conservative management (drainage, antibiotics, stent) for iatrogenic perforations remains the treatment of choice, if possible. Airway compromise most often occurs in the context of a large upper or mid-mediastinal tumor burden, wherein the lack of space results in airway compression when the esophageal stent is deployed. Likewise, a common complication following placement of a SEMS is chest pain or tightness, which is thought to be associated with the radial pressure from stents placed in a tight compartment (upper mediastinum) and has been shown to be more common when larger diameter stents are placed. Globus sensation is another complication observed soon after stent placement—in particular, when the stent is placed close to the upper esophageal sphincter. It is unclear whether this sensation is directly associated with the distance from the upper sphincter or whether proximal esophageal stent placement can inherently cause globus sensation, but some recommend that, to minimize risk, the proximal end of the stent be placed at least 3–4 cm distal to the sphincter.

Beyond a week after stent placement, the most common complications are stent migration, food bolus impaction, reflux, tumor ingrowth or overgrowth (see **Figure 28.7**), and fistula formation. These complications, which have been reported to occur at an incidence of 30%–50% in some series, require repeated intervention. These complications have been variably attributed to stent location and stent diameter (proximal location and larger stent diameter are associated with fistula formation), type of stent (fully covered and plastic stents are more likely to migrate), and stent location (placement across the hiatus can lead to high reflux rates and increased aspiration risks). Although a stent with a "valve" has been developed to minimize the problem of reflux in stents placed across the hiatus (Cook Esophageal Z-Stent), the benefits of this stent have not been consistently demonstrated.

SUMMARY

Esophageal stents have become the primary means of managing local problems that arise in patients with locally-regionally advanced and advanced stage esophageal cancer. SEMS are the treatment of choice for patients with advanced stage disease with an obstruction or fistula and are increasingly being used to treat complications following the surgical treatment of esophageal cancer. Problems persist primarily with migration, but technological advances have decreased the incidence of placement-related complications, as well as problems that arise after their placement.

FURTHER READING

Dasari BV, Neely D, Kennedy A et al. The role of esophageal stents in the management of esophageal anastomotic leaks and benign esophageal perforations. *Annals of Surgery.* 2014; 259: 852–60.

Hindy P, Hong J, Lam-Tsai Y, Gress F. A comprehensive review of esophageal stents. *Gastroenterology and Hepatology.* 2012; 8: 526–34.

Hürtgen M and Herber SC. Treatment of tracheoesophageal fistula. *Thoracic Surgery Clinics.* 2014; 24: 117–27.

Irani S and Kozarek R. Esophageal stents: past, present, and future. *Techniques in Gastrointestinal Endoscopy.* 2010; 12: 178–90.

Sharma P and Kozarek R. Role of esophageal stents in benign and malignant diseases. *American Journal of Gastroenterology.* 2010; 105: 258–73.

Shenfine J, McNamee P, Steen N, Griffin SM. A randomized controlled clinical trial of palliative therapies for patients with inoperable esophageal cancer. *American Journal of Gastroenterology.* 2009; 104: 1674–85.

29

Esophageal anastomoses: sutured and stapled

JON SHENFINE AND GLYN G. JAMIESON

PRINCIPLES AND JUSTIFICATION

The penalties of anastomotic leak from an esophageal anastomosis can be severe. They vary from mortality to a prolonged and traumatic hospital stay or considerable postoperative morbidity, particularly with respect to dysphagia from strictures. This interferes with postoperative quality of life. The causes of anastomotic dehiscence are undoubtedly multifactorial, with both local and systemic factors playing a role. The esophagus itself has no serosa and longitudinal muscles hold sutures poorly. Surgical exposure may also be awkward and gastric fundal perfusion can be compromised through a number of factors. Surgeons have striven to reduce anastomotic-related complications through a variety of surgical approaches and techniques. The fact that most of these variations persist suggests that debate continues over the optimum technique and even the optimum site of the anastomosis.

SITE AND APPROACH

Reconstruction of the continuity of the alimentary tract following esophagectomy is typically completed in the neck or the chest. It is generally perceived that cervical anastomoses are associated with lower mortality if a leak occurs, since drainage through an opened cervical wound is regarded as less life-threatening than a leak in the chest. However, not infrequently, a cervical leak passes through the thoracic inlet, and cervical anastomoses are thought to be associated with a higher risk of leak, anastomotic stricture, and recurrent laryngeal nerve injury than intrathoracic reconstructions. Therefore, the main factor that drives the operative approach should be oncological necessity. For example, a cervical approach and anastomosis may be required to provide adequate longitudinal clearance of an upper third esophageal squamous cell carcinoma; equally, a transthoracic approach and anastomosis may be necessary for a type III junctional

adenocarcinoma where the proximal gastric resection might compromise conduit length. Thereafter, the site of anastomosis is dependent on surgical preference, experience, and the proposed radicality of the associated nodal dissection. In addition, there has been a recent and dramatic expansion in minimally invasive surgical approaches to esophagectomy. These approaches employ similar anastomotic techniques but the literature suggests that they are associated with a higher rate of postoperative gastric necrosis. Robot-assisted surgery with improved optics and articulated instruments that allow fine control within a confined space is now an option and should in theory complement a minimally invasive approach. However, there have been reports of increased airway injuries, long operating times, and an extremely high cost. The potential benefits of these new approaches and technology are still being evaluated.

Essentially, both hand-sewn and stapled anastomotic techniques can be applied equally to either neck or chest with minor variations. The variety of surgical techniques for anastomosis makes it difficult to compare them. In addition, the underlying clinical heterogeneity of patients in most cases requires an individualized approach to surgical treatment.

CONDUIT

The stomach is the most commonly used organ for reconstruction following esophagectomy (see Chapter 30, "Use of the stomach as an esophageal substitute"). It is flexible and has a plentiful blood supply, allowing for ease of construction of a well-vascularized, tension-free conduit. This approach is uncomplicated and associated with an excellent long-term functional result. There are a number of circumstances where a colonic or jejunal interposition may be used and more appropriate (refer to Chapter 31, "Use of the colon as an esophageal substitute"), but this chapter will only focus on an esophagogastric anastomosis. One very important point is that the gastric conduit should be fashioned such that it retains as much width as possible (at least 5–6 cm). This has been shown to reduce the risk of gastric ischemia and necrosis, by preserving the intramural vascular arcades.

HAND-SEWN TECHNIQUES

Thoracic

The anastomosis should be undertaken in the apex of the thoracic cavity, above the level of the azygos vein. The esophagus is transected and the specimen resected for histology (and "back table" dissection of nodal stations). Four full-thickness stay sutures are placed at 3, 6, 9, and 12 o'clock positions in the esophagus, to aid safe manipulation and prevent retraction of layers (see **Figure 29.1**). The gastric conduit is checked for vascularity and length. The conduit is brought up to the apex of the chest lying posterior to the esophagus. Two nonabsorbable sutures are used to anchor the apex of the conduit to the esophagus as high as is practicable. An "esophageal lumen"-sized gastrotomy is made on the anterior stomach wall, a minimum of 2 cm from the newly sutured or stapled margin of the tubularized conduit to minimize the risk of angle of sorrow gastric necrosis (see **Figure 29.2**). The authors favor a single-layer continuous anastomosis but there are other excellent alternative suturing techniques that can be employed, such as a two-layer interrupted closure. In all cases, full-thickness stitches are taken, ensuring at least 4–5 mm of tissue in each bite, and moving around the span by 3–4 mm.

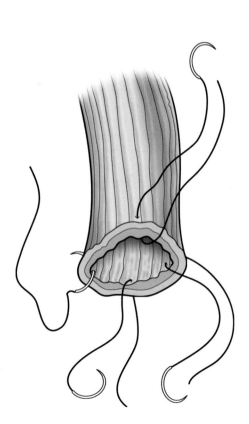

29.1

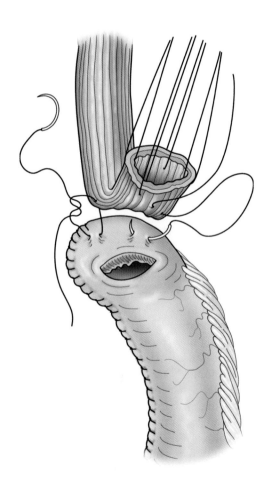

29.2

The anastomosis is started in the posterior midline using a double-ended needled 3-0 monofilament absorbable suture. The knot is thrown intraluminally and midlength so that equal spans of suture are available for each needle (see **Figure 29.3**). Care should be taken to draw the gastric conduit up to the esophagus rather than the other way around, otherwise there is risk of the sutures cutting out through the serosa-less longitudinal muscles of the esophageal wall. An over-and-over running suture is fashioned "inside out" on the stomach and "outside in" on the esophagus. Once one side of the posterior wall is completed, the suture is left "outside" the stomach and the other suture commenced but going inside out on the esophagus and outside in on the conduit, with the last throw situated on the outside of the esophagus.

The sutures are then completed anteriorly, over and over, so that when they meet they can be tied securely across the suture line (see **Figure 29.4**). If there is any concern about the anastomotic integrity, further "external" horizontal mattress sutures may be placed to buttress the anastomosis. The nasogastric tube is readvanced through the join and into the distal stomach and secured at the nose.

There is often a reasonable amount of redundant greater curve fat/omentum. The authors recommend placing this between the conduit and the airway, and then wrapping the omentum over the anastomosis. Some surgeons perform a modified loose fundoplication over the anterior surface of the anastomosis using interrupted nonabsorbable sutures, believing it reduces reflux.

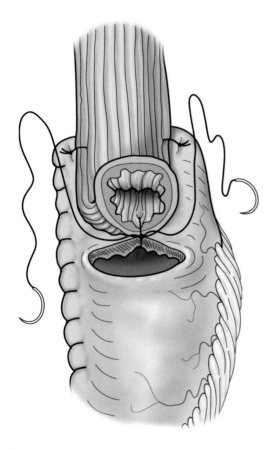

29.3

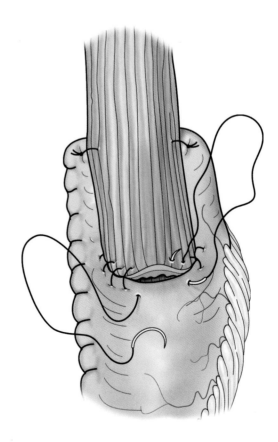

29.4

Cervical

The cervical hand-sewn anastomosis bears similarities to the thoracic approach. However, the anastomosis is usually constructed on the posterior aspect of the gastric conduit rather than anteriorly. The authors prefer to use a longitudinal gastrotomy rather than transverse to minimize ischemia. As well, the authors perform a single-layer join with full-thickness interrupted absorbable sutures, as this uses less gastric conduit length (see **Figures 29.5 through 29.7**). Care should be taken when transecting the esophagus to ensure that enough esophagus is present to facilitate the anastomosis. A simple rule to follow is to ensure there is enough esophagus to reach the skin for esophagostomy should this be required. Once completed, the anastomosis is gently returned into the wound so that the join sits neatly in the lower part of the wound. The wound is drained and closed.

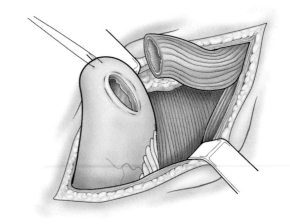

29.5

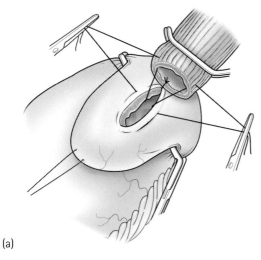

(a)

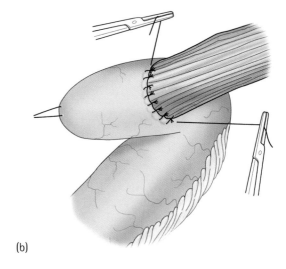

(b)

29.6a–b

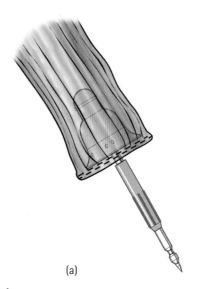

(a)

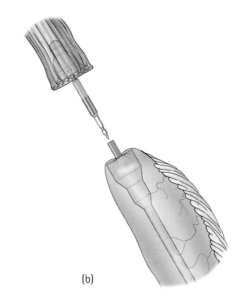

(b)

29.7a–b

STAPLED TECHNIQUES

Thoracic (circular)

There are two main stapling techniques: circular and linear. The majority of thoracic-stapled anastomoses are performed using the circular stapler, whereas the linear partial-stapled technique, described by Collard and popularized by Orringer, is more frequently used in a cervical approach. However, either may be employed the other way around and the linear technique is gaining increasing popularity for an intrathoracic anastomosis. Regardless, these will be separately described and the steps are easily substituted for site. In all descriptions, it is imperative to withdraw all indwelling catheters, such as decompressing nasogastric tubes and nasoenteric temperature probes, to a safe distance, as these are easily and disastrously incorporated into a stapled anastomosis.

An anvil is sited in the proximal esophagus. There are three techniques for this. The first two involve the placement of a purse string, while the other technique is an emerging one using an orogastric anvil:

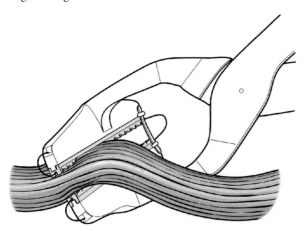

29.8

1. If an automatic purse-string device is used this should be applied prior to esophageal transection (see **Figure 29.8**). The distal esophagus is encircled with a heavy suture to prevent spillage and the esophagus transected flush with the purse string. Esophageal contents are suctioned out. The authors place a single over-and-over suture laterally to incorporate the purse string to prevent slippage when this is tightened (see **Figure 29.9**).

2. A 0 monofilament polypropylene-type suture on a round-bodied needle is used to site the purse string by hand. The distal esophagus is held in a large-jawed right-angle clamp (e.g., Hayes anterior resection or vascular Satinsky clamp), two lateral stay sutures are placed proximally for manipulation, and the esophagus is transected. Esophageal contents are sucked out, being careful not to "push" back the mucosa with the suction device. Using the lateral stay sutures to manipulate the esophagus, six or eight full-thickness 4-0 absorbable stay sutures are placed around the circumference taking at least 5 mm of esophageal wall to control the mouth of the esophagus. The purse-string suture then begins anteriorly at the 12 o'clock position, passing from outside to inside, with a hemostat clip placed on the end of this suture. The authors secure this clip to the drapes to give a slight tension on the thread. The assistant is then simply able to follow the stitch as this is run around the esophagus over and over, taking bites of 4–5 mm in depth and distance. The stay sutures facilitate the accuracy of this purse string. The final suture is brought from within out and reclipped to the end of the suture using the same hemostat (see **Figure 29.10**). The esophagus is dilated with a large Foley catheter with a 25 mL balloon. The catheter is well lubricated and inserted well into the esophagus, slowly inflated, then withdrawn using suction to prevent soiling of the surgical field.

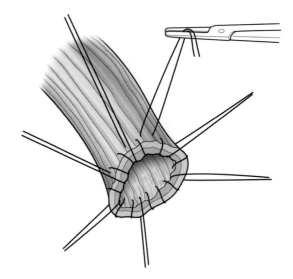

29.9

29.10

By whichever method, once the purse string is in place, an appropriately sized staple anvil is sited. If too small, this will cause "bunching" of the esophageal wall, jeopardize the join, or lead to stricturing, so this should be no smaller than 25 mm. Once in position, the purse-string suture is tied snugly and firmly to the shaft of the anvil with flat half-hitch knots. If there is any concern over the purse string at this point, a second purse string is easily placed with the anvil in situ.

3. The third alternative is the use of the OrVil device (Medtronic, Minneapolis, US). This consists of a tilted circular anvil head, which is supplied attached to an orogastric tube. The esophagus is mobilized above the intended point of transection to allow the anvil to sit comfortably in the esophageal stump. Stay sutures are not necessary. The esophagus is divided with a single-use reloadable linear stapler with a 4.8 mm staple load. The anesthetist inserts a well-lubricated 25 mm OrVil (Medtronic) per oral, ensuring that the black line of the orogastric tube remains posterior at all times. This places the anvil in the correct orientation to allow smooth passage through the pharynx and cricopharyngeus. The operating surgeon watches carefully to ensure that the tip of the tubing comes to lie centrally over the anterior staple line of the esophageal stump. Diathermy is then used to open the esophagus just over the tip of the tube. The tube is grasped and gently pulled down as the anesthetist guides the anvil over the back of the tongue and into the pharynx. Resistance is felt as the anvil crosses both cricopharyngeus and as it descends past the endotracheal tube cuff. A jaw thrust maneuver and slight deflation of the cuff may also help passage. The anvil is pulled through until it is sitting in the esophageal stump. One limb of the suture attached to the anvil can now be cut, allowing the orogastric tubing to detach and be discarded (see **Figure 29.11**).

Whichever technique is used, once the anvil has been sited, the main staple gun device is introduced into the conduit (see **Figure 29.12**). This can be through the gastric transection line, which has been left open for this purpose—this being later resected to tubularize the stomach. Alternatively, an already placed stapled gastrotomy line is partially reopened or a separate gastrotomy is made (again, preferably in an area that will be resected). Or, finally, if access allows, the pyloroplasty can be used for access prior to its closure. The stapler is opened, turning the button on the stapler anticlockwise, to allow the spike to perforate the wall of the conduit, usually on the greater curve at the fundus, ensuring there is no twist or tension on the conduit and that there is at least 3 cm distance from the margin of the anastomosis to the gastrotomy line—this space is the so-called angle of sorrow and is at the highest risk for ischemic necrosis. The anvil is engaged to the circular stapler with an audible click. The button on the stapler is turned clockwise to oppose the stapler head with the anvil, until the tissue tension marker lies within the "green zone." Care should be taken to ensure that no extraneous tissue is caught between the jaws. The safety catch is released and the gun fired firmly to result in an end-to-side anastomosis. The stapler is opened with anticlockwise turns,

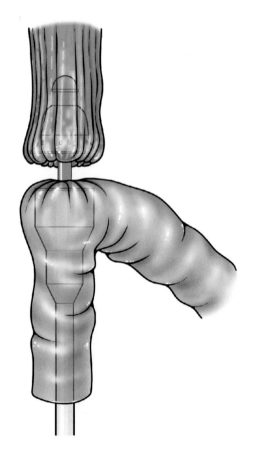

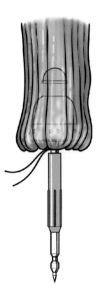

29.11

29.12

and removed with a gentle rocking motion while the anastomosis is supported with the other hand. The "doughnuts" are checked to ensure that they are complete and sent for histology as the esophageal resection margin. If not complete or if there is doubt about the integrity of the anastomosis, then a few mattress sutures should be placed to reinforce the anastomosis. The authors do not routinely perform a leak test. The nasogastric tube is then readvanced back into the distal gastric conduit and secured at the nose. The resection is completed where appropriate or the gastrotomy closed using staplers or sutures. The authors' preference is to oversew the gastrotomy line. Again, any redundant vascularized greater curve omental fat should be used to protect the airways from the conduit and to wrap around the anastomosis. Finally, any redundant posterior gastric wall may be used to fashion a modified loose fundoplication to prevent reflux.

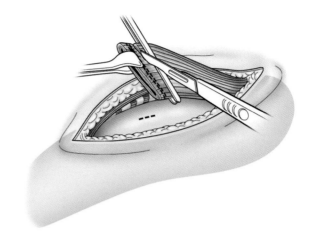

29.13

Cervical (linear)

Full mobilization of the stomach should allow for 4–5 cm of gastric tip lying within the cervical dissection field and above the level of the clavicles. The esophagus is transected with a linear stapler and the end is grasped gently with Babcock forceps and elevated away from the conduit. The anterior wall of the conduit is grasped, elevated, and rotated medially so that the gastrotomy staple line is turned away from the site of the anastomosis toward the patient's right shoulder. A 3-0 suture should be placed inferiorly on the stomach to facilitate traction. The site of the anastomosis is determined by lying the transected esophagus down onto the gastric wall and a small gastrotomy made at this point, taking care to ensure that there is sufficient room in the proximal conduit to accommodate the linear stapler. The esophagus is pulled inferiorly and the staple line excised obliquely so that the posterior margin is shorter than the anterior one. Care should be taken not to overshorten the esophageal remnant (see **Figure 29.13**). The excised portion is sent for histology as the esophageal resection margin. Stay sutures are placed both in the apex of the esophageal remnant and through the posterior esophageal wall, also taking the apex of the gastrotomy (see **Figure 29.14**). While applying traction on these stay sutures, the linear stapler is introduced into both lumens (the thinner blade is introduced into the conduit) (see **Figure 29.15**). The blades are approximated, taking care to align the gastric and esophageal walls accurately. It may be necessary to rotate the stapler toward the patient's left ear to straighten the join and distance this from the gastrotomy line. Before firing, two absorbable sutures are placed across the conduit and the esophagus on either side of the anastomosis to reduce any traction. The staple gun is fired and removed (see **Figure 29.16**). The nasogastric tube is readvanced and guided into the distal stomach. The esophagogastric defect is closed with two layers of absorbable monofilament sutures (see **Figure 29.17**). The authors' preference is a continuous full-thickness suture then a few interrupted sutures. Both layers attempt to invert the anastomotic lip (see **Figure 29.18**).

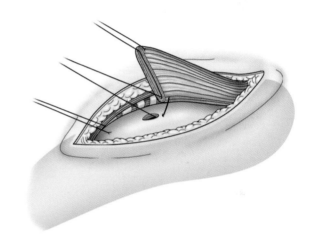

29.14

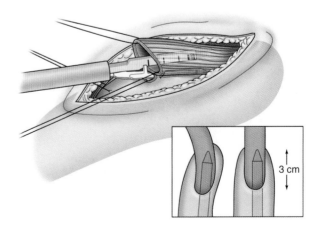

29.15

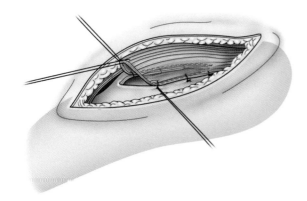

29.16

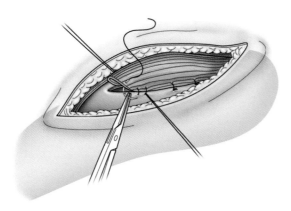

29.17

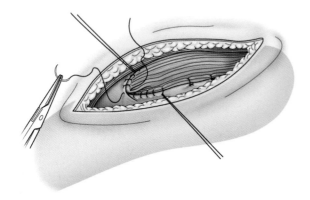

29.18

The anastomosis is gently relaxed back into the depths of the wound with removal of the traction suture. The wound is irrigated. The use or not of a soft drain remains the surgeon's preference.

MINIMALLY INVASIVE TECHNIQUES

The uptake of minimally invasive approaches to esophageal resection has been rapid, but benefits have been slow to emerge and there is still no consensus that the outcomes are superior to conventional open surgery. In addition, questions have been raised over the safety of the anastomosis and, specifically, the higher risk of gastric necrosis. A variety of combinations of approaches are possible, from a totally minimally invasive esophagectomy to hybrid resections where one or more phases of the operation are performed in an open manner. It appears that minimally invasive techniques are feasible and safe but that there is a marginally higher rate of postoperative gastric necrosis. Preconditioning of the conduit does not appear to improve this, but using a wide gastric conduit and placing the anastomosis in the chest do. In the neck, the anastomotic techniques are identical to those already described, as these are always performed in an open manner, whether hand sewn or stapled. A thoracoscopic hand-sewn anastomosis is more difficult, so staplers are usually employed, being introduced through widened port sites. Classically, a circular stapling technique is used either with placement of a hand-sewn purse string (this is facilitated with the Endo Stitch device (Medtronic, Minneapolis, US)) or using the OrVil device (Medtronic) approach.

TECHNIQUE: HAND–SEWN SUTURED VERSUS STAPLED

Consistent outcome differences between one anastomotic technique over another have not been identified in numerous studies and randomized comparisons. In the hands of less experienced and lower volume operators, there is much to recommend a stapled technique due to its consistency and reproducibility. Regardless, good preparation is key to any gastrointestinal anastomosis and using staplers is not an excuse for sloppy technique; meticulous attention to detail applies to any anastomosis.

SUMMARY

Reconstructive options following esophagectomy are greatly varied. Not only is there is a choice of conduit, but the route of the conduit, the site of the anastomosis, and the technique of anastomosis are all variables that could influence outcome. Technical proficiency and experience probably account for any outcome differences in studies to date, so that no single technique has demonstrated significant or definite advantages over any other.

FURTHER READING

Aly A, Jamieson GG, Watson DI, Devitt PG, Ackroyd R, Stoddard CJ. An antireflux anastomosis following esophagectomy: a randomized controlled trial. *J Gastrointest Surg.* 2010 Mar; 14(3): 470–5.

Beitler AL, Urschel JD. Comparison of stapled and hand-sewn esophagogastric anastomoses. *Am J Surg.* 1998 Apr; 175(4): 337–40.

Goldsmith HS, Kiely AA, Randall HT. Protection of intrathoracic esophageal anastomoses by omentum. *Surgery.* 1968; 63(3): 464–6.

Kim RH, Takabe K. Methods of esophagogastric anastomoses following esophagectomy for cancer: A a systematic review. *J Surg Oncol.* 2010; 101(6): 527–33.

Knight BC, Rice SJ, Devitt PG, Lord A, Game PA, Thompson SK. Proximal anastomosis using the OrVil circular stapler in major upper gastrointestinal surgery. *J Gastrointest Surg.* 2014; 18(7): 1345–9.

Law S, Fok M, Chu KM, Wong J. Comparison of hand-sewn and stapled esophagogastric anastomosis after esophageal resection for cancer: a prospective randomized controlled trial. *Ann Surg.* 1997 Aug; 226(2): 169–73.

Orringer MB, Marshall B, Iannettoni MD. Eliminating the cervical esophagogastric anastomotic leak with a side-to-side stapled anastomosis. *J Thorac Cardiovasc Surg.* 2000; 119(2): 277–88.

Xu QR, Wang KN, Wang WP, Zhang K, Chen LQ. Linear stapled esophagogastrostomy is more effective than hand-sewn or circular stapler in prevention of anastomotic stricture: a comparative clinical study. *J Gastrointest Surg.* 2011 Jun; 15(6): 915–21.

Zhang J, Wang R, Liu S, Luketich JD, Chen S, Chen H, Schubert MJ. Refinement of Minimally minimally invasive Esophagectomy esophagectomy techniques after 15 years of experience. *J Gastrointest Surg.* 2012; 16(9): 1768–74.

30

Use of the stomach as an esophageal substitute

ARNULF H. HÖLSCHER AND J. RÜDIGER SIEWERT

HISTORY

The use of the stomach as an esophageal substitute was introduced by Kirschner in 1920 as a nonresectional operative bypass. His operation consisted of skeletonization of the greater curvature of the stomach, and the mobilized stomach was then brought subcutaneously up to the divided cervical esophagus. The application of this procedure using either the orthotopic or the retrosternal route after esophagectomy and the standardization of this method was largely due to the work of Ong, Nakayama, and Akiyama.

PRINCIPLES AND JUSTIFICATION

The reconstruction of intestinal transit after esophagectomy is normally made using stomach or colon. The small bowel is used much less frequently for complete substitution of the esophagus. Small bowel interposition does have a place, however, for partial esophageal replacement of both proximal and distal esophagus.

Gastric interposition is the simplest form of esophageal replacement. Furthermore, as it guarantees good long-term functional results, it has become the method of first choice as an esophageal substitute, especially after esophagectomy for cancer. Only when the stomach is not available because of previous operations or in benign esophageal diseases is colonic interposition used.

An important question to be answered in planning an esophageal replacement is where to site the esophagoenteral anastomosis. If intrathoracic anastomoses are performed, they should be carried out near the apex of the pleura. Anastomotic leakage is less likely to occur with intrathoracic anastomosis than with cervical anastomosis, but the consequences of such a leak are much more serious. With regard to oncologic radicality (remaining esophagus) and long-term results, both types of anastomosis are similar.

Finally, the site for the esophageal substitute must be chosen. Antesternal subcutaneous placement is usually not indicated. This leaves the posterior and anterior mediastinal routes available.

Swallowing, at least in the early postoperative phase, is more normal when the interposition is in the posterior mediastinum. One should also note that the distance through the posterior mediastinum is the shortest. If an intrathoracic anastomosis is performed in the upper thorax, the gastric conduit can only be placed in the posterior mediastinum. In case of cervical anastomoses, both routes are possible. The posterior mediastinal route should be avoided for reconstruction if a high risk for local recurrence exists, especially after R1 or R2 resection. If a postoperative radiotherapy of the former tumor site is planned, the anterior mediastinum should be preferred for reconstruction in order to avoid radiation damage of the gastric conduit.

PREOPERATIVE ASSESSMENT AND PREPARATION

The stomach may be used as an esophageal substitute only if it has not previously been operated on. After gastric resections, the length will be insufficient, and after vagotomy procedures, the vascularization is doubtful. If lesser procedures (such as suturing of a bleeding ulcer or closure of a perforation) have been performed, then a transposition of the stomach may be possible, but the vascularity should be checked at the beginning of the operation. A preoperative gastroscopy should be carried out to exclude any mucosal pathology and to confirm the borders of the esophageal tumor. If the cancer is infiltrating the cardia or the subcardial area, the safety margin between the lower edge of the tumor and the resection line of the gastric tube may not be sufficient. Lymph node metastases to the lesser curvature (compartment I according to the classification in gastric cancer) and the celiac trunk (compartment II) should be detected by preoperative endoscopic ultrasonography.

In all cases, the colon should be prepared by bowel lavage and colonoscopy so that it may be used if the stomach should prove unusable.

Anesthesia

The type of anesthesia used depends more on the type of esophagectomy than on the method of reconstruction. If an intrathoracic anastomosis is to be performed, a double lumen endotracheal tube should be used.

Anatomical points

1. A knowledge of the arterial blood supply of the stomach is essential for its use as an esophageal substitute. The arterial supply of the stomach originates from the celiac trunk. This vessel has a short stem that immediately divides into three branches. The left gastric artery runs in a cranial ventral direction, covered by the peritoneum of the posterior wall of the lesser sac. Subcardially, it turns to the lesser curvature in an aboral direction, where it supplies the anterior and posterior gastric wall by small branches. The left gastric artery has anastomoses with the right gastric artery, which originates from the common hepatic artery and approaches from the region of the pylorus. By these means, an arterial ring along the lesser curvature is completed, with its strongest inflow being from the left gastric artery.

   The second vessel of the celiac trunk is the splenic artery, which runs along the upper border of the pancreas behind the posterior wall of the omental bursa to the hilum of the spleen. At the splenic hilum, the short gastric vessels originate; they proceed to the fundus and the cranial third of the greater curvature of the stomach. The left gastroepiploic artery arises from the splenic artery and runs through the gastrocolic ligament parallel to the greater curvature of the stomach in a caudad direction. This artery gives gastric branches to both walls of the stomach and epiploic branches to the greater omentum. It anastomoses with the right gastroepiploic artery, which comes from the region of the pylorus. Thus, the greater curvature also has a vascular ring, with its strongest supply being from the right gastroepiploic artery. This artery has a number of anatomical variations, which may be relevant to gastric interposition.

   The third vessel of the celiac trunk, the common hepatic artery, turns to the right, in the direction of the hepatoduodenal ligament of the small omentum. There it divides into the hepatic and gastroduodenal arteries. The hepatic artery runs through the hepatoduodenal ligament to the liver and usually gives rise to the right gastric artery, which proceeds to the lesser curvature of the stomach. The right gastric artery may also originate from the gastroduodenal artery. The gastroduodenal artery runs posterior to the superior part of the duodenum distal to the pylorus and comes out caudad to the duodenum, where it divides into the right gastroepiploic and superior pancreaticoduodenal arteries. All gastric arteries anastomose between themselves directly or indirectly by intramural or extramural branches. Therefore, the ligation of two or even three gastric arteries preserves the blood supply of the stomach under normal circumstances.

   The veins of the stomach lead the blood to the portal vein. With only minor exceptions they correspond in their courses to the four gastric arteries. From the gastric fundus, the short gastric veins run through the gastrosplenic ligament to the splenic vein. The left gastroepiploic vein from the greater curvature also proceeds in this direction to the left side. It reaches the splenic vein through the gastrosplenic ligament. The right gastroepiploic vein accompanies its artery to the area of the pylorus. At this point, the vein turns in a posterior direction and flows into the superior mesenteric vein. At the lesser curvature, a venous arch runs along both arteries (coronary or left gastric vein). This vein flows near the right gastric artery into the portal vein or splenic vein within the hepatoduodenal ligament. At the cardia, the venous arch follows the left gastric artery up to the area of the celiac trunk. (See **Figure 30.1a through d.**)

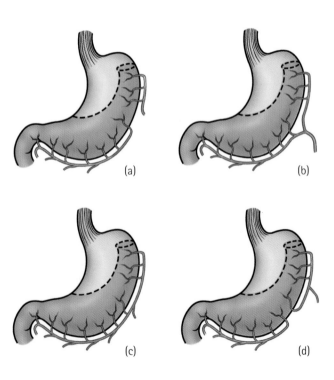

(a) (b)

(c) (d)

30.1a–d

OPERATION (OPEN TECHNIQUE)

The laparoscopic technique for preparation of the gastric conduit is described in Chapter 35, "Thoracoscopic and laparoscopic esophagectomy."

Position of patient

2. The patient lies in a supine position with the head turned to the right to provide a free approach to the left side of the neck. A rolled-up towel or a sandbag is placed behind the shoulders to facilitate the approach to the anterior mediastinum, and under the lumbar region to facilitate access to the stomach. (See **Figure 30.2**.)

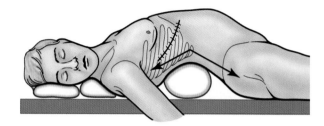

30.2

Incision

3. The abdomen is opened by a transverse incision extended by an upper midline incision in the direction of the xiphoid process. This ensures a good view of the epigastric area. (See **Figure 30.3**.)

Preparation of the stomach

Skeletonization of the stomach begins along the greater curvature outside the gastroepiploic arch. It is performed stepwise in the direction of the fundus. Although the supply to the stomach from the right gastroepiploic artery shows variations (as illustrated in **Figure 30.1**), it is sufficient in nearly all cases to guarantee a blood supply to the gastric tube. After division of the left gastroepiploic artery, the preparation of the upper third of the gastric fundus may be performed close to the stomach wall.

4. In an aborad direction, the preparation must be done very carefully outside the gastroepiploic arch to the origin of the right gastroepiploic artery from the gastroduodenal artery (see **Figure 30.4**.)

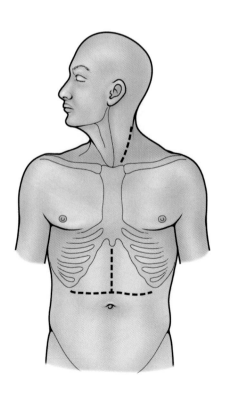

30.3

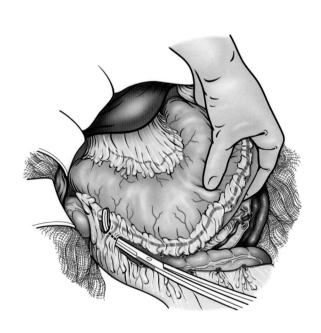

30.4

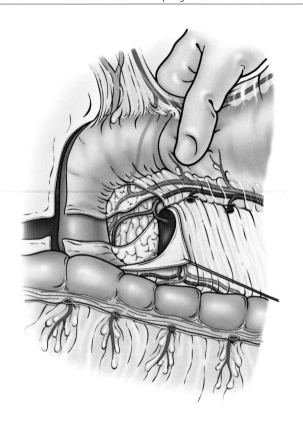

30.5

5. Maintaining the venous drainage via the right gastroepiploic vein is also important (see **Figure 30.5**.)

Lymph node dissection

The gastroduodenal artery is dissected immediately distal to the pylorus. This allows the common hepatic artery to be easily identified. Dissection proceeds in a medial direction to preserve the origin of the right gastric artery from the common hepatic artery. The right gastric artery may aid the vascularization of the gastric tube, and it should be spared if possible.

6. The lymph nodes are dissected in a manner similar to that used in gastric cancer, which means that all lymph nodes along the common hepatic artery, the celiac trunk, and the medial part of the splenic artery are dissected and taken with the specimen. The ligation of the left gastric artery is performed near its trunk of origin.

    After dissection of the lesser omentum, the esophagus, which has previously been dissected by a transthoracic or transmediastinal approach, is pulled out of the esophageal hiatus for the final preparation of the gastric tube (see **Figure 30.6**).

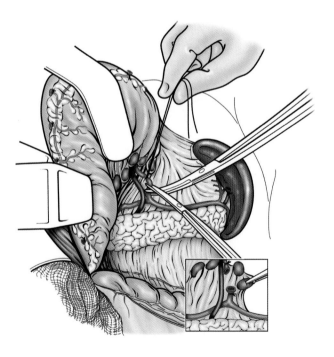

30.6

Formation of the gastric tube

7. Akiyama recommends that the highest point of the stomach be marked by two stay sutures. This point is located quite a long way to the left of the cardia. The skeletonization of the lesser curvature involves approximately two-thirds of the lesser curvature, which means it starts distal to the third or fourth branch of the left gastric artery, at the region of the "crow's foot," and continues close to the gastric wall in the direction of the cardia. (See **Figure 30.7**.)

8. The lesser omentum should be divided in this area and the vascular arcade suture ligated. The stomach now can be cut in an oblique direction, from the distal point of skeletonization to the highest point of the gastric fundus (the interrupted line in **Figures 30.7 and 30.8**). This means that approximately half of the gastric fundus, including the lymphatic drainage along the left gastric artery (compartment I), is removed. The resulting gastric tube has a width of 3–4 cm.

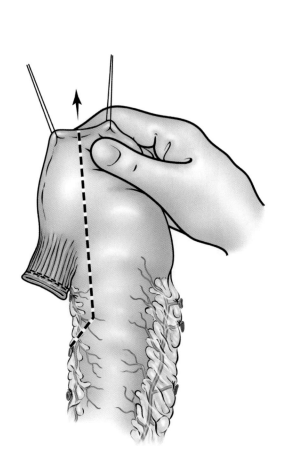

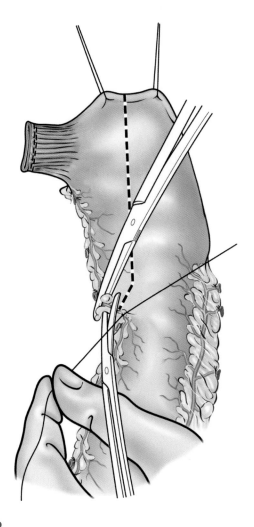

30.7   30.8

9. Before the stomach is finally cut along this line, the gastric fundus should be opened near the cardia and a pair of long forceps inserted to carry out an intraluminal pyloric dilatation. This helps to avoid early postoperative pylorospasm. The best way to divide the stomach is to use a linear stapler (TA 90). Two applications of this stapler are usually required to close the quite long resection line. (See **Figure 30.9a through c.**)

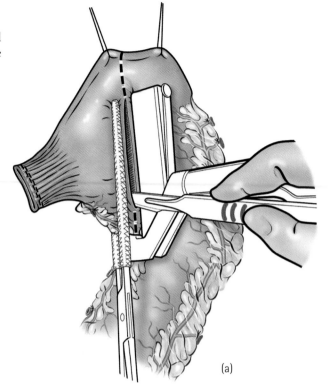

(a)

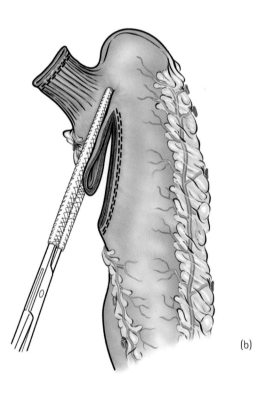

(b)

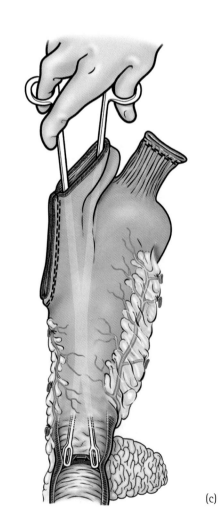

(c)

30.9a–c

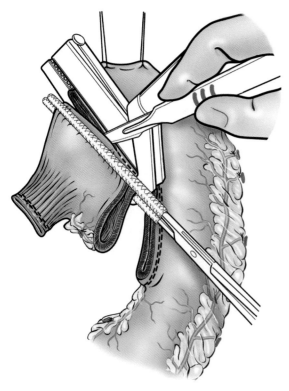

30.10

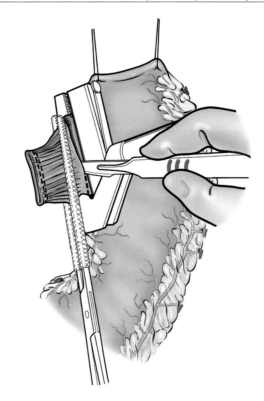

30.11

10. If the stomach appears too short for elevation to the neck, cutting the seromuscular layer with a scalpel and then closing the mucosa by stapler results in greater elasticity of the gastric tube (see **Figure 30.10**).
11. If additional suturing of the staple line is undertaken, interrupted rather than running sutures are best used to avoid shortening of the tube by a purse-string effect (see **Figure 30.11**).

Interposition of the whole stomach

The whole stomach, rather than a gastric tube, can be used as the esophageal interposition. This can be done only if the tumor is not infiltrating the gastroesophageal junction. The skeletonization should start at the same point and in the same manner as for the formation of the gastric tube. However, it is continued along the lesser curvature up to the cardia.

12. The staple line (using a TA 55 stapler) is then placed directly below the cardia to preserve the whole gastric fundus.

    Pyloric dilatation can be performed through the cardia before stapling.

    The advantage of using the whole stomach as the esophageal substitute is that the gastroesophageal anastomosis does not include the tangential staple line at the highest point of the gastric fundus. This may avoid a *locus minoris resistentiae* of such an anastomosis. (See **Figure 30.12**.)

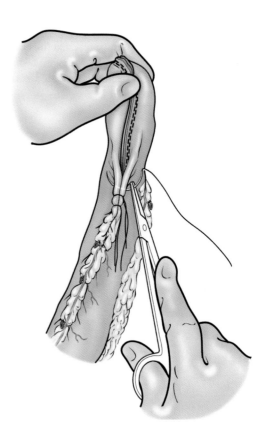

30.12

Duodenal mobilization

An essential prerequisite for a tension-free stomach interposition is a careful and extensive duodenal mobilization. This Kocher maneuver is performed in the usual way from the right side and should be continued until the vena cava and the aorta up to the superior mesenteric artery are freed. This means that the duodenum and the head of the pancreas are quite mobile.

Another important step is to separate the right colonic flexure from the head of the pancreas and the duodenum. This mobilization should be performed up to the middle colic vein. After this maneuver, the pylorus can easily be moved up to the esophageal hiatus or even higher.

Preparation of the tunnel for the interposition

13. If the interposition is to be placed in the posterior mediastinum, some form of tape or Penrose tubing must be drawn down as the esophagus is removed. This is attached to the stomach so that the gastric tube can be pulled upward without further preparation, in the bed of the former esophagus. If the plan is for the interposition to be placed in the anterior mediastinum, a retrosternal tunnel is prepared by blunt dissection. (See **Figure 30.13**.)

14. This blunt dissection can be performed with the help of a swab in sponge-holding forceps. It is essential to limit this preparation strictly to the midline and always with contact to the posterior part of the sternum. Once the sponge-holding forceps have reached the cervical incision, the channel is dilated in a stepwise fashion so that the interposition can be accommodated without compression. (See **Figure 30.14**.)

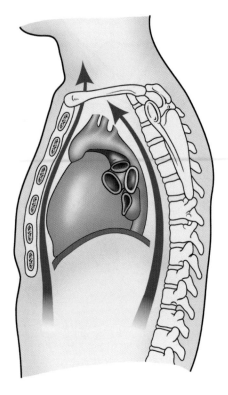

30.13

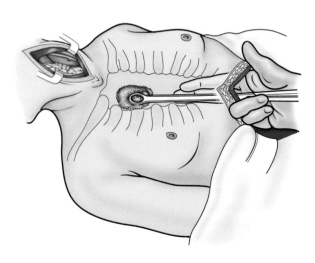

30.14

Elevation of the stomach and cervical anastomosis

15. While the abdominal team is operating, another team starts the cervical part of the operation using a left lateral incision along the sternocleidomastoid muscle. The omohyoid muscle and the inferior thyroid artery are ligated and divided, the left thyroid lobe is mobilized, and the recurrent laryngeal nerve is dissected and preserved.

    After transthoracic esophagectomy, mobilizing the esophageal remnant and extracting it from the posterior mediastinum is usually easy. The preparation of the esophagus should be extended in the direction of the hypopharynx until it is completely free so that the esophagus passes directly to the anastomosis without kinking.

    If the interposition is placed in the anterior mediastinum, the retrosternal space must also be opened from the cervical incision to complete the tunnel from the abdominal and cervical directions. It is a good idea to place the stomach in a plastic bag when drawing it through the tunnel to avoid any trauma to the organ. This part of the operation is facilitated by placing a tube via the cervical incision through the anterior or posterior mediastinum. (See **Figure 30.15**.)

16. The stomach is then sutured to the lower tip of the tube. The stomach can be slowly pulled through the mediastinum in an upward direction. It is important to push the stomach upward from the abdomen as well. (See **Figure 30.16**.)

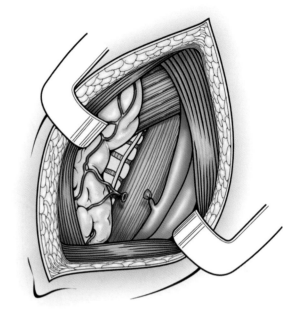

30.15

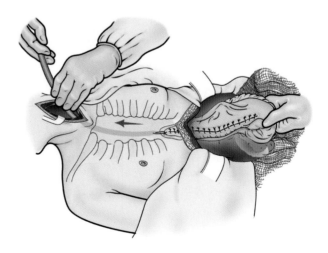

30.16

17. The gastric interposition usually has sufficient (and sometimes even excessive) length and reaches the neck without tension. Often, the cervical esophageal stump overlaps the gastric tube, and an additional resection of the stomach can be performed. The vascularization of the top of the fundus is unreliable and should be resected. The anastomosis with the cervical esophagus is performed in the upper part of the gastric corpus. The anastomosis is usually located just above the clavicle. Before the anastomosis is performed, the back wall of the stomach is fixed to the neck by two or three sutures. The back wall of the anastomosis is constructed using interrupted sutures, which emerge between the mucosa and muscularis; the anterior wall is completed using all-layer interrupted sutures. (See **Figure 30.17a through c**.)

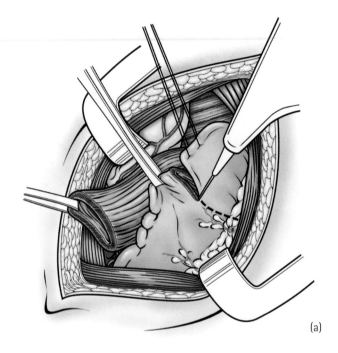

(a)

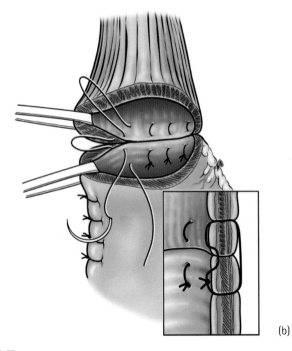

(b)

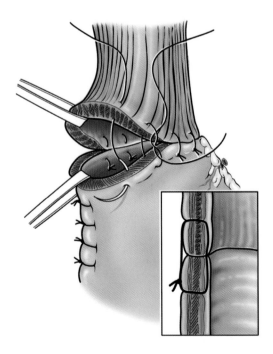

(c)

30.17a–c

Elevation of the stomach and intrathoracic anastomosis

If an intrathoracic anastomosis is planned, it should be performed toward the apex of the pleura. It is important for the postoperative long-term results that the stomach be completely transferred into the thorax. This means that the preparation of the stomach is identical to the preparation for an abdominocervical interposition. When the preparation of the stomach has been finished, the gastric tube is pushed through the esophageal hiatus into the posterior mediastinum and the right pleural cavity. The abdominal approach is closed, and the patient is turned for a right thoracic approach to the esophagus. The anastomosis is now performed directly between the esophageal stump and the stomach, either end to end, or as an implantation of the esophageal remnant on the front wall of the stomach. The suture technique can either be performed by hand or by stapling. If the gastric tube is long enough to preserve a blind oral part of the stomach above the anastomosis, then this can be used to cover the front wall suture line of the esophagogastrostomy. This procedure also has an antireflux effect.

Drainage

The cervical anastomosis is drained by a Penrose or other soft drain. In an intrathoracic anastomosis, the pleural cavity is drained by a thoracic tube.

Finishing of the abdominal operation

After the esophagogastric anastomosis in the neck is finished, the abdominal operation should be completed. The operative field is checked for hemostasis. Drainage of the peritoneal cavity is not necessary. When the gastric interposition is positioned well, the pylorus should be located in the area of the diaphragm. The abdomen is closed in layers.

POSTOPERATIVE CARE

Postoperative care should follow the course described for gastroesophagectomy for adenocarcinoma of the cardia in Chapter 32, "Abdominal and right thoracic esophagectomy."

Complications

The most common complication of gastric interposition is leakage from the cervical anastomosis. In the authors' experience, this complication is unlikely if the gastric tube is elevated as proximally as possible so that the end-to-end anastomosis is performed in a well-vascularized area of the stomach. Other kinds of cervical anastomoses cannot be

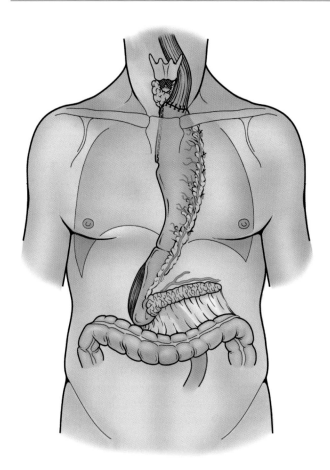

30.18

18. The anastomosis is splinted by a transnasal gastric tube to guarantee postoperative decompression of the stomach. The wound is closed by subcutaneous and skin sutures. (See **Figure 30.18.**)

As an alternative, the cervical anastomosis can be performed using a stapling technique (see Chapter 29, "Esophageal anastomoses: sutured and stapled"). The detachable head of the end-to-end anastomosis (EEA) stapler is introduced into the esophageal stump, which is closed around the mandrel by a purse-string suture. The most appropriate size of stapler is usually size 28; smaller staplers tend to induce postoperative anastomotic stenosis. The recommendation is that the specially designed shorter head of the EEA stapler be used for introduction into the cervical esophagus because it can more easily be placed into the esophageal stump. The stapler is inserted through an incision at the top of the stomach, and the central spike is driven out 5–7 cm aborad through the stomach front wall. After the stapler is turned in the direction of the esophageal remnant, the central pin is connected with the mandrel, and the stapler is closed, fired, and removed. The site of introduction into the stomach is closed using a TA 55 linear stapler.

recommended, as often the gastric part orad to the anastomosis develops necrosis.

If leakage does develop, a salivary fistula results, which usually heals without complications provided sufficient external drainage is present. If drainage is insufficient, a phlegmon may develop in the cervical soft tissue. Therefore, whenever a fever of unknown origin develops postoperatively, the cervical anastomosis should be checked. This can be performed radiologically using contrast medium, but sometimes a safer method is to check the anastomosis directly by opening the cervical incision.

If leakage has occurred, open treatment of the cervical wound is appropriate. Early and adequate external drainage of a cervical leak is necessary to avoid spread of infection into the mediastinum.

More major (or even complete) necrosis of the interposed stomach is extremely rare, as the gastric tube usually has a very good blood supply. Very occasionally, postoperative pylorospasm may occur that leads to clinically relevant delay in gastric emptying. Such a situation can easily be treated by a careful endoscopic dilatation of the pylorus. Gastric dilatation as a consequence of postoperative paralysis is extremely rare after gastric tube formation by this technique. A dislocation of the interposed stomach from the mediastinum into one of the pleural cavities is also very rare. If the stomach is shown to be distended with air on postoperative thoracic radiography, temporary placement of a nasogastric tube is suggested. This avoids compression of mediastinal organs and also avoids aspiration.

The most important long-term complication is the development of an anastomotic stricture. This is usually caused by scarring as a result of anastomotic vascular insufficiency, but use of a stapler that is too small could also cause dysphagia from anastomotic stenosis. In either case, the problem can be solved by endoscopic dilatation. If it has no lasting effect, resection of the stenosis and reanastomosis is recommended.

OUTCOME

Functional studies of patients with intrathoracic stomach as esophageal replacement have shown good long-term results. Despite a persistent acid secretion of the vagotomized thoracic stomach, no pathological gastroesophageal reflux or esophagitis was found proximal to the cervical anastomosis. Gastric biopsies mostly reveal mild gastritis of the antral mucosa, and metaplasia is rare. The intrathoracic stomach needs no drainage to facilitate emptying. Postoperative reflux esophagitis is prevented by complete intrathoracic stomach transposition with cervical esophagogastrostomy.

In young patients with benign esophageal diseases requiring an esophagectomy, the authors prefer to use the colon as an esophageal substitute to preserve the gastric reservoir.

FURTHER READING

Aly A, Jamieson GG, Pyragius M, Devitt PG. Antireflux anastomosis following esophagectomy. *Australian and New Zealand Journal of Surgery.* 2004; 74: 434–8.

Atkins BZ, Shah AS, Hutcheson KA et al. Reducing hospital morbidity and mortality following esophagectomy. *Annals of Thoracic Surgery.* 2004; 78: 1170–6.

Collard JM, Romagnoli R, Otte JB, Kestens PJ. The denervated stomach as an esophageal substitute is a contractile organ. *Annals of Surgery.* 1998; 227: 33–9.

Hölscher AH, Bollschweiler E, Bumm R, Bartels H, Höfler H, Siewert JR. Prognostic factors of resected adenocarcinoma of the esophagus. *Surgery.* 1995; 118: 845–55.

Hölscher AH, Schröder W, Bollschweiler E, Beckurts KT, Schneider PM. Wie sicher ist die hoch intrathorakale Ösophagogastrostomie? [How safe is high intrathoracic esophagogastrostomy?] *Chirurg.* 2003; 74: 726–33. German.

Law S, Fok M, Chu KM, Wong J. Comparison of hand-sewn and stapled esophagogastric anastomosis after esophageal resection for cancer: a prospective randomized controlled trial. *Annals of Surgery.* 1997; 226: 169–73.

Siewert JR, Stein HJ, Feith M, Bruecher BL, Bartels H, Fink U. Histologic tumor type is an independent prognostic parameter in esophageal cancer: lessons from more than 1,000 consecutive resections at a single center in the Western world. *Annals of Surgery.* 2001; 234: 360–9.

31

Use of the colon as an esophageal substitute

BENJAMIN KNIGHT AND GLYN G. JAMIESON

PRINCIPLES AND JUSTIFICATION

The colon as a viable conduit after esophageal resection has been used for over a hundred years and was first described separately by Kelling and Vulliet. Its use gained favor over the next 30 years or so as a durable well-functioning substitute for the esophagus in benign and malignant disease. However, the stomach has become the favored conduit for most surgeons due to perceived lower rates of anastomotic complications and the technical ease of the operation.

The colon was routinely used to bypass the esophagus for palliation, but the advent of self-expanding metal stents means that this is rarely performed nowadays. As such, experience in colonic interposition has dwindled. Even so, the colon is considered a suitable replacement when the stomach is unusable as a conduit or has failed. With meticulous attention to detail, good long-term results using the colon as a conduit can be achieved with low mortality and morbidity and it should at least be considered as the primary conduit in the young and those with benign disease. Some believe the colon to be the conduit of choice in patients with benign esophageal disease and a long life expectancy.

Quality of life after esophagectomy is of paramount importance and is often overlooked, especially in the setting of malignant disease. Patients enjoy eating and want to do it without symptoms of fullness, pain, reflux, regurgitation, or aspiration. Therefore, the conduit must function well and have the capability of propelling food from the pharynx to the stomach. The colon is suited for this and, in experienced hands, colonic interposition has low rates of anastomotic complications and good long-term quality of life.

INDICATIONS

There are few absolute indications to use the colon as an esophageal substitute. If the stomach is unavailable due to

previous surgery or a jejunal graft too short to bridge the gap, then perhaps the colon is the only option. Situations in which the colon might be used include: surgeon preference and expertise (rare today); restoration of gastrointestinal continuity after gastroesophageal resection for a long tumor extended well beyond the cardia; when it is deemed that the conduit must last over 10 years or so; when only the substernal route is available for reconnection—previous lung disease or thoracic sepsis may make the posterior mediastinal route impossible; and following vagal-sparing esophagectomy. Vagal-sparing esophagectomy is rarely performed these days and is reserved for benign disease. Functional results with a colonic interposition in this setting are very good, as the stomach and duodenum remain innervated.

CONTRAINDICATIONS

Severe intrinsic disease of the colon will preclude its use. Absolute contraindications include colorectal malignancy, polyposis coli, inflammatory bowel disease, severe diverticular disease, and inadequate blood supply due to atherosclerotic disease. The colon can still safely be used in mild diverticular disease with the right colon being used as opposed to the left. Scattered colonic polyps do not prohibit the colon as a graft, as these can be removed safely at colonoscopy prior to interposition. Patient factors such as extremes of age and cardiorespiratory fitness are relative contraindications. Often in these patients, the extra rigors of colonic dissection and interposition do not outweigh the benefit of needing a conduit to last more than a decade or so.

EMERGENCY VS. ELECTIVE

Colonic interposition requires meticulous surgical technique and is demanding on both the patient and surgeon.

An experienced theater and anesthetic team is crucial, all of whom should be well briefed prior to surgery. There are times when an "unplanned" colonic interposition may be considered. This can occur if the gastric conduit has been deemed unsuitable intraoperatively—perhaps due to a damaged arcade, or tumor burden, or after gastric conduit necrosis. While feasible, we do not recommend an emergency colonic interposition. In this situation, it is far safer to deal with the immediate issue, and create a de-functioning esophagostomy in the left cervical region and place a feeding jejunostomy. In this way, the colon can be prepped prior to its use and the correct resources mobilized for a planned staged procedure.

ADVANTAGES OF THE COLON AS A CONDUIT

Increased incidence of duodenogastric reflux is common when transposing the stomach into the thoracic cavity. Excessive reflux and regurgitation lead to heartburn symptoms, dental decay, and silent aspiration, as well as the development of esophagitis and Barrett's esophagus. Acid exposure at the anastomosis may also lead to stricture formation and dysphagia. As a consequence, studies have shown a significantly lower incidence of stricture formation when the colon is used compared with when the stomach is used. Patients also experience postprandial fullness and bloating with a gastric pull-up and this is probably due to the impaired reservoir function of the stomach. In colonic interposition, the remnant stomach remains in the abdomen and functions as an additional reservoir for gastric and biliary secretions. Not surprisingly, studies have shown better weight gain as a consequence of improved satisfaction and pleasure when eating 15 months postinterposition.

PATIENT PREPARATION

All patients should undergo endoscopic assessment of the colon prior to using the colon as a conduit to rule out occult malignancy, diverticular disease, colitis, or polyposis coli. Any scattered polyps can be excised and sent for histology and any worrying areas tattooed for future reference.

Mesenteric angiograms were used routinely to assess anatomical variations in blood supply and to identify atherosclerotic lesions, which might impede blood flow to the conduit. However, the invasive nature of angiography and its ability to predict clinical outcome has been called into question recently. In an angiographic series, McDermott et al. showed that only 65% of patients met angiographic criteria for colonic interposition. Despite this, there was no significant difference in ischemic complications and leak rate between those who underwent angiography and those who did not. As such, many centers have stopped routinely using angiography. High resolution computed tomography (CT) with arterial phase contrast is noninvasive and easy to perform and has superseded routine angiography.

Colonic blood supply is highly variable, with classic branches of the superior mesenteric artery only present 70% of the time. Attention should be given to the middle colic artery and the marginal artery arcade at the splenic flexure. Both of these areas have variable anatomy and the latter arcade is absent in 5% of patients. Multiple middle colic arteries make for a tenuous distal graft and difficult dissection. Similarly, an absent middle colic artery or middle colic artery originating from the coeliac trunk makes for dubious blood supply to the distal end of the graft and often precludes using the colon. Interruption of the marginal arcade at the splenic flexure is well reported on angiographic series, but, in practice, it rarely appears to be of clinical importance.

Cardiopulmonary fitness is assessed with lung function tests and echocardiogram or cardiopulmonary exercise testing. Smoking cessation is imperative and a planned, structured preoperative exercise program is desirable.

Prior to surgery, patients are fasted from solid food from 14:00 hours the day before surgery and given an osmotic electrolyte bowel preparation (ColonLYTELY or equivalent). Low molecular weight heparin is prescribed for the day of surgery. Intraoperatively, we use an enhanced recovery-based protocol with goal-directed fluid therapy, prophylactic antibiotics 6 hourly that continue for 3 days postoperatively, and pneumatic calf compression devices. Patients are prescribed a clear carbohydrate drink the night before and 2 hours prior to surgery to help prevent insulin resistance.

SURGICAL TECHNIQUE

The choice of colonic segment to be used is based on surgeon preference and experience, adequate vascular supply of the segment to be used, and any intrinsic colonic factors, which favor one segment over another. Of these, surgeon experience of one particular technique is probably of most importance.

There is no level-one evidence that favors the right, left, or transverse colon for interposition and data published are based mostly on personal series. For instance, in a combined analysis of results, a more reliable vascular supply of the inferior mesenteric artery has been shown with subsequent lower leak rates using the left colon (4.6% vs. 10.8%). However, similar leak rates and ischemic complications have also been reported whichever segment of colon is used. Whichever segment is chosen, it should be placed in an isoperistaltic fashion, as this allows a better functional outcome and lower rates of aspiration.

Left colon

Standard esophageal mobilization is first performed either open (see Chapter 32, "Abdominal and right thoracic esophagectomy") or thoracoscopically (see Chapter 35, "Thoracoscopic and laparoscopic esophagectomy").

The entire colon is mobilized from ascending colon to the sigmoid colon. The omentum is dissected from the transverse colon. Great care is taken not to damage any mesenteric

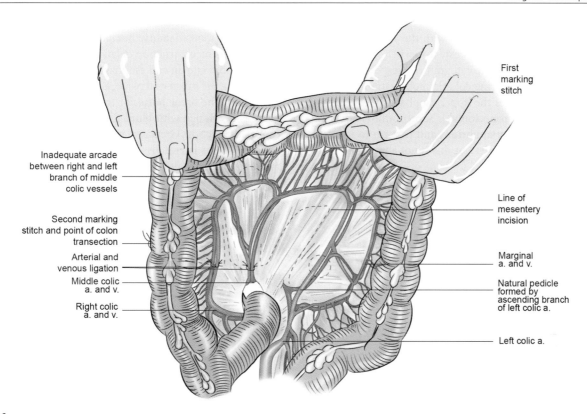

Inadequate arcade between right and left branch of middle colic vessels

Second marking stitch and point of colon transection

Arterial and venous ligation

Middle colic a. and v.

Right colic a. and v.

First marking stitch

Line of mesentery incision

Marginal a. and v.

Natural pedicle formed by ascending branch of left colic a.

Left colic a.

31.1

vessels. The colon is mobilized in a cephalad direction so that the colon tethers on the ascending branch of the inferior mesenteric artery (see **Figure 31.1**).

The length of the colonic graft is measured by the aforementioned tethering (see **Figure 31.2**). It usually reaches to just about the xiphoid process and this area is marked on the chest. A marking stitch can be used on the colonic apex as this will be the site of division of the colon distally. The distance from the chest mark to the mandible is measured and this distance is then measured out on the colon in a proximal direction toward the ileocecal valve. A further marking stitch is placed on the colon at this point, usually around the midpoint of the ascending colon, just distal to the right colonic artery (see **Figure 31.1**). The marginal artery is ligated. Prior to division, bulldog clamps are used to occlude the middle colic artery below its left and right branches to assess the integrity of the vascular supply. If adequate, the middle colic pedicle is divided proximal to its first divisions (see **Figure 31.1**). The segment of colon between the two marking stitches is now exclusively fed by the left colonic artery. If a short graft only is required, then often only the left branch of the middle colic needs division.

If the conduit is to be placed at the time of esophageal resection, it is easier to use the posterior mediastinal route and place the conduit in the esophageal bed (orthotopic). Depending on the shape of the patient, this is probably the shortest of all the routes and the easiest to create. If a staged procedure is being undertaken, the substernal route

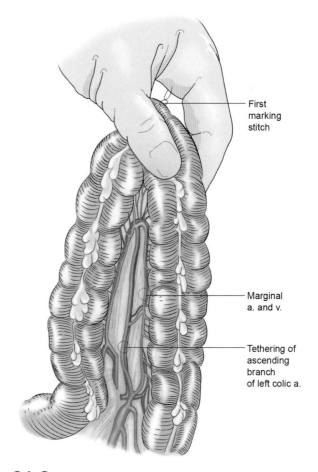

First marking stitch

Marginal a. and v.

Tethering of ascending branch of left colic a.

31.2

is preferred. This route has the advantage of not requiring a thoracotomy. The biggest risk with the substernal route is conduit compression. At best, this will result in poor functional results and, at worst, graft congestion, ischemia, and conduit failure. During colonic mobilization, a second surgical team mobilizes the upper esophagus (see Chapter 34, "Transhiatal esophagectomy"). Some authors advocate removing part of the manubrium and first rib to increase the size of the thoracic inlet but this is not always necessary (see **Figure 31.3**).

At this point, the colon is reassessed for vascularity. If there is any doubt about viability, the colon is returned to the abdomen and the reconstruction delayed. A feeding jejunostomy is then placed and an end esophagostomy fashioned.

To create the substernal plane, a small pocket is developed by dividing the tissue posterior to the xiphoid process. This plane is developed with blunt dissection and extended in a cephalad direction. Great care is taken to stay directly behind the sternum, as lateral dissection risks injury to the internal mammary arteries and pleura. In the neck, dissection is commenced directly behind the manubrium in a similar fashion. It should be possible to connect both substernal tunnels using finger dissection. The colon is then divided with a linear stapler at the second marking stitch at the proximal colonic end. The colon is brought up and laid on the chest to ensure adequate length and nontwisted mesentery (see **Figure 31.4**). A wire is passed from the neck in a caudal direction with either a tape or Foley catheter attached. To allow atraumatic passage of the conduit and mesentery, the conduit is placed in a laparoscopic camera sleeve and then ligated to the distal end of the Foley catheter. Historically, Mousseau–Barbin tubes have been used with good effect but are no longer readily available. The sleeve is lubricated with warm water and then the conduit and sleeve are pulled up into the neck using gentle traction.

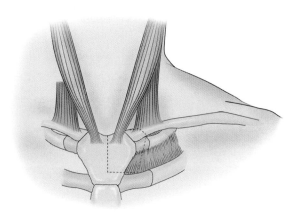

31.3

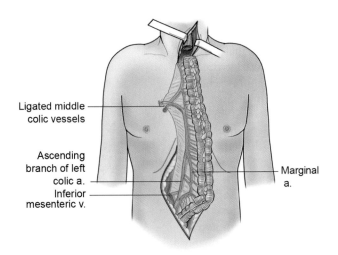

Ligated middle colic vessels

Ascending branch of left colic a.

Inferior mesenteric v.

Marginal a.

31.4

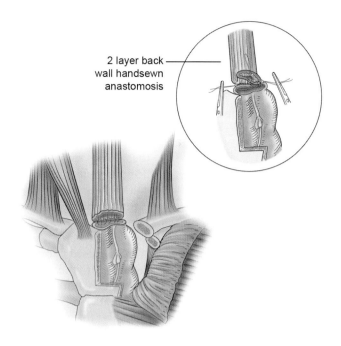

2 layer back wall handsewn anastomosis

31.5

The proximal anastomosis is fashioned. There are many reported techniques and none has shown favor over another. Hand sewn interrupted end-to-side stitches with 3-0 absorbable monofilament suture is safe and reliable and is our anastomosis of choice if access is challenging (see **Figure 31.5**). If access permits, we often employ a side-to-side anastomosis for better blood supply and this mitigates the size discrepancy between the esophagus and colon (see Chapter 29, "Esophageal anastomoses: sutured and stapled").

For improved functional results, the conduit is placed under gentle caudal traction, as a redundancy will lead to a tortuosity and the conduit will not empty well. This is particularly a problem with the posterior mediastinal route. For this route, the colon is anchored to the left side of the diaphragmatic opening semicircumferentially to keep it straight and prevent "bow stringing" (see **Figure 31.6**). The remaining hiatal defect is closed to prevent herniation of abdominal contents.

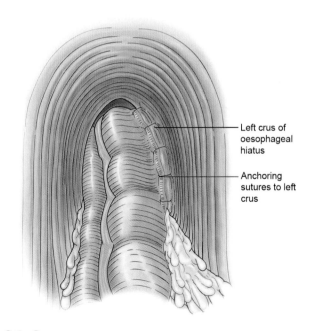

Left crus of oesophageal hiatus

Anchoring sutures to left crus

31.6

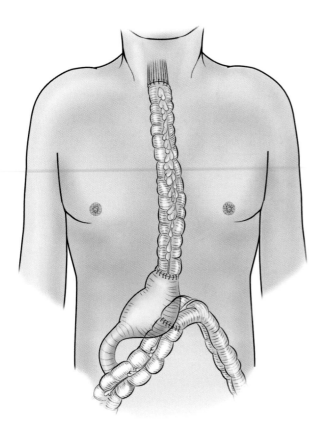

31.7

The colon is then divided distally approximately 8–10 cm from its emergence through the diaphragm. The mesentery is divided flush with the colonic wall for approximately 2 cm. Great care is taken to preserve and protect the marginal artery. An end-to-side anastomosis is fashioned to the remnant one-third of the stomach using a two-layer hand sewn technique. This anastomosis is generally placed posteriorly on the stomach, as the weight of the fluid-filled stomach can act as an antireflux mechanism. The right colon is brought across and anastomosed to the remnant left colon (see **Figure 31.7**). Again, we prefer here to use a stapled side-to-side anastomosis, as there is less risk of damaging the marginal artery with sutures. The mesentery of the descending and sigmoid colon remains intact and is sutured to the mesentery of the right to prevent internal hernia. We routinely insert a feeding jejunostomy at this point.

Right colon

The capacious nature of the cecum and antiperistaltic contractions maximize right colonic function, but this can be a detriment to its use as an esophageal replacement. Several techniques have been described, with none showing superiority.

The standard operation commences in a similar fashion as described earlier. The omentum is dissected free but vessels from the stomach and around the splenic flexure are preserved. The origins of ileocolic artery, marginal artery, and right colic artery are cleanly exposed and atraumatic vascular bulldog clamps placed. The entire right colon is now supplied by the middle colic. The length of colonic conduit required is measured again as for the left colon. Once vascularity is assured, the vessels are divided at their origin, proximal to the arcades supplying the marginal artery. The terminal ileum is divided and the desired length of colon measured and divided at the appropriate position. An appendectomy is performed. Again, the substernal or posterior mediastinal route can be used. The esophagogastric anastomosis is performed as described previously. Commonly, the esophagus is anastomosed to the terminal ileum, as the esophagus and ileum are of similar caliber and the ileocecal valve can act as an antireflux mechanism, although it can cause dysphagia, necessitating dilatations at a later date. If there are any concerns over the vascularity of the terminal ileum at this stage, the anastomosis should be made onto the cecum.

POSTOPERATIVE CARE

We cannot overemphasize the meticulous attention to detail this operation requires in the perioperative period. We recommend that a planned colonic interposition should be the only case listed on a theater list for that day. This removes any unnecessary time pressures and distractions from the theater team. During the operation, patients receive goal-directed fluid therapy measured against real time cardiovascular analysis. This is crucial because there is a risk patients may not receive appropriate fluid replacement, as blood loss during this procedure has become less major with the advent of new hemostatic devices and agents. There is still considerable third-space loss and fluid shift and these must not be underestimated.

Our preference is to wake the patient after the procedure and stabilize in recovery prior to transfer to the intensive care unit at a sensible hour. However, if the procedure has been challenging and lengthy or there are any signs of physiological instability, the patient should be left intubated overnight and be considered for extubation the next morning. Chest X-ray (CXR) is taken in recovery to ensure that any drains are in the correct position and that the lungs are expanded. It is vital that pain is well controlled and that a thoracic epidural is working effectively. If not, this must be addressed prior to transfer. Arterial saturations above 96% should be maintained and mean arterial pressures above 70 mmHg with vasopressor support if necessary. We encourage early mobilization. Nasogastric tubes are left on suction for 5 days and then removed if there is no evidence of conduit dilation on the CXR.

COMPLICATIONS

The most feared complication is graft ischemia and necrosis but this is fortunately uncommon, with reported rates from 0% to 9%. If this occurs early in the first 24- to 48-hour period, it is usually the result of a technical problem. Graft tension, twisting, or kinking of the colonic mesentery or venous congestion at the hiatus are common causes. Venous congestion is the most probably cause of graft ischemia and it is why particular attention to detail is required to ensure there is no kinking of the graft or compression at the hiatus and why the left colonic mesentery is not dissected to allow maximal drainage into the sigmoidal and hemorrhoid veins.

Low flow states, such as hypotension, hypovolemia, and embolic events, are often the cause of late graft ischemia. These events can be mitigated to a degree by strict attention to detail perioperatively and ensuring cardiovascular support is optimal. Early graft ischemia is difficult to detect, and while a rising lactate and persistent base deficit are often an early sign, graft ischemia can often be corrected with judicious intravenous fluids. Graft ischemia eventually leads to anastomotic failure and mediastinal sepsis, which is the entity that poses the most risk to the patient. Early intervention and an open mind to serious complications are paramount. Any suspicion of sepsis or graft ischemia should be investigated with CT imaging and bedside endoscopy. It is not uncommon for the mucosa to look ischemic with green/brown mucus. This does not necessarily mean the graft will fail, as it often recovers. With high definition endoscopy, it is possible to see the healthy submucosa underneath and this is reassuring. Daily bedside endoscopy should be performed until the surgeon is reassured there is no infarction.

If infarction is suspected or sepsis from an anastomotic leak is identified, prompt salvage surgery is key. With a leak from an infarcted graft, the graft will need to be disconnected and removed, with an esophagostomy performed on the left side of the neck and thorough lavage and debridement of any contaminated material. The cologastric anastomosis should be stapled off and closed. If the conduit is viable and the leak contained, then a washout and esophagostomy can suffice. Often, anastomotic leaks are identified late (day 10–14) on CT or esophagogram without signs of systemic sepsis. In this situation, control of infected collections is required either percutaneously or transnasally. We have found endoscopic placement of nasomediastinal drains on low pressure wall suction effective at draining contained leaks and collapsing abscess cavity. Broad-spectrum antibiotics should be prescribed along with antifungals and high dose proton pump therapy and the patient should remain on jejunal feeding for 2–4 weeks until the leak has sealed.

QUALITY OF LIFE OUTCOMES

Quality of life after colonic interposition is not routinely reported. However, good results from colonic interposition can be achieved in 75%–85% of patients and this is most noted in those with benign disease. In a review of 45 patients with benign disease, 34% had no gastrointestinal symptoms. Revision surgery or some other form of intervention can be high and has been reported in up to 45% of patients at some point in their life. In a more recent paper by Greene et al., long-term quality of life after colonic interposition was assessed in 63 patients. Reoperation rate in the surviving group was 11% (mostly for redundancy), while 89% had no dysphagia and over 90% could eat three meals a day, with a median alimentary satisfaction of nine out of ten.

FURTHER READING

Ahmad SA et al. Esophageal replacement using the colon: is it a good choice? *J Pediatr Surg.* 1996; 31(8): 1026–30; discussion 1030–1.

Briel JW et al. Prevalence and risk factors for ischemia, leak, and stricture of esophageal anastomosis: gastric pull-up versus colon interposition. *J Am Coll Surg.* 2004. 198(4): 536–41; discussion 541–2.

Cerfolio RJ et al. Esophageal replacement by colon interposition. *Ann Thorac Surg.* 1995; 59(6): 1382–4.

Davis PA et al. Colonic interposition after esophagectomy for cancer. *Arch Surg.* 2003; 138(3): 303–8.

DeMeester TR et al. Indications, surgical technique, and long-term functional results of colon interposition or bypass. *Ann Surg.* 1988; 208(4): 460–74.

Furst H et al. Colon interposition for esophageal replacement: an alternative technique based on the use of the right colon. *Ann Surg.* 2000; 231(2): 173–8.

Greene CL et al. Long-term quality of life and alimentary satisfaction after esophagectomy with colon interposition. *Ann Thorac Surg.* 2014. 98(5): 1713–19; discussion 1719–20.

Gupta S. Surgical management of corrosive strictures following acid burns of upper gastrointestinal tract. *Eur J Cardiothorac Surg.* 1996; 10(11): 934–40.

Isolauri J et al. Gastrointestinal symptoms after colon interposition. *Am J Gastroenterol.* 1986; 81(11): 1055–8.

Kent MS et al. A new technique of subcutaneous colon interposition. *Ann Thorac Surg.* 2005; 80(6): 2384–6.

Kolh P et al. Early stage results after esophageal resection for malignancy: colon interposition vs. gastric pull-up. *Eur J Cardiothorac Surg.* 2000; 18(3): 293–300.

McDermott S et al. Role of preoperative angiography in colon interposition surgery. *Diagn Interv Radiol.* 2012; 18(3): 314–18.

Motoyama S et al. Surgical outcome of colon interposition by the posterior mediastinal route for thoracic esophageal cancer. *Ann Thorac Surg.* 2007; 83(4): 1273–8.

Oida T et al. Anterior vs. posterior mediastinal routes in colon interposition after esophagectomy. *Hepatogastroenterology,* 2012; 59(118): 1832–4.

Peters JH et al. Arterial anatomic considerations in colon interposition for esophageal replacement. *Arch Surg.* 1995; 130(8): 858–62; discussion 862–3.

Yildirim S et al. Colonic interposition vs. gastric pull-up after total esophagectomy. *J Gastrointest Surg.* 2004; 8(6): 675–8.

32

Abdominal and right thoracic esophagectomy

S. MICHAEL GRIFFIN AND SHAJAHAN WAHED

HISTORY

Before 1946, the only widely practiced approach to the thoracic esophagus had been described by Sweet using a left-sided thoracotomy. Although this operation permitted relatively good access to the lower third of the esophagus, cancers of the middle and upper third of the esophagus were dissected with greater difficulty because of the overlying aortic arch. In 1946, Ivor Lewis described the abdominal and right thoracic approach for subtotal esophagectomy. This operation was adopted by Tanner in the United Kingdom (Lewis–Tanner operation) and by Santy in France (Lewis–Santy operation). This has remained the favored operation for an abdominal and right thoracic subtotal esophagectomy.

PREPARATION

A two-stage resection with a two-field lymphadenectomy is the procedure of choice for lower and middle third esophageal cancers, and types I and II junctional cancers. Prophylactic antibiotics are administered. A pneumatic calf compression device is used to reduce to the risk of venous thromboembolism. It is our practice to ask the radiologists to insert an inferior vena cava filter preoperatively in patients who already have proven venous thromboembolism on staging imaging. This is more likely after neoadjuvant chemotherapy. Epidural analgesia is established before anesthetizing the patients. A double lumen endotracheal tube and a nasogastric tube are inserted after induction. The patient is positioned supine with both arms extended and catheterized. A headlight is used routinely to improve visualization. The operation should be performed with minimal blood loss; precise dissection and meticulous hemostasis are crucial.

ABDOMINAL APPROACH

Access and exposure

Access for the gastric mobilization and abdominal lymphadenectomy is achieved with an upper midline incision skirting the umbilicus and extending to the xiphisternum (see **Figure 32.1a**). Excision of the xiphisternum improves access. A rooftop incision is a suitable alternative strategy particularly in patients with a wide angle at the costal margin. A wide exposure is achieved by using a retraction device fixed to the table such as the Omni-Tract® (see **Figure 32.1b**). A careful laparotomy is performed to exclude the presence of abdominal metastases. The ligament attaching the tip of the left lobe of the liver to the diaphragm is occasionally divided. One blade of the retractor is used to retract the left and caudate lobes of the liver once the pars flaccida has been divided close to the liver edge. This provides full access to the lesser curve and the right crus.

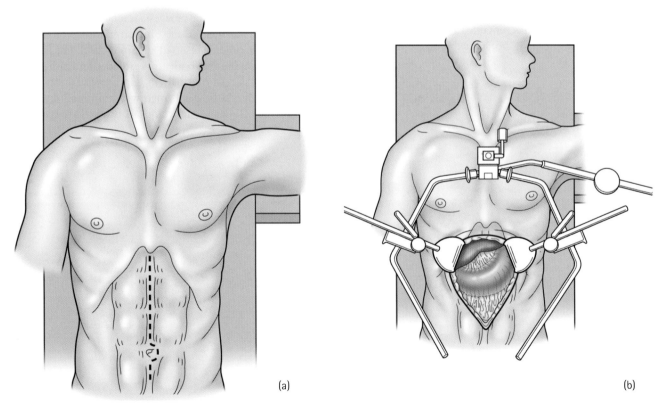

(a)

(b)

32.1 (a) Midline incision. (b) Abdominal exposure using a fixed table retractor.

Gastric mobilization

The stomach is the standard conduit used to replace the resected esophagus (see Chapter 30, "Use of the stomach as an esophageal substitute"). It is imperative that the right and left gastroepiploic vascular arcades are identified before any dissection commences. The operator needs to be aware of the variations in the extramural anastomoses between the two gastroepiploic arteries so that these can be identified. All vessels associated with the greater curve are preserved to optimize the vascularity of the gastric conduit.

The initial dissection releases any adhesions from the gastrosplenic ligament to the lower pole of the spleen, as this reduces the risk of an inadvertent traction injury. The authors use bipolar diathermy for this and much of the rest of the dissection. Placing the patient in a reverse Trendelenburg position will aid exposure. The dissection of the greater curve must always maintain a safe distance away from the arcade (see **Figure 32.2**). The authors advocate the preservation of omental fat along the greater curve. This fat can be used to cover the anastomosis and gastrotomy in the chest, and protect the membranous part of the trachea from the anastomosis. This precaution reduces the chance of a fistula. Avoid taking excessive amounts of omentum, as this will make subsequent delivery of the stomach through the hiatus difficult.

Once the window between the left gastroepiploic and short gastric arteries is identified, the dissection can migrate closer to the stomach. The short gastrics can be individually dissected, ligated, and divided. The use of a right-angled clip helps isolate and circumvent the vessels before ligation. Division of the short gastric vessels in this way can be difficult and time-consuming, particularly in the obese patient. The newer ultrasonic energy devices can make the dissection and division easier, although use of such devices should not be an excuse for poor dissection and isolation of the vessels. An inadequate dissection and subsequent use of the device on only part of a vessel can lead to troublesome bleeding. The dissection is continued on to the left crus. It is usual practice to take part of both crura *en bloc* with the specimen. The pars flaccida is dissected up to the right crus.

The duodenum is kocherized and the adhesions between the hepatic flexure and duodenum divided. The "C" of the duodenum is mobilized. These three maneuvers reduce the tension on the stomach and allow the stomach to be delivered easily into the chest with the pylorus positioned at or above the level of the hiatus.

The dissection along the greater curve is taken distally as far as the origin of the right gastroepiploic vessels. It is not necessary to completely skeletonize these vessels, as any inadvertent injury may jeopardize the blood supply to the conduit.

En bloc abdominal lymphadenectomy

The stomach can now be lifted cranially or retracted caudally to allow dissection of the common hepatic nodes. The tissues can be grasped gently with Wangensteen forceps to minimize bleeding. The dissection can be performed with a variety of techniques but the use of forceps diathermy or bipolar diathermy scissors allows for precise dissection and reduces the risk of bleeding from small vessels. The dissection follows closely the line of the common hepatic artery back to its origin and the proximal splenic artery is also dissected in

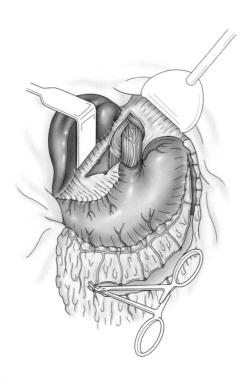

32.2

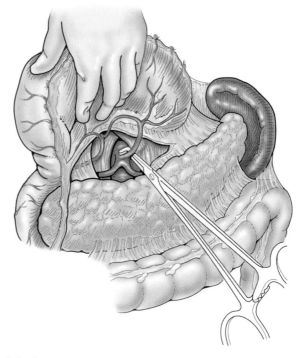

32.3

the same way. The left gastric vein is isolated and ligated in continuity with a 2-0 absorbable suture. The dissection leads on to the left gastric artery and celiac axis. All nodes around the left gastric artery and celiac trunk are removed *en bloc*. The left gastric artery is ligated in continuity then divided (see **Figure 32.3**). The suture on the specimen side is cut long to help with identification of the left gastric nodes when the specimen is dissected *ex vivo*. The remainder of the tissue from the left gastric territory up to the hiatus is dissected upward onto the stomach until it is completely mobilized (see **Figure 32.4**).

The dissection should continue through the hiatus, removing all the fat from the posterior aspect of the pericardium. The assistant could use a copper blade retractor or a renal vein retractor to provide optimum exposure. Both pleurae are dissected and the para-aortic tissue dissected off the aorta. Care needs to be taken not to damage the cisterna chyli. This is particularly vulnerable in thin patients.

Pyloroplasty

A pyloroplasty is routinely performed by the authors to improve gastric emptying and reduce the risk of aspiration. The authors use 3-0 PDS (polydioxanone) stay sutures inserted either side of the center of the pylorus. A small (1 cm) incision is made using diathermy to divide the pylorus longitudinally (see **Figure 32.5**). Suction is applied to remove bile or gastric juices through the pyloroplasty. The pyloroplasty is closed transversely with 3-0 PDS sutures, ensuring the corners are inverted. Each bite should incorporate a small amount of mucosa. A Gambee-type suture incorporating a circle of the mucosa and submucosa reduces the risk of bleeding. Often, only three sutures are required to close the pyloroplasty.

Feeding jejunostomy

It is the authors' practice to routinely insert a feeding jejunostomy. This is an important procedure and meticulous attention to detail is crucial to minimize complications. It allows for early enteral nutrition but, most important, allows for postoperative feeding in the event of complications preventing oral intake. A suitable loop of proximal jejunum is identified by tracing distally away from the duodenal-jejunal flexure. The loop should reach the left side of the abdominal wall without tension. The authors' preference is to use a 14 Fr MIC feeding tube (Kimberly-Clark, Ballard Medical Products, USA). The jejunostomy is flushed through with sterile saline. A small stab incision in the skin is made and a clip passed from the peritoneal side to exit through this incision. The tip of the feeding tube is grasped and pulled through to the peritoneal side. The tube is much longer than required so it can be shortened so that it is approximately 30 cm in length. A seromuscular purse-string suture is inserted into the chosen loop of jejunum on the antimesenteric aspect.

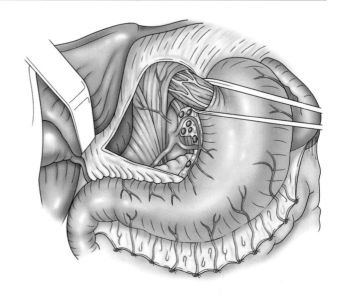

32.4 View of the completely mobilized stomach with preservation of all vessels along the greater curve and the right gastric vessels.

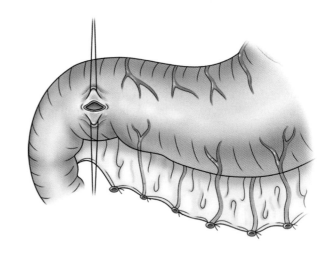

32.5 A small pyloroplasty is routinely performed to improve gastric emptying and reduce the risk of aspiration.

An absorbable suture such as a 2-0 Vicryl should be used. Diathermy is used to make a stab incision into the jejunal lumen and this is widened just enough with a mosquito forceps or small artery clip to allow insertion of the feeding tube. The tube is inserted and advanced along the jejunum, ensuring that the tip is in the lumen and not within the wall of the jejunum. Slow flushing of the tube during this stage aids in the smooth passage of the tube and reduces the risk of coiling. A distance of approximately 2 cm is left between the distal end of the jejunostomy balloon and the entry point in the lumen. The purse-string suture is ligated and then the suture ends are wrapped around the tube itself and retied. This prevents slippage of the jejunostomy tube out of the jejunal lumen.

A Witzel tunnel is created using seromuscular 2-0 Vicryl sutures either side of the tube to cover the length between the distal balloon end and the entry point. It is important not to narrow the jejunal lumen when doing this. Interrupted 2-0 Vicryl sutures are inserted to secure the peritoneum to the jejunal wall all around the start of the Witzel tunnel. The lateral suture is inserted first and clipped. At least one more of the sutures is inserted before pulling the feeding tube back so that the balloon sits within the abdominal wall. The sutures can now be tied and a total of three or four sutures are used to secure the peritoneum to the jejunal wall. A slit is made in the omentum so that it can lie either side of the jejunostomy. A further 2-0 Vicryl suture is inserted above the jejunostomy site incorporating peritoneum, omentum,

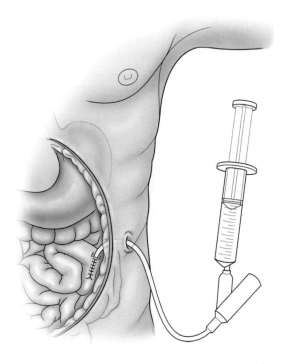

32.6 A feeding jejunostomy is routinely inserted. The jejunostomy is secured with a purse-string suture. A Witzel tunnel is created and it is anchored to the abdominal wall with a surrounding omental wrap.

jejunum, omentum and then tied. A similar suture below the jejunostomy site ensures that there is no fulcrum around which the jejunum can kink or twist and that the omentum is anchored in place. Creating this omental wrap reduces the possibility of infracolic bowel herniating through the widened hiatus. The jejunostomy is flushed to ensure there is free flow (see **Figure 32.6**). The bolster is secured loosely to the skin with interrupted 3-0 Ethilon sutures and the balloon is filled with 1–4 mL of water.

The abdominal cavity is washed with water and hemostasis checked, particularly around the lymph node dissection sites. The authors' preference is for 1 nylon sutures to close the midline and 3-0 subcuticular Monocryl sutures for the skin.

THORACIC APPROACH

Right posterolateral thoracotomy

The patient is secured in a left lateral decubitus position with the right arm rotated forward across an arm support. A posterolateral incision following the line of the ribs is made, skirting below the tip of the scapula, aimed toward the nipple, and terminating at the anterior axillary line. Diathermy and a bipolar electrosurgical tissue-sealing device are used to dissect through the tissues and divide the latissimus dorsi and serratus anterior muscles. The rib spaces are counted after insertion of the hand anterior to the scapula and pushed toward the apex. The 4th intercostal space should be used to allow for an anastomosis toward the apex of the thoracic cavity and permit a supra-azygos dissection if required. For middle-third squamous lesions, the 3rd rib space may be needed. Too low an incision makes this part of the operation difficult. The intercostal muscles are dissected off the top of the rib for the identified rib space with diathermy. A small incision is made to breach the pleura, ensuring the underlying lung is not damaged. At this stage, the anesthetist should be asked to deflate the right lung. The remainder of the pleura in the rib space is opened while a retractor is used to protect the underlying lung. One centimeter of the neck of the rib is excised to allow improved exposure and retraction while reducing the risk of uncontrolled rib fractures. The intercostal nerve is stripped along the rib, ligated, and excised. It is the authors' experience that this reduces the incidence of postthoracotomy wound pain. The rib space is gradually opened using a rib spreader. A retraction device such as the Omni-Tract® or a Finochietto is used to gain exposure.

The authors use bipolar diathermy for the dissection in the chest. Monopolar diathermy increases the risk of inadvertent collateral injury, particularly to the airways. The first step is to divide the pulmonary ligament as far as the inferior pulmonary vein. The parietal pleura above and below the arch of the azygos vein is incised and the azygos is ligated with 2-0 Vicryl before being divided (**Figure 32.7a and b**). It is imperative to ensure that the knots sit square on the vein to avoid the vein twisting and the suture subsequently twisting off. There are smaller vessels posterior to the azygos arch to be aware of that

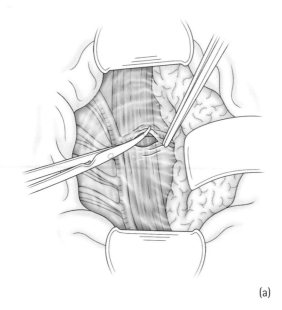

(a)

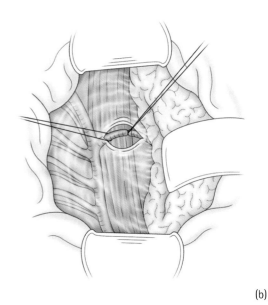

(b)

32.7a–b Dissection (a) and ligation (b) of the azygos arch.

most of the time can be preserved. The pleura is dissected superiorly off the esophagus as a flap. This can subsequently be used as a "pleural hood" to cover the anastomosis along with the omentoplasty.

The dissection follows the line of the azygos vein caudally as far as the hiatus (see **Figure 32.8**). The thoracic duct lies in the groove between the azygos vein and aorta at this level. The medial para-aortic tissue is dissected so that a plane of dissection flush on the aorta is entered. At this level, the tissues are dissected and the thoracic duct identified, ligated, and divided (see **Figure 32.9**). It is important to be aware that some individuals will have a second or even a third large lymph channel (more common in females).

All the para-aortic tissue is dissected *en bloc* with the esophagus. The retracting hand is crucial in making this step easier and safer. Any vessels coming off the aorta are tied with 2-0 Vicryl before division. It is common to have larger branches toward the upper part of the dissection, especially near the aortic arch. The esophagus and para-aortic tissue are retracted and the dissection continued to create a window in the preaortic plane. A nylon tape can be passed through this window to help with retraction as the dissection is continued in the cranial direction. The tissue from the back of the pericardium is dissected. The esophagus should become more mobile and the dissection continued cranially from both sides until the esophagus with the *en bloc* tissue is fully

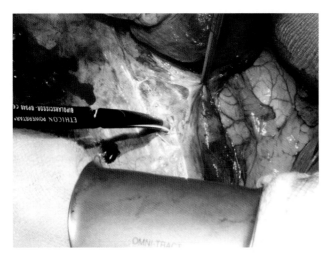

32.8 Dissection alongside the azygos vein.

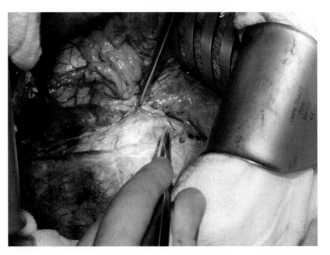

32.9 Identification of the thoracic duct in the groove between the azygos vein and aorta, close to the hiatus.

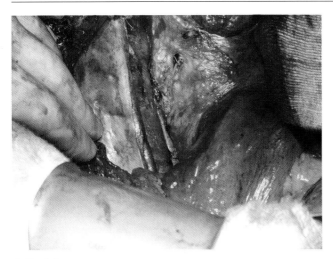

32.10 View of the completed dissection with *en bloc* dissection of the para-aortic tissue and tracheobronchial lymphadenectomy.

mobilized to a level above the azygos arch. The cranial end of the thoracic duct is ligated and divided. When dissecting the tissue posterior to the trachea and bronchi, it is vital to ensure the membranous parts of the airways are not damaged. Dissecting onto the fingers of the operating surgeon helps to protect the airways from any damage.

The right bronchial, subcarinal, and left bronchial lymph node groups are all resected *en bloc*. Gentle retraction on the nodes with an atraumatic grasper such as Wangensteen forceps helps delineate the tissue planes. There is often a feeding vessel that requires ligation before division at the carina (see **Figure 32.10**).

The dissection is completed cranially to include the right paratracheal lymph nodes and ensuring that the entire esophagus is mobile. The vagus nerve is divided without diathermy to prevent retrograde current passing to the right recurrent laryngeal nerve. An appropriate transection point in the apex of the thorax well above the aortic arch is chosen. Stay sutures (2-0 Monocryl) are inserted on either side of the esophagus above this level. The nasogastric tube is withdrawn to a level above the transection site and an angled esophageal clamp is placed just distal to the intended transection line. The esophagus is cleanly divided with a fresh scalpel blade, with a copper retractor placed posteriorly for protection.

Esophagogastric anastomosis

The authors' preference is for a stapled circular end-to-end anastomosis (CEEA) (described in further detail in Chapter 29, "Esophageal anastomoses: sutured and stapled"). Full-thickness 2-0 Monocryl stay sutures are inserted and clipped to hold the esophageal lumen open. Up to eight sutures are usually required (see **Figure 32.11**). The two original stays that were inserted before the transection are removed. A 0 Prolene purse-string suture is inserted around these stay sutures. The esophagus is dilated with up to 20 mL

of water in the balloon of 22 Fr Foley catheter. This is left in place for several seconds while a staple gun of appropriate size is chosen (see **Figure 32.12**). The authors' current preference is to use a 28 mm (or 25 mm) CEEA stapler. The lightly lubricated anvil (no lubrication should be on the actual staples) is inserted into the proximal esophagus immediately after removing the Foley. The Prolene suture is pulled so that it runs freely before tying. The tension is gradually increased when tying the first throw on the purse-string suture to ensure the anvil is securely tied in. The knot of the purse string should lie such that it falls inside the circular staples when they are fired.

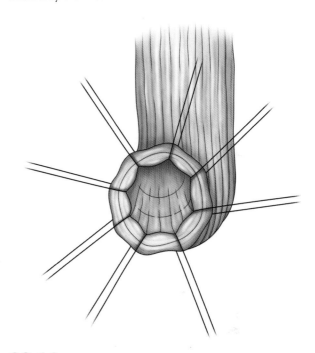

32.11 The proximal esophagus after insertion of full-thickness stay sutures.

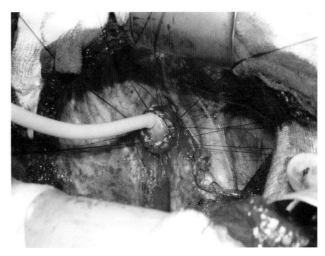

32.12 Dilatation of the proximal esophagus with the balloon of a Foley catheter after insertion of the stay Monocryl sutures and Prolene purse-string suture.

Gastric conduit formation

The stomach is delivered into the chest by gentle traction along the greater curve side, taking care to avoid any twisting. The entire stomach should lie within the chest with the sutures of the pyloroplasty palpable at the level of the hiatus. The lesser curve fat is dissected at an appropriate location on to the lesser curve, where the left and right gastric arteries connect, with any vessels encountered ligated or sealed. The high point of the stomach is identified by lifting the stomach up and ensuring this will reach the proximal divided esophagus (see **Figure 32.13**). This will be the point of the anastomosis. A long esophageal clamp is used to delineate the line of transection that removes the proximal half of the lesser curve and cardia. It is vital at this stage to ensure that the distance between the gastrotomy and the intended point for the anastomosis is not too short (the "angle of sorrow"). It is also vital not to narrow the conduit too much (the authors use a width of at least 5 cm) to reduce the risk of ischemia in the conduit. The stomach is divided with diathermy just below the clamp, using Babcock graspers to hold the gastrotomy as the dissection continues. The specimen with the two clamps attached at either end is removed.

The circular stapler is inserted and checked so that the point will exit at the predetermined high point. The distance along the angle of sorrow between the anastomosis and the proximal edge of the gastrotomy is rechecked. With two fingers firmly holding the stomach against the stapler, the point of the stapler is advanced through before a 3-0 PDS pursestring suture is placed to hold the stomach in place against the anvil and prevent any splitting. The stapler is engaged and tightened while checking to ensure no other tissue is drawn in between the esophagus and stomach (see **Figure 32.14**). The stapler is deployed, unlocked, and carefully removed.

The donuts on the stapler anvil are inspected to ensure they are completely intact and the anastomosis is gently inspected. The nasogastric tube is advanced over the anastomosis under vision and positioned in the distal stomach at the hiatus. The nasogastric tube is secured to the nose with a "bull ring" method. Commercial kits are available for this although simple use of a narrow caliber Foley is equally effective and considerably cheaper.

The gastrotomy is closed with a stapler. The authors' preference is for a Covidien DST Series TA 90 mm stapler (see **Figure 32.15**). If a long section of lesser curve is resected, a TCT 75 cutting stapler is used to divide the stomach inferiorly before using the TA 90 to close the remainder. The staple line is checked for hemostasis before being inverted with a continuous 3-0 PDS suture starting at the proximal end (see **Figure 32.16**). Omental fat is used to wrap around the conduit, covering the gastrotomy and anastomosis and buttressing the airways. The "pleural hood" is sutured over the anastomosis. The chest cavity is washed out and two chest drains inserted. A soft 20 Fr drain is inserted more anteriorly and positioned to lie at the apex alongside the anastomosis (anterior–apex) and a posterior 24 Fr chest drain to sit in the base (back–basal). A mattress suture through the incision for the chest drains is placed so that it can be used to close when the drains are removed. The authors use a 1 silk suture for this. Interrupted 1 Vicryl sutures are used to close the intercostal space. The assistant can draw the two ribs together with fingers or by crossing one of the sutures over to make tying the sutures easier. The lung is now reinflated under vision so that reexpansion of all lobes of the right lung can be witnessed and the drains held in place just before tying these sutures. The muscles are reapproximated in two layers with 1 PDS and the skin closed with 3-0 Monocryl.

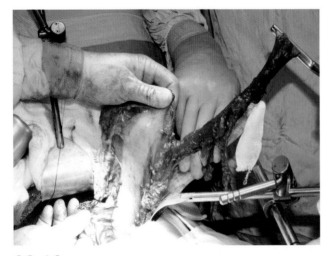

32.13 Preparation of the gastric conduit starts by identifying the high point of the stomach.

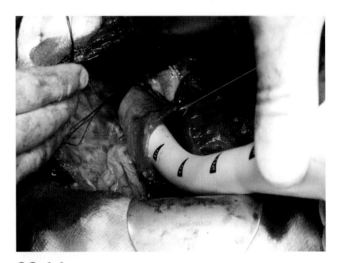

32.14 Formation of a circular stapled esophagogastric anastomosis.

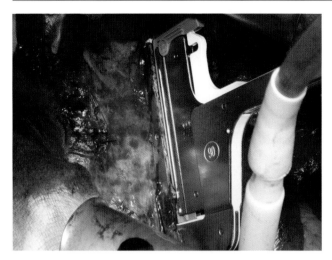

32.15 Linear stapler closure of the gastrotomy after completion of the circular stapled esophagogastric anastomosis.

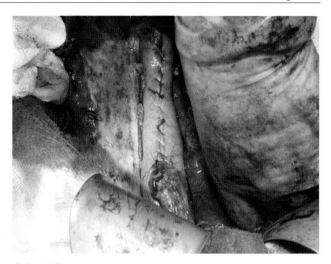

32.16 The gastrotomy staple line is inverted with 3.0 PDS sutures.

POSTOPERATIVE CARE

The patient is extubated in the operating theater and recovered in a high dependency or intensive care unit. The patient follows the protocol according to our Enhanced Recovery After Surgery (ERAS) Program described elsewhere. If their clinical condition is satisfactory and their mean blood pressure is greater than 70 mmHg, they are mobilized on the evening of operation. Walking the following morning is commenced, and the patient is returned to our dedicated esophagogastric ward the following morning. Analgesia is provided by a thoracic epidural at the level of T4. Nasogastric suction is applied for 1 to 4 days. Antibiotics are given for 24 hours, and thromboembolic prophylaxis is achieved with subcutaneous heparin/tinzaparin together with thromboembolic disease stockings. Since 1997, the use of a nonionic contrast swallow on day 5 has been abandoned due to its false negative results in a small number of anastomotic and gastric conduit leaks. Our unit has had no leak-associated mortality in over 500 consecutive esophagectomies. Chest drains are removed from day 3. Nutrition is administered from day 1 by a formal feeding jejunostomy. Blood transfusion is avoided unless serum hemoglobin persistently falls below 6 g/dL because of its potentially adverse immunomodulatory effects. The patient is discharged when mobile and tolerating a modified oral diet, usually between days 7 and 9.

OUTCOMES

The approach described provides excellent exposure and allows a safe radical *en bloc* lymphadenectomy. We performed over 1100 esophagectomies between 1989 and 2014 using the approach described. Our median lymph node yield using this approach was 30. Surgical outcomes have improved significantly over time: in the most recent 5-year cohort, 90-day operative mortality was 2.1% and overall 5-year survival for patients with invasive cancer was 46.6%.

FURTHER READING

Allum WH, Blazeby JM, Griffin SM, Cunningham D, Jankowski JA, Wong R et al. Guidelines for the management of oesophageal and gastric cancer. *Gut.* 2011; 60: 1449–72.

Couper G. Jejunostomy after oesophagectomy: a review of evidence and current practice. *Proc Nutr Soc.* 2011; 70: 316–20.

Griffin SM & Berrisford RG. Surgery for cancer of the oesophagus. In *Oesophagogastric Surgery: a companion to specialist surgical practice*, 5th edition, 2014. Eds.: Griffin SM, Raimes SA & Shenfine J. Philadelphia: Saunders Elsevier; pp. 81–106.

Omloo JMT, Lagarde SM, Hulscher JBF, Reitsma JB, Fockens P, van Dekken H et al. Extended transthoracic resection compared with limited transhiatal resection for adenocarcinoma of the mid/distal esophagus: five-year survival of a randomized controlled trial. *Ann Surg.* 2007; 246: 992–1000.

Peyre CG, Hagen JA, DeMeester SR, Altorki NK, Ancona E, Griffin SM et al. The number of lymph nodes removed predicts survival in esophageal cancer: an international study on the impact of extent of surgical resection. *Ann Surg.* 2008; 248: 549–56.

33

Left thoracic subtotal esophagectomy

JUN-FENG LIU

HISTORY

More than 100 years ago, esophagectomy began to be used for obstructive esophageal diseases. Czerny resected the cervical esophagus for a 50-year-old woman with esophageal cancer in 1877, and she survived for 15 months. Jejunal interposition was performed in a patient with benign esophageal stricture by Roux and Herzen in 1907. Kelling was the first to use colon as a substitute for the esophagus in 1911. The first successful thoracic esophagectomy was undertaken by Torek in 1913. No attempt was made to perform a reconstruction and the patient fed herself through a gastrostomy until she died from a stroke 13 years later. Ohsawa performed a gastroesophagostomy using an abdominal approach after resection of a cardiac cancer in 1932. Adams and Phemister performed a left thoracic subtotal esophagectomy for cancer in 1938 and undertook an esophagogastric anastomosis in the thorax. A combined left thoracoabdominal subtotal esophagectomy for cancer was initially reported by Sweet in 1945. Lewis undertook a three-stage esophagectomy first in 1946, and three-field esophagectomy was first used in the treatment for esophageal cancer by Akiyama in 1981.

PRINCIPLES AND JUSTIFICATION

Indications

This operation provides a means for resecting the thoracic esophagus, with anastomosis of the esophagus to the fundus of the stomach in the thorax or in the neck from the left side. The principal indication for this approach is resection of tumors of the thoracic esophagus and cardia, but it is also applicable to resection of a benign esophageal stricture. The main advantages of this method of subtotal esophagectomy are that it permits exploration of the tumor, dissection of the esophagus, and mobilization of the stomach through a single thoracotomy incision. This is quicker and simpler than a right-sided three-stage approach—that is laparotomy, right thoracotomy, and right neck incision—and it permits dissection of the tumor and its lymphatic or other extensions under direct vision. In general, indications for surgical therapy of esophageal carcinoma are dictated by cancer stage and fitness of patients for surgery. The stages 0, I, II, and $T_3N_1M_0$ of stage III disease can be radically resected. Palliative resection is usually performed for a T_3 intrathoracic esophageal cancer, but with supraclavicular and/or upper abdominal lymph node metastasis. Although there is a steady increase in surgical mortality with advancing age and a precipitous rise in mortality over the age of 75, left thoracic subtotal esophagectomy can be well tolerated by patients whose age is close to 80 years if they have no obvious cardiopulmonary problems.

Contraindications

The contraindications to this approach are when a tumor is located at the cervical esophagus (judged by barium swallow and not endoscopy) and when the upper part of the stomach is involved by tumor and there is insufficient stomach to reach the anticipated anastomotic site. It is also contraindicated when patients are cachectic, or have significant comorbid disease and are judged unfit to withstand the operation. Clinical factors, which indicate an advanced stage of carcinoma, are recurrent laryngeal nerve paralysis, Horner's syndrome, persistent spinal pain, paralysis of the diaphragm, fistula formation, and malignant pleural effusion, and these indicate inoperability. Factors that make surgical cure unlikely are a tumor greater than 8 cm in length, abnormal axis of the esophagus on barium roentgenograph, enlarged lymph nodes, invasion of aorta or trachea on computed tomography (CT), and a weight loss greater than 20%.

PREOPERATIVE ASSESSMENT

Routine investigations

Investigations before operation are designed to assess the patient's fitness for operation and to determine whether there is spread of the tumor beyond the limits of surgical resection. Routine investigations include hematological and biochemical tests and measurement of renal and hepatic function. Cardiac status is assessed by chest radiography, electrocardiography, and additional tests if indicated. Respiratory assessment includes routine spirometry, with full tests of respiratory function and blood gases if significant abnormalities are found. Possible spread of the tumor is investigated by barium swallow, esophagoscopy, and biopsy, CT, and/or ultrasonography in all cases, as well as positron emission tomography scan if available, and bronchoscopy, indirect laryngoscopy, lymph node biopsy, cytology of effusions, and other tests as indicated by symptoms or the findings on physical examination.

Nutritional assessment

Since the predominant symptom of esophageal carcinoma is difficulty in swallowing, most patients are nutritionally depleted. The nutritional status of the patients is important in predicting the outcome. A poor nutritional status decreases host resistance to infection and affects healing of an anastomosis. Physical examination should look for peripheral edema, specifically in the feet and flanks which, if present, gives an initial clue for very poor nutritional status of the patient. Measurement of the serum albumin is a more objective estimate of the status of the patient. A low value of serum albumin (<34 g/L) increases the risk of surgical complications, including anastomotic leakage. A positive nitrogen balance is important for the patient's safe passage through the rigors of this major operation and postoperative stress. Hyperalimentation may be necessary for patients with poor nutritional status before surgery. Albumin or blood plasma can be given to supplement nutrition in patients with hypoproteinemia.

Pulmonary assessment

In addition to the effects of thoracotomy on pulmonary function, the intrathoracic stomach takes up room in the thorax after esophagectomy, and this adversely affects pulmonary function. Thus, pulmonary function should be meticulously assessed before resection of the esophagus. Pulmonary complications, including retained secretions, atelectasis, pneumonia, and respiratory failure, are the most severe problems following thoracic surgical procedures. Patients who are heavy smokers have a significantly increased risk of postoperative complications. The ability to cough is important because cough helps avoid postoperative atelectasis. Preoperative pulmonary function testing is undertaken routinely. The tests range from the simplest medical assessment (history taking, particularly of past pulmonary disease; physical examination; and stair climbing) to the most sophisticated exercise testing, and even analysis of blood gases. After deep inspiration, the ability to breath hold for more than 30 seconds suggests normal lung function. A value less than 20 seconds implies a high risk for thoracotomy. After climbing stairs of three stories, a pulse rate of more than 120 beats per minute indicates a high risk for esophagectomy. In my experience, a patient with a maximum volume ventilation (MVV) and vital capacity (VC) more than 70% of predicted values will tolerate a transthoracic esophagectomy; however, if the MVV and VC are less than 50% of predicted values, forced expiratory volume in 1 second (FEV1)/forced vital capacity less than 60%, and oxygen saturation (SO_2) less than 90% after exercise, surgery is contraindicated.

Cardiovascular assessment

The risk of both morbidity and mortality from thoracic surgery increases exponentially in patients with respiratory and significant cardiovascular disease. It is important to have an accurate cardiac history and know all cardiovascular medications used. If there is concern, a detailed assessment of the cardiac state should be undertaken in consultation with a cardiologist within a formal risk assessment protocol, such as the New York Heart Association (NYHA) Functional Classification published in 1928 (see **Table 33.1**)

In general, patients with class I or II cardiac function can tolerate esophagectomy well. Class III cardiac function

Table 33.1   NYHA Functional Classification of cardiac function

NYHA class	Symptoms
I	Cardiac disease, but no symptoms and no limitation in ordinary physical activity, e.g. shortness of breath when walking, climbing stairs, etc.
II	Mild symptoms (mild shortness of breath and/or angina) and slight limitation during ordinary activity
III	Marked limitation in activity due to symptoms, even during less-than-ordinary activity, e.g. walking short distances (20–100 m). Comfortable only at rest
IV	Severe limitations. Experiences symptoms even while at rest. Mostly bedbound patients

is a relative contraindication for esophagectomy and such patients need to be prepared meticulously to recover their cardiac function to class II before surgery. Class IV cardiac function is a contraindication for esophagectomy. In our experience, heart infarction is a contraindication for the surgery except for inferior wall myocardial infarction, which can tolerate the surgery if more than half a year has elapsed since the heart incident. Although angina rarely undermines heart function, it should be stable for at least 3 months before the surgery. Hypertension and heart arrhythmias are not contraindications for esophageal resection, but should be effectively controlled before surgery.

Preparation

Adequate preoperative management will improve the ability of the patient to tolerate the operation. Smoking is stopped for at least 2 weeks before the operation, and all patients are instructed by an experienced respiratory physiotherapist in the breathing and coughing techniques that will be required after operation and in the use of incentive spirometry. Cessation of smoking, aggressive bronchopulmonary toilet, and bronchodilators may improve a marginal FEV1. Patients with chronic lung disease do better if their operations are scheduled for the afternoon, thus allowing them to ambulate and cough up secretions that have accumulated in the lung overnight. For the patients complicated with infectious respiratory diseases such as asthma or chronic obstructive pulmonary disease, intravenous use of antibiotics and mucus thinner—Ambroxol—and inhalation of bronchodilator and inhaled corticosteroids are needed. As discussed earlier, most esophageal cancer patients have difficulty swallowing, so preoperative nutritional support is important. Oral intake is usually inadequate in patients with advanced esophageal cancer, and hyperalimentation may be necessary. Enteral alimentation via a nasogastric tube and intravenous hyperalimentation are selected according to the status of the patients.

In resection of the esophagus, the mediastinum is extensively dissected and the bacteriologically contaminated esophagus is opened. Therefore, it is necessary to use prophylactic antibiotics to reduce the incidence of wound infection and anastomotic breakdown. Adequate doses of a broad-spectrum antibiotic with adequate Gram-positive and Gram-negative coverage is prescribed intravenously. A nasogastric tube is placed before surgery. Washout of esophageal content through the nasogastric tube is necessary for patients who have severe obstruction of the esophagus.

ANESTHESIA

After the administration of general anesthesia and endotracheal intubation with a single- or double-lumen tube (the latter is preferable), the patient is placed in the right lateral decubitus position with the arm flexed at the elbow and shoulder. The table is flexed or a soft pad is placed under the right chest to widen the operative field.

OPERATION

Incisions

1. The site of the incision is decided according to the anatomical level of the tumor and the anticipated site of anastomosis. If the tumor is in the cardia or the lower third of the esophagus and the anastomosis is constructed below the aortic arch, the incision is made through the seventh intercostal space or by resection of the seventh rib. When the tumor is in the middle or upper third of the esophagus and the anastomosis is to be constructed above the aortic arch or in the neck, the incision is made through the sixth intercostal space or by resection of the sixth rib. Usually, the sixth or seventh rib is identified as the standard left thoracotomy incision, including anterior and posterior extensions when necessary. The basic incision is made from the level of the costal cartilage in front to the paravertebral region at the angle of the scapula behind. It may be extended upward between the scapula and the vertebral column to the level of the posterior end of the fourth rib. This allows the transaction of a higher rib, usually the fifth at the costal end, giving access for a supra-aortic dissection of the esophagus, and it also permits an easier high intrathoracic anastomosis. A left thoracoabdominal incision is usually used for resection of the proximal stomach or for obese patients. With the patient in the right lateral position, an oblique lateral incision is made, starting in the left hypochondrium and continuing over the costal margin and along the line of the seventh rib to the angle of the rib posteriorly. The incision on the abdomen is the oblique extension of the thoracic incision to the edge of the rectus sheath. The peritoneum is opened in the line of the incision, which provides excellent access to the upper abdominal organs (see **Figure 33.1**.)

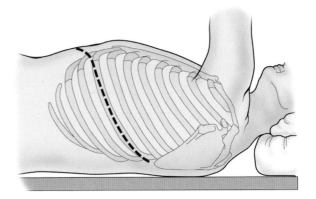

33.1

Dissection of the esophagus

For resection of the gastric cardia, the dissection of the esophagus needs to be carried out to the level of the inferior pulmonary vein. For cancer arising from the lower third of the esophagus, the dissection of the esophagus should be conducted to the level of the bifurcation of the trachea. The whole of the thoracic esophagus should be dissected for cancers that occur in the middle or upper third of the esophagus and also for cancers involving the cervical esophagus.

2. After a thorough exploration of the pleural cavity, the mediastinal pleura overlying the esophagus is incised posterior to the aorta and anterior to the pleural reflection at the pericardium, and the tumor is identified and assessed for resectability. If resection of tumor is thought possible, a tape is placed around the esophagus just below the tumor to lift the esophagus for facilitating its dissection. The inferior pulmonary ligament is mobilized to the level of the inferior pulmonary vein,

and the lymph nodes within it are removed. The esophagus is dissected from the hiatus below to a level above or at least 5 cm proximal to the tumor. To avoid dissection too close to the tumor, the descending aorta and pericardium are completely bared. The esophageal arterial branches and the bronchial artery on the adventitia of the aorta are divided. Paraesophageal adipose tissue and all mediastinal lymph nodes are completely removed with the esophagus. If invaded by tumor, resection of pulmonary ligament, pericardium, azygos vein, the right mediastinal pleural membrane, and even a wedge of the lung can be undertaken.

For patients with a middle or upper third esophageal cancer, the whole of the thoracic esophagus is usually mobilized for a curative resection. The technique of esophageal dissection at the aortic arch is critical, particularly for cancers located at this level. The esophagus is freed from behind the aortic arch by blunt dissection in the plane between the esophageal muscle and the adventitia of the aortic arch. A finger is passed

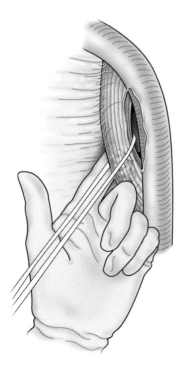

33.2a

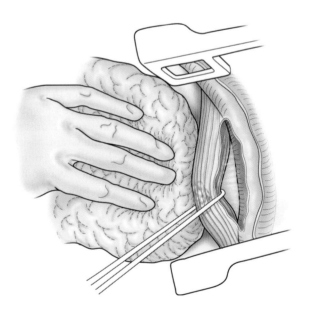

33.2b

behind the aortic arch so that the fingertip appears beneath the mediastinal pleura above the arch. At the level of the upper edge of the aortic arch, the thoracic duct runs from the posterior mediastinum to behind the subclavian artery on the left of the esophagus posteriorly. Therefore, a longitudinal incision of the pleura over the upper mediastinum is made along the front edge of the thoracic spine to prevent damage to the thoracic duct. After the pleura is opened, a tape is passed around the esophagus above the aortic arch. This facilitates mobilization of the upper esophagus into the root of the neck, the level of which is identified by palpation of the inner border of the first rib. If tumor adheres to the arch of the aorta, and blind dissection is not possible, division of the uppermost intercostal aortic arterial branches may be necessary to help in the mobilization of the arch itself, but care must be taken not to divide more than three branches to prevent the possibility of spinal cord ischemia. The left recurrent laryngeal nerve is carefully preserved to avoid being injured. As the nerve passes by the side of the aortic arch, loops below it, and ascends behind the aortic arch to the left tracheoesophageal groove, mobilization of the upper thoracic esophagus should be close to its adventitia. The thoracic duct is usually protected beyond the descending aorta, using the left transthoracic approach, but chylothorax can ensue if the dissection is carried out widely and toward the right pleura. It is always wise to check for possible damage to the duct. If the thoracic duct is injured, it is ligated below the point of injury. In the author's unit, the thoracic duct is routinely ligated at a lower site, usually the level of the ninth or tenth thoracic vertebra. The azygos arch can also be injured from the left side, and this must be carefully avoided. The left main bronchus is examined to make sure there is no injury to its membranous portion. (See **Figure 33.2a through d.**)

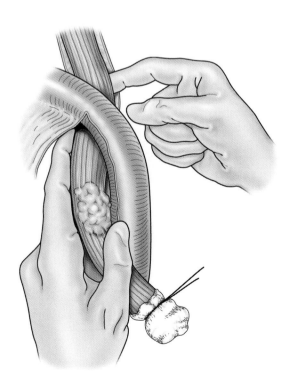

33.2c

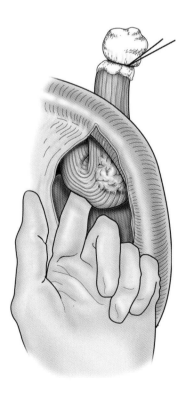

33.2d

Incision of the diaphragm

3. Based on the anatomy, incision of the diaphragm should preserve the branches of the phrenic nerve in the diaphragm. For the transthoracic approach, a radial diaphragmatic incision between the spleen and the liver is commonly used in our unit. The incision is extended from the esophageal hiatus through the aponeurotic portion to the muscular portion of the diaphragm. If the diaphragm is involved by tumor, the affected portion is resected with the tumor. In general, the length of the diaphragm incision is approximately 10 cm, but it can be extended to 15 cm for obese patients or for large tumors in the gastric cardia. Traction sutures are placed through the cut edges of the diaphragm to aid exposure. The blood vessels in the cut edges are sutured and ligated. For a combined thoracoabdominal approach, the diaphragm is divided peripherally from its origin on the ribs, around to the hiatus, leaving the phrenic nerve undamaged. (See **Figure 33.3a and b.**)

Mobilization of the stomach

4. For gastric mobilization, the essential principles are the preservation of a blood supply by preserving the right gastric and right gastroepiploic vessels and arcades and obtaining maximal length by using the greater curvature for the positioning of the anastomosis.

   Before mobilization of the stomach, the abdominal cavity is thoroughly inspected. The liver, pancreas, and lymph nodes of the upper abdominal region are inspected and palpated to determine if potential metastases have occurred to these organs and tissues. The initial step in detachment of the stomach is division of the phrenoesophageal ligament. Next, the greater omentum is divided outside the arch of the gastroepiploic vessels. Care is taken to preserve the gastroepiploic arcade when separating the greater omentum and the spleen from the stomach. The dissection of the greater omentum is carried out to the level of the pylorus, and the rather small omental branches from the epiploic vessels are clamped and divided. The dissection is then directed toward the spleen, where the left gastroepiploic artery is ligated above its uppermost branch to the stomach wall. The short gastric arteries are divided carefully between hemostatic forceps and are ligated securely. The proximal branches of these vessels may be very short and require the application of suture ligatures. Ligatures on the stomach side must be tied securely because these ties can slip off the stomach if distension of the stomach in the thorax occurs. Elevation of the stomach to the right by the assistant permits exposure of the left gastric artery and facilitates celiac lymph node dissection from behind the stomach. Much attention should be directed toward exposure of the origin of the left gastric artery

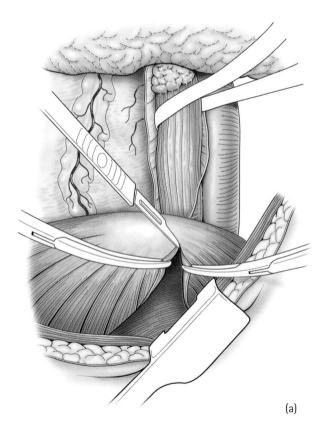

(a)

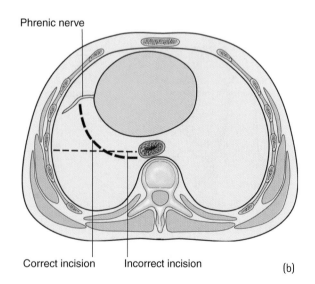

Phrenic nerve

Correct incision   Incorrect incision

(b)

33.3a–b

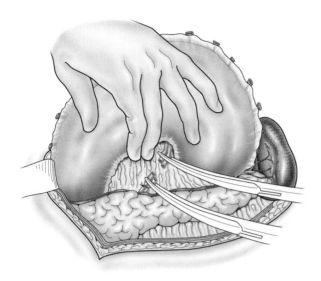

33.4

at the trifurcation of the celiac axis. It is necessary to divide the filmy, avascular adhesions between the back of the stomach and the retroperitoneum. The left gastric artery is exposed by the surgeon, whose thumb and forefinger encircle the lesser curvature attachments. The fat tissue and lymph nodes around the left gastric artery are dissected carefully, starting from the upper edge of the pancreas. Then two hemostatic clamps are applied to the proximal side of the vessel and one to the distal side. The left gastric artery is divided between the second and third clamps. The left gastric artery is doubly ligated at its origin from the celiac axis with a heavy nonabsorbable silk suture. The first ligature is placed and firmly tied proximal to the first clamp, and the clamp is removed. The second tie is then placed on the left gastric artery distal to the first tie. The artery on the gastric side is best managed with a secure suture ligature. (See **Figure 33.4**.)

5. Lymph nodes and fat tissue along the left gastric artery and around the gastric cardia are dissected to remain with the resected specimen. For cardia cancer, the transaction of the proximal stomach is performed with a linear stapler, and the esophagus is mobilized up to the level of the inferior pulmonary vein. The incision of the stomach is then strengthened with interrupted 4-0 silk sutures placed in the seromuscular layer. For cancer of the esophagus, the stomach itself is transected at, or just below, the esophagogastric junction. The stapler is usually used to close the incision of the stomach, and reinforced with interrupted 4-0 silk sutures in the seromuscular layer. The stump of the esophagus is covered with a sterilized condom to prevent contamination.

After completion of the detachment of the stomach and its transection, further mobilization of the

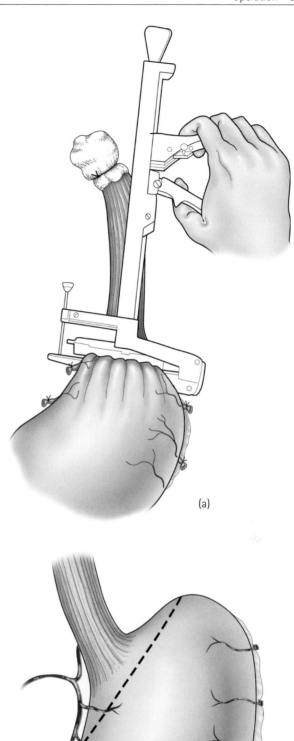

(a)

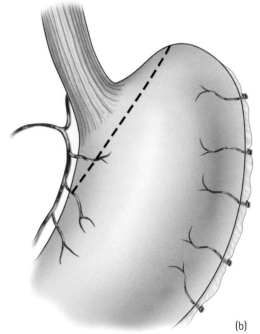

(b)

33.5a–b

postesophageal region up to the level of the carina is carried out. Upward lift of the esophagus by an assistant helps resection of subcarinal lymph nodes and freeing of the esophagus from the arch of the azygos vein. Then the total esophagus is pulled to the supra-aortic arch region. The next step is anastomosis in the thorax. However, if an anastomosis in the neck is necessary, the stump of the esophagus is connected to the uppermost region of the stomach with four interrupted stitches to aid pulling the stomach into the neck. (See **Figure 33.5a and b**.)

The anastomosis

Although a variety of anastomotic methods have been reported, these can be classified as hand-sewn anastomoses and stapled anastomoses (see Chapter 29, "Esophageal anastomoses: sutured and stapled"). This chapter describes the anastomotic methods most commonly used in China.

HAND-SEWN ANASTOMOSIS

6. After completion of the mediastinal dissection and gastric mobilization, the stomach can be brought to any level within the thorax by gentle traction on the upper end of the greater curvature. This is where the maximal length of the viscus can be obtained. Traction on the esophageal specimen upward as a sort of handle permits an end (esophagus)-to-side (stomach) esophagogastric anastomosis. The first row of 4-0 silk sutures is placed in a horizontal mattress fashion between the muscular layer of the esophagus and the seromuscular layer of the uppermost stomach wall. Approximately three or four stitches are placed first. These form the outer posterior row. At 2.5 cm from the first row of sutures, an incision of the gastric wall to fit the diameter of the esophagus is made, and the intramural plexus of vessels is suture-ligated. Then the sutures forming the first row are tied carefully by the surgeon, who always draws the stomach upward to the esophagus by positioning the tying forefinger above the point of the actual approximation of tissue. The esophagus is a fixed structure that cannot be brought down distally; its serosa-less muscular coat is more fragile and does not hold sutures as well as the stomach. The outer posterior row of sutures covers about a half of the circumference, and the corner ties are left long and marked with hemostats. After completion of the first row of sutures, a soft clamp is applied proximal to the first row of sutures to stop bleeding from the upper stump of the esophagus.

The esophagus is transected 3 cm distal to the first row of sutures and the specimen is removed. Then posterior inner sutures, also 4-0 silk, are placed and tied with care so as not to cut the tissue with the suture. Each stitch is placed about 1 cm from the cut margin, with the stitches 0.3 cm apart from each other. The needle is pulled through each edge separately, to make sure whole layers of the esophagus and stomach are sutured. The gastric and esophageal mucosa are picked up with a similar bite of tissue. When the suture is tied, it is necessary to press the muscular layer with the tip of a clamp, held by an assistant, to approximate the mucosa of the esophagus and stomach. The anterior inner row is continued in an interrupted fashion; the stitches are placed and tied as the posterior inner row. Whole layers of the esophagus and stomach are sutured. The assistant holds the previous sutures up to facilitate the surgeon placing subsequent stitches. As each suture is tied, the assistant inverts muscular and mucosal layers into the lumen when necessary. This method allows complete inversion of the mucosal layer. This row of sutures is tied from either end toward the middle so that a final suture can be placed anteriorly, which is an easy way to complete the anterior row. After all stitches are tied, sutures are then cut.

A nasogastric tube is directed downward through the anastomosis to the level of the gastric antrum and is fixed by the anesthetist to the patient's nose to prevent later inadvertent withdrawal.

The anterior outer row is placed in a horizontal mattress fashion over the remaining half of the circumference of the esophagus. As the anastomosis has been placed 2.5 cm down from the apex of the stomach, this row should bring the anterior wall of the stomach up to the same level as the posterior wall. Three to four horizontal mattress stitches are put between the muscular layer of the esophagus and the seromuscular layer of the stomach, which brings it upward circumferentially. This constructs a valve-like luminal orifice, which helps to minimize the possibility of gastroesophageal reflux.

The anterior aspect of the anastomosis may further be buttressed by a flap of omentum, which remains at the upper end of the gastroepiploic arcade. The stomach is suspended by a series of nonabsorbable sutures to the fascia that overlies the thoracic spine. This helps to avoid downward traction on the anastomosis. (See **Figure 33.6a through e**.)

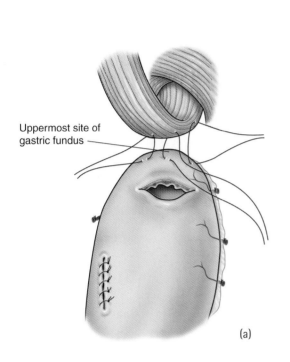

Uppermost site of
gastric fundus

(a)

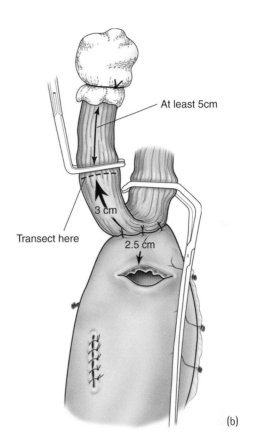

At least 5cm

3 cm

Transect here

2.5 cm

(b)

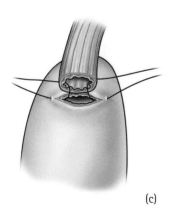

(c)

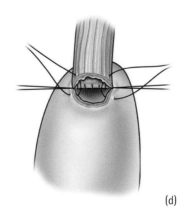

(d)

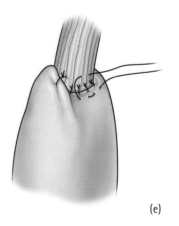

(e)

33.6a–e

ANASTOMOSIS WITH A CIRCULAR STAPLER

To simplify the anastomotic process, an anastomotic stapler was invented in the former Soviet Union in the 1950s. Since then, the apparatus has been greatly improved. The currently available circular anastomotic stapler has become safe.

7. If an anastomosis using a stapler is planned, the incision in the stomach is left open after transection at the esophagogastric junction for the later placement of a stapler. A purse-string applicator is put on the anticipated site of the anastomosis in the esophagus. After a purse-string suture is applied, the esophagus is transected distal to the clamp. Three Allis forceps are used to grasp the stump of the esophagus at 120 degrees

apart after removal of the purse-string applicator, and the anvil is put into the lumen of the esophagus before the purse-string suture is tied. The head of the circular stapler is then put into the cavity of the stomach through the gastric cardia and applied against the gastric wall at the fundus. The turn button at the distal end of the stapler is rotated anticlockwise to allow the tip of the central pole to puncture the gastric wall and connect into the central pole of the anvil. Then the turn button is rotated clockwise to approximate the stomach wall to the esophageal stump, to the extent as indicated in the scale plate of the stapler. Examination of the closed stapler is carried out to make sure surrounding structures and tissues (including pleura, the subclavian

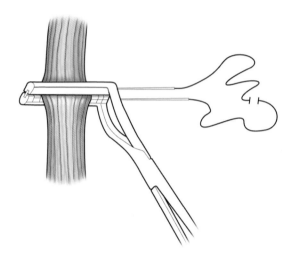

33.7a

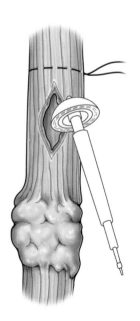

33.7b

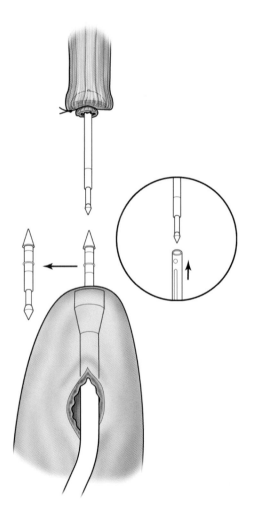

33.7c

artery, and foreign bodies such as gauze) have not been caught. The stapler is fired and the turn button rotated anticlockwise. The stapler, with anvil, is pulled out through the cardia. Check that two complete circular "doughnuts" from the esophageal and gastric ends are present. If there is any doubt as to the integrity of the doughnuts, the anastomosis is reinforced with interrupted nonabsorbable sutures. The incision in the stomach is closed with a linear stapler and strengthened by oversewing the seromuscular layer with interrupted 4-0 silk sutures. A nasogastric tube is placed into the intrathoracic stomach to decrease postoperative gastric distension. (See **Figure 33.7a through d.**)

Folding suture of the stomach

8. After completion of the anastomosis, the lesser curvature of the stomach is oversewn. This minimizes the size of the intrathoracic stomach and prevents compression of the stomach on the intrathoracic organs, especially the lung and heart. Interrupted 4-0 silk sutures are put on the anterior and posterior walls, which are adjacent to the lesser curvature, at 2 cm apart from each other. After each suture is tied, the stomach is folded in along the lesser curvature. (See **Figure 33.8.**)

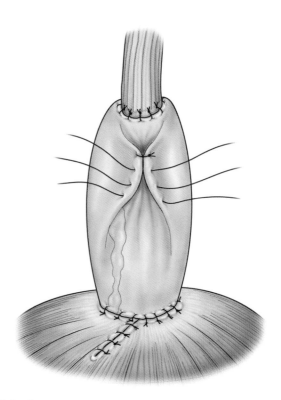

33.8

Closure of the diaphragm incision and the chest

The incision of the diaphragm is closed with 7-0 interrupted silk sutures and is also sutured to the wall of the stomach with 4-0 thread to prevent prolapse of intra-abdominal contents into the thorax. The space between the edge of the diaphragm incision and the stomach should be snug enough to prevent an index finger passing after completion of the closure of the diaphragm. The pulse in the right gastroepiploic artery is checked. A No. 28 Argyle chest catheter is placed through the eighth intercostal space in the axillary line, for drainage. The chest wall is closed with interrupted heavy nonabsorbable silk sutures and careful approximation of the muscles of the chest wall is undertaken to avoid interference with postoperative shoulder function. Fine interrupted silk sutures are used to suture the skin.

33.7d

Left cervical approach

The left thoracic or thoracoabdominal cervical approach is an additional procedure for the treatment of carcinoma of the esophagus. The major difference between this method and the classic left thoracic approach is the level of anastomosis. For cancers located in the upper thoracic esophagus, there is not enough length of normal esophagus to construct an anastomosis in the thoracic cavity according to oncological principles. The left cervical approach is therefore carried out in most of these patients.

LEFT NECK INCISION

9. When the thoracoabdominal incision has been closed, the patient is placed in the supine position with a pad under the left shoulder. An oblique incision no more than 8 cm in length is made along the anterior border of the left sternocleidomastoid muscle.

   The omohyoid muscle is divided together with the middle thyroid vein and the inferior thyroid artery if these are in the way of the exposure. The carotid artery and jugular vessels are retracted laterally, and the trachea is retracted medially to expose the already mobilized esophagus. The esophagus and fundus of the stomach are delivered through the wound, the stomach being held with a pair of Duval forceps to prevent it slipping back into the chest. (See **Figure 33.9a through c.**)

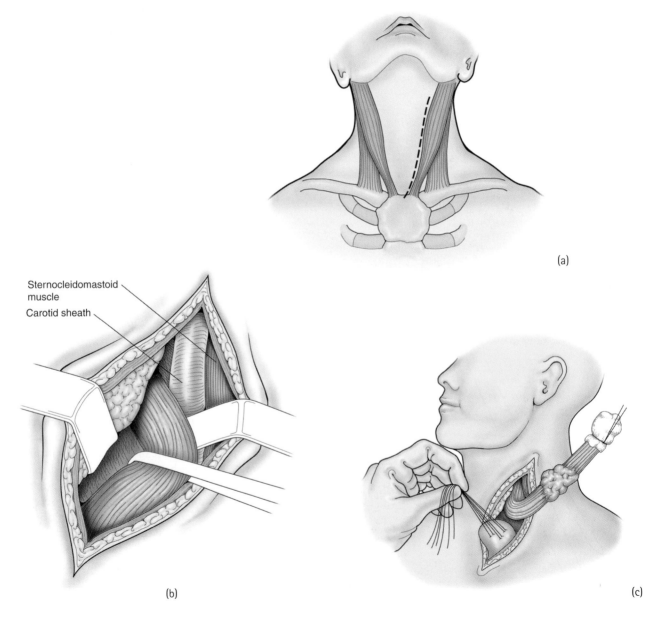

(a)

Sternocleidomastoid muscle

Carotid sheath

(b)

(c)

33.9a–c

ANASTOMOSIS IN THE NECK

10. A small incision is made in the fundus of the stomach and the esophagus is transected at an adequate level. An end-to-side anastomosis is performed between the two organs, using two layers of interrupted 4-0 silk sutures, as described earlier. The fundus of the stomach is then returned to the chest so that the completed anastomosis lies comfortably in the lower part of the incision. The stomach is anchored to surrounding tissue with three stitches at the lowest level of the incision to lessen tension on the anastomosis and to prevent gastric content entering the thorax if leakage should occur. A soft drainage tube is put around the anastomosis before the neck is closed in layers with silk sutures. (See **Figure 33.10a through c.**)

POSTOPERATIVE CARE AND OUTCOME

A nasogastric tube is placed and kept until the fourth or fifth postoperative day, when gastrointestinal function usually recovers. Artificial ventilation is not used routinely unless respiratory failure occurs. Intravenous fluids are limited to 3 L every 24 hours. The chest drain is removed on the third day. Oral fluids are commenced on the fifth or sixth day, with 100 mL water every second hour, followed by 200 mL on the eighth day when the intravenous infusion is discontinued. Feeding then progresses gradually to semisolid and solid diets, and a routine barium swallow is obtained before discharge, which is usually on the tenth postoperative day.

Complications related to the reconstruction are uncommon, but include leaks and, occasionally, complete disruption. Anastomotic leakage is easily demonstrated by swallowing methylene blue, which can be seen to drain from the drainage tube. Fasting is not considered necessary for patients with cervical leaks. The area of leakage is dressed, applying mild local pressure to prevent the further leakage of swallowed food and gastric juice. By contrast, intrathoracic leakage usually leads to severe infection, fluid imbalance, and malnutrition. Treatment usually involves adequate control of infection, thorough drainage of the thoracic cavity, maintenance of nutrition, and correction of fluid imbalance. Although parenteral nutrition has been used increasingly in recent years, the preferred current method is feeding jejunostomy.

Another complication related to the operation is chylothorax. The management of chylothorax is still a challenge, although it is an uncommon complication. Chylous output of less than 1000 mL/d is managed conservatively by drainage of the thorax and maintenance of nutrition. When daily output of chyle is more than 1000 mL, with no decrease after 4–5 days' observation, reoperation is performed with ligation of the thoracic duct. Supradiaphragmatic ligation of the main thoracic duct is undertaken routinely in Fourth Hospital, Hebei Medical University, as part of esophagectomy for cancer to prevent postoperative chylothorax.

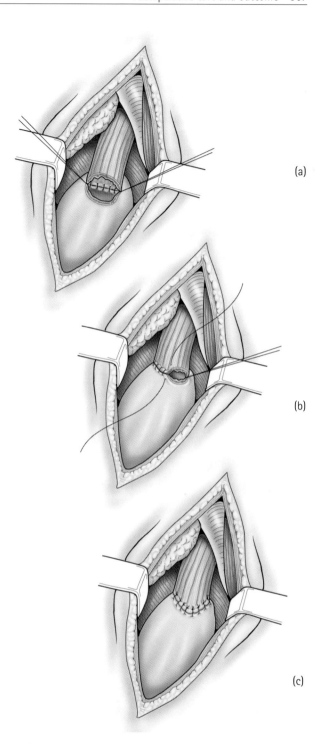

(a)

(b)

(c)

33.10a–c

Other common complications occurring before discharge are pulmonary infections, cardiovascular complications, and emphysema. These complications are easily diagnosed and the patients are likely to recover with appropriate treatment. Late complications are uncommon, but include anastomotic stricture and recurrence, which are treated by dilatation, intubation, or radiotherapy, as appropriate.

Using the approach described here, the author's unit has undertaken 20 000 esophagectomies in the past 53 years, in which the postoperative mortality rate was 2.0%. In the past 5 years, the author's unit has undertaken 4337 esophagectomies and the postoperative mortality rate was 0.76%.

FURTHER READING

Liu JF, Wang QZ, Hou J. Surgical treatment for cancer of the esophagus and gastric cardia in Hebei, China. *Br J Surg.* 2004; 91: 90–8.

Ma J, Zhan C, Wang L, Jiang W, Zhang Y, Shi Y, Wang Q. The Sweet approach is still worthwhile in modern esophagectomy. *Ann Thorac Surg.* 2014; 97: 1728–33.

Song L, Liu Y, Wang Z, Ren WG, Liu XY. Curative effect comparison between Ivor-Lewis esophagectomy and left transthoracic esophagectomy in treatment of middle thoracic esophagus carcinoma. *Hepatogastroenterology.* 2012; 59: 738–41.

Stiles BM, Altorki NK. Traditional techniques of esophagectomy. *Surg Clin North Am.* 2012; 92: 1249–63.

Takeno S, Takahashi Y, Ono K, Moroga T, Yamana I, Maki K, Shiroshita T, Kawahara K, Yamashita Y. Surgical resection for cancer located mainly in the lower esophagus. *Hepatogastroenterology.* 2013; 60: 1955–60.

34

Transhiatal esophagectomy

BRECHTJE A. GROTENHUIS, BAS P. L. WIJNHOVEN, AND J. JAN B. VAN LANSCHOT

INTRODUCTION

It is widely recognized that a surgical procedure such as esophagectomy has lower mortality and morbidity rates when performed in high volume centers. Nevertheless, esophagectomy is still associated with a substantial operative risk. For a continuous improvement of outcomes, optimization of the surgical approach for patients with esophageal cancer has been the focus of many studies over the last years.

Two major surgical approaches in case of esophagectomy for cancer have emerged in the past decades: (1) a more limited surgical procedure with regional lymphadenectomy only (transhiatal esophagectomy—THE), and (2) radical esophagectomy with extended lymphadenectomy (transthoracic esophagectomy—TTE). THE was first performed in 1933 by the British surgeon Turner, by blunt dissection and pull-through of the esophagus. In the decades thereafter, THE was not popularized because the transthoracic approach was preferred after the introduction of general anesthesia and artificial ventilation techniques that made chest surgery feasible. In 1978, Orringer and Sloan described their initial series of blunt THE, after which interest in the procedure was rekindled.

WHEN TO PERFORM A TRANSHIATAL ESOPHAGECTOMY

THE, with regional lymphadenectomy only, primarily aims for minimal surgical trauma and thus for improvement of short-term outcome by means of decreased morbidity and mortality. On the contrary, TTE aims to improve locoregional control and long-term survival by performing a wide excision of the tumor in combination with an *en bloc* lymph node dissection in both the posterior mediastinum and the upper abdomen. A well-recognized advantage of an extended resection is improved pathological lymph node

staging, leading to a potential shift from falsely node-negative patients to correctly node-positive patients: the so-called stage migration. Many studies have been published comparing the two open procedures (THE versus TTE) with regard to postoperative morbidity and mortality, long-term survival, and staging of the tumor.

Short–term outcome: postoperative morbidity and mortality

RANDOMIZED CONTROLLED TRIALS

Few randomized studies have been conducted comparing both open surgical techniques for esophageal cancer. Most studies included a limited number of patients (between 29 and 67 subjects). However, Hulscher et al. performed a large randomized two-center trial (the "Dutch trial"). Patients with adenocarcinoma of the mid-/distal esophagus or adenocarcinoma of the gastric cardia substantially involving the distal esophagus were randomly assigned to TTE with two-field lymphadenectomy (N = 114) or limited THE (N = 106). Perioperative morbidity was higher after TTE; in particular, pulmonary complications were seen more often in patients who underwent TTE (57% after TTE versus 27% after THE, $p < .001$). There was no difference with regard to in-hospital mortality (4% after TTE versus 2% after THE, $p = .45$).

META-ANALYSES

Three meta-analyses of the English-language literature comparing TTE with THE for carcinoma of the esophagus and/or the gastroesophageal junction have been published. These studies give an overview of the randomized controlled trials (RCTs), comparative cohort studies, and case series. The meta-analyses are summarized in **Table 34.1**.

In the most recent meta-analysis, studies until 2010 were analyzed, including the Dutch RCT. According to this review, TTE took a mean of 85 minutes longer than THE ($p < .001$).

Table 34.1 The results of three meta-analyses with regard to the short- and long-term outcome after esophagectomy for cancer

Meta-analysis	Rindani et al.	Hulscher et al.	Boshier et al.	
Pulmonary complications				
TTE	25%	18.7%	35.7%	OR 1.32; *p* = .02
THE	24%	12.7%	28.0%	CI 1.05–1.66
Cardiac complications				
TTE	10.5%	6.6%	–	OR 1.03; *p* = .86
THE	12.4%	19.5%	–	CI 0.77–1.37
Anastomotic leakage				
TTE	10.0%	7.2%	10.6%	OR 0.69, *p* = .005
THE	60.0%	13.6%	16.9%	CI 0.53–0.89
Vocal cord paralysis				
TTE	4.8%	3.5%	5.6%	OR 0.57, *p* = .005
THE	11.2%	9.5%	10.9%	CI 0.38–0.84
*Mortality**				
TTE	9.5%	9.2%	10.6%	OR 1.48, *p* = .001
THE	6.3%	5.7%	7.2%	CI 1.20–1.83
*Survival***				
TTE	26.0%	23.0%	26.6%	OR = 1.03, *p* = .84
THE	24.0%	21.7%	25.8%	CI 0.80–1.32

Notes: *Mortality rate is defined as either <30 days postoperatively or in-hospital mortality. **Survival is defined as overall 5-year survival. OR, odds ratio; CI, confidence interval.

There was no significant difference in blood loss. The postoperative length of hospital stay in patients who underwent THE was, on average, 4 days less than in patients who underwent TTE ($p < .01$). TTE was associated with a higher risk of respiratory complications (36% after TTE versus 28% after THE, $p = .02$), but not with an increased cardiac risk ($p = .86$). Vocal cord paralysis and anastomotic leakage were more frequent after THE. The mortality rate, defined as 30-day mortality or in-hospital mortality, was significantly higher after TTE (odds ratio 1.48, 95% confidence interval 1.20–1.83, $p = 0.001$).

Long-term outcome: survival

RANDOMIZED CONTROLLED TRIALS

The Dutch trial did not detect a statistically significant difference in survival, but it is possible this was a type II statistical error. After TTE and THE 5-year survival rates were 36% and 34%, respectively ($p = 0.71$). In a subgroup analysis based on the location of the primary tumor, no overall survival benefit for either surgical approach was seen in 115 patients with a type II junctional tumor (TTE 27% versus THE 31%, $p = 0.81$). However, although not statistically significant, an absolute survival benefit of 14% was seen in patients with a type I esophageal tumor with the transthoracic approach (51% versus 37%, $p = 0.33$). In patients (N = 55) without positive nodes, locoregional disease-free survival after THE was comparable to that after TTE (86% and 89%, respectively). The same was true for patients (N = 46) with more than eight

positive nodes (0% in both groups). However, patients (N = 104) with one to eight positive lymph nodes in the resection specimen showed a 5-year disease-free survival advantage if operated via the transthoracic route (TTE 64% versus THE 23%, $p = 0.02$). It was concluded that there was no significant overall survival benefit for either approach, but TTE with extended lymphadenectomy for patients with type I esophageal adenocarcinoma, particularly when there were a limited number of positive lymph nodes in their resection specimen, showed an ongoing trend toward better 5-year survival.

META-ANALYSES

There was no significant difference in long-term survival between TTE and THE resections in all three meta-analyses (see **Table 34.1**).

Effect on staging and the role of neoadjuvant chemoradiotherapy

TTE with extended lymphadenectomy may offer better insight in the lymphatic dissemination of tumor cells. Dissecting more lymph nodes increases the chance of finding a tumor-positive node, which may influence pathological staging (stage migration). On the contrary, due to a limited regional lymphadenectomy with the inferior pulmonary veins as the most cranial extension of the mediastinal lymphadenectomy, patients who undergo THE may be falsely staged as node-negative when positive nodes in the upper and middle part of the chest have not been dissected. The

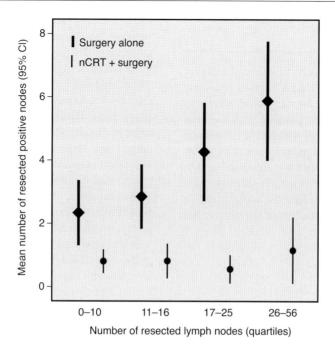

34.1 Correlation between number of resected nodes (quartiles) and mean number (95% confidence interval [CI]) of resected positive nodes in patients who underwent surgery alone (N = 161) or neoadjuvant chemoradiotherapy (nCRT) followed by surgery (N = 159). (Adapted from Talsma AK, Shapiro J, Looman CW, van Hagen P, Steyerberg EW, van der Gaast A, van Berge Henegouwen MI et al. *Ann Surg.* 260, 786–793, 2014. With permission.)

diagnostic yield of an extended lymphadenectomy has been studied. Some 37% of patients who underwent TTE showed tumor-positive nodes in extended fields. Extended resection led to tumor upstaging in 23% of patients; however, this was mainly due to positive nodes at the celiac trunk (20%), which can also be effectively resected during THE.

Proponents of an extended resection with *en bloc* lymphadenectomy argued that the number of removed lymph nodes appeared to be an independent predictor of survival after esophagectomy for cancer. However, in the light of the recently published large multicenter RCT by van Hagen et al., which showed that preoperative chemoradiotherapy (CRT) improves survival, one can question whether these findings are still valid. Besides a high pathologically complete response rate of 29% and a significantly higher rate of complete R0 resection after preoperative CRT, it was found that this neoadjuvant regime frequently leads to sterilization of locoregional lymph nodes. Lymph node positivity in the resection specimen was found in 50 patients (31%) after CRT, as compared with 120 patients (75%) in the surgery-alone group ($p < .001$).

Since this trial was published, it has been questioned whether extended lymphadenectomy after neoadjuvant CRT is still indicated for prognostic and/or therapeutic reasons. A more recent study in the same randomized study population explored the association between the total number of resected nodes and survival in patients with or without

neoadjuvant CRT. In the surgery-alone group, a positive association was identified between number of resected nodes and number of resected positive nodes. However, this association was absent in patients treated with neoadjuvant CRT followed by surgery (see **Figure 34.1**). More important, total number of resected nodes was significantly associated with survival for patients in the surgery-alone arm (hazard ratio [HR] = 0.76; $p = .007$), but not in the multimodality arm (HR = 1.00; $p = .98$). These data question the indication for maximization of lymphadenectomy after neoadjuvant CRT.

Conclusion

After the Dutch RCT (TTE versus THE), transthoracic resection has been considered the standard surgical treatment, especially for type I esophageal tumors in patients who are fit to undergo a transthoracic dissection and who have suspected lymph nodes on clinical pretreatment staging. However, after the publication of the latest meta-analysis, in which no differences were shown with regard to long-term survival between TTE and THE, and after the implementation of neoadjuvant CRT with its sterilizing effect on locoregional lymph nodes, the indication for extended lymphadenectomy by means of TTE is again open to debate. Therefore, THE may reattain its popularity in the near future.

HOW TO PERFORM A TRANSHIATAL ESOPHAGECTOMY

Preoperatively, the anesthetist places an epidural catheter and intravenous antibiotic prophylaxis is given routinely between 15 and 30 minutes before the start of the operation. The patient is placed in the supine position with the neck slightly extended and the head tilted toward the right. Both arms are padded and placed at the patient's side. The sterile field extends from the mandibles to the pubic bone and to both midaxillary lines. THE is performed in three separate phases: the abdominal, the cervical, and the anastomotic or completion phases. Note that this section of the chapter has partly been adapted from Orringer.

Abdominal phase

The abdominal phase of the operation is performed through a midline supra-umbilical incision (see **Figure 34.2**). After exploring the abdomen to exclude metastases that would preclude resection, the left triangular ligament of the liver is divided, and the left liver lobe is retracted to the right to allow exposure of the diaphragmatic hiatus. The location of the tumor is checked and the stomach is assessed for its suitability as an esophageal substitution. Gastric mobilization begins by gently retracting the greater omentum downward, away from the stomach, and by gently pulling the greater curvature (using the nasogastric tube) in order to facilitate

identification of the gastroepiploic vessels. The lesser sac is entered through an avascular area of the omentum. The left gastroepiploic and short gastric vessels are divided between long clamps or high energy devices (LigaSure or Ultracision) and ligated along the high greater curvature of the stomach. Care is taken to stay as high as possible in the splenic hilum to prevent serosal lesions of the fundus. As the omentum is then separated from the lower half of the greater curvature, clamps are applied at least 2 cm below the right gastroepiploic artery and vein to ensure that these vessels are not injured during gastric mobilization. Then attention is directed toward the lesser curvature. The gastrohepatic part of the lesser omentum is incised; caution is taken of an aberrant left hepatic artery, which must be sacrificed if present. The left gastric vein and artery are identified and ligated, the latter is ligated at its origin from the celiac trunk, while carefully dissecting lymph nodes along the common hepatic artery and splenic artery. The first part of the right gastric artery is identified and protected during mobilization of the lesser curvature. Sometimes it is necessary to mobilize the duodenum by the Kocher maneuver to obtain maximum upward reach of the mobilized stomach. In some patients, it can be easier to first create the gastric tube prior to peritumoral dissection

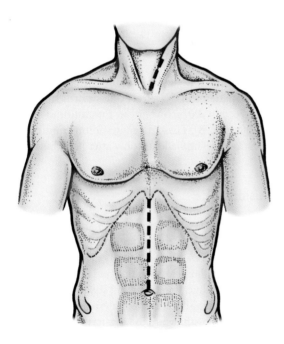

34.2 The abdominal phase of the operation is performed through a midline supra-umbilical incision; the cervical phase through an oblique incision parallel to the anterior border of the left sternocleidomastoid muscle.

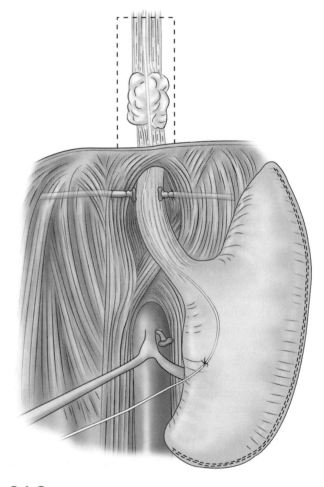

34.3 After widening of the esophageal hiatus, the lower esophagus is mobilized under direct vision up to the level of the inferior pulmonary vein (dotted line).

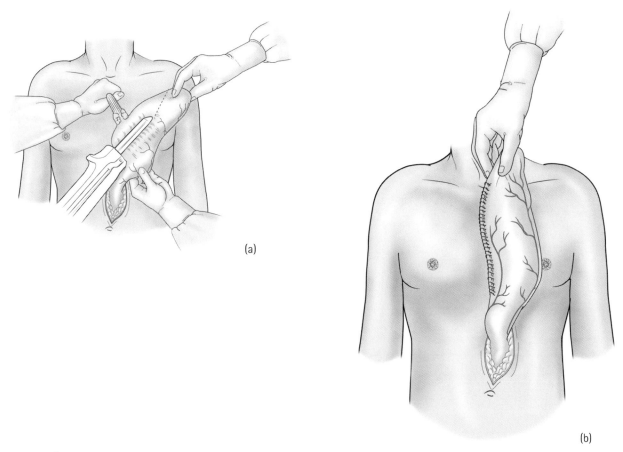

(a)

(b)

34.4a–b Creation of a 3–5 cm wide gastric tube by using a longitudinal stapling device (a). The gastric staple line is oversewn with running sutures, especially to cover the fragile sites between the applied stapler cartridges (b).

(see later in section). However, this should only be done in patients in whom local irresectability is not suspected, based on preoperative clinical staging.

The peritoneum overlying the gastroesophageal junction is next incised and the left and right pillar of the right crus are identified. The left diaphragmatic vein is ligated and the hiatus is widened by incising the fibrous central part of the diaphragm anteriorly. A narrow Deaver retractor placed into the hiatus anteriorly and a Mark retractor placed behind the right pillar facilitate exposure of the lower esophagus, which is mobilized under direct vision along with all periesophageal fatty tissue and adjacent lymph nodes. The distal 10 cm of the esophagus and paraesophageal soft tissues are progressively mobilized from the pericardium and bilateral pleurae under direct vision. While retracting the esophagus downward by one hand, sharp mobilization of the esophagus to the level of the inferior pulmonary vein is performed (dotted line in **Figure 34.3**). Mobility of the esophagus within the posterior mediastinum is assessed through the hiatus by moving the esophagus from side to side to determine if fixation to the prevertebral fascia, aorta, or adjacent mediastinal tissues is present. With the left hand inserted through the widened hiatus behind the esophagus, sharp dissection of the dorsal interpleural ligament is performed. In this stage of the

operation, the thoracic duct can be encountered; to avoid injury to the thoracic duct, one should operate on the ventral side of the aorta only. At a higher level, a clamped small gauze into the inferior mediastinum may facilitate dissection, gently sweeping away periesophageal attachments. Dissection from below is continued up to at least 2–3 cm above the proximal border of the tumor. During this mediastinal part of the operation, careful monitoring of the blood pressure is necessary to avoid prolonged hypotension that can result from cardiac displacement and obstructed venous return. Vagal branches can now be palpated along the mid-esophagus, and, either bluntly or under direct vision, they are transected, allowing further longitudinal mobilization of the esophagus.

Attention is then turned toward preparing the stomach for its transposition into the chest. The lesser curvature of the stomach is cleared by dividing the right gastric vessels and fat 1–2 cm below the level of the crow's foot. A longitudinal stapling device with a 60 mm cartridge is then applied, beginning at this point on the lesser curvature and proceeding toward the gastric tip, thereby preserving the gastric fundus. Each time the stapler is removed, traction is applied to the gastric fundus to allow the stomach to be straightened progressively so that its cephalad reach is maximized. A 3–5 cm wide gastric tube is now created (see **Figure 34.4a and b**).

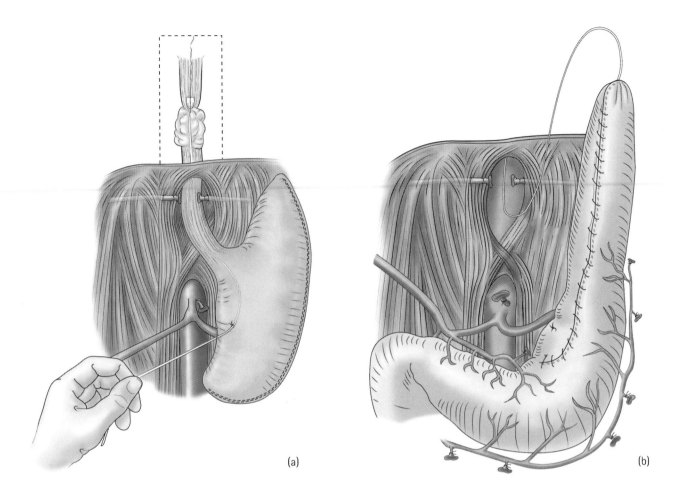

(a)   (b)

34.5a–b   After transection of the cervical esophagus, a vein stripper is inserted into the distal part of the cervical esophagus and pushed downward, until its tip can be released from the intra-abdominal cardia. A shoelace is fixed to the distal part of the transected esophagus, followed by stripping of the thoracic esophagus. The esophagus invaginates while pulling the stripper distally (a). Fixation of the shoelace to the tip of the gastric tube, after which the gastric tube will be pulled/pushed up into the neck. The gastric tube receives its vascularization from the right gastroepiploic artery and vein (b).

The gastric staple suture line is oversewn with running PDS (polydioxanone) sutures, especially to cover the fragile sites between the applied stapler cartridges.

Cervical phase

An 8 cm oblique cervical incision parallel to the anterior border of the left sternocleidomastoid muscle is performed (see **Figure 34.2**). The platysma is incised and the sternocleido-mastoid muscle, internal jugular vein, and carotid sheath are gently retracted laterally. The omohyoid muscle is transected. The larynx and trachea are retracted medially using the fingers of the assistant or a clamped small gauze only; no metal retractor is placed against the tracheoesophageal groove so that the risk of recurrent laryngeal nerve injury is minimized. The middle thyroid vein and inferior thyroid artery are identified and ligated. The dissection is carried out directly posteriorly on to the prevertebral fascia, which is followed

bluntly with the index finger into the superior mediastinum. Then the plane between trachea and esophagus is developed further. The cervical esophagus is bluntly mobilized from adjacent tissues circumferentially, with particular care taken not to injure the posterior membranous part of the trachea, and encircled with a vessel loop. With upward traction on this vessel loop, blunt mobilization of the upper esophagus from the superior mediastinum is carried out, with the fingers kept at the esophagus at all times. A clamped small gauze can be helpful for onward blunt dissection. No formal cervical lymphadenectomy is carried out. The cervical esophagus is transected and a vein stripper is inserted and pushed downward until the tip can be released from the intra-abdominal cardia. A shoelace is fixed to the distal part of the transected cervical esophagus (see **Figure 34.5a**). A gallbladder clamp is placed on the distal margin of the cardia and is gently pulled downward to induce a slight tension on the specimen.

Stepwise, the normal part of the thoracic esophagus proximal to the tumor (the tumor itself has already been fully

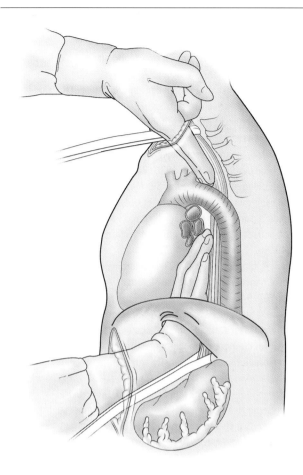

34.6 In case more length of the esophageal remnant is needed, a complete manual mobilization of the esophagus is required.

dissected from below under direct vision) is now invaginated by gentle traction with the right hand on the distal end of the stripper (see **Figure 34.5a**). Meanwhile, the left hand is put into the mediastinum for tactile control. If still intact, both vagal trunks are cut with a long pair of scissors at the level of the carina. In case of an obstructive tumor, the tip of the stripper should be kept above its proximal border to prevent rupture with potential spill. Finally, the specimen can be removed and sent out for histopathological examination. If the left and/or right pleural cavity have been opened, uni- or bilateral chest tubes are inserted with the tips dorsocaudally in the pleural sinus. The distal end of the shoelace is now fixed to the tip of the gastric tube (see **Figure 34.5b**). However, if a side-to-side semimechanical cervical anastomosis is preferred, more length of the esophageal remnant is needed, requiring a complete manual mobilization of the esophagus rather than using the vein stripper (see **Figure 34.6**).

Completion of the operation

By pulling the shoelace, the gastric tube is pushed upward in the prevertebral plane and brought out in the cervical wound.

Esophagogastrostomy is performed in the neck, and either an end-to-end, an end-to-side, or a side-to-side anastomosis is accomplished. With regard to the detailed operation technique required for this anastomosis, we refer readers to Chapter 29, "Esophageal anastomoses: sutured and stapled." The construction of the anastomosis can be hand sewn, stapled, or semimechanical. Until recently, the hand-sewn end-to-end anastomosis was our standard of care; however, results of our currently underway RCT comparing the semimechanical side-to-side anastomosis with the hand-sewn end-to-end anastomosis are awaited. A nasojejunal feeding tube, as well as a nasogastric decompression tube, are inserted and their correct position verified. The diaphragmatic hiatus is again narrowed by a couple of stitches to prevent intrathoracic herniation of the bowel. Final inspection for bleeding is recommended. Closure of the abdominal and cervical incisions will end the operation. Preferably, the patient is extubated in the operating theatre, which is almost always feasible.

Postoperative course

In general, patients are admitted to the intensive care unit (ICU) for early postoperative monitoring. After 24 hours in ICU, patients can usually be transferred to the ward, where early mobilization is commenced under the guidance of a physiotherapist. Analgesia is taken care of by the thoracic epidural catheter; its main goal, besides sufficient pain management, is to prevent respiratory complications such as pneumonia. Enteral feeding via the nasojejunal feeding tube is started slowly and is increased daily. The nasogastric tube is removed at day 2 postoperatively if its production is less than 200 mL/24 h. Chest tubes are removed when the production is below 150 mL/24 h. After 5 days, the patient is allowed to drink water, and if there are no clinical signs of leakage, diet is progressively advanced from a liquid to a soft diet. A radiological oral contrast examination or an endoscopy is only performed when anastomotic leakage is suspected clinically.

A recent development in gastrointestinal surgery is the implementation of enhanced recovery after surgery (ERAS) programs. Evidence regarding the benefit of these programs in patients undergoing esophageal surgery is scarce; one study showed that the implementation of ERAS items (preoperative nutrition, early extubation, early removal of nasogastric tube, and early mobilization) was feasible, but did not lead to a significant reduction in overall morbidity in that cohort of patients.

VIDEO LINK

Link to a video providing a summary of an open THE performed in the Erasmus University Medical Center, Rotterdam, The Netherlands: http://www.erasmusmc.nl/chirurgie/AbdominaleChirurgie/ziektebeeldenabdominalechirurgie/slokdarm/4774709/.

FURTHER READING

Blom RL, van Heijl M, Bemelman WA, Hollmann MW, Klinkenbijl JH, Busch OR, van Berge Henegouwen MI. Initial experiences of an enhanced recovery protocol in esophageal surgery. *World J Surg.* 2013; 37: 2372–8.

Boshier PR, Anderson O, Hanna GB. Transthoracic versus transhiatal esophagectomy for the treatment of esophagogastric cancer: a meta-analysis. *Ann Surg.* 2011; 254: 894–906.

Grey Turner GG. Excision of thoracic esophagus for carcinoma with construction of extrathoracic gullet. *Lancet.* 1933; 222: 1315–16.

Hulscher JB, Tijssen JG, Obertop H, van Lanschot JJ. Transthoracic versus transhiatal resection for carcinoma of the esophagus: a meta-analysis. *Ann Thorac Surg.* 2001; 72: 306–13.

Hulscher JB, van Sandick JW, de Boer AG, Wijnhoven BP, Tijssen JG, Fockens P, Stalmeier PF et al. Extended transthoracic resection compared with limited transhiatal resection for adenocarcinoma of the esophagus. *N Engl J Med.* 2002; 347: 1662–9.

Hulscher JB, van Sandick JW, Offerhaus GJ, Tilanus HW, Obertop H, van Lanschot JJ. Prospective analysis of the diagnostic yield of extended en bloc resection for adenocarcinoma of the oesophagus or gastric cardia. *Br J Surg.* 2001; 88: 715–19.

Nederlof N, Tilanus HW, Tran TC, Hop WC, Wijnhoven BP, De de Jonge J. End-to-end versus end-to-side esophagogastrostomy after esophageal cancer resection: a prospective randomized study. *Ann Surg.* 2011; 254: 226–33.

Omloo JM, Lagarde SM, Hulscher JB, Reitsma JB, Fockens P, van Dekken H, Ten Kate FJ, Obertop H, Tilanus HW, van Lanschot JJ. Extended transthoracic resection compared with limited transhiatal resection for adenocarcinoma of the mid/distal esophagus: five-year survival of a randomized clinical trial. *Ann Surg.* 2007; 246: 992–1000.

Orringer MB. Transhiatal esophagectomy. In: Kaiser LR, Jamieson GG, eds., *Operative Thoracic Surgery*, 5th edition. Transhiatal esophagectomy. CRC Press (Boca Raton, Florida), 2006; pp. 397–412.

Orringer MB, Sloan H. Esophagectomy without thoracotomy. *J Thorac Cardiovasc Surg.* 1978; 76: 643–54.

Peyre CG, Hagen JA, DeMeester SR, Altorki NK, Ancona E, Griffin SM, Hölscher A et al. The number of lymph nodes removed predicts survival in esophageal cancer: an international study on the impact of extent of surgical resection. *Ann Surg.* 2008; 248: 549–56.

Rindani R, Martin CJ, Cox MR. Transhiatal versus Ivor-Lewis oesophagectomy: is there a difference? *Aust N Z J Surg.* 1999; 69: 187–94.

Talsma AK, Shapiro J, Looman CW, van Hagen P, Steyerberg EW, van der Gaast A, van Berge Henegouwen MI et al. Lymph node retrieval during esophagectomy with and without neoadjuvant chemoradiotherapy; prognostic and therapeutic impact on survival. *Ann Surg.* 2014; 260: 786–93.

van Hagen P, Hulshof MC, van Lanschot JJ, Steyerberg EW, van Berge Henegouwen MI, Wijnhoven BP, Richel DJ et al. Preoperative chemoradiotherapy for esophageal or junctional cancer. *N Engl J Med.* 2012; 366: 2074–84.

Thoracoscopic and laparoscopic esophagectomy

B. MARK SMITHERS, IAIN THOMSON, AND ANDREW BARBOUR

INTRODUCTION

Minimally invasive esophagectomy (MIE) has become an established option in the approach to esophageal resection and reconstruction for cancer. Technical and oncological outcomes are similar to those of open surgery, with evidence for improved respiratory outcomes with the MIE approach. The resection may be performed as a total MIE or there may be a combination of open and minimally invasive approaches (hybrid). The approach is used for cancers of the esophagus and gastroesophageal junction (GEJ). In our unit, the decision with respect to approach relates to the site of the primary cancer. The three-field dissection is suitable for cancers restricted to the esophagus. The two-field, Ivor Lewis, approach is used for cancers of the mid/lower and GEJ where there is gastric involvement that requires a proximal gastric resection that will not leave enough stomach for a neck anastomosis. The open approaches to the thoracic esophagus, including mobilization of the stomach to construct the gastric conduit, are described elsewhere (see Chapter 32, "Abdominal and right thoracic esophagectomy" and Chapter 33, "Left thoracic subtotal esophagectomy").

The laparoscopic gastric mobilization can be performed as the first phase of an Ivor Lewis approach with the chest performed open or thoracoscopically. It can be performed as the second phase of a three-field resection when the thoracoscopic component is the first phase and a cervical anastomosis is performed. Initially, we will describe laparoscopic gastric mobilization as the first phase of an Ivor Lewis resection, and then, as part of a three-phase thoracoscopic esophageal mobilization with a gastric conduit taken to the neck. Then we will describe the prone thoracoscopic approach used for a three-phase procedure and finally the thoracoscopic approach for an Ivor Lewis procedure with an intrathoracic anastomosis.

Patients have a double lumen endotracheal tube inserted to allow single-left lung ventilation, although a single lumen endotracheal tube may be used with carbon dioxide (CO_2) pneumothorax, with the insufflation pressures set at 7 mmHg.

LAPAROSCOPIC GASTRIC MOBILIZATION
(see **Figure 35.1**)

The patient is positioned in the reverse Trendelenburg position, with the table tilted 20–30 degrees head up. The legs are extended in stirrups with minimal hip flexion. The surgeon

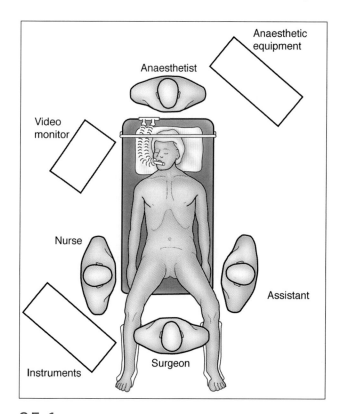

35.1

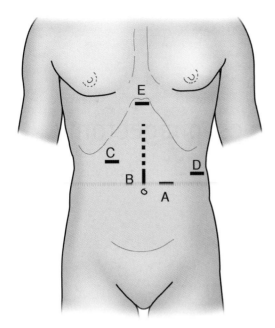

35.2

and Fridley, Minnesota, United States) to identify and enter the lesser sac. Visualizing the gastroepiploic arcade, the dissection is taken proximally, maintaining the arcade. Short gastric branches are taken, leaving a minimum of a 3 cm cuff of omentum to ensure collateral vessels to the fundus are preserved. We also prefer to leave sufficient omentum to wrap the anastomosis if it is to be performed in the chest. The gastric fundus is mobilized to the right, identifying the left crus of the diaphragm. A cuff of crural muscle is taken if the cancer is in the lower esophagus or GEJ. This dissection also clears the tissue above the pancreas toward the left side of the left gastric artery.

Now the dissection is taken distally. The right gastroepiploic origin will become obvious along the inferior margin of the pancreas. Omental branches are divided to allow the duodenum to become mobile. The posterior stomach is mobilized and the posterior pylorus mobilized to the gastroduodenal artery. Adhesions around the duodenum are divided to ensure that the pylorus will mobilize to the hiatus.

stands between the legs and there is an assistant who holds the camera standing on the patient's left. The video monitor is to the left of the head of the table at the level of the patient's shoulder.

Trocar placement (see Figure 35.2)

The initial port is either a 12 mm Hasson cannula placed by a cut down or an optical port placement in the midclavicular line between the umbilicus and the left costal margin. The abdomen is insufflated to a pressure of 12 mmHg. Following the insertion of a 30-degree laparoscope, a 12 mm port is inserted above the umbilicus (B). Two 5 mm ports are placed in the right upper quadrant (C), the left lateral abdomen (D), and a 5 mm incision is made in the epigastrium to place a Nathanson liver retractor (Cook Group Incorporated, Bloomington, Indiana, United States). If the gastric tube is to be fashioned intracorporeally, then the right upper quadrant port (C) should be 12 mm, rather than 5 mm. The dotted line on **Figure 35.2** is the site of an incision if the plan is to create a gastric tube extracorporeally. The supra-umbilical port incision is extended as a midline incision, measuring 6 cm.

Mobilization of the greater curve of the stomach

The gastroepiploic arcade is identified and carefully preserved. Omental branches are divided with either the Harmonic scalpel (Ethicon, U.S., LLC, Somerville, New Jersey, United States) or LigaSure (Covidien, Medtronic, Dublin, Ireland,

Dissection of the hiatus and division of the left gastric vascular pedicle

The gastro-hepatic ligament is divided and the right crus of the diaphragm incised, leaving crural muscle and pleura on the esophagus if a lower or GEJ cancer. The dissection is carried anteriorly to dissect the fat pad from the pericardium.

Now attention returns to the posterior stomach and the left gastric pedicle is defined. The nodal tissue over the common hepatic artery (station 8a) is mobilized from the artery with the Harmonic shears (Ethicon, U.S., LLC). This is dissected toward the vascular pedicle to define the left gastric vein, which is divided between clips. The nodal tissue is dissected proximally (station 9), and the left gastric artery is defined. It is dissected clear on the left side. The nodal tissue above the proximal splenic artery (station 11) is dissected to expose the left side of the left gastric artery. This is divided between clips or by using a laparoscopic stapling device. A pyloromyotomy can be performed if considered necessary.

The dissection returns to the hiatus and is carried proximally into the mediastinum. If required, the pleura on one or both sides can be removed. The anesthetist should be informed that the pleura has been breached, as tension pneumothorax can occur when there is only a small hole made in the pleura (due to flap valve formation), prior to more formal pleural resection. The dissection will meet a prior thoracoscopic dissection if a three-phase procedure, or alternatively, if this is the first phase of a two-phase dissection, the dissection is taken as high as possible around the esophagus under direct vision. An intercostal catheter with underwater sealed drainage may be necessary if the pleura on the left side is resected. Tube drainage of the left chest is often not necessary and the use of left chest drainage can be guided by surgeon preference.

Gastric conduit construction as phase one of two-phase procedure (Ivor Lewis) (see Figure 35.3)

The lesser curve is cleared by the shears above the level of the vascular "crow's foot" and the stomach is divided by endo-staplers, aiming for a 4–5 cm margin distal to the cancer. At this stage, the gastric conduit can be formed totally intra-corporeally or via a small midline laparotomy abdominal incision (see **Figure 35.2**). If intracorporeal, the division is taken toward the greater curve but not completed to allow the stomach to be pulled into the mediastinum. The gastric tube should be at least 6 cm in diameter. Care should be taken to preserve all attached omentum so that it may be used later to wrap around the anastomosis in the chest. A feeding jejunostomy can be constructed laparoscopically or via a small 3–4 cm incision having identified the appropriate jejunal segment laparoscopically.

If the conduit is formed via a midline minilaparotomy, a 5–6 cm incision is extended from the supra-umbilical port (see **Figure 35.2**). This minilaparotomy is used to fashion the feeding jejunostomy. A nylon tape (or equivalent) should then be sutured to the proximal end of the gastric conduit (fundus) with a heavy suture (such as 0 Monocril). The conduit is then placed back into the abdomen, paying careful attention to maintain normal anatomical lie of the stomach. The nylon tape is then placed high into the right chest through the hiatus for retrieval during the thoracoscopic chest phase.

The feeding jejunostomy is then formed and secured to the abdominal wall, and the incision is closed.

Gastric mobilization as phase II of a thoracoscopic, laparoscopic mobilization with cervical anastomosis (see Figure 35.4)

If the patient is having a three-field resection, the esophagus will have been divided in the neck and a tape will have been attached. The esophagus is pulled into the abdomen with the attached tape. A small epigastric incision is made above the umbilicus (see **Figure 35.2**—dotted line) and a retraction device is placed to retract and to protect the wound. The stomach and esophagus are delivered to construct the gastric tube. The gastric tube is constructed by dividing the tissue on the lesser curve above the crow's foot region. The stomach is extended and divided with a linear stapling device, allowing a suitable margin from the tumor if lower esophagus, and a tube 5–6 cm wide is constructed with multiple staple applications. The staple line is inverted with sutures. Bulky omental attachments are reduced, ensuring vascularity to the fundus. The tape from the neck is attached to the apex of the fundus and the gastric tube returned to the abdomen. A feeding jejunostomy can be performed at this stage through the small laparotomy wound. The abdominal wound is closed and the abdomen is inflated once more.

The gastric tube is gently fed into the hiatus while traction is placed on the tape at the neck. It is advisable to extend the crural dissection if difficulties are encountered feeding the stomach and omental attachments through the hiatus. Care is taken to ensure the gastric tube is not twisted. The gastric tube is delivered to the neck, ensuring the pylorus is just below the level of the hiatus. The cervical anastomosis is performed (see Chapter 29, "Esophageal anastomoses: sutured and stapled").

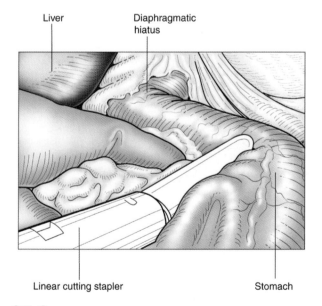

35.3

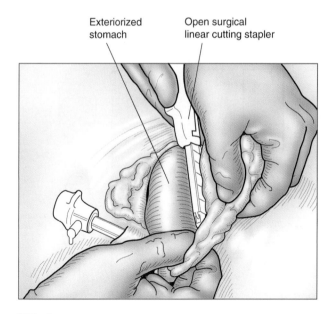

35.4

THORACOSCOPIC ESOPHAGEAL MOBILIZATION (PRONE POSITION) FOR THREE-FIELD DISSECTION

Positioning (see Figure 35.5)

The patient is positioned prone with both arms placed forward on padded arm supports. The patient's head is placed in a Mayfield headrest, two pillows placed under the shoulders and the hips with the abdomen free between. Further pillows are placed under the knees and legs to prevent any pressure areas. The surgeon stands on the patient's right side with the assistant standing on the surgeon's left-hand side. The monitor and stack are placed on the patient's left-hand side, opposite the surgeon.

Trocar placement (see Figure 35.6a and b)

A 10 mm 30-degree camera port is placed at the inferior border of the angle of the scapula. Blunt dissection is used to enter the thoracic cavity once lung deflation has been achieved via the double lumen endotracheal tube. A 10 mm port is then placed at approximately the level of the azygos arch, medial to the border of the scapula. This is the main working port for the surgeon. A 10 mm port is then placed

in the 9th or 10th intercostal space, near the post axillary line, sliding over the dome of the diaphragm—this will be the surgeon's left-hand working port and enables a stapling device to be deployed to divide the azygos arch. A further 5 mm port can be placed inferior to the superior 10 mm port to allow the assistant to retract or suction if required.

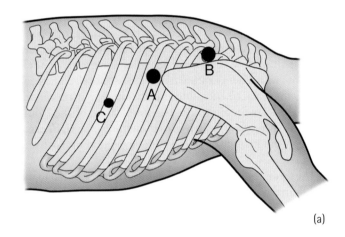

(a)

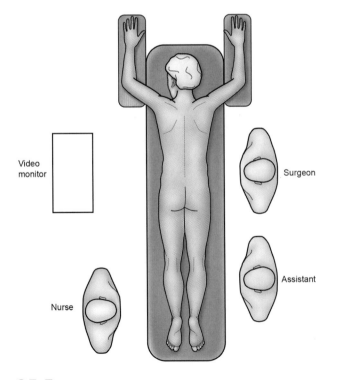

35.5

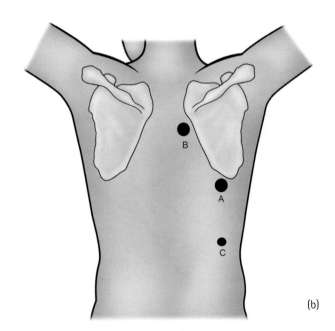

(b)

35.6a–b

Identification of landmarks and dissection of azygos arch (see Figure 35.7a and b)

The right lung should be deflated. It may be necessary to use gentle compression with blunt instruments to aid in full lung deflation. Any pleural adhesions restricting deflation need to be divided at this stage. The surgeon identifies the azygos arch, remembering the orientation in the prone position places the vertebral column superiorly, followed by the azygos vein and then the esophagus, with airway structures and the pericardium most inferior. The pleura is divided parallel to the line of the azygos arch overlying the esophagus both inferiorly and superiorly. Careful blunt dissection behind the azygos vein arch is performed, paying close attention to any small venous tributaries or bronchial vessels. Once a tunnel is developed under the vein, a laparoscopic stapling device using a vascular cartridge is placed through port C and the azygos arch is divided.

Division of pleural attachments and inferior pulmonary ligament (see Figure 35.8)

Using a hook diathermy placed through the working port (port A) and a blunt grasper through port C, the pleura is divided. The line of dissection commences at the azygos dissection toward the diaphragm. The posterior line of dissection is in the groove that lies between the superior border of the esophagus, and the azygos vein and vertebral column. The anterior line of dissection is along the pleural reflection on the lung and pericardium. This will lead to the inferior pulmonary ligament, which is divided, allowing the right lower lobe to fall away out of the field. If the dissection is to include the thoracic duct and para-aortic tissue, then the posterior line of dissection is immediately along the anterior border of the azygos vein down to the plane along the anterolateral aspect of the thoracic aorta.

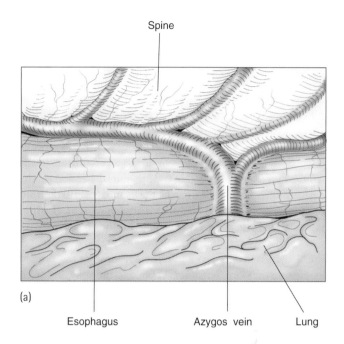

(a)

Spine

Esophagus   Azygos vein   Lung

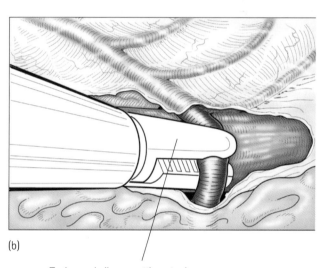

(b)

Endoscopic linear cutting stapler

35.7a–b

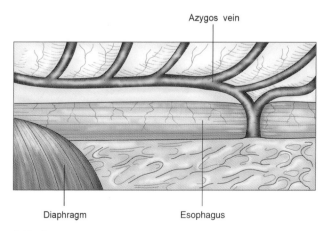

Azygos vein

Diaphragm   Esophagus

35.8

Esophageal dissection and sling retraction (see Figure 35.9)

Inferior to the subcarinal nodal package at the level of the inferior pulmonary vein, the esophagus is mobilized superiorly to identify the glistening pericardium and the dissection progresses toward the left. Between the esophagus and the aorta, with instrument retraction (not grasping) of the esophagus and a combination of hook diathermy, blunt dissection, and vascular clips to aortic arterial branches, a window is created by meeting the previous dissection on the pericardium. This space dissects the esophageal tissue from the thoracic aorta, thoracic duct, and azygos vein. A 5 mm Portex tube is then placed as a sling around the esophagus, with both ends of the sling taken out the 10 mm camera port site. The port is removed and replaced, allowing the sling to lie outside the port. Tension is applied to the sling and fixed with artery forceps.

Esophageal and subcarinal node dissection (see Figure 35.10)

The dissection around the esophagus continues distally toward the hiatus both anteriorly and posteriorly. Care is taken posteriorly to identify arterial branches from the aorta and the thoracic duct. If the thoracic duct tissue is taken *en bloc* with the specimen, it is controlled with endoscopic clips before being divided just superior to the diaphragm. The

fat pad on the pericardium is dissected to remain with the esophagus.

The dissection then continues proximally along the inferior aspect of the esophagus, with identification of the right main bronchus and trachea. There will be branches of the vagus nerve and small vessels crossing the right main bronchus. These fibers along with vessels are divided between endoscopic clips. The dissection proceeds proximally to the main trunk of the right vagus nerve, which is divided. The nodes along the medial side of the right main bronchus are mobilized away from the bronchus with a hook diathermy and vascular clips to vessels. Care is taken to avoid diathermy beside the airway structures. The dissection is extended toward the carina.

Now the esophagus is retracted toward the floor with a grasper in the surgeon's left hand. The dissection is taken proximally to mobilize the azygos vein away from the esophagus. With further deeper retraction pushing the esophagus downward, vessels and left vagal branches sweeping posterior to the left main bronchus are divided to identify the bronchus. The left main bronchus will be distended with the balloon of the endobronchial tube. Care must be taken to ensure no injury to this structure. The nodal tissue is swept away from the left main bronchus and the apex of the subcarinal nodal package is identified. This is best divided by lifting the esophagus toward the spine, placing the final strands of subcarinal tissue under tension to allow division between endo-clips.

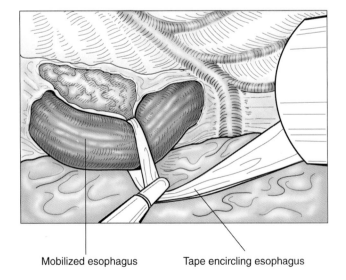

Mobilized esophagus   Tape encircling esophagus

35.9

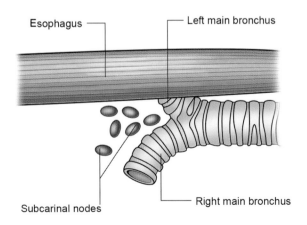

Esophagus — ⎤   ⎡ — Left main bronchus

Subcarinal nodes   Right main bronchus

35.10

Superior mediastinal dissection

The esophagus is then dissected clear in the superior mediastinum using a combination of sharp and blunt dissection. Avoiding pressure or diathermy near the membranous section of the trachea is vital. The esophagus is rolled out from under the azygos arch. If taking the thoracic duct tissue *en bloc*, the duct needs to be clipped and divided at this location; otherwise, care is taken to ensure it is not injured at this site. The pleura is divided proximally and the esophagus retracted away from the trachea being mobilized to the thoracic inlet. This dissection is performed close to the esophageal wall. A few centimeters' extra dissection superiorly, at this stage, will enable an easier dissection at the cervical stage. To assist the cervical phase, a Penrose drain can be introduced and wrapped around the proximal esophagus and stapled to form a collar. When this is identified at the time of the cervical dissection, it allows an easier delivery of the esophagus into the neck incision.

A careful inspection is performed to ensure complete dissection with no esophageal attachments, the presence of hemostasis, and the absence of chyle (which will be a clear fluid pooling in the subcarinal region). A single chest drain is then placed via the camera port or port C and placed with the tip in the superior mediastinum while the lung is reinflated under vision. The drain is secured and the port sites closed.

CERVICAL DISSECTION AND ANASTOMOSIS
(see **Figure 35.11a and b**)

The neck is approached per the description in Chapter 34, "Transhiatal esophagectomy." Once the esophagus has been mobilized, it is divided with a tape attached to the section that will be delivered to the abdomen. Once the gastric tube has been brought to the neck, an end to side anastomosis is performed on the upper greater curve, with a single layer of interrupted absorbable sutures ensuring complete inversion of the mucosa. A nasogastric tube is passed once the posterior layer of sutures has been placed in the anastomosis. The site of the suture used to secure the tape used to pull the gastric tube to the neck is oversewn or removed if there is significant redundancy. The anastomosis is returned to the mediastinum with the small blind apex secured either to a strap muscle or behind the sternomastoid muscle to stop it from falling into the thoracic cavity.

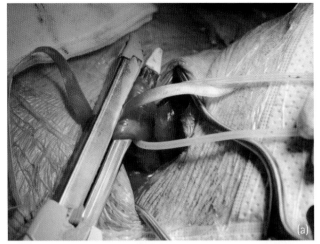
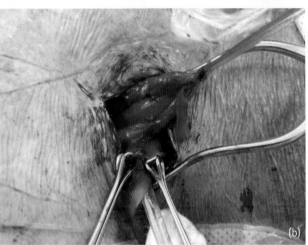

35.11a–b

THORACOSCOPIC MOBILIZATION WITH INTRATHORACIC ANASTOMOSIS

Port site placement (see Figure 35.12)

The patient is in the left lateral position with a double lumen endotracheal tube in place to allow deflation of the right lung. A 10 mm port is placed in the 5th intercostal space in the anterior axillary line using blunt dissection. This port is initially used as the camera port until all ports are placed, and then serves as the port for a "fan-type" retractor used for lung retraction. Subsequent ports are inserted under thoracoscopic vision. A 5 mm port is placed one rib space cephalad to the inferior border of the angle of the scapula, in the anterior axillary line. This will be used by the assistant. A 10 mm 30-degree camera port is placed in the 9th or 10th intercostal space in the midaxillary line, sliding over the dome of the diaphragm. A 10 mm port is placed in the 9th or 10th intercostal space near the postaxillary line, sliding over the dome of the diaphragm—this will be the surgeon's left-hand working port and enables a stapling device to be deployed to divide the azygos arch, and will be extended as a minithoracotomy to allow access for the circular stapler into the chest. A 10 mm port is placed at approximately the same transverse level as the previous port in the anterior axillary line. This is the main working port for the surgeon.

Division of azygos vein arch and esophageal mobilization

The right lung should be deflated. It may be necessary to use gentle compression with blunt instruments to aid in full lung deflation. Any pleural adhesions restricting deflation need to be divided at this stage. The lung is retracted anteriorly using a fan retractor. The surgeon identifies the azygos arch. The pleura is divided parallel to the line of the azygos arch overlying the esophagus both inferiorly and superiorly. Careful blunt dissection behind the azygos vein arch is performed as previously described, a stapling device using a vascular cartridge is placed through port C, and the azygos arch is divided.

Division of pleural attachments and inferior pulmonary ligament

Inferiorly the dissection from the abdomen should be seen and the nylon tape attached to the gastric conduit, if placed, should be identified early and placed on the diaphragm away from the dissection.

Through working ports A or C, a hook diathermy or Harmonic scalpel are used to divide the pleura to meet the inferior mediastinal dissection, with the line of dissection commencing at the upper limit of the abdominal dissection, just above the diaphragm, toward the azygos dissection.

Patient in the left lateral position

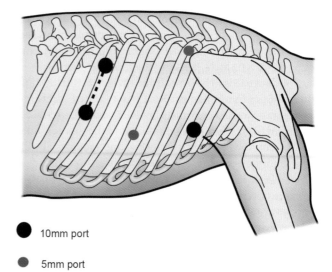

● 10mm port

● 5mm port

35.12

This will allow division of the inferior pulmonary ligament, allowing the right lower lobe of the lung to drop out of the field. The posterior line of dissection is in the groove that lies between the superior border of the esophagus, and the azygos vein and vertebral column. The anterior line of dissection is along the pleural reflection on the lung and pericardium. If the dissection is to include the thoracic duct and para-aortic tissue, then the posterior line of dissection is immediately along the anterior border of the azygos vein, extending onto the plane along the anterolateral aspect of the thoracic aorta, using vascular clips to control major vessels

Esophageal dissection and sling retraction

The glistening white pericardium is defined anterior to the esophagus, and posteriorly, the plane between the aorta and periesophageal fat is dissected. Between the esophagus and the aorta, with instrument retraction (not grasping) of the esophagus and a combination of a hook diathermy or Harmonic shears, blunt dissection, and vascular clips to aortic arterial branches, a window is created by meeting the previous dissection on the pericardium, allowing circumferential clearing of the esophagus.

The distal esophagus and proximal stomach are free of attachments below this point and ideally should not be drawn into the chest at this early stage of the dissection, as the specimen is often bulky and obscures the operative field. A Penrose drain or similar type of drain may be placed around the esophagus and knotted or stapled into a circle to be grasped for retraction in order to avoid grasping the specimen itself. Then the esophagus and periesophageal tissue are dissected from the thoracic aorta, thoracic duct, and azygos vein, although the thoracic duct may be resected *en bloc*. If the thoracic duct is to be included in the resection, the caudal end must be secured with clips or an endo-loop just superior to the diaphragm. The fat pad on the pericardium is dissected free with the esophagus.

Dissection of the subcarinal lymph nodes

The dissection continues superiorly toward the thoracic inlet both anteriorly and posteriorly. Care is taken posteriorly to identify arterial branches from the aorta.

Anterior to the esophagus, the dissection continues proximally with identification of the right main bronchus and trachea. Care is taken to identify vagal nerve branches that cross the right main bronchus. These nerves along with vessels are divided between endoscopic clips. The dissection proceeds proximally to the main trunk of the right vagus nerve, which is divided. The nodes along the medial side of the right main bronchus are mobilized from the bronchus with a hook diathermy and vascular clips to vessels. Care is taken to avoid diathermy beside the airway structures. The dissection is extended toward the carina as previously described.

Now the esophagus is retracted anteriorly and the azygos vein is mobilized from the esophagus. With further retraction pushing the esophagus anteriorly, vessels and left vagal branches sweeping posterior to the left main bronchus are divided to identify this structure. As previously described, the left main bronchus will be distended with the balloon of the endobronchial tube, so care must be taken to ensure no injury occurs to this structure. The nodal tissue is swept away from the left main bronchus and the apex of the subcarinal nodal package is identified. This is best divided by lifting the esophagus toward the spine, placing the final strands of subcarinal tissue under tension to allow division between endo-clips.

Once the esophagus has been mobilized to a point 2 cm above the planned level of esophageal transection above the azygos vein, the 12 mm port site in the posterior axillary line in the 9th intercostal space is extended anteriorly for 6 cm as a minithoracotomy. It is advisable to divide the parietal pleura as far anteriorly and posteriorly as possible to facilitate widening the intercostal space for passing the stapler. A small wound retractor is then placed and a small rib retractor is slowly opened in the intercostal space, taking care not to break the ribs.

The esophagus is divided above the azygos vein with laparoscopic scissors and the specimen is removed via the minithoracotomy. The previously placed nasogastric tube should be withdrawn at least 5 cm above the line of transection.

Esophagogastric stapled anastomosis (see Figure 35.13a and b)

After division of the esophagus above the level of the azygos, a purse string suture of 2-0 Prolene is placed in the esophagus, ensuring all layers are included with the suture bites. The head of the 25 mm diameter circular stapling device is placed into the esophagus and the purse string tied. An endo-loop is also applied to ensure all layers are included and there is appropriate inversion of the esophagus. The nylon tape attached to the gastric conduit is identified and gentle traction applied in a cephalad direction to deliver the conduit into the chest, and it is then delivered through the minithoracotomy. At the apex, the last 3 cm of the staple line is excised to open the conduit. Three stay sutures are placed evenly around the circumference at the opening of the conduit to keep the conduit in position after the stapler has been inserted and during subsequent maneuvers. The conduit is returned to the chest, ensuring it is not twisted. The stapling device is placed into the opening in the conduit and the sharp process of the stapling device is wound out to pierce the greater curve of the conduit. The stapler is coupled to the head to create the anastomosis.

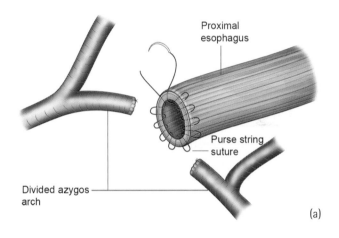

(a)

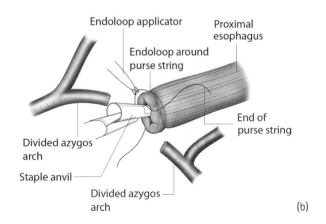

(b)

35.13a–b

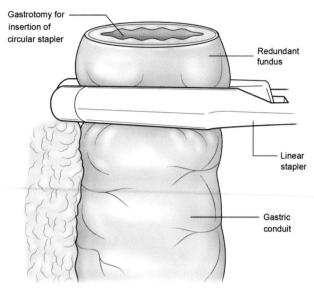

Gastrotomy for
insertion of
circular stapler

Redundant
fundus

Linear
stapler

Gastric
conduit

Resection of redundant fundus

35.14

The redundant fundus, including the gastrotomy used to insert the stapling device, is removed using a linear endoscopic stapling device (see **Figure 35.14**).

The excess omentum is then used to wrap and seal around the anastomosis. This may be fixed with sutures. An intercostal drain is inserted up to the apex of the chest and a second is placed beside the conduit near the anastomosis site.

POSTOPERATIVE CARE

The aim is to have the patient extubated immediately or soon after the operation, with management in a high dependency or intensive care unit. The patients will typically have a thoracic epidural, which is removed after 3–4 days. The apical intercostal drain is removed on day 2. Jejunostomy feeds commence on postoperative day 1 and progress to 80 mL/h by day 3. A blue dye swallow is performed on day 5 and oral intake is commenced if the patient is well and there are no signs of infection. The patient is discharged when mobile and tolerating a modified oral diet. The jejunostomy tube is removed after 10 days, either in hospital or at the first postoperative visit to the clinic.

OVERVIEW

We have preferred the thoracoscopic approach with a cervical anastomosis due to the ease with which the anastomosis is performed and the reduced morbidity from a leak at this site. From 1993 to June 2014, we performed 623 three-field thoracoscopic-assisted esophagectomies and 25 two-field thoracoscopic/laparoscopic esophagectomies for cancer. For the three-field approach, we converted to open surgery in 11

patients (1.8%) and had in-hospital operative mortality in 14 patients (2.2%). The technical complications included: chyle leak, 33 (5%); vocal cord palsy, 15 (2.4%); conduit necrosis, eight (1.3%); anastomotic leak, 68 (11%); tracheoesophageal fistula, four (0.6%). We found that significant respiratory complications, such as severe pneumonia, delay to discharge, return to intensive care, and prolonged ventilation support are reduced in patients having total MIE (4%) and hybrid MIE (7%) when compared with an open approach (12%). There is one randomized controlled trial (Biere et al, *Lancet* 2012) of total MIE compared with the open approach to an esophagectomy that confirms the reduction in respiratory complications from the MIE approach.

Following our experience with the three-field approach, we evolved to perform the two-field Ivor Lewis approach as a hybrid (laparoscopic gastric mobilization and open chest) approach, and then to a total MIE Ivor Lewis approach. A major difficulty with the thoracoscopic component is the challenge of performing the anastomosis between the gastric conduit and the esophagus in the chest. There are a number of approaches that include direct suturing, a combination of staples and suturing, the use of a circular stapling device (as we have described), and the use of a double stapled technique. The technique used will depend on the experience of the surgeon and their favored approach, with the aim that the outcomes will be equal to what is seen as gold standard—an open thoracotomy and anastomosis.

FURTHER READING

Biere SS, van Berge Henegouwen MI, Maas KW, Bonavina L, Rosman C, Garcia JR et al. Minimally invasive versus open oesophagectomy for patients with oesophageal cancer: a multicentre, open-label, randomised controlled trial. *Lancet.* 2012; 379: 1887–92.

Campos GM, Jablons D, Brown LM, Ramirez RM, Rabl C, Theodore P. A safe and reproducible anastomotic technique for minimally invasive Ivor Lewis esophagectomy: The circular stapled anastomosis with Transoral anvil. *Eur J Cardiothorac Surg.* 2010; 37: 1421–6.

Leibman S, Smithers BM, Gotley DC, Martin I, Thomas J. Minimally invasive esophagectomy: short- and long-term outcomes. *Surg Endosc.* 2006; 20: 428–33.

Luketich JD, Pennathur A, Awais O, Levy RM, Keeley S, Shende M et al. Outcomes after minimally invasive esophagectomy: review of over 1000 patients. *Ann Surg.* 2012; 256: 95–103.

Nguyen NT, Hinojosa MW, Smith BR, Chang KJ, Gray J, Hoyt D. Minimally invasive esophagectomy: lessons learned from 104 operations. *Ann Surg.* 2008; 258: 1081–91.

Pennathur A, Awais O, Luketich JD. Technique of minimally invasive Ivor Lewis esophagectomy. *Ann Thorac Surg.* 2010; 89: S2159–S2162.

Smithers BM, Gotley DC, McEwan D, Martin I, Bessell J, Doyle L. Thoracoscopic mobilization of the esophagus: a 6 year experience. *Surg Endosc.* 2001; 15: 176–82.

36

Thoracoscopic removal of benign esophageal tumors

DAVID IAN WATSON

PRINCIPLES AND JUSTIFICATION

The application of thoracoscopic techniques to the excision of benign esophageal lesions provides a minimal access approach to these lesions that avoids the need for an open thoracotomy incision. Benign esophageal lesions, which are usually leiomyomata, or less commonly esophageal wall (bronchogenic) cysts or gastrointestinal stromal tumors, are found within the esophageal wall musculature. In the case of leiomyoma, the tumor can at times be densely adherent to the underlying esophageal mucosa. Thoracoscopic excision entails dissecting the tumor from the surrounding esophageal wall muscle, while at the same time taking care to avoid opening the mucosa if possible. As this is not always feasible, the mucosa, if breached, can be repaired by thoracoscopic suturing.

The indications for surgical removal of lesions using a thoracoscopic approach include:

- Lesions more than 2 cm in diameter
- Enlarging lesions
- Symptomatic lesions

Malignant transformation in leiomyomata is very rare, and there is no indication for prophylactic removal to prevent this problem.

Before thoracoscopic techniques were developed, it was generally accepted that lesions that exceeded 5 cm in diameter should be removed in fit patients, irrespective of symptoms. However, with the development of less "invasive" thoracoscopic approaches, the size cut-off has been reduced to 2 cm, with lesions less than 2 cm in diameter generally managed conservatively.

Endoscopic ultrasound (EUS) facilitates accurate measurement of size and is the preferred follow-up method. Leiomyomata tend to grow very slowly and often remain stable for many years, but if they enlarge progressively, resection is indicated. Very large tumors require more extensive dissection and may not be suitable for thoracoscopic enucleation.

When tumors exceed 7–8 cm there is a much greater chance that resection will entail esophagectomy. At the other end of the size spectrum, some very small lesions (<1 cm) confined to the submucosal layer of the esophageal wall can be dealt with by endoscopic techniques using an intraluminal approach.

Tumors that cause symptoms such as dysphagia are usually large (>5 cm), whereas smaller tumors are usually asymptomatic. Surgeons need to be aware that dysphagia in patients with a small tumor is often due to a different problem.

PREOPERATIVE ASSESSMENT AND PREPARATION

Patients should undergo full cardiorespiratory evaluation, if necessary with the addition of pulmonary function testing and echocardiography. Patients unsuitable for an open thoracotomy approach should not undergo thoracoscopic surgery, as conversion to an open procedure is occasionally necessary if significant intraoperative difficulties are encountered. Computed tomographic scanning and endoscopy provide important information that helps determine the location of the tumor and ascertains the presence or absence of mucosal involvement or ulceration. If feasible, EUS should also be performed, as it will provide additional diagnostic information and confirm which layers of the esophageal wall are affected. EUS-guided needle biopsy can also be used to obtain a tissue diagnosis, but as the needle crosses the mucosa, needle biopsy can render dissection in the plane between the tumor and mucosa more difficult, thereby increasing the risk of mucosal perforation during surgical enucleation. In addition, as a tissue diagnosis usually does not change surgical decision-making, biopsy is probably best avoided in most patients with these tumors. However, if a very large lesion is present and not suitable for enucleation, then needle biopsy can be considered to confirm the diagnosis before esophagectomy.

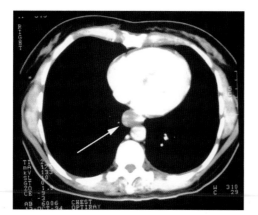

36.1

Unlike traditional open surgical approaches via a left thoracotomy, thoracoscopic excision can be performed through either a right- or left-sided approach to the esophagus. The choice is determined by the anatomy demonstrated preoperatively by computed tomographic scanning (i.e., if the lesion is in the right esophageal wall, then a right thoracoscopic approach is easiest). For example, for the leiomyoma of the esophagus shown in **Figure 36.1**, the best access for thoracoscopic excision entailed a right thoracoscopic approach (the arrow shows the direction of access for the endoscopic dissecting instruments). If the tumor is within the anterior or posterior esophageal wall (i.e. potentially suitable for either left or right thoracoscopic resection), the choice of approach is influenced by the proximity of the tumor to the esophageal hiatus and the aortic arch. Distal lesions (within 5 cm of the hiatus) may best be approached from the left, as the elevation of the right hemidiaphragm can restrict access from the right. On the other hand, more proximal lesions are often better accessed from the right side, as the heart and aortic arch can restrict access from the left. From the right side, these structures do not encroach on the operative field.

OPERATION

Anesthesia and position of patient

Two patient positions for thoracoscopic esophageal surgery can be used. Based on open surgical experience, many surgeons position their patients in the lateral position. This necessitates the placement of a double-lumen endotracheal tube to enable the lung to be collapsed. The alternative patient position (which the author prefers) is the prone position. This position provides excellent access to the posterior mediastinum and enables thoracoscopic surgery to be performed without the need for lung retraction. In addition, good access to the esophagus can be obtained in this position using low-pressure (8 mmHg) insufflation of the pleural cavity without collapse of the lung. This allows thoracoscopic surgery to be performed while using a single-lumen endotracheal tube if it is known preoperatively that the lung will not need to be collapsed. Low-pressure insufflation rarely creates anesthetic difficulties. (See **Figure 36.2**.)

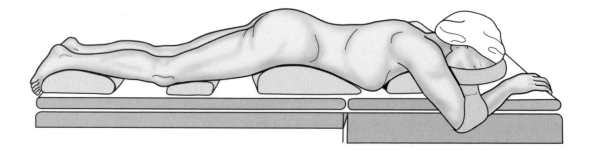

36.2

Operating theater set-up

When the patient is positioned prone, both the surgeon and assistant stand on the side of the patient that will provide access for thoracoscopy (i.e., right side for right thoracoscopic approach, and left for left thoracoscopy). The video monitor is positioned directly opposite the surgical team. When the lateral position is used, the surgeon and assistant stand in front of the patient, with the video monitor located opposite. (See **Figure 36.3.**)

Thoracoscopic access

For the remainder of this description, a right thoracoscopic approach with the patient positioned prone is assumed. Access to the thoracic cavity is obtained using an open dissection technique. Initially, an 11 mm port is placed through the sixth intercostal space in the midaxillary line to provide access for a conventional 10 mm laparoscope (port A). The port is placed using a blunt dissection technique in which a conventional artery clip is used to open into the pleural cavity before blunt-ended trocars are passed through the chest wall. The right lung is then collapsed either by using insufflation to a maximum pressure of 8 mmHg or by selectively collapsing the right lung while at the same time letting room air passively enter the pleural cavity. (See **Figure 36.4.**)

Three ports in total provide access for surgery. All of these are placed using blunt dissection. The passage of sharp trocars or trocars with "ribbed" shafts should be avoided, as the intercostal vessels can be easily lacerated or torn, resulting in troublesome hemorrhage. Placement of the secondary trocars is facilitated by thoracoscopic vision. Two 5 mm ports (ports B and C) are sited in the posterior axillary line in the fifth and seventh intercostal spaces to provide access for dissecting instruments. Once dissection is completed, one of the 5 mm ports can be exchanged with an 11 mm port (port B) to facilitate retrieval of the specimen at the completion of the procedure. Alternatively, if a 5 mm laparoscope is available, the specimen can be removed via the original 11 mm port (port A).

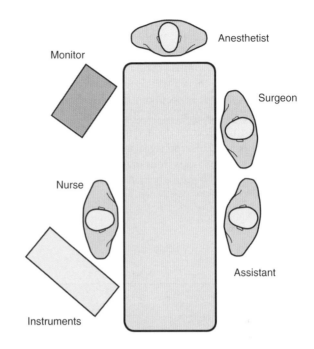

36.3

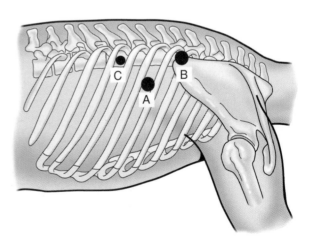

36.4

Thoracoscopic dissection

Providing the thoracoscopic approach is from the same side of the esophagus that the tumor arose from, it can usually be easily seen through the intact mediastinal pleura. If it is not immediately visible, then it will probably become apparent after initial esophageal dissection. Alternatively, intraoperative endoscopy can be used to localize the tumor accurately.

The mediastinal pleura is divided to expose the tumor and adjacent esophagus. Full esophageal mobilization is unnecessary unless the tumor arises from the esophageal wall on the opposite side to the operative field. (See **Figure 36.5.**)

If, however, the esophagus is fully mobilized, exposure of the tumor can be assisted by passing a tape behind the esophagus. This is used to elevate the esophagus from its bed. (See **Figure 36.6.**)

As benign esophageal tumors usually arise within the muscle wall of the esophagus and often do not involve mucosa, dissection close to the tumor, by separating it from adjacent muscle and the underlying mucosa, will usually be successful. Dissection is performed using a combination of diathermy hook and endoscopic scissor dissection. (See **Figure 36.7.**)

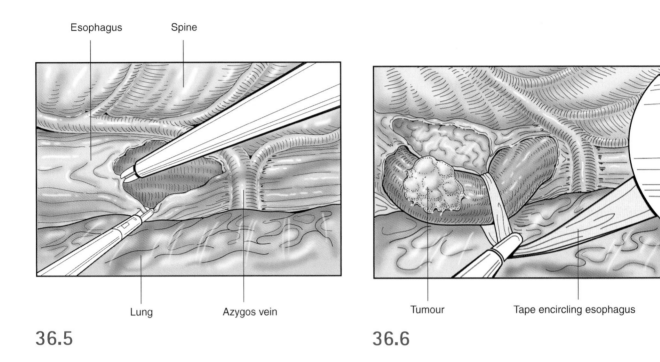

36.5

36.6

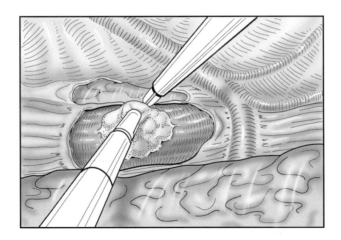

36.7

Determination of the integrity of esophageal mucosa

It is important to ensure that the underlying esophageal mucosa is intact. Leakage of luminal contents may not occur during thoracoscopic surgery, particularly if positive pressure insufflation is used. Hence, a high index of suspicion is essential to avoid postoperative problems from esophageal leakage. The mucosa should be carefully inspected visually. If there is any doubt about its integrity, careful intraoperative endoscopy with a flexible gastroscope can reveal whether the mucosa is intact.

Repair of esophageal mucosa

Perforation (deliberate or inadvertent) of esophageal mucosa is repaired by suturing the mucosal edges. This is performed using standard laparoscopic suturing methods (with intracorporeal or extracorporeal knotting). The author's preference is to use interrupted sutures, placed using a small needle attached to 4-0 polypropylene suture material, with the knots tied intracorporeally. (See **Figure 36.8**.)

Specimen retrieval and closure

The dissected specimen is placed in a specimen retrieval bag, which is introduced through one of the 10 mm ports, and is delivered through this port wound. Use of a bag is essential to prevent wound seeding of the tumor. Small tumors can be removed without the need to enlarge the wound. Larger tumors can only be removed after widening the wound to an appropriate extent.

An intercostal drain is placed with its tip near the excision site to drain any possible mucosal leak.

POSTOPERATIVE CARE

Patients are not allowed oral intake until after a radiological contrast examination has been performed on the first postoperative day. If mucosal integrity is confirmed, oral fluids are commenced and the drain is removed. A pureed diet is commenced on the second postoperative day. Patients are discharged after the second postoperative day and are maintained on a soft food diet for 2 weeks.

OUTCOME

Surgery for benign esophageal tumors is uncommon. For this reason, most reports of thoracoscopic techniques are limited to small case series or case reports. In general, these reports describe technical success and good short-term outcomes. The postoperative recovery appears to be substantially faster than following thoracotomy, and the hospital stay is shorter. It is therefore reasonable to attempt the removal of benign esophageal tumors using the thoracoscopic approach, although the operating surgeon should not hesitate to convert to an open thoracotomy if the procedure is difficult.

FURTHER READING

Jiang G, Zhao H, Yang F, Li J, Li Y, Liu Y, Liu J, Wang J. Thoracoscopic enucleation of esophageal leiomyoma: a retrospective study on 40 cases. *Dis Esophagus.* 2009; 22: 279–83.

Roviaro GC, Maciocco M, Varoli F, Rebuffat C, Vergani C, Scarduelli A. Videothoracoscopic treatment of oesophageal leiomyoma. *Thorax.*1998; 53: 190–2.

Taniguchi E, Kamiike W, Iwase K, Nishida T, Akashi A, Ohashi S, Matsuda H. Thoracoscopic enucleation of a large leiomyoma located on the left side of the esophageal wall. *Surg Endosc.* 1997; 11: 280–2.

von Rahden BH, Stein HJ, Feussner H, Siewert JR. Enucleation of submucosal tumors of the esophagus: minimally invasive versus open approach. *Surg Endosc.* 2004; 18: 924–30.

Watson DI, Britten-Jones R. Thoracoscopic excision of bronchogenic cyst of the esophagus. *Surg Endosc.* 1995; 9: 824–5.

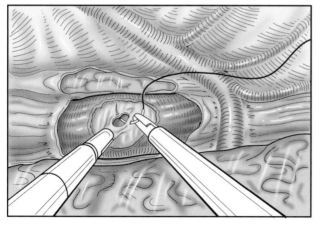

36.8

37

Perforation of the esophagus

AARON M. CHENG, DOUGLAS E. WOOD, AND CARLOS A. PELLEGRINI

HISTORY

The first reported spontaneous rupture of the esophagus was described by Herman Boerhaave, a "leading physician of the age," in early mid-eighteenth century Germany. His patient, the Baron de Wassenaer, consumed a large meal and subsequently "strove to excite vomiting by tickling his fauces," resulting in a postemetic esophageal perforation. Not unexpectedly, the baron died within 24 hours, and his postmortem revealed a linear esophageal perforation that had ruptured into both pleural spaces. A number of similar reports followed Boerhaave's seminal description. Attempted suture repair was only contemplated in the mid-twentieth century, and initial attempts in the United States (1944) and England (1946) were unsuccessful. Successful suture repair was performed by Norman Barrett in 1947, the year following his insightful and comprehensive review of the subject. Although postemetic perforation is no longer the principal etiology for esophageal perforation, it is notable that successful surgical repair followed two centuries later.

PRINCIPLES AND JUSTIFICATION

Despite improvements in the management of critically ill patients, perforation of the esophagus can be fatal unless diagnosed promptly and treated effectively. Most esophageal perforations today are caused by instrumentation (usually therapeutic) of the esophagus, especially during forced dilatation of an esophageal stricture. Injury to the cervical esophagus can occur during endoscopy and endotracheal intubation, and, together, these iatrogenic events account for 60% of cervical perforations. External trauma due to stab or gunshot wounds is the second most common cause of cervical and thoracic perforations of the esophagus. Other etiologies include the "spontaneous" or emetogenic disruption of the esophagus (Boerhaave's syndrome), perforation

of an esophageal cancer, sloughing of the esophageal wall after injection sclerotherapy or caustic injury, foreign body impaction, surgical injury, and infectious processes.

A very important consideration in the management of esophageal perforation is the evaluation and management of underlying esophageal pathology. It is critical to obtain an accurate history that may identify symptoms or signs of pre-existing abnormalities, such as esophageal stricture or cancer, which may require different or concomitant treatment.

Historically, mortality associated with esophageal perforation has been reported as high as 80%. However, with modern improvements in diagnosis and management, the current overall mortality rate for patients who develop esophageal perforation is 18%. The risk of dying from an esophageal perforation varies markedly with the location and extent of the perforation, the time elapsed prior to treatment, the age and general condition of the patient, and the presence of intrinsic esophageal disease. Key to understanding the pathophysiology of esophageal perforation is the recognition that it causes a rapidly evolving infection of the mediastinum, with substantial spread and necrosis of poorly vascularized mediastinal fat tissue. In addition, and particularly pertinent to treatment options, there is prompt deterioration of the esophageal wall at the site of the rupture. Thus, ideally, an esophageal perforation should be treated within 12 hours of its occurrence—attempts at primary repair after the first 24–48 hours are more challenging.

PREOPERATIVE ASSESSMENT

Clinical diagnosis

The most common symptom is *pain*. When the perforation is iatrogenic, patients may attest to pain symptoms during, or immediately after, completion of the instrumentation. Pain is constant, most often radiates to the back, and may be felt in the upper abdomen and chest, particularly when the perforation involves the thoracic esophagus. Perforations in the neck often present with pain on neck flexion or manipulation of the thyroid cartilage. *Subcutaneous* emphysema and crepitation are often evident following cervical perforation and are present in approximately 20% of thoracic esophageal perforations. Many patients also complain of *dysphagia*, *odynophagia*, and *profuse salivation*. *Fever* and *leukocytosis* are common within the first 4–6 hours after perforation and some patients rapidly develop features of *systemic shock* (hypotension, tachycardia, sweating). *Airway compromise* is uncommon following injury to the esophagus, but may be of concern in the case of a cervical perforation.

The commonly quoted triad of symptoms described by Mackler—thoracic pain, followed by vomiting associated with cervical emphysema—is only present in approximately 40% of patients. These findings are only relevant to postemetic esophageal perforation.

Radiological diagnosis

Chest and abdominal radiography are routinely obtained when the diagnosis of esophageal perforation is suspected but are usually insufficient to confirm the diagnosis, in particular the location of the perforation. Nonetheless, a perforation may be suspected from plain films, as free air may dissect adjacent tissues, creating subcutaneous emphysema, pneumomediastinum, pneumoperitoneum, or even pneumothorax. Cervical perforation may present with subtle

findings such as air in fascial planes, widening of the retroesophageal space, and loss of cervical lordosis. Thoracic perforations often demonstrate widened mediastinal silhouette and air–fluid levels within the mediastinal space. A left pleural effusion is also an indirect sign of esophageal perforation. In the experience of the authors and of others, however, these signs are present only in approximately 30% of cases.

A contrast esophagogram will reliably confirm an esophageal perforation and is the most useful diagnostic test (see **Figure 37.1**). The esophagogram will define the site and extent of the perforation, the amount of extravasation, the communication with the pleural or peritoneal cavity, and the presence of distal obstruction. Thus, a contrast study is not only important for the diagnosis of esophageal perforation but is essential to correct planning of surgery.

The authors prefer to use diatrizoate meglumine 66% and sodium diatrizoate 10% (Gastrografin), as the contrast medium in the initial investigation. This water-soluble material is rapidly absorbed from the gastrointestinal tract and from the pleural or peritoneal cavity if extravasated. It allows even small amounts of extravasation to be detected by a follow-up computed tomography (CT) scan. Gastrografin may be more caustic to the airway if aspirated and generates a false negative study in approximately 20% of cervical esophageal perforations and 10% of intrathoracic perforations. In cases where aspiration is a concern or a false negative is suspected, a thin barium study may be more informative.

A CT scan is a useful adjunct to an esophagogram, predominantly to identify the extent of pleural and mediastinal fluid and contamination that may require debridement and drainage (see **Figure 37.2**). However, CT scanning is neither a sufficient nor appropriate modality for guiding clinical management of an esophageal perforation, and is definitely not an alternative or replacement for an esophagogram. Often the CT scan is the first study that is performed, and may reveal subtle signs of perforation. In these cases, the CT scan should be followed by an appropriate contrast study of the esophagus.

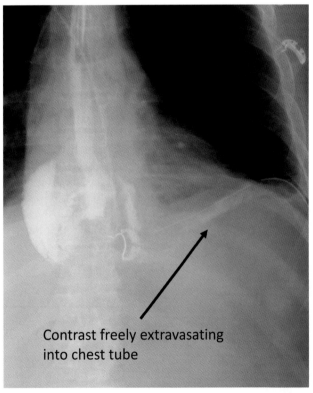

Contrast freely extravasating into chest tube

37.1

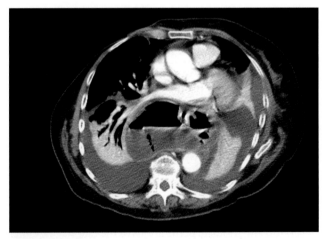

37.2 Esophageal perforation with mediastinal abscess and bilateral pleural contamination.

A CT scan provides invaluable information on patients who present with delayed perforations. These are patients who survived the initial insult and who have developed an abscess that effectively contains the perforation and prevents further mediastinal or pleural soiling. To plan adequate drainage, one must define the site, the extent, and the relation of the abscess to adjacent structures, and CT scanning is the test of choice.

Endoscopic diagnosis

Endoscopic examination often adds little information to that obtained from a high-quality contrast esophagogram. In some patients, however, particularly those suffering from foreign body perforation or penetrating trauma, endoscopy may help to identify and characterize the injury (see **Figure 37.3**). For example, a patient who has stab or gunshot wounds may also have a perforated esophagus, and, due to other concomitant injuries, the patient may be hemodynamically unstable to undergo a contrast esophagogram. The overall sensitivity of esophagoscopy in detecting subtle injuries is inferior to a contrast study, and, not unexpectedly, it is operator dependent. Therefore, we recommend that in trauma patients with penetrating injuries where there is high suspicion for esophageal injury, a contrast esophagogram be performed once the patient is stabilized, even if endoscopy is unrevealing.

Endoscopic examination may be helpful in those patients that have intrinsic esophageal disease and esophageal perforation. In these cases, discovery of a cancer, stricture, or other underlying esophageal pathology will affect planning of the operation. For this reason, the authors routinely perform endoscopy immediately following induction of anesthesia in all patients with symptoms or signs of preexisting esophageal pathology who are undergoing an operation for esophageal perforation.

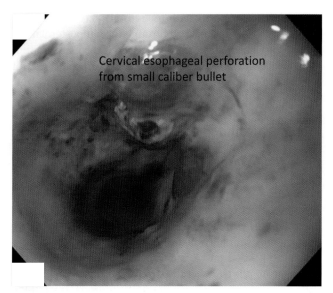

Cervical esophageal perforation from small caliber bullet

37.3

INITIAL MANAGEMENT

The initial management of an esophageal perforation involves several steps.

Aggressive resuscitation

These patients suffer rapid dehydration and overwhelming contamination if there is free perforation involving the mediastinum and pleural space. Large bore intravenous access or central access is warranted. A secure airway is also paramount in patients requiring large volume resuscitations and who have compromised ventilation. Early pleural drainage may be required to evacuate a pneumothorax or drain a large pleural fluid collection.

Antibiotic administration

As soon as a perforation is suspected, the patient should be started on broad-spectrum antibiotics directed against oral flora to adequately cover aerobic Gram-positive and Gram-negative bacteria, as well as anaerobic microorganisms. Antifungal coverage is also routinely administered at our institution because of the high incidence of pathologic oral fungal flora.

Assessment of the perforation

The surgeon should ask the following before deciding on the approach and treatment strategy:

- Is the perforation contained or free? Contained esophageal perforations are often incomplete intraluminal injuries without true mediastinal contamination, or limited to soilage of the tissue immediately adjacent to the esophagus. Free perforations with extravasation of esophageal contents into the neck, the pleural cavity, or the peritoneal space are the most common type of perforations and those that require intervention.
- How much time has elapsed since the perforation occurred?
- What is the location and the extent of the perforation?
- What is the etiology of the perforation? Is the perforation iatrogenic, spontaneous, traumatic, etc.?
- Is there preexisting underlying esophageal disease?
- Is there an obstruction distal to the perforation site?
- What is the general health and functional status of the patient? What is the patient's current hemodynamic stability?

Traditional management of esophageal perforations relied on open operative repair; however, the contemporary role of esophageal stenting has gained prominence in the management paradigm for select esophageal perforations and will be discussed in the section on "Alternative approaches."

Contained perforations

Contained perforations, which may be partial thickness or localized injuries without extensive contamination, may be treated without surgery, provided that: the perforation is small, the contrast material flows immediately back into the esophagus and distally into the stomach, no underlying esophageal disease is present distal to the perforation (i.e., stricture), and the clinical manifestations are minimal (i.e., low-grade fever, minimal pain, etc.). Such nonoperative management is the exception, not the rule, when treating esophageal perforation. In fact, in some instances, the surgeon ought to look "beyond the horizon" in making the decision, as may be the case for a patient who has achalasia and has a "minimal" perforation. It is unlikely that anyone will attempt subsequent dilatation of this achalasia; thus, operating early, closing the perforation, and performing a myotomy will address both aspects of the problem: the underlying disease and the complication of the dilation.

One perforation that may be treated successfully with conservative (nonoperative) management is that which occurs a few weeks after injection sclerotherapy. The inflammatory reaction caused by the sclerosing agent adheres the periesophageal tissues to the wall of the esophagus, effectively blocking the perforation and decreasing the chance of mediastinal spread of infection. Furthermore, the underlying general state of the patient (cirrhosis) and the esophagus (varices) would make any attempt at open repair very difficult. When this strategy is followed, the patient should be given enteral or parenteral nutrition, and broad-spectrum antibiotics should be administered for 7–10 days. The most important aspect of management is close clinical observation, as any clinical deterioration or recurrence of symptoms (e.g., pain) warrants reevaluation and consideration of surgical intervention. The esophagus should be evaluated periodically with contrast radiography and CT scanning to monitor the progress. Any evidence of spread of infection or lack of adequate response to this treatment should elicit an immediate change of treatment, prompting more aggressive intervention.

Free perforations

Free perforations are much more common than contained perforations, and almost always require intervention, regardless of location or size. Traditionally, open surgical repair was the mainstay of treatment, but, more recently, esophageal stenting has become an important alternative treatment modality. Regardless of which interventional approach is undertaken, the principles of treating free perforations are control/drainage of the esophageal leak, eradication of mediastinal and pleural sepsis, and reexpansion of the lung.

Time elapsed since perforation

The time elapsed since the perforation determines, to some extent, the intervention to be used. Patients who suffered their perforation 24–72 hours previously should undergo an exploration of the area, and, if possible, the perforation should be closed with buttressing. The mediastinal and pleural spaces should be debrided and drained and the lung decorticated. Patients who present several days after perforation are likely to have a periesophageal abscess. In these cases, primary closure of the perforation may no longer be possible; if mediastinal and pleural sepsis is controlled and the lung is reexpanded, interventional radiological techniques, plus or minus esophageal stenting, may be used to drain the infected areas.

Location and extent of perforation

Injuries to the esophagus above the thoracic inlet should be treated by neck incision on the side of the extravasation, or on the left side (the esophagus is easier to access from the left). Occasionally, cervical esophageal perforations will extend into the mediastinum or right chest and require open mediastinal and pleural debridement through a right fifth intercostal posterolateral thoracotomy. Nonoperative treatment of perforations in the neck has been advocated, on the basis that most heal by apposition of adjacent tissue (no "real" space is present around the esophagus in the neck). The authors believe that early closure or drainage of these injuries accelerates recovery and allows for treatment of associated injuries, which are common when external trauma is the cause of the perforation. If the perforation has occurred in a Zenker's diverticulum, resection of the diverticulum, and a concomitant cricopharyngeal myotomy are recommended. Most other esophageal perforations should be approached through a thoracotomy. Upper thoracic and mid-esophageal injuries are best approached by thoracotomy in the right posterolateral fourth to sixth intercostal space. Most distal lesions should be approached through the left posterolateral seventh or eighth intercostal space, even if the extravasation is in the abdomen. Occasionally bilateral thoracotomies will be required to decorticate both pleural spaces.

Presence of underlying esophageal disease

Underlying esophageal disease plays a critical role in determining the kind of procedure to be performed. As perforation occurs most commonly during dilatation of strictures, and because the mechanism of injury is such that the wall of the esophagus is injured at or just above the stricture, therapy should be planned accordingly. If the stricture is chronic, fibrotic, and recalcitrant to previous dilations, the best treatment is to resect the stricture and perforated area, and immediately reconstruct the gastrointestinal tract. If the perforation is caused by dilatation for achalasia, closure of the perforation and a Heller myotomy on the other side of the esophagus are recommended. Likewise, if an early stage or locally advanced esophageal cancer is perforated and promptly identified, immediate esophagectomy and primary reconstruction should be considered if the patient is a candidate for esophagectomy. Whatever the choice, the key surgical principle is to *never* close primarily a perforation above an esophageal obstruction.

General health and condition of the patient

Unfortunately, early discovery of a free perforation mandates treatment intervention, regardless of the fitness of the patient. The intervention may be operative surgical repair or endoscopic stenting, dependent on the extent of injury, timing of the procedure, and experience of the managing team.

OPERATIVE PROCEDURES

Repair of perforation of the unobstructed esophagus

Most spontaneous and instrumental perforations occur in the distal esophagus. The best way to approach these lesions is by thoracotomy through the left posterolateral seventh or eighth intercostal space (see **Figure 37.4**). We routinely harvest an intercostal muscle flap on entry into the chest. The pedicle is then wrapped in a warm saline sponge and left in the chest until it is required for buttress of the perforation. The parietal pleura overlying the esophagus should be opened at a site near the perforation. Occasionally, the esophageal lesion has lacerated the pleura, and the site of perforation is obvious from the beginning. If the perforation is not evident, the chest can be filled with saline while the anesthetist blows air through the esophageal lumen. Bubbles of air will appear at the site of perforation. Alternatively, an endoscope can be passed transorally and an examination performed while the patient is anesthetized and the chest is open. Most often, the perforation is easily identified by surrounding inflammation as well as the presence of Gastrografin or thin barium in the esophageal lumen.

With care taken not to injure the contralateral mediastinal pleura, the esophagus is encircled (see **Figure 37.5**); the plane of dissection on the esophagus is on the longitudinal muscular coat and not in the periesophageal tissue. Adequate mobilization of the esophagus may require moderate dissection, particularly if the perforation has occurred in the right side of the esophagus. The extent of injury must be clearly identified, as well as the normal esophagus above and below. The mucosal edges of the perforation are usually healthy and normally do not require significant debridement. Often the muscular layer of injury requires additional myotomy to clearly define the proximal and distal extent of the mucosal injury. Failure to demonstrate the entire extent

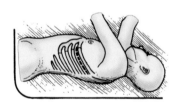

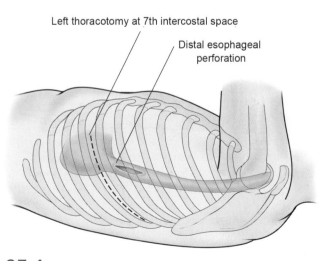

Left thoracotomy at 7th intercostal space

Distal esophageal perforation

37.4

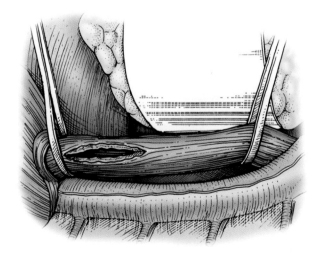

37.5

of the mucosal injury will lead to inadequate closure of the esophageal perforation. The mucosa should be approximated using an interrupted suture of 4-0 silk or polyglyconate, and the muscular coat closed with interrupted sutures of 4-0 silk or similar nonabsorbable sutures (see **Figure 37.6**).

Whenever possible, the esophageal closure should be buttressed with the previously harvested intercostal muscle pedicle or, less optimally, by a flap of pleura (see **Figure 37.7**). The buttress should be securely sutured to the esophagus to provide an additional layer of tissue to secure the closure, similarly to a third layer of an anastomosis with multiple, well-placed sutures. The intercostal flap should be placed parallel on the repair and sutured to a healthy muscular layer with interrupted sutures. Other possible options for buttressing the repair are stomach, muscle flap, or omentum. Finally, any fibrinous and necrotic tissue is debrided and the lung should expand or pleural decortication should be performed to allow for its full expansion. The control of mediastinal and pleural sepsis is a critical aspect of the care of esophageal perforation, and this aspect of the patient's operative management cannot be overlooked. The chest is drained with multiple large bore chest tubes (usually two to three) to accomplish both pleural and mediastinal drainage. One of the tubes should be near but not directly against the area of surgical repair. The proximity of this chest drain to the repair allows adequate drainage of the esophagus if the repair is unsuccessful. The chest is then irrigated and closed.

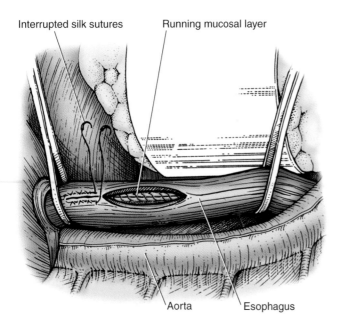

37.6

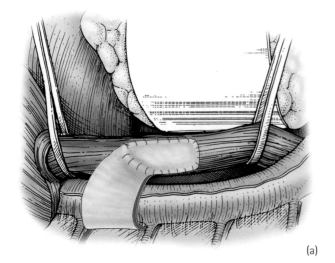

(a)

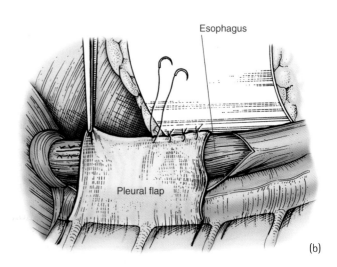

(b)

37.7a–b

Repair of perforation of the obstructed esophagus

The two most common conditions are perforation occurring during pneumatic balloon dilatation of a patient with achalasia and perforation occurring during instrumentation of a benign or malignant stricture.

PERFORATION FROM PNEUMATIC DILATATION FOR ACHALASIA

The approach and the initial procedure are similar to those described for the treatment of the unobstructed esophagus. This perforation always affects the lower esophagus and is approached from the left side of the chest with a seventh or eighth posterolateral intercostal space thoracotomy. Simply closing the perforation may result in early dehiscence (because of the concomitant obstruction) and leaves the patient with untreated achalasia. Thus, after closing the perforation in a manner similar to that described earlier, the opposite side of the esophagus is exposed, exactly 180 degrees from the perforated area, and a longitudinal myotomy approximately 6–8 cm along the esophagus is performed (see **Figure 37.8**). After the phrenoesophageal ligament is divided, the fundus of the stomach is brought up and the myotomy is extended 1–2 cm onto the stomach. A partial fundoplication (Dor, Thal, Belsey) over the area of the perforation is made. The wrap is secured with interrupted sutures to each side of the myotomy. This not only buttresses the repair well but also acts as an antireflux procedure and helps to keep the edges of the myotomy far apart, which minimizes recurrence of achalasia obstruction. The 360-degree plication, as described by Nissen, should not be used as it is contrary to the principle of diminishing the lower esophageal sphincter pressure.

PERFORATION OF A BENIGN OR MALIGNANT STRICTURE

Whenever possible, resection of the esophagus by the transhiatal approach and esophagogastrostomy at the neck are recommended (see Chapter 34, "Transhiatal esophagectomy"). This treats the perforation and underlying disease and brings a graft of well-vascularized tissue into the posterior mediastinum that fills the space and helps treat the mediastinal infection.

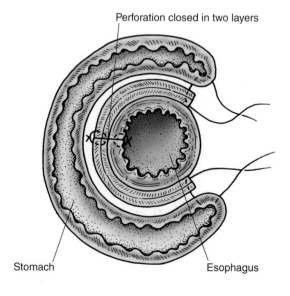

Perforation closed in two layers

Stomach   Esophagus

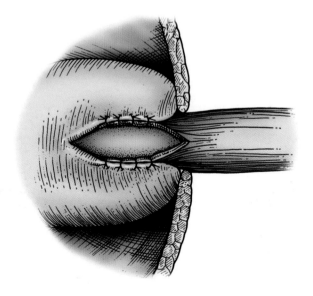

37.8

Repair of perforation of the cervical esophagus

Surgical exposure of the cervical esophagus is usually on the left side and the incision follows along the anterior aspect of the left sternocleidomastoid muscle, similar to performing an esophagogastrostomy in the neck for a transhiatal esophagectomy (see **Figure 37.9**). A similar approach to thoracic esophageal injury is undertaken, including debridement of muscular tissue to identify the mucosal rent and closure in two layers. The repair may be buttressed with strap muscle, but this aspect is less critical in the neck. In fact, many authors advocate simple drainage of cervical esophageal perforations because of the tendency of these injuries to heal without direct suture repair. Adequate drainage can be provided with either closed suction drains or Penrose drains. Debridement of the mediastinal space through a right thoracotomy should be considered if there is significant undrained abscess on CT scan.

Perforation diagnosed several days after occurrence

Patients in whom the perforation is diagnosed several days after occurrence are treated primarily by interventional radiological techniques, although some authors have used operative techniques. The strategy is to drain the cavity adjacent to the perforation and the abscesses as adequately as possible. This involves placing a transthoracic CT-guided drainage tube to aspirate the cavity. In addition, a percutaneous gastrostomy is performed. Another option for drainage occasionally used is advancing a retrograde intraluminal catheter from the gastrostomy access to the esophagus and into the cavity. As the patient will not be able to eat for some time, a feeding jejunostomy catheter should be placed. This can be done laparoscopically to obviate the need for laparotomy.

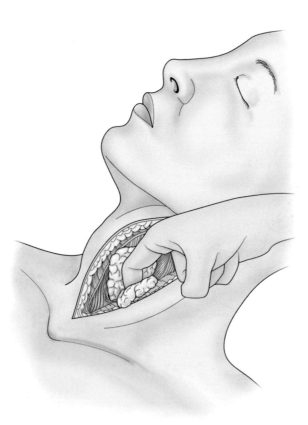

37.9

ALTERNATIVE APPROACHES

T–tube drainage of an esophageal perforation

In some patients it may not be possible to close the perforation because of a delay in diagnosis, because the patient is too sick to undergo primary repair, or because sepsis persists after interventional radiological management or dehiscence of a previous closure. A preferred therapy for an esophageal perforation that is not amenable to primary repair is the insertion of a T-tube, as this allows maintenance of the native esophagus. Moreover, the subsequent steps of management and reestablishment of gastrointestinal continuity is far simpler than esophageal reconstruction after diversion and exclusion (see following). Placement of an esophageal T-tube essentially creates a controlled esophagocutaneous fistula and a "stent" or "scaffold" for secondary esophageal closure over the tube. The appliance favored by the authors are large bore silicone tracheal T-tubes of 14, 16, or 18 mm (E. Benson Hood Laboratories, Inc., Pembroke, Massachusetts, United States). The T-tube is inserted into the esophagus and an appropriate-sized cut chest tube with the distal holes removed is inserted into the side limb of the T-tube to complete the transthoracic drainage of the esophagocutaneous fistula (see **Figure 37.10**). A nasogastric tube is passed through the T-tube into the stomach. After the resolution of sepsis, and 2–3 weeks to establish a mature drainage tract, the esophagus can be restudied by esophagogram to confirm a controlled fistula without other extravasation. The external chest tube can then be slowly withdrawn (2–3 cm every 3–4 days) until out and the track drainage and/or esophagogram confirms closure. The T-tube itself can be removed transorally with rigid esophagoscopy. Although this strategy has been used successfully by a number of surgeons, it is only recommended when the esophagus cannot be resected, reconstructed, or closed in a poor risk patient.

Diversion and exclusion

When there are no feasible options for primary repair or T-tube, a management strategy of last resort is esophageal diversion and exclusion. This involves division of the esophagus in the neck, creation of an end-esophagostomy (spit fistula), and closure of the distal thoracic esophagus as low as possible in the neck (see **Figure 37.11**). It is useful to tag the distal esophagus with long permanent suture and to tack it to the underside of the sternocleidomastoid muscle. This allows ease of identification during the reconstruction procedure and limits contraction of the distal esophageal segment into the mediastinum, maintaining length if it is possible to perform direct esophageal reconstruction at the later stage. The stoma can be tunneled onto the anterior chest wall and matured at an appropriate location. The cardio-esophageal junction should not be closed with a stapling device as is often proposed, as this creates obstruction distal to the injury and unnecessarily complicates later reconstructive options. A draining gastrostomy allows decompression of the perforated segment and stops mediastinal and pleural soiling.

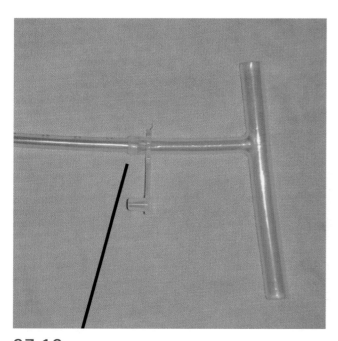

37.10 Chest tube with distal holes cut inserted into tracheal T-tube.

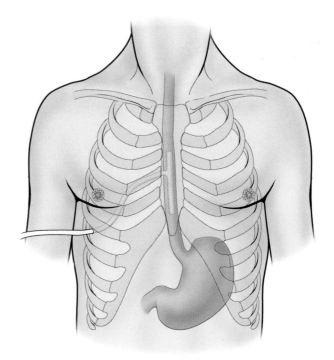

37.11

Unfortunately, this procedure requires a second operation to reestablish continuity of the gastrointestinal tract. This is best accomplished several months later via primary reconstruction with a cervical esophago-esophageal anastomosis or a total esophagectomy by the transhiatal approach and a gastroesophageal anastomosis at the neck. The advantages of the former approach are that it maintains the native esophagus (always the best in absence of esophageal pathology) and accomplishes reconstruction with a relatively minor neck operation rather than an extensive transthoracic and/or transabdominal procedure. If the latter approach is necessary, high mortality and significant morbidity exist.

Esophageal stenting

In the last decade, the advent of a number of stents with different characteristics and the development of appropriate safe deployment devices have made stenting a much more attractive method to treat many esophageal perforations that, in the past, would have only been considered for surgical therapy (refer to Chapter 28, "Esophageal stents"). Fully covered self-expanding stents are now commercially available in a variety of lengths and diameters and, once deployed, remain in place by exerting radial force (see **Figure 37.12**). For an esophageal perforation, the covered stent traverses and covers the perforation site, effectively prevents ongoing

contamination of the mediastinum and pleural cavities from gastric and enteral contents, and provides a scaffold for esophageal healing that minimizes secondary esophageal stricture. As the inflammatory process surrounding the perforation leads to scarring of the area, the esophageal perforation is sealed by the adjacent tissue. This contemporary hybrid strategy of deploying fully covered esophageal stents to exclude perforations and subsequently managing associated pleural and mediastinal contamination with less invasive drainage procedures has been widely reported by many centers to successfully treat esophageal perforations.

Esophageal stenting for esophageal perforations should be used in select patients and, ideally, should be reserved for patients with esophageal perforations who do not have underlying esophageal pathologies that could be treated in the same surgical procedure—for example, leak associated with dilated esophagus from end-stage achalasia or a perforation due to malignancy in an operable patient. In general, we reserve the use of esophageal stenting for patients with limited perforation of the intrathoracic esophagus or when surgical repair has failed, or, more frequently, when there is a small leak associated with a previous anastomosis (esophagogastrostomy). If a patient presents with significant hemodynamic instability due to septic shock from the esophageal perforation, we also will readily favor deploying an esophageal stent in order to prevent further mediastinal and pleural contamination while resuscitating the patient

Plastic stents

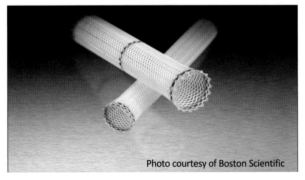

Photo courtesy of Boston Scientific

Fully covered metal stents

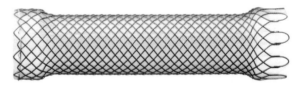

Photo courtesy of Boston Scientific

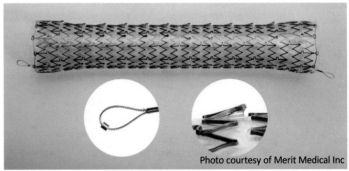

Photo courtesy of Merit Medical Inc

37.12

and widely draining the contaminated pleural and mediastinal spaces.

Technique is covered in Chapter 28, "Esophageal stents." For the particular indication of esophageal perforation, it is important to use a fully covered stent that is designed to be removed and choose a stent with a large enough diameter that will exert sufficient radial force to seal the perforation and avoid undesired stent migration. Depending on specific surgeon preference, we prefer either a self-expanding silicone-covered polyester braided stent (Polyflex™; Boston Scientific, Marlborough, Massachusetts, United States) or a fully covered double-flared metal stent (ALIMAAX™ or EndoMAXX™; Merit Medical Systems, Inc., South Jordan, Utah, United States; WallFlex™, Boston Scientific).

POSTOPERATIVE CARE

Postsurgical repair management

The patient often remains intubated for the first 12–24 hours. Good ventilation and full lung expansion are essential to prevent atelectasis and pneumonia. Full expansion of the lung will prevent further accumulation of pleural fluid, and hopefully the development of an empyema. We are conservative with regards to extubation; if emergency reintubation is necessary, forceful mask ventilation before reintubation increases esophageal pressure and can jeopardize the integrity of the closure at the site of the perforation. Depending on the hemodynamic status of the patient, intensive care management may be required during the first few days or for a prolonged length of stay. The nasogastric tube must be carefully cared for and routinely flushed, as draining the stomach and esophagus is imperative. To decrease gastric acid secretion, proton pump inhibitors are administered.

Antibiotics and antifungals are generally continued for 7–10 days, depending on the degree of contamination: in patients with positive results on preoperative blood cultures, antibiotics should be continued for 14 days. Enteral nutrition via a feeding jejunostomy is started 48 hours after surgery and, once a patient is stabilized, hemodynamically. If no feeding tube is inserted, parenteral nutrition is initiated if the patient has evidence of preexisting malnutrition or if the patient is anticipated to be unable to initiate enteral nutritional therapy within the initial 7- to 10-day postoperative period.

Seven to eight days after surgery, a barium swallow examination should be performed (water-soluble material should be used if there is any suspicion of dehiscence). If this study demonstrates no extravasation, the patient is started on a mechanically soft diet. Patients are discharged home as soon as they can eat and have no evidence of residual infection. If dehiscence is noted and it is contained or well drained and asymptomatic, they are kept on enteral or parenteral nutrition for an additional 10 days and the study is then repeated. If symptoms of abscess are present, treatment should be the same as if a delayed perforation is discovered.

Postesophageal stent management

Following placement of the stent, we perform an endoscopic examination to ensure that the perforation is fully covered, to ensure the stent has fully has expanded radially, and to determine the appropriate location of the nasogastric tube in the stomach. An esophagogram is not routinely performed immediately after stenting but is useful during the ensuing few days, as it provides accurate information with regards to potential continuing extravasation. Although we choose as large a stent diameter as reasonable (usually 21–25 mm), stent migration can occur, especially when there is no underlying esophageal stricture. Therefore, we obtain daily chest radiographs to monitor for migration. If the stent has migrated, we promptly return to the operating room and are prepared with full endoscopy and fluoroscopy capabilities in order to reposition or to remove and/or replace the stent as required.

Generally, we avoid leaving the esophageal stent in place longer than 4 weeks, and once enough time has elapsed for the esophageal perforation to heal, and the systemic infection has resolved, we remove the stent by endoscopy in the operating room under general anesthesia. Again, we perform esophagogastroscopy both before and after stent removal to thoroughly evaluate the esophagus and obtain a contrast esophagogram before any oral intake is resumed.

CONCLUSION

Successful management of the perforated esophagus remains a formidable challenge and requires a high index of clinical suspicion, prompt and efficient diagnosis, and frequently aggressive surgical intervention. Choosing the best operative strategy to treat an esophageal perforation depends on the location and the extent of the perforation at the time of diagnosis, the underlying integrity of the esophagus, and the overall status of the individual patient. Esophageal stenting offers an attractive alternative to traditional open surgical techniques in appropriately selected cases. However, for the contemporary surgeon, time-honored surgical principles for treating esophageal perforations remain: eradication and control of any present and ongoing source of sepsis from the site, repair and preservation of the native esophagus whenever possible, and meticulous attention to the postoperative care and nutritional management of the patient.

FURTHER READING

Abbas G, Schuchert MJ, Pettiford BL et al. Contemporaneous management of esophageal perforation. *Surgery.* 2009; 146: 749–56.

Biancari F, D'Andrea V, Paone R et al. Current treatment and outcome of esophageal perforations in adults: systematic review and meta-analysis of 75 studies. *World J Surg.* 2013; 37: 1051–9.

Cameron JL, Kieffer RF, Hendrix TR et al. Selective nonoperative management of contained intrathoracic esophageal disruptions. *Ann Thorac Surg.* 1979; 27: 404–8.

D'Cuntha J, Rueth NM, Groth SS et al. Esophageal stents for anastomotic leaks and perforations. *J Thorac Cardiovasc Surg.* 2011; 142: 39–46.

Dasari BV, Neely D, Kennedy A et al. The role of esophageal stents in the management of esophageal anastomotic leaks and benign esophageal perforations. *Ann Surg.* 2014; 259: 852–60.

Flynn AE, Verrier ED, Way LW et al. Esophageal perforation. *Arch Surg.* 1989; 124: 1211–15.

Freeman RK, Ascioti AJ, Giannini T et al. Analysis of unsuccessful esophageal stent placements for esophageal perforation, fistula, or anastomotic leak. *Ann Thorac Surg.* 2012; 94: 959–65.

Keeling WB, Miller DL, Lam GT et al. Low mortality after treatment for esophageal perforation: a single-center experience. *Ann Thorac Surg.* 2010; 90: 1669–73.

Madhukar SP, Malinoski DJ, Zhou L et al. Penetrating oesophageal injury: a contemporary analysis of the National Trauma Data Bank. *Injury.* 2013; 44: 48–55.

Maroney TP, King EJ, Gordon RL et al. Role of interventional radiology in the management of major esophageal leaks. *Radiology.* 1989; 170: 1055–7.

Orringer MB, Stirling MC. Esophagectomy for esophageal perforationdisruption, *Ann Thorac Surg.* 1990; 49: 35–42.

Sauer L, Pellegrini CA, Way LW. The treatment of achalasia: a current perspective. *Arch Surg.* 1989; 124: 929–32.

38

Laparoscopic antireflux surgery

SARAH K. THOMPSON AND GLYN G. JAMIESON

HISTORY

Rudolph Nissen popularized a fundoplication that bears his name in 1956, following the discovery that a fundal patch, used to reinforce an esophageal suture line, also corrected gastroesophageal reflux. In 1991, two almost simultaneous publications were released describing the adaption of Nissen's technique laparoscopically. The principles of the operation closely followed the open technique, with division of the short gastric vessels, posterior closure of the diaphragmatic hiatus, and creation of a 1–2 cm 360-degree wrap, calibrated by *at least* a 52 Fr bougie. Although the initial reports included very good levels of reflux control, adverse effects—such as dysphagia, inability to belch, gas bloat, and increased flatulence—were not uncommon.

In an attempt to achieve an effective antireflux barrier with fewer side effects, a number of partial fundoplications have been proposed over the years. We will concentrate on the two most popular of these: the posterior 270-degree fundoplication and the anterior 180-degree fundoplication. The laparoscopic posterior 270-degree wrap was first described by Cushieri et al. in 1993, closely mimicking Toupet's original description in 1963. Reports of laparoscopic anterior 180-degree wrap began to emerge in the early to mid-1990s, from our group in Adelaide, Australia, based on Dor's reports, in 1962, of an anterior 180-degree wrap designed to control reflux in patients undergoing cardiomyotomy for achalasia.

Minimally invasive techniques have revolutionized surgery. Comparisons between open and laparoscopic fundoplication have conclusively demonstrated that a laparoscopic approach has clear advantages in terms of reduced complications and quicker recovery. Furthermore, this is not at the cost of less durable reflux control. It is now the standard surgical approach, and most large medical centers offer laparoscopic fundoplication.

PRINCIPLES AND JUSTIFICATION

The ideal antireflux operation would alleviate reflux by replicating normal physiological function of the lower esophageal sphincter. Surgery creates a mechanical barrier to reflux between the stomach and the esophagus, which is independent of the constituent of the refluxate, whether this is acid based or duodeno-gastric in nature. The effect is immediate and does not limit normal activity and is often permanent, but is not without consequences. Although the operative risks are low and laparoscopic approaches have lessened the insult to the abdominal wall, which in turn reduces postoperative pain, surgery is never painless and comes with the potential for morbidity. Also, the surgical reflux barrier sometimes works in both directions, so that patients can develop dysphagia: limiting diet in one direction and gas release in the other—that is, belching and vomiting may not be possible.

The aims of surgery include the following:

- To reduce a hiatal hernia (for large hiatal hernia, see Chapter 39, "Laparoscopic large hiatus hernia repair")
- To repair a hiatal defect by tightening the diaphragmatic crural pillars
- To restore 3–4 cm of the esophagus below the diaphragm
- To create a valve at the gastroesophageal junction to prevent acid reflux

How does it work?

As stated, most surgeons now perform a variant of one of three eponymous abdominal operations: a Nissen 360-degree fundoplication, a Dor 180-degree anterior fundoplication, and a Toupet 270-degree posterior fundoplication. The exact mechanism of action of all three antireflux operations is not completely clear but they all bear similarities. The main reason is probably the creation of a "physical" valve. Surgery ensures that the distal esophagus is placed intra-abdominally, at the same time exaggerating the sharpness of the angle between it and the adjacent gastric fundus. This forms a flap-like valve that closes in two situations: (1) a rise in intragastric pressure, which leads to gastric fundal expansion and thus compression of the adjacent esophagus, and (2) a rise in intra-abdominal pressure, which directly collapses the intra-abdominal esophagus. As well, repair of the diaphragm allows it to contribute to its normal antireflux activity via contraction of the crura.

PREOPERATIVE ASSESSMENT AND PREPARATION

History and workup

It is important to take a careful history for reflux. "Reflux" can mean a great many things to patients. One common approach is to divide presenting symptoms under *typical* and *atypical* headings. Typical (or classic) symptoms include retrosternal burning or pain and acid regurgitation (also referred to as "water brash" or "volume reflux"). Atypical symptoms (considered extra-esophageal manifestations of reflux) include cough, hoarseness, aspiration pneumonia, dental erosions, and globus. It is important to define response of symptoms to antireflux medication, and to document type of medication, amount, and timing of medication.

With a goal of 100% satisfaction among our patient population (however unattainable!), potential candidates for antireflux surgery must be properly assessed. In our opinion, this involves a minimum of endoscopy, ambulatory pH monitoring (in the absence of Grade II esophagitis or higher on endoscopy), and esophageal manometry. In our practice, the operating surgeon generally repeats the endoscopy to look at the gastroesophageal junction and anatomy, rule out Barrett's esophagus/peptic stricture, and document the presence/absence of esophagitis (see Chapter 27, "Endoscopy"). If esophagitis is present, a postoperative endoscopy is prudent to rule out subsequent development of Barrett's esophagus. The surgeon should document the percentage of time acid is in the lower esophagus, and, in particular, the temporal correlation between symptoms and episodes of reflux (either reported as the symptom index or symptom association probability). A barium swallow is a useful adjunct in a patient with a hiatus hernia.

Selection criteria for surgery

Classic teaching dictates that a patient with *typical* symptoms of reflux, a good response to antireflux medication and a positive 24-hour pH study will have a good result with 90% certainty. So, who are the 10% of patients who will do poorly? Studies have shown that the following patient characteristics are associated with poorer outcomes:

- Female
- Atypical symptoms, especially the patient with cough as their sole symptom
- Poor response to antireflux medication
- Low symptom index or symptom association probability on 24-hour pH study
- No hiatus hernia
- Poor esophageal motility
- Public hospital treatment

TAILOR THE WRAP TO THE PATIENT

The Nissen 360-degree fundoplication is termed a "total" fundoplication as the wrap completely encircles the distal esophagus. This offers good and durable reflux control but this sometimes comes at the expense of an "overcompetent" barrier; that is, one that is too tight and leads to dysphagia with solids, and/or gas bloat and increased flatulence from an inability to belch and release swallowed air. Partial repairs, both anterior 180 degree and posterior 270 degree, are cited as causing fewer of these competency problems. A number of randomized studies have attempted to clarify this. The evidence to date suggests that "wind"-related side effects and postfundoplication dysphagia are less common following a partial fundoplication but that this may be offset by a slightly higher risk of recurrent reflux.

In the authors' practice, young patients with good esophageal motility are offered a 360-degree fundoplication, with the knowledge that adverse effects will be better tolerated in these individuals, and then subside over time. A 360-degree fundoplication is also used in patients with Barrett's esophagus, and in those with a peptic stricture from severe reflux. In most other patients, especially elderly patients with a primary complaint of large hiatus hernia, a partial fundoplication is performed. In our institutions, this tends to be a 180-degree fundoplication.

Preoperative preparation

The vast majority of our patients undergo 3–4 weeks of a very low calorie diet prior to surgery. The reason for this is a dramatic reduction in liver volume, which optimizes the surgeon's access to the hiatus for successful laparoscopic surgery. Patients also meet a dietician prior to surgery for education regarding a suitable postfundoplication diet. In general terms, this is a minced and moist diet and excludes foods likely to obstruct at the gastroesophageal junction, such as bread, pasta, and chunky pieces of meat.

The anesthetic is tailored to minimize postoperative nausea and/or vomiting. This involves avoidance of volatile agents (e.g., isoflurane, sevoflurane, nitrous oxide) and morphine. In our institution, the anesthetists prefer total intravenous anesthesia with propofol infusion. Dexamethasone 4 mg intravenous (IV) is administered, and a 5-HT3 antagonist (e.g., ondansetron) is commenced. All patients wear stockings in addition to pneumatic compression stockings, and receive appropriate antibiotic prophylaxis.

OPERATIVE TECHNIQUE

Position of patient and port placement

We prefer to work between the patient's legs (with the patient in lithotomy), with the right arm tucked, and left arm abducted. A pneumoperitoneum is established using a Veress technique under the left subcostal margin. Carbon dioxide is insufflated to a maximum pressure of 14 mmHg. A 10–12 mm port is then placed just to the left of midline, 15 cm from the xiphoid process. A 30-degree camera is inserted and all ports thereafter are placed under direct vision: 10–12 mm port in the left upper quadrant (11 cm from xiphoid under the left subcostal margin) and a further two 5 mm lateral ports and a subxiphoid Nathanson retractor to retract the left lobe of the liver. The patient is tilted in a steep reverse Trendelenburg position prior to positioning of the liver retractor. The surgeon moves between the patient's legs, the assistant sits on a stool to the patient's left side, and the monitor is positioned over the head of the patient with an extra monitor (if available) to the right side of the patient's head. (See **Figure 38.1**.)

Dissection and identification of esophagus

The pars flaccida of the lesser omentum is opened and dissected down to the right crus with diathermy, avoiding damage to the hepatic branches of the vagus nerve. The peritoneum overlying the right pillar is divided and blunt dissection with a Hunter bowel grasper opens the esophago-hiatal groove to expose the esophagus. The phrenoesophageal ligament is then divided with cautery and the left pillar is identified, taking care to avoid trauma to the anterior vagus nerve. The left pillar is now dissected using blunt technique, and the angle of His is taken down. (See **Figure 38.2**.)

The surgeon then exposes the "V" of the crural pillars posteriorly. A window can then be made posterior to the esophagus, taking care to preserve the posterior vagus nerve. The esophagus is slung with an infant feeding tube (5 Fr) to aid retraction, and the esophagus is mobilized to allow 3–4 cm to sit within the abdominal cavity without traction. Any remaining posterior attachments to the left pillar are divided. (See **Figure 38.3**.)

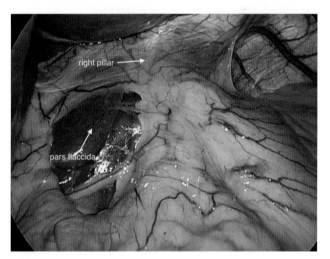

38.2

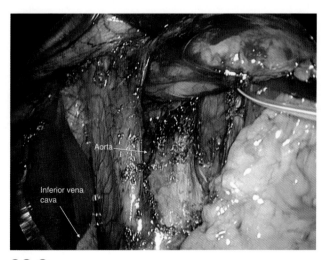

38.3

38.1

Closure of hiatus

By retracting the esophagus to the patient's left, the hiatal pillars are exposed and approximated with interrupted non-absorbable sutures (we use 2-0 Novafil [Covidien, Medtronic, Dublin, Ireland, and Fridley, Minnesota, United States]), taking bites incorporating the epimysium/endoabdominal fascia. Care is taken not to injure the aorta posteriorly or the inferior vena cava laterally. Gauging how "tight" to close the hiatus can be aided by the use of an intraesophageal 54 Fr bougie. We do not believe in the use of mesh to reinforce diaphragmatic closure for a straightforward antireflux procedure (i.e., no large hiatal defect). (See **Figure 38.4**.)

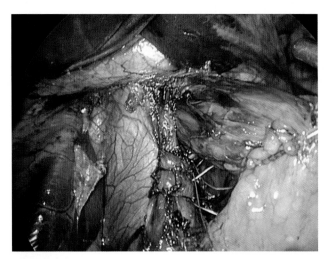

38.4

Laparoscopic Nissen 360-degree fundoplication

The anterior gastric fundus is passed posterior to the esophagus from left to right and the position checked by a "shoe-shine" maneuver to ensure that the wrap is not twisted or under tension (see **Figure 38.5**).

If the wrap is under tension, the short gastric vessels may need to be divided. In our experience, this is a very rare occurrence indeed. We accept that many surgeons feel that division of the short gastric vessels is essential to ensure a "floppy," tension-free fundoplication. However, we find that nondivision simplifies the dissection, as long as careful judgement is made to select the correct piece of stomach to use for the construction of a sufficiently loose fundoplication. There is now good randomized evidence to back this up, with a poorer outcome in three of six trials due to an increase in the incidence of bloating symptoms when the short gastric vessels were divided. Nevertheless, if necessary, the surgeon retracts the stomach to the patient's right, and the assistant retracts the gastrosplenic ligament to the patient's left. The short gastric vessels are divided with ultrasonic shears from the inferior pole of the spleen toward the left pillar. The lesser sac is entered and care is taken to avoid injury to a tortuous splenic artery. There are usually one or two posterior gastric vessels, which require division toward the left pillar.

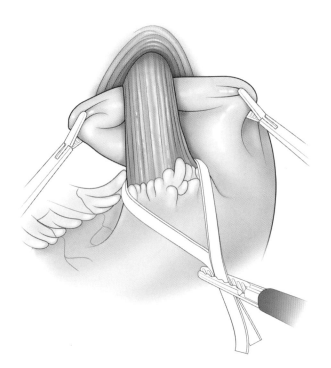

38.5

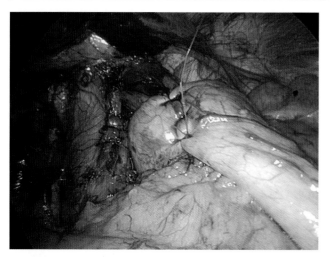

38.6

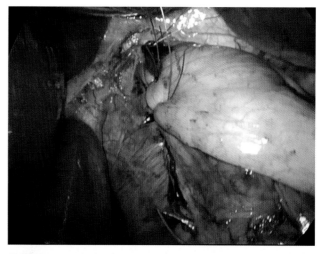

38.7

The gastric fundus is sutured to itself and the anterior wall of the esophagus over a 54 Fr bougie. A 2 cm wrap is created with three separate nonabsorbable sutures approximately a centimeter apart. The esophageal sling is removed, the bougie removed, and the liver retractor removed under direct vision. The ports are removed, the wounds closed, and dressings applied. (See **Figure 38.6**.)

Anterior partial 180-degree fundoplication

The angle of His is recreated by suturing the medial gastric fundus to the left lateral esophagus with two nonabsorbable sutures. The lateral gastric fundus (adjacent to the short gastric vessels) is then folded over the intra-abdominal esophagus, and sutured to the right crus, at the 11 o'clock position. As per Dor's original description, the short gastric vessels are not divided, as this is never necessary with a primary 180-degree wrap. Two further sutures are placed into the gastric fundus, the right lateral esophagus, and right diaphragmatic crus to secure the fundus over the esophagus, as a 180-degree wrap. Care is taken not to create a "waist," which may cause dysphagia with compression of the intra-abdominal esophagus. At times, a "crown stitch" is placed between the gastric fundus and diaphragmatic hiatus at the 1 or 2 o'clock position to avoid herniation of a floppy gastric fundus above the diaphragm. (See **Figure 38.7**.)

Posterior partial 270-degree fundoplication

Similar to the Nissen fundoplication, the anterior gastric fundus is passed posterior to the esophagus from left to right and the position checked by a shoe-shine maneuver to ensure that the wrap is not twisted or under tension (see **Figure 38.5**). The assistant holds the fundus in place posterior to the esophagus, while the primary surgeon places three nonabsorbable sutures into the posteriorly held fundus and right crus. Three further sutures are placed into the posteriorly held fundus and the anterior esophagus (10 o'clock position) approximately 1 cm apart. Finally, three more sutures are placed into the anterior gastric fundus and anterior esophagus (2 o'clock position) to create a 2 cm 270-degree wrap. This is best done over a 54 Fr bougie to prevent a tight wrap. (See **Figure 38.8**.)

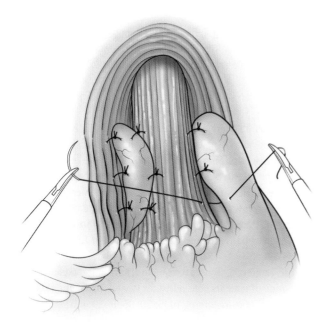

38.8

POSTOPERATIVE CARE

Aggressive anti-emesis is administered postoperatively to prevent vomiting. We use an intravenous 5-HT3 antagonist (e.g., ondansetron) at regular time periods over 48 hours. Other anti-emetics are charted, including droperidol 0.5 mg, metoclopramide 10–20 mg, and cyclizine 50 mg. Patients are given regular IV paracetamol, and low dose opioid (e.g., fentanyl) if needed. Clear fluids are allowed the same day, with a contrast swallow performed on postoperative day 1. If the wrap is subdiaphragmatic and no leak is identified (see **Figure 38.9**), free fluids are commenced, with an upgrade to a minced/pureed diet that evening. A soft diet is commenced the following day, either as an outpatient or prior to discharge.

All patients are counselled to refrain from heavy lifting (anything over 10 kg) for 8 weeks, and to avoid constipation or any other type of strain on the hiatal repair. If a patient is worried about the flu season or exposure to illness, a prescription is given for ondansetron 4 mg wafers (every 6 hours as needed). Patient are reviewed at 4–5 weeks postoperatively, and once more at 3 months.

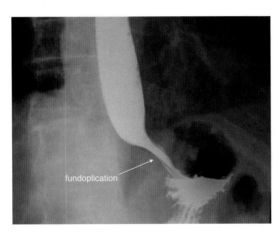

fundoplication

38.9

Early problems

As stated previously, early problems are probably more accentuated in patients with a total wrap. Nevertheless, all patients experience some discomfort and often experience varying degrees of dysphagia, gas bloat, the inability to belch, and increased flatulence. These problems are most pronounced in the first 3 months following surgery, necessitating a strict postfundoplication diet for at least 4–6 weeks. If gas bloat is moderate to severe, a gastric motility agent (e.g., domperidone) may help until the swelling at the gastroesophageal junction settles down.

Later problems

Refer to Chapter 40, "Revisional antireflux surgery" for a detailed discussion regarding appropriate history, workup, and investigation of recurrent or new symptoms postlaparoscopic fundoplication.

OUTCOMES

Over 1991 to 2016, over 2800 consecutive patients have undergone laparoscopic antireflux surgery in South Australia. All patients are captured on a National Health and Medical Research Council-funded database, and fill out prospective questionnaires at 3 and 12 months, and annually thereafter. In 2012, we published our experience on 2261 patients followed over 20 years. We had a 3.2% conversion rate (zero for the last 5 years), and 9.6% of patients underwent revisional surgery (the majority within the first year of surgery, and some probably secondary to a steep learning curve in the early 1990s). Satisfaction rates were close to 90% for both 360-degree and 180-degree fundoplication patients at late follow-up, confirming that, *in the carefully selected patient*, laparoscopic fundoplication is a durable, effective treatment for gastroesophageal reflux.

FURTHER READING

Broeders JA, Roks DJ, Ahmed Ali U, Watson DI, Baigrie RJ, Cao Z, Hartmann J, Maddern GJ. Laparoscopic anterior 180-degree versus Nissen fundoplication for gastroesophageal reflux disease: systematic review and meta-analysis of randomized clinical trials. *Ann Surg.* 2013; 257: 850–9.

Dallemagne B, Weerts JM, Jehaes C, Markiewicz S, Lombard R. Laparoscopic Nissen fundoplication: preliminary report. *Surg Laparosc Endosc.* 1991; 1: 138–43.

Engström C, Cai W, Irvine T, Devitt PG, Thompson SK, Game PA, Bessell JR, Jamieson GG, Watson DI. Twenty years of experience with laparoscopic antireflux surgery. *Br J Surg.* 2012; 99: 1415–21.

Geagea T. Laparoscopic Nissen's fundoplication: preliminary report on ten cases. *Surg Endosc.* 1991; 5: 170–3.

Hunter JG, Trus TL, Branum GD, Waring JP, Wood WC. A physiologic approach to laparoscopic fundoplication for gastroesophageal reflux disease. *Ann Surg.* 1996; 223: 673–85.

Lewis MC, Phillips ML, Slavotinek JP, Kow L, Thompson CH, Toouli J. Change in liver size and fat content after treatment with Optifast very low calorie diet. *Obes Surg.* 2006; 16: 697–701.

Thompson SK, Watson DI. What is the best anti-reflux operation? All fundoplications are not created equal. *World J Surg.* 2015; 39: 997–9.

Waring JP, Hunter JG, Oddsdottir M, Wo J, Katz E. The preoperative evaluation of patients considered for laparoscopic antireflux surgery. *Am J Gastroenterol.* 1995; 90: 35–8.

Watson DI, Jamieson GG, Pike GK, Davies N, Richardson M, Devitt PG. Prospective randomized double blind trial between laparoscopic Nissen fundoplication and anterior partial fundoplication. *Br J Surg.* 1999; 86: 123–30.

39

Laparoscopic large hiatus hernia repair

ALEX NAGLE, GEOFFREY S. CHOW, AND NATHANIEL J. SOPER

INTRODUCTION

The diaphragm is both a muscular and tendinous tissue that begins to bear mechanical pressure from the abdominal viscera during the tenth week of life. Abnormal diaphragmatic development can lead to large congenital diaphragmatic hernias present at birth, while other smaller areas of diaphragmatic weakness can enlarge over time and become apparent later in life. Hiatal hernias result from a widening of the diaphragmatic crura and a weakening of the phrenoesophageal membrane. This results in a protrusion of a hernia sac containing intra-abdominal organs through the diaphragmatic hiatus and into the mediastinum. The prevalence of large hiatal hernias increases with age, suggesting that environmental and tissue-aging factors are involved in the pathophysiology. In addition, there is a positive association between the presence of hiatal and inguinal hernias, suggesting either a genetic predisposition affecting tissue integrity or some other common factor, such as increased intra-abdominal pressure.

A large hiatal hernia can result in a wide range of symptoms and potentially lead to gastric incarceration and strangulation, a life-threatening emergency. For this reason, hernia repair is generally indicated for most patients with symptomatic hernias. The technical aspects of such operations have undergone significant evolution in the last century and laparoscopy is now considered the preferred approach. When compared with laparotomy or thoracotomy, laparoscopy offers reductions in pain, convalescence, hospital length of stay, and morbidity. However, many controversies still remain, including whether to reinforce the crural closure with mesh, how frequently an esophageal lengthening procedure is necessary, and the role of a concomitant antireflux procedure. This chapter will address the work-up and preoperative evaluation of patients with a large hiatal hernia, describe the technical aspects of a laparoscopic repair as we perform it, and review the literature regarding the unresolved debates over optimal technique.

HERNIA CLASSIFICATION

Hiatal hernias are subclassified into four types (see Table 39.1). In a type I hiatal hernia, the esophagogastric junction (EGJ) migrates cephalad to the crura, resulting in a portion of intrathoracic stomach. As the EGJ forms the lead-point of herniation between the abdomen and mediastinum, type I hiatal hernias are also termed "sliding hernias." Type I hernias are by far the most common form of hiatal hernia, making up 95% of the total prevalence. Type II, III, and IV hernias are together termed "paraesophageal hernias" (PEHs) and combined account for the remaining 5% of

Table 39.1 The four types of hiatal hernias

Hiatal hernia type	Anatomy
I	The EGJ herniates above the diaphragmatic crura, often moving transiently from the abdomen into the mediastinum
II	A portion of the stomach is herniated into the mediastinum alongside the esophagus, with the EGJ in normal (i.e., intra-abdominal) position
III	The EGJ is above the hiatus and a portion, or the entirety, of the stomach is folded alongside the esophagus
IV	An intra-abdominal organ other than the stomach is additionally herniated through the hiatus

hiatal hernias. Type II anatomy consists of a hernia in which a portion of the stomach (usually the fundus) has migrated through the hiatus and into mediastinum, but with an EGJ that remains below the diaphragm. A true type II hiatal hernia is rare. In a type III hernia, the EGJ is above the diaphragm and a portion of the stomach is additionally present within the chest and alongside the esophagus. Type III hernias are typically caused by a large crural separation, which can result in a large portion, or the entirety, of the stomach lying intrathoracically. For this reason, type III hernias are often referred to as "giant" PEHs. A type III hiatal hernia is the most common type of PEH. Type IV is defined as any hiatal hernia in which an intra-abdominal organ other than the stomach has also migrated through the crura. Common examples are the omentum, small bowel, transverse colon, spleen, and/or pancreas.

PRESENTING SYMPTOMS

Patients with PEHs commonly present with symptoms due to either intermittent obstruction or gastroesophageal reflux. Obstruction is caused by a kinking of the esophagus and/or stomach, and results in episodes of dysphagia, early satiety, regurgitation, nausea, vomiting, and/or chest pain. The anatomic distortion of PEHs often leads to an incompetence of normal EGJ function. This in turn causes gastroesophageal reflux, with its characteristic symptom of intermittent retrosternal heartburn, which is often postprandial and exacerbated when supine. PEHs can also result in erosions of the gastric mucosa, termed "Cameron ulcers." These ulcers can cause anemia from chronic bleeding and their exact etiology has not been conclusively determined. Friction from repeated passage of the stomach through the hiatus, increased acid exposure from stasis of gastric juices, and ischemia have all been proposed as causal mechanisms. Larger type III and IV hernias can additionally cause respiratory and cardiac impairment via direct compression of the lungs and left atrium of the heart.

The symptoms discussed so far are usually subacute, and patients can suffer for prolonged periods of time while being evaluated, and often incorrectly treated, for more common conditions such as non-hernia-related gastroesophageal reflux, peptic ulcer disease, angina, and biliary colic. This scenario of clinical manifestation is distinct from patients who present acutely with an incarcerated PEH. Acute PEH incarceration is a life-threatening surgical emergency, as it can lead to gastric ischemia and, if not alleviated, necrosis. The classic presenting symptoms and signs of an acute incarceration are together known as "Borchardt's triad": chest pain, the urge but inability to vomit, and failure of nasogastric tube passage below the diaphragm. Immediate reduction of the hernia is required to restore blood flow to the stomach, and a laparotomy or thoracotomy is often necessary to achieve this. The remainder of this chapter will address only the evaluation and management of patients with PEH in an elective setting.

INDICATIONS FOR SURGERY

Based on the potential for gastric incarceration, it was a long accepted surgical principle that PEHs should be repaired on an elective basis when discovered, regardless of the patient's symptoms. This traditional assumption was challenged by a landmark study by Stylopoulos and colleagues in 2002. The authors constructed a Markov Monte Carlo analytic model using pooled outcomes data to estimate quality of life years for patients with asymptomatic PEH treated with either laparoscopic repair or watchful waiting. This analysis showed that watchful waiting resulted in a yearly acute incarceration rate of only 1.1%, and was superior to surgery for 83% of patients. Based on these findings, expectant management is now considered a reasonable option in patients with truly asymptomatic PEH. On the other hand, the presence of any symptoms related to a PEH is considered an indication for laparoscopic repair, as long as the patient is of reasonable operative risk.

PREOPERATIVE EVALUATION

In addition to a thorough history and physical examination, several tests are indicated preoperatively to secure the diagnosis of PEH and help define the anatomy and physiology of the esophagus and stomach. Contrast esophagram, or an "upper GI (gastrointestinal) study," forms the basis for diagnosis of a PEH and description of its anatomy (see **Figure 39.1**). The location of the esophagus, EGJ, stomach, and pylorus can all be assessed. This secures the diagnosis and subclassification within hiatal hernia type, and allows the surgeon to approximate the size of the hernia sac and width of the crural defect. The distance between the EGJ and hiatus can also be measured, which, if greater than 5 cm, serves as a predictor

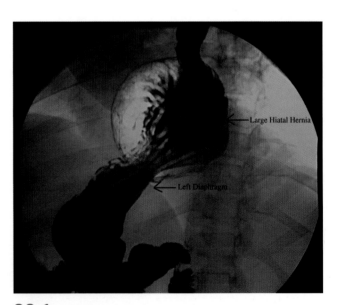

39.1 A preoperative barium esophagram demonstrating a typical PEH.

that an esophageal lengthening procedure may be required. The use of fluoroscopy to obtain multiple images over time allows for an assessment of esophageal function. Pooling of a contrast column within the esophagus and a delay in contrast transit through the EGJ indicate a functional obstruction as a result of the hernia. Conversely, reflux of contrast material from the stomach back into the esophagus is indicative of an incompetent EGJ, resulting in gastroesophageal reflux.

Upper endoscopy is mandatory in the preoperative evaluation of patients prior to planned PEH repair (refer to Chapter 27, "Endoscopy"). The primary purpose is to rule out a malignancy near the EGJ, which can present with the same obstructive symptoms as a PEH. It is also important to check for the presence of esophagitis or gastritis, Barrett esophagus, Cameron ulcers, and/or peptic ulcer disease.

Although not universally adopted, we routinely perform an esophageal manometry study on patients being evaluated for PEH. This study is often technically difficult to perform in these patients and it is often easiest to place the manometry catheter during endoscopy. Patients with a PEH often have abnormal esophageal motility, and these impairments can improve after surgery. However, in patients with complete aperistalsis on preoperative manometry, or those who have weak peristalsis and dysphagia that cannot be explained by the anatomy seen on esophagram, we will tailor our operation to include a partial, rather than complete 360-degree, fundoplication.

A 24-hour pH monitoring study is not necessary, as the results will not change the need for surgery or alter the surgical approach.

OPERATIVE TECHNIQUE

Patient positioning and set-up

Laparoscopic PEH repair is performed under general anesthesia with endotracheal intubation and full paralysis. Patients are positioned supine with legs abducted. We tuck the right arm and abduct the left arm, and use a vacuum beanbag mattress to support the patient's sides and perineum. This positioning provides stability when the table is shifted into a steep reverse Trendelenburg position and helps to prevent neuropathy during what may be a lengthy operation. Pneumatic compression stockings and a urinary catheter are placed, and patients receive appropriate antibiotic prophylaxis prior to the initial incision.

Trocar placement

Five trocars are utilized: one for the laparoscope, two for the operating surgeon, one for the assistant, and one for a liver retractor (see **Figure 39.2**). We begin by placing a 10 mm trocar slightly to the left of midline and superior to the umbilicus, approximately 12–15 cm from the xiphoid process. This is typically done using a Veress technique in patients without prior upper abdominal surgery, but an open Hasson technique may be used as well. Once this trocar is inserted and the abdomen insufflated, a 30- or 45-degree laparoscope is inserted and an initial diagnostic laparoscopy is performed. Use of an angled laparoscope during PEH repair is essential so that unobstructed views can be obtained when working in the confined space of the hiatus and mediastinum.

A 5 mm trocar for the liver retractor is then placed just below the right costal margin, approximately 15 cm from the xiphoid. We use a self-retaining retractor to elevate the left lateral segment of the liver and expose the hiatus. A 5 mm port for the assistant's instrument is then placed in the right upper abdomen, approximately midway between the liver retractor and laparoscope ports. A common alternative is to place the assistant's trocar in a lateral position below the left costal margin.

The two trocars for the operating surgeon's instruments are then placed. The positioning of these ports is intended to create a triangulation effect, in which the two instruments enter the operative field at a 30- to 60-degree angle from either side of the laparoscopic image. The esophagus enters the abdomen through the hiatus at a right-to-left angle, so the surgeon's two working trocars are also arranged "off center" toward the patient's left side. For the surgeon's right hand, a 10 mm trocar (to accommodate a curved needle) is inserted just inferior to the left costal margin, approximately 10 cm from the xiphoid process. We lastly place the surgeon's

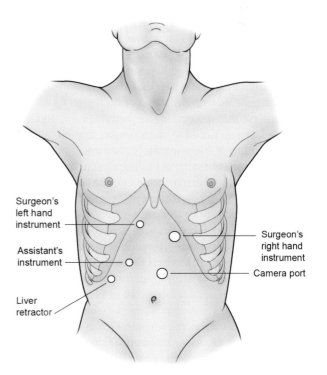

39.2 Trocar positioning for laparoscopic PEH repair.

left-hand 5 mm trocar slightly inferior and to the right of the xiphoid process. Depending on the size and anatomy of the liver, this trocar may need to be placed more inferiorly on the abdominal wall. For this reason, once the liver retractor has been secured, we test potential locations for this trocar by first passing a Veress needle through the abdominal wall to ensure that the working instrument will have a clear path to the hiatus.

Once the trocars have been placed, the patient is tilted to a steep reverse Trendelenburg position to shift the abdominal contents inferiorly, away from the hiatus, and to bring the patient's upper abdomen closer to the surgeon, thereby improving ergonomics. This should be done slowly, and in coordination with the anesthesiologist, as this maneuver can significantly reduce venous return. The operating surgeon then moves to a position between the patient's legs with the laparoscopic monitor placed directly over the head of the patient. The assistant stands to the patient's right and the camera operator is seated on a stool to the patient's left.

Dissection and reduction of the hernia sac

An initial diagnostic laparoscopy is performed, focusing on delineating the hernia and relevant anatomy. Specific attention is paid to the positions of the pylorus, left gastric artery, spleen, and short gastric vessels, as well as the width of the crural defect. An attempt is made to reduce the stomach from the hernia sac and into the abdominal cavity. This helps to facilitate the remainder of the operation by creating additional working space in the mediastinum. A hand-over-hand technique is used to gently pull the stomach inferiorly using atraumatic graspers. Excessive force should never be applied to the stomach during this initial maneuver. Significant adhesions often exist between the stomach and the hernia sac, and excessive traction can result in gastric injury. If the stomach does not reduce easily, this step should be abandoned and the operation proceed with dissection of the hernia sac.

To initiate this dissection, the hepatogastric ligament is divided to gain access to the lesser sac and mobilize the lesser curvature of the stomach. In the case of a large type III PEH, a significant portion of the lesser curvature may lie intrathoracically and extreme care must be taken to identify the location of the left gastric artery, right gastric artery, and even porta hepatis, prior to dividing the hepatogastric ligament, as these structures can be shifted toward the hiatus. Once the lesser sac is entered, division of the lesser omentum continues superiorly to the level of the right crus. We use an ultrasonic dissector to accomplish this, although bipolar or monopolar energy devices can also be employed. The hepatic branch of the vagus nerve can be divided without physiologic consequence, as long as the surgeon has confirmed that an aberrant left hepatic artery is not present alongside it.

The next step is to enter the mediastinum and develop a plane on the outside of the hernia sac. The importance of this maneuver cannot be overemphasized, and the relative ease or difficulty of the remainder of the operation often

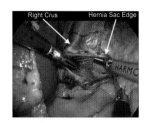

39.3 Dissection of the hernia sac begins at the medial border of the right crus. The hernia sac and sac contents are swept to the right of the laparoscopic image and the right crus is swept to the left in order to enter the mediastinum on the outside of the sac. The assistant provides retraction inferiorly on the hernia sac.

hinges upon it. To achieve this, the surgeon grasps the right crus with a blunt grasper and then incises the peritoneal layer at its medial aspect (see **Figure 39.3**). The hernia sac is an extension of this peritoneal membrane, and therefore, if it is divided at the medial edge of the right crus, the mediastinum can be entered external to the sac. Opening this plane will allow carbon dioxide to help dissect the space exterior to the sac and limit the "spinnaker effect" caused by the pneumoperitoneum. Blunt dissection is used to sweep the sac and its contents medially and inferiorly, separating them from the rest of the mediastinal structures. The assistant forcibly retracts the hernia sac inferiorly in order to continuously reduce the hernia contents as the dissection proceeds. It should be noted that neither the surgeon nor assistant should grasp the esophagus directly, as it can be injured easily. During this portion of the procedure, the use of cautery should also be limited so as to not inadvertently cause a tear in the hernia sac or thermal injury to the esophagus or vagus nerves.

If the correct plane has been entered, the hernia sac should separate relatively easily, revealing the right-sided mediastinal pleura laterally, pericardium anteriorly, and vertebrae and aorta posteriorly. The anterior and posterior vagus nerves should be identified as well, and kept alongside the esophagus. As this mediastinal working space is enlarged, the edge of the hernia sac is sequentially divided at its junction with the crura. This is done in a clockwise direction, starting at the point of mediastinal entry and proceeding toward the left crus. Blunt dissection of the hernia sac then proceeds to the patient's left, and the left pleura is exposed. During this mediastinal dissection, tears in the pleura and resulting capnothorax can occur. This usually does not result in adverse physiologic consequences, but the anesthesiologist should be immediately informed. In the case of capnothorax that results in hypotension or increased airway pressures, a reduction in insufflation pressure, or complete deinsufflation of the abdomen, will almost always correct these abnormalities. Insertion of a chest tube is rarely, if ever, required.

Once the dissection reaches the left crus, we next divide the short gastric vessels and gastrosplenic ligament. This mobilization will be required eventually to perform the fundoplication, and when performed at this point in the operation, it allows for easier access to the posterior aspect

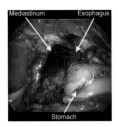

39.4 The anatomy seen after completion of hernia sac dissection and esophageal mobilization. The entire stomach and EGJ lie intra-abdominally and the esophagus is mobilized off of the crura circumferentially.

of the hiatus and hernia sac. We prefer to mobilize the entire fundus, starting at the point at which the vessels begin to run perpendicularly to the greater curve (i.e., the short gastric vessels). The assistant retracts the stomach medially, while the surgeon uses his or her left hand to retract the omentum laterally. This aligns the short gastric vessels horizontally in the laparoscopic view. Division with an ultrasonic dissector, or other energy device, then proceeds proximally up the greater curvature until the stomach is separated completely from the left crus and posterior hiatal attachments. The posterior hernia sac, arising from the lesser peritoneal sac, is divided at the base of the crura.

At this point, the esophagus should be circumferentially mobilized away from the crura. Blunt dissection of any remaining hernia sac off of the mediastinal structures and into the abdomen continues until the sac is completely freed and reduced (see **Figure 39.4**). At this point, we prefer to excise as much of the hernia sac as possible. This allows for accurate identification of the EGJ and prevents incorporation of remaining sac tissue into the eventual fundoplication. Care must be taken to identify and trace both vagal trunks prior to sac excision, as there can be dense adhesions between the vagi, sac, and stomach.

Esophageal mobilization and lengthening

Once the sac is excised and removed though a trocar, the intra-abdominal length of the esophagus is measured. We prefer to have an esophageal segment of at least 2.5 cm below the diaphragm, with no axial traction exerted, so that a 2 cm long Nissen fundoplication can be comfortably constructed around it. Failure to achieve this length will predispose to reherniation of the wrap into the chest, which can cause obstructive symptoms, and may necessitate reoperation. To measure this length accurately, we use the distance between the open jaws of an atraumatic grasper (2.5 cm in our instrument set). It is critical that no caudad traction is placed on the stomach while obtaining these measurements, as this can falsely lengthen the intra-abdominal distance.

If there is less than 2.5 cm of esophagus below the crura, the mediastinal esophagus is mobilized further cephalad to gain additional length. During this dissection, the posterior

vagal trunk is used as a landmark while bluntly mobilizing the esophagus anteriorly away from the spine and aorta, leaving the posterior vagal trunk attached to the posterior wall of the esophagus. This circumferential dissection can be taken to the level of the inferior pulmonary veins and is successful in achieving the desired intra-abdominal segment in the majority of cases. However, even after meticulous dissection, in 3%–14% of cases, the EGJ remains close to or above the crura, resulting in a "short esophagus." Preoperative risk factors that predispose to the occurrence of short esophagus include long-standing gastroesophageal reflux or reoperation, an EGJ that is greater than 5 cm above the hiatus on esophagram or manometry, or the presence of peptic strictures or Barrett esophagus on endoscopy. However, even when taken in combination, these risk factors do a poor job of predicting which patients will ultimately require esophageal lengthening, and the final diagnosis is always made intraoperatively after a complete esophageal mobilization has been performed.

If a short esophagus still exists after the previously described maneuvers, an esophageal lengthening procedure should be performed so that a completely intra-abdominal fundoplication can be created. We prefer a stapled wedge-gastrectomy technique that creates a length of "neo-esophagus" from the proximal gastric cardia. This is performed using a standard laparoscopic linear cutting-stapler that is capable of articulation. First, a 50 Fr bougie is passed into the stomach along the lesser curve. A marking stitch is placed on the left edge of the bougie at a distance approximately 3 cm inferior to the hiatus, at the point that will become the new "EGJ." The stapler is then used to divide the fundus from the greater curvature to this marked point. The stapler is then articulated and fired alongside the left lateral aspect of the bougie to create a length of neo-esophagus and resect a small wedge of fundus (see **Figure 39.5**). Other techniques for accomplishing a similar gastroplasty have been described, including introduction of the stapler through a right-sided thoracoscopy port, which eliminates the need to resect a portion of fundus.

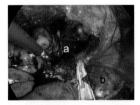

39.5 A Collis gastroplasty is completed by firing an endoscopic stapler in parallel with the esophagus (a) to resect a "wedge" of fundus (b). A 50 Fr bougie is placed down the esophagus and into the gastric body prior to performing the gastroplasty to prevent creation of an overly narrow (or large) neo-esophagus.

Crural closure, relaxing incisions, and options for mesh reinforcement

Once an adequate intra-abdominal esophageal length has been established (via dissection or lengthening procedure), the crura are then closed in order to repair the hernia defect. Interrupted 2-0 nonabsorbable braided sutures are placed at 1 cm intervals, beginning at the posterior crural junction and working anteriorly (see **Figure 39.6**). The use of pledgeted sutures has been described, but we prefer not to leave any synthetic material in this closure, as it may come in contact with the esophagus. It is important to incorporate intact crural fascia, along with muscle, into these bites so they do not pull through. This relies on meticulous preservation of this fascia throughout the prior hernia sac dissection. Often only posterior sutures are necessary, but if this configuration creates an abnormal anterior angulation (speed-bump effect) at the EGJ, then one or more anterior sutures may be needed. Once the closure is completed, a final inspection is performed to ensure that the crural closure is not too tight and that a 5 mm instrument can pass between the crura and esophagus.

As the role of synthetic mesh in reinforcing inguinal and ventral hernia repairs became firmly established, its use in hiatal hernia repair gained considerable attention. Several early series, and even randomized controlled trials, appeared to indicate that routine reinforcement of hiatal hernia repairs with synthetic mesh resulted in lower recurrence rates when compared with primary closure alone. However, a number of serious, and potentially life-threatening, complications have been described as a result of mesh erosion into the esophagus, and even aorta and bronchi. For this reason, the use of synthetic mesh for PEH repair has largely been abandoned.

Biologic meshes used in this context have the potential to provide structural support with less theoretical risk for erosion, as they result in a less severe inflammatory response and are eventually incorporated and absorbed. A trial by Oelschlager and colleagues (2011) randomized patients undergoing PEH repair to crural reinforcement with a biologic mesh (porcine intestinal submucosa) or primary closure only. While rates of recurrent hiatal hernia at 6 months were lower in the mesh group (9% vs. 23%), this advantage was no longer present at 5-year follow-up (54% vs. 59%). However, despite the fact that both groups had high radiologic recurrence rates, they had relatively

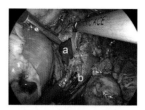

39.7 A relaxing incision (a) is created in the right hemidiaphragm, just lateral to the right crus (b) and medial to the IVC.

minor symptoms and improvements in quality of life, and reoperation was rarely needed. Based on these results, there is insufficient evidence currently to support the routine use of biologic mesh during PEH repair.

However, if the hiatal defect is too large to allow approximation of the crura, or if there is significant tension when attempting primary closure of the crura, then a relaxing incision of the diaphragm is indicated. Crural tension will contribute to the risk of hernia recurrence, and a relaxing incision will allow for crural approximation without undo tension. A diaphragmatic relaxing incision can be performed either on the right or left hemidiaphragm or bilaterally. Our current approach is to create a "relaxing incision" on the right hemidiaphragm just medial to the inferior vena cava (IVC) (see **Figure 39.7**). However, if a right-sided relaxing incision is inadequate, or if the right crus is simply too thin, then a left-sided relaxing incision can be used. When performing a left-sided diaphragmatic relaxing incision, caution must be taken to avoid injury to the phrenic nerve. As described by DeMeester et al., the left-sided incision should not be made radially on the diaphragm but instead should follow the inferior margin of the rib and extend laterally behind the spleen. The resultant diaphragmatic defect is then repaired with a synthetic mesh, typically polytetrafluoroethylene (PTFE), to prevent herniation at the site of the relaxing incision.

The right-sided relaxing incision is performed with the active blade of the ultrasonic shears to incise the diaphragm full-thickness approximately 1 cm medial to the IVC. The pleural cavity is entered and the incision is carried anteriorly and then curves medially at the top of the hiatus. The right crus is thereby mobilized toward the patient's left side, thus allowing the two crura to come together without undue tension. The diaphragmatic defect is covered with either a biologic or nonbiologic absorbable mesh. An off-centered U-shaped patch is used to cover both the diaphragmatic defect and reinforce the posterior crural closure (see **Figure 39.8**). This is performed by positioning the base of the mesh posterior to the esophagus and the right upright limb of the mesh covering the relaxing incision defect. The right lateral aspect of the mesh extends laterally beyond the IVC and is tucked beneath the caudate lobe of the liver. The mesh is secured with 2-0 permanent sutures at the two top inside (medial) corners and at the base of the mesh. In addition, the mesh is affixed to the diaphragm with fibrin glue. Alternatively, the right lateral edge of the mesh can be sutured

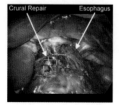

39.6 After completion of a posterior crural repair with interrupted sutures. The esophagus has been sufficiently mobilized so that a segment longer than 2.5 cm lies intra-abdominally.

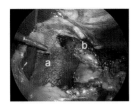

39.8 An absorbable mesh (a) is positioned and sutured in a U-shape configuration, posterior and lateral to the esophagus (b). The mesh serves to buttress the crural repair and cover the relaxing incision defect.

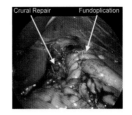

39.9 The final anatomy after completion of crural repair and Nissen fundoplication. The fundoplication is created around the intra-abdominal esophagus, rather than the stomach body.

to the residual cuff of tissue medial to the IVC. We do not advocate the use of tacking devices, such as a titanium helical tack, to secure the mesh to the diaphragm, as reports have described cardiac injury and cardiac tamponade. Compared with the left side, the right-sided relaxing incision is advantageous because it does not require a synthetic mesh and there is less concern for hernia formation at the relaxing incision defect, given its protected location behind the liver. The long-term results of this technique have not been established.

Fundoplication

Once the hiatus has been closed, a functional antireflux barrier is constructed. We perform a 360-degree Nissen fundoplication regardless of the presence of preoperative heartburn or objective evidence of gastroesophageal reflux (e.g., esophagitis on upper endoscopy). However, we modify this to a partial fundoplication if preoperative manometry shows complete aperistalsis, or severely impaired peristalsis that is associated with dysphagia. Other authors have contended that these markers are poor predictors of postoperative function and advocate for use of a complete fundoplication in all cases.

To create the fundoplication, the surgeon first passes his or her left-hand instrument posterior to the esophagus and grasps the most superior aspect of the fundus along the greater curvature. The instrument is then pulled back behind the esophagus in order to wrap the fundus around the esophagus posteriorly. With the right hand, the surgeon then grasps the anterior fundus that remains to the left of the esophagus and performs a "shoe-shine" maneuver, sliding the fundus back and forth with both hands, to check for twists in the wrap and abnormal angulation of the esophagus. It is essential that the wrap be situated entirely around the esophagus, rather than the stomach. This is because a low-lying fundoplication at the level of the gastric body can cause pooling of acidic secretions proximal to the wrap, which can then reflux into the esophagus. Additionally, this anatomy recreates that of a "slipped wrap," which is generally associated with significant dysphagia.

After the fundus is deemed to be in an acceptable location, a 60 Fr bougie is passed into the gastric body under direct laparoscopic vision. The wrap is secured in place

with interrupted seromuscular bites of 2-0 nonabsorbable, braided suture (see **Figure 39.9**). Typically, three sutures are required to create a wrap that is approximately 2 cm in length. We incorporate the most proximal suture into the muscle of the esophageal body to prevent wrap slippage. We do not anchor the fundoplication to the crura, although other authors have described doing so to prevent wrap migration into the chest. Some surgeons add a gastropexy to the anterior abdominal wall, although we have not found this to be routinely necessary (for further detail on the technique of laparoscopic fundoplication, please see Chapter 38, "Laparoscopic antireflux surgery").

After completion of the fundoplication, the abdomen is aspirated and checked for hemostasis. If any questions exist regarding esophageal or gastric injury, or wrap malformation, an upper endoscopy and insufflation leak test are performed. The liver retractor and trocars are then removed under direct vision. The fascia of trocar sites greater than 5 mm is closed and the skin is closed with absorbable suture.

POSTOPERATIVE CARE

Patients are started on scheduled anti-emetics and intravenous ketorolac, with intravenous narcotics as needed for breakthrough pain. Unless the mediastinal dissection was difficult and required extensive esophageal and gastric manipulation, patients are allowed sips of liquids on the day of surgery and then full liquids the following morning. A routine esophagram is not obtained, unless an esophageal lengthening procedure was performed. If advancing as expected, a soft diet is initiated for lunch and patients are discharged home in the afternoon of the first postoperative day. If an esophageal lengthening procedure has been performed the patient is discharged on a proton-pump inhibitor.

Retching occurs not infrequently in the early postoperative period and can cause wrap herniation above the crural repair. For this reason, any nausea should be treated aggressively with additional anti-emetics and an esophagram should be performed after any episode of vomiting to check for anatomic disruption. Any significant deviation from the normal postoperative course, such as severe nausea, significant abdominal or chest pain, fever, or tachycardia, should be assumed to be a leak from an esophageal or gastric perforation until proven otherwise. Such patients should be investigated immediately with an esophagram using water-soluble contrast, with a low threshold for diagnostic laparoscopy if the results are inconclusive.

After hospital discharge, patients are maintained on a soft diet until their first postoperative visit at 2 weeks, and then solid foods are slowly reintroduced as tolerated. Additional tests are not needed unless the patient complains of significant symptoms. Symptoms that are potentially related to either obstruction or gastroesophageal reflux are first investigated with an esophagram to confirm the anatomy of the repair and fundoplication, and then an upper endoscopy. Long-term, approximately 30%–50% of patients will ultimately develop a small recurrent sliding hiatal hernia on repeat imaging. These are managed symptomatically and may require initiation of PPIs. The need for reoperation in most series is less than 5% and is usually only performed for a large recurrent paraesophageal hiatal hernia that is markedly symptomatic (see Chapter 40, "Revisional antireflux surgery").

CONCLUSION

Laparoscopic PEH repair is a complex operation that presents a unique challenge with each case due to the anatomic variation inherent to the disease. A detailed understanding of esophageal physiology and the ability to safely perform a thorough upper endoscopy in the context of distorted anatomy are essential in the preoperative work-up of these patients. Intraoperatively, patience and adaptability are required when formulating strategies to achieve adequate intra-abdominal esophagus length and a durable (tension-free) crural repair. The optimal techniques for accomplishing these aspects of PEH repair have not been conclusively defined and further research is needed.

FURTHER READING

DeMeester SR. Laparoscopic paraesophageal hernia repair: critical steps and adjunct techniques to minimize recurrence. *Surg Laparosc Endosc Percutan Tech.* 2013; 23: 429–35.

Nason KS, Luketich JD, Witteman BP et al. The laparoscopic approach to paraesophageal hernia repair. *J Gastrointest Surg.* 2012; 16(2): 417–26.

Nguyen NT, Christie C, Masoomi H et al. Utilization and outcomes of laparoscopic versus open paraesophageal hernia repair. *Am Surg.* 2011; 77(10): 1353–7.

Oelschlager BK, Pellegrini CA, Hunter JG et al. Biologic prosthesis to prevent recurrence after laparoscopic paraesophageal hernia repair: long-term follow-up from a multicenter, prospective, randomized trial. *J Am Coll Surg.* 2011; 213(4): 461–8.

Roman S, Kahrilas PJ, Kia L et al. Effects of large hiatal hernias on esophageal peristalsis. *Arch Surg.* 2012; 147(4): 352–7.

Stylopoulos N, Gazelle GS, Rattner DW. Paraesophageal hernias: operation or observation? *Ann Surg.* 2002; 236(4): 492–500; discussion 500–1.

Stylopoulos N, Rattner DW. The history of hiatal hernia surgery: from Bowditch to laparoscopy. *Ann Surg.* 2005; 241(1): 185–93.

Swanstrom LL, Jobe BA, Kinzie LR et al. Esophageal motility and outcomes following laparoscopic paraesophageal hernia repair and fundoplication. *Am J Surg.* 1999; 177(5): 359–63.

Swanstrom LL, Marcus DR, Galloway GO. Laparoscopic Collis gastroplasty is the treatment of choice for the shortened esophagus. *Am J Surg.* 1996; 171(5): 477–81.

Zehetner J, Demeester SR, Ayazi S et al. Laparoscopic versus open repair of paraesophageal hernia: the second decade. *J Am Coll Surg.* 2011; 212(5): 813–20.

40

Revisional antireflux surgery

PETER G. DEVITT, ARAVIND SUPPIAH, AND SARAH K. THOMPSON

INTRODUCTION

Antireflux surgery is a well-established treatment for gastroesophageal reflux disease, with long-term success rates in the region of 80%–90%. Perhaps some 1% of individuals with troublesome symptoms undergo surgery and of these, a further 1%–5% will have recurrent or persistent symptoms that lead to some form of revisional surgery.

Symptomatic problems after antireflux surgery can be associated with a poor quality of life, making revisional surgery an attractive proposition for some. Although not as effective as primary repair, revisional antireflux surgery is associated with good outcomes, with patient satisfaction rates of 70%–85%. Revisional antireflux surgery may remain the only meaningful therapeutic measure for symptom relief for some patients—provided they are carefully selected and thoroughly evaluated.

The potential benefit must be balanced against the known risks. These include the operative risks of an increased conversion rate (1.5%–10.0%), increased operating time (up to 180 minutes), and a recognized complication rate in terms of bleeding and gastric and/or esophageal perforation (5%–10%). Patients also need to be aware of the higher rate of persistence or recurrence of symptoms compared with a first-time antireflux procedure. These rates can be as high as 15%–30%. While difficult to quantify, patients' expectations of any planned revisional surgery must be considered.

A laparoscopic approach is the standard of care for most patients contemplating primary antireflux surgery. Similarly, laparoscopic intervention is the first choice for revisional surgery—even for those patients whose initial operation was done through an open approach. Adhesion formation is variable and a previous laparotomy does not necessarily preclude a laparoscopic approach for revisional surgery—although these patients should be warned about the increased risk of conversion. The obvious advantages of laparoscopic revision include decreased pain scores, fewer wound complications, reduced postoperative morbidity, shorter hospital stay, and more rapid resumption of normal duties.

PREOPERATIVE ASSESSMENT AND PREPARATION

Symptom evaluation

A careful symptom assessment must be made in any patient contemplating revisional antireflux surgery. The most common symptom is recurrent reflux, occurring in 50%–70% of patients seeking revisional surgery. Some 30%–50% of patients will have dysphagia, with an overlap of 10%–30% having both reflux and dysphagia.

With regards to reflux symptoms, clarification must be sought in terms of:

- Details of presenting symptoms and their relief by the initial operation
- Duration of current symptoms
- Similarity of current symptoms to those that led up to the initial procedure
- Possible reasons for return of symptoms
- Expectations of the patient

Persistence or recurrence or new symptoms after antireflux surgery does not necessarily equate with a failure of the initial procedure and may reflect an initial misinterpretation by both patient and surgeon as to the origin of the symptoms. Supporting this is the observation that most patients who take a proton pump inhibitor after antireflux surgery do not have objective evidence of reflux.

Patients presenting with recurrent reflux have better outcomes than those presenting with dysphagia with no anatomical or manometric abnormality. Patients who had primary surgery for atypical symptoms (e.g., voice change or cough) are unlikely to have a satisfactory outcome from revisional antireflux surgery, particularly if the initial operation did not provide any symptomatic relief.

Patients with new symptoms typically complain of dysphagia or gas bloat. Both of these symptoms are common after fundoplication and are usually transient. The patients should have been warned about their occurrence prior to initial surgery and these problems are best dealt with by reassurance and managing patient expectations. However, any persistence or worsening of symptoms may require investigation. Obviously, complete dysphagia will demand early laparoscopic reoperation.

The possible reasons for recurrence of symptoms must be considered and they include:

- The hiatus:
  - Too tight (dysphagia)
  - Too loose (recurrence of hernia and/or reflux)
- The wrap:
  - Too tight (dysphagia)
  - Slipped in position (reflux and/or dysphagia)
  - Intact fundoplication migrated into chest (reflux and/or dysphagia)
  - Undone (reflux)
- Other:
  - Vagal damage with gastric stasis (bloating)
  - Poor esophageal motility (dysphagia)
  - Inappropriate initial operation (persistence of original symptoms)

Perhaps the last reason is the most important to consider if the current symptoms are persistence or rapid reappearance of symptoms after the initial operation. In other words, although the patient might have had objective evidence of gastro-esophageal reflux, this might not have been the cause of the symptoms or the patient might have had unrealistic expectations of what surgery would achieve.

Objective assessment

Persisting or recurrent reflux symptoms require further investigation and this includes 24-hour pH studies, esophageal manometry, endoscopy, and contrast evaluation. All patients require this full work-up. Many patients with recurrent reflux symptoms will be found to have normal pH studies. Patients with pathologic acid exposure on postoperative pH studies and/or positive symptom correlation are more likely to benefit from revisional antireflux surgery than those with normal studies. Patients with persistent dysphagia are associated with poor postrevisional surgery outcomes.

Some patients who do not demonstrate pathologic overall acid exposure time (due to the wrap) but have good symptom correlation (symptom index and symptom association probability) and/or endoscopic esophagitis may be reasonable candidates for revisional antireflux surgery. Predictors for poor outcome in revisional antireflux surgery performed for reflux symptoms are persistent (not recurrent) symptoms after primary surgery and normal pH exposure with poor symptom correlation.

Endoscopy

Ideally, the upper gastrointestinal endoscopy should be performed by the operating surgeon. This is done to assess wrap position and presence of any hiatal hernia (better seen on a contrast study). Evidence of reflux should be sought in terms of esophageal mucosal erosion. Other causes for the symptoms might be identified, such as gastritis (acid or bile induced) or peptic ulcer, which would then dictate alternate therapies. Refer to Chapter 27, "Endoscopy," for further information on endoscopic assessment of prior antireflux surgery.

Contrast study

A contrast study may be performed to determine any anatomical anomaly in terms of:

1. Intact wrap migration. This can be defined as partial (Type I) defect in which the wrap has partially migrated into the chest, with the gastro-esophageal junction remaining below the diaphragm (see **Figure 40.1**) or a total (Type II) migration where the entire gastro-esophageal wrap complex has migrated up into the chest (see **Figure 40.2**).
2. Wrap slippage (intact wrap which has slipped in position down onto the stomach leading to "gastric band effect" or "bilobed" stomach).
3. Primary wrap unwrapping.

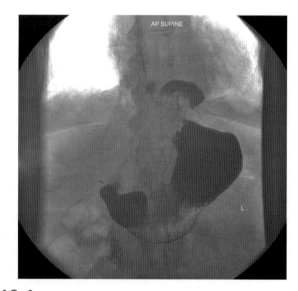

40.1 Barium swallow images of anterior 180 degrees fundoplication wrap with Type I migration (wrap migration without gastro-esophageal junction). (From Raeside, M.C., Madigan, D., Myers, J.C., Devitt, P.G., Jamieson, G.G., Thompson, S.K. *Br J Radiol.*, 85, 792–9, 2012. With permission.)

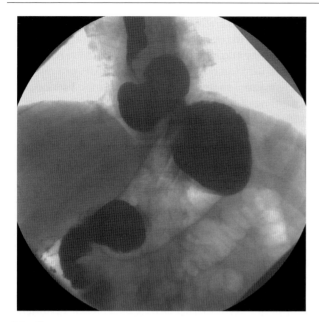

40.2 Barium swallow images of Nissen 360 degrees wrap with Type II migration (wrap migration with gastro-esophageal junction). (From Raeside, M.C., Madigan, D., Myers, J.C., Devitt, P.G., Jamieson, G.G., Thompson, S.K. *Br J Radiol.*, 85, 792–9, 2012. With permission.)

The most common anatomical indication for recurrent reflux surgery is intrathoracic migration of the fundoplication. The presence of these abnormalities alone is often sufficient to proceed to revision surgery. Input from an experienced gastrointestinal radiologist is essential, as there can be poor correlation in radiology reporting with subsequent operative findings. Radiological opinion should be sought on contraction, motility, reflux, and gastric emptying.

Esophageal manometry

The initial manometry (prior to primary laparoscopic fundoplication) should be reviewed for evidence of esophageal dysmotility/spasm or missed achalasia, which will be found in up to 1% of cases being considered for further surgery. Subsequent manometry can then be compared with the preoperative study. Esophageal pressures and peristalsis can help the surgeon determine the best option for the revisional wrap. This is relatively straightforward in patients whose sole symptom is recurrent reflux. In these cases, the same type of wrap can be refashioned (if the primary wrap had become undone), or tightened (anterior 180 degrees to posterior 270 degrees or total 360 degrees) if reflux is present and/or there are pathologic 24-hour pH studies despite an apparently intact wrap. Extra thought is required if dysphagia is the predominant symptom with no other abnormalities, as this can be associated with poor outcome. In such cases, consideration might need to be given to widening the esophageal hiatus.

Timing of revision surgery

Any planned revisional surgery should be deferred for an absolute minimum of 6 months from the original operation for the following reasons:

1. To allow resolution and settling of postsurgical edema, inflammation, and scarring. As most operations for gastro-esophageal reflux are now performed laparoscopically, it is quite reasonable to consider the same approach for any planned revisional surgery. In general, there will be less trouble with dense adhesions, although the possibility of conversion to an open procedure must be discussed with the patient—particularly when there is a Type I or II migration, with stomach potentially adherent within the thoracic cavity.

2. To facilitate accurate assessment of symptoms. In the first few months after fundoplication, up to 25% of patients complain of "persistent" symptoms that will, given time, resolve spontaneously. Most of these cases require little more than alleviation of patient anxiety and management of patient expectations. Likewise, apparently new symptoms of nonsignificant dysphagia and gas bloat should be similarly managed. Investigations are rarely required in this group of patients.

3. To allow time for appropriate management of patients with persistence or worsening of symptoms and/or the development of significant new symptoms. This management might involve further investigation (endoscopy, contrast study, manometry, 24-hour pH studies) and/or trials of conservative treatment. These might involve prokinetics if the predominant symptom is dysphagia, or acid suppression if the predominant symptom is reflux.

4. Early surgery should be considered for aphagia or severe dysphagia, where there has been a substantial intrathoracic migration of the wrap and/or the stomach. Another indication for early surgical intervention is impending gastric volvulus, which might be suggested by intermittent severe upper abdominal pain or persistent vomiting.

Summary

Anatomical abnormalities on contrast study will often require revisional laparoscopic fundoplication. Where no abnormalities are seen, the best outcomes are expected in those patients presenting with:

- Recurrent rather than persistent or new symptoms
- Reflux-predominant symptoms
- Pathologic reflux or positive symptom correlation on 24-hour pH studies

Revisional antireflux surgery can produce good results, particularly when the main indication for intervention is recurrent reflux.

INFORMED CONSENT

The patient must understand the increased risk of conversion to an open procedure, the risks of tissue injury, particularly gastric and/or esophageal perforation, and that there will still be a failure rate associated with reoperation.

ANESTHESIA

The general anesthetic technique is the same as for any laparoscopic procedure, but there must be an emphasis on minimizing the risk of patient straining, coughing, or vomiting during the surgery and in the immediate postoperative period.

OPERATION

The patient is placed in lithotomy with reverse Trendelenburg position and intermittent pneumatic calf compression is instituted. Broad-spectrum antibiotics are administered on induction. Pneumoperitoneum is usually maintained at 14 mmHg and reduced to 8 mmHg if there is any difficulty undertaking crural narrowing or the pleura is inadvertently opened. Port site placement and access is similar to that used for primary laparoscopic fundoplication (see Chapter 38,

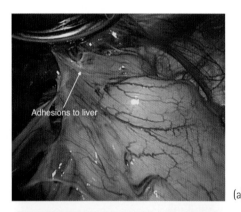

(a)

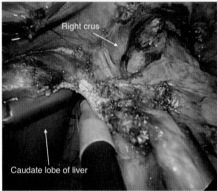

(b)

40.3a–b Adhesions to liver taken down, liver retractor replaced in correct position (against diaphragm) and right pillar exposed by dividing scar tissue over caudate lobe of the liver.

"Laparoscopic antireflux surgery"). The operative approach will vary with the degree of adhesion formation and the surgical anatomy encountered. The basic principles remain the same and focus on restoration of the normal anatomy (with sufficient intra-abdominal esophagus), mobilization, and dismantling of the old wrap and creation of a new tension-free wrap.

The first step is to restore the normal anatomy. Our initial approach is the right pars flaccida approach to the right crus, curving around the anterior esophagus and onto the left crus (see **Figure 40.3a,b**). Full hiatal dissection and sac mobilization are necessary to reduce any migrated wrap back into the abdomen with sufficient intra-abdominal esophageal length. To achieve this, it is often necessary to extend the peri-esophageal dissection 5–6 cm up into the chest. The esophagus is slung around by a tape or plastic catheter, lifted, and held anteriorly by the assistant's grasping forceps (see **Figure 40.4**). Every effort is made to identify and preserve the posterior vagus, particularly as the anterior vagus tends to be bound down by adhesions and may be inadvertently damaged when the existing wrap is dismantled. Visualization of the esophagus can occasionally be difficult and sometimes illumination of the structure with an endoscope can help identify planes for dissection. The right and left hiatal pillars must be fully displayed down to the crural decussation (see **Figure 40.5**). This will facilitate an accurate approximation and narrowing of the hiatal defect.

The second step is to identify and undo the wrap. Old sutures often provide helpful landmarks to start dissection. Dissection is done with combination of sharp and blunt dissection. Use of diathermy should be minimal to reduce the risk of unobserved thermal injury to the esophagus. Likewise, heat and ultrasound hand-held laparoscopic devices should be used with caution. The risk of gastro-esophageal perforation is highest at this stage. It is imperative for the wrap to be completely mobilized in order to recreate a new tension-free wrap.

To create a completely tension-free wrap with a totally mobile fundus, it might be necessary to divide some or most

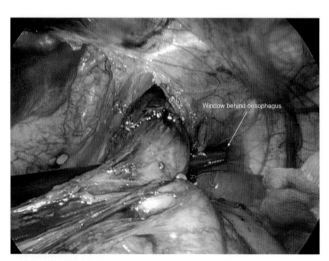

40.4 Passage of grasper behind esophagus.

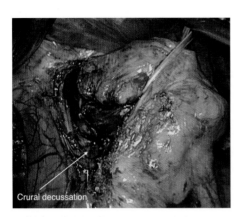

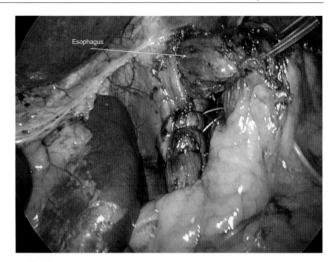

40.5 Sling around esophagus and old wrap to identify the crural decussation.

40.6 Approximation of right and left pillars with non-absorbable sutures.

of the short gastric vessels—particularly if these were not divided at the time of the initial fundoplication. In such circumstances, there is an increased risk of hemorrhage from these vessels or the spleen.

Once the esophagus has been mobilized, the hiatus defined, the wrap dismantled, and the fundus mobilized, the repair can begin. With the right and left hiatal pillars clearly identified, the hiatus is narrowed. Ideally, this is achieved by approximating the right and left pillars posteriorly with one or two nonabsorbable sutures (see **Figure 40.6**). Provided that the pillars have been mobilized satisfactorily with division of all scar tissue, approximation without any undue tension is usually a fairly straightforward exercise. Access is facilitated by the assistant exposing a window with an instrument passed behind the esophagus, pressing gently on the diaphragm and lifting the esophagus anteriorly and to the patient's left. While the use of various forms of mesh has been described, these materials do not appear to provide any superiority in terms of integrity of the hiatal repair. A

52 Fr esophageal bougie is passed to calibrate the size of the hiatus. While this is often left to fine judgement, the narrowed hiatus should fit comfortably around the esophagus, leaving sufficient gap to allow easy passage of the tip of a laparoscopic grasper between hiatus and esophagus.

The now floppy and completely mobile fundus should be manipulated into position to ensure a tension-free wrap, as described in Chapter 38, "Laparoscopic antireflux surgery." The type of wrap to be created will have been determined preoperatively and based on the patient's symptoms and the manometry/24-hour pH studies. For example, if the predominant problem is one of obstruction, with symptoms of dysphagia, supported by findings of hold-up on contrast study and/or high pressures on manometry, a 360 degrees wrap could be revised to a 180 degrees anterior wrap. Conversely, a less constricting wrap, such as a 180 degrees anterior fundoplication might be converted to a posterior 270 degrees or 360 degrees wrap if recurrent reflux is the primary problem (see **Figure 40.7a–b**).

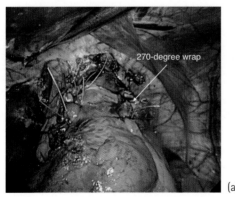

(a)

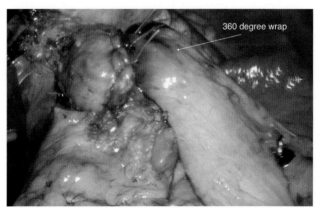

(b)

40.7a–b Creation of a tension-free wrap.

POSTOPERATIVE CARE

Unless there has been an esophageal or gastric perforation during the procedure, further antibiotics are not required. A key component of postoperative management is minimizing the risk of undue strain being placed on the hiatal repair. In the immediate postoperative period, the patient must be given adequate analgesia to reduce the risk of respiratory complications, yet opiates and other emetogenic agents must be avoided. Liberal use should be made of agents to reduce nausea and vomiting. Patients remain nil-by-mouth until a postoperative contrast study is performed. This study is performed to check for positioning of the wrap and stomach and to look for any perforations that might have been missed during the operation. Following a normal study, patients are started on clear fluids and over the next 2 or 3 days built up to a smooth pureed diet. Patients are discharged home on a soft fundoplication diet for 6 weeks until review in clinic. Appropriate pain relief and anti-emetics are provided on discharge, along with clear instructions that the patient is to avoid doing anything strenuous that might put undue strain on the surgical repair.

OUTCOME

The incidence of immediate postoperative dysphagia (3%–10%) is similar to that of primary laparoscopic fundoplication. The overall morbidity associated with a revisional procedure is about 15%, which is higher than that for primary antireflux surgery. While the commonest postoperative problems are respiratory, other complications, including gastro-esophageal perforation (5%–10%), pneumothorax (3%), and bleeding (2%), are more likely to occur in this group of patients. Overall patient satisfaction following revisional antireflux surgery ranges between 70% and 90%. While further revisional surgery might be contemplated for some patients, the risks of ongoing failure of relief of symptoms and added surgical complications must be considered.

FURTHER READING

Awais O, Luketich JD, Schuchert MJ et al. Reoperative antireflux surgery for failed fundoplication: an analysis of outcomes in 275 patients. *Ann Thorac Surg.* 2011; 92: 1083–9.

Frantzides CT, Madan AK, Carlson MA et al. Laparoscopic revision of failed fundoplication and hiatal herniorraphy. *J Laparoendosc Adv Surg Tech A.* 2009; 19: 135–9.

Furnée EJB, Draaisma WA, Broeders IAMJ, Gooszen HG. Surgical reintervention after failed antireflux surgery: a systematic review of the literature. *J Gastrointest Surg.* 2009; 13: 1539–49.

Furnée EJB, Draaisma WA, Broeders IAMJ et al. Surgical reintervention after antireflux surgery for gastresophageal reflux disease: a prospective cohort study in 130 patients. *Arch Surg.* 2008; 143: 267–74.

Khajanchee YS, O'Rourke R, Cassera MA et al. Laparoscopic reintervention for failed antireflux surgery: subjective and objective outcomes in 176 consecutive patients. *Arch Surg.* 2007; 142: 785–91.

Lamb PJ, Myers JC, Jamieson GG et al. Watson. Long-term outcomes of revisional surgery following laparoscopic fundoplication. *Br J Surg.* 2009; 96: 391–7.

Raeside MC, Madigan D, Myers JC et al. Post-fundoplication contrast studies: is there room for improvement? *Br J Radiol.* 2012; 85: 792–9.

Society of American Gastrointestinal and Endoscopic Surgeons. *Guidelines for Surgical Treatment of Gastroesophageal Reflux (GERD).* Accessed July 2014, http://www.sages.org/publications/guidelines/guidelines-for-surgical-treatment-of-gastroesophageal-reflux-disease-gerd/

Symons NRA, Purkayastha S, Dillemans B et al. Laparoscopic revision of failed antireflux surgery: a systematic review. *Am J Surg.* 2011; 202: 336–43.

Thompson SK, Jamieson GG, Myers JC et al. Recurrent heartburn after laparoscopic fundoplication is not always recurrent reflux. *J Gastrointest Surg.* 2007; 11: 642–7.

41

Laparoscopic cardiomyotomy for achalasia

SHERAZ MARKAR AND GIOVANNI ZANINOTTO

INTRODUCTION AND HISTORICAL NOTES

Esophageal achalasia, albeit a rare disease with an incidence ranging from 0.4 to 1.5 per 100 000 inhabitants/year, is the most characterized esophageal motor disorder and it is defined by the failure of the lower esophageal sphincter to relax at swallowing and by the absence/impairment of peristaltic contractions along the esophageal body. As a direct consequence, a residual pressure gradient between the esophagus and the stomach remains after swallowing, causing a functional obstruction at the gastro-esophageal junction. Dysphagia, regurgitation of undigested food, respiratory symptoms (nocturnal cough, recurrent aspiration, pneumonia), chest pain, and weight loss are the most common symptoms experienced by the patients. Present understanding suggests that achalasia results from the disappearance of the myenteric neurons that coordinate esophageal peristalsis and lower esophageal sphincter relaxation. It is believed the myenteric neurons disappear due to chronic ganglionitis, with experimental data suggesting that in genetically predisposed patients, an aberrant autoimmune response to the herpes simplex virus may be the trigger leading to achalasia.

Due to the absence of an etiologic therapy, the medical community has focused treatment around how to palliate dysphagia, the main symptom of achalasia. This is done by lowering the lower esophageal sphincter pressure, either by forceful dilatation, by sectioning the lower esophageal sphincter muscle, or by paralyzing it with Botulinum toxin.

For many years, surgery has represented the most effective therapy for achalasia. The original treatment was proposed by a German surgeon, Heller, in 1914. The myotomy as described by Heller was performed in April 1913 on a 49-year-old patient who had been suffering from dysphagia for more than 30 years. It consisted of two separate longitudinal incisions 8 cm long on the anterior and posterior sides of the esophagus and cardia, through a left subcostal approach. Some years later, a Dutch surgeon, de Bruyn Grenwaldt,

limited the procedure to the anterior myotomy (though this adaptation is attributed to another Dutch surgeon, Zaaijer). The modified technique with only the anterior myotomy has remained substantially unchanged ever since and the procedure has continued to be linked to the name of Heller. After the advent of thoracic surgery, the operation was performed in English-speaking countries through a thoracotomy, while in continental Europe and South America, the abdominal approach continued to be preferred. In the 1960s, a French surgeon, Dor, suggested adding a partial anterior gastric fundoplication to the myotomy to prevent acid reflux.

In the following years, the preferred treatment for achalasia shifted toward the less invasive option, endoscopic pneumatic dilatation (PD), but the advent of mini-invasive surgery in the early 1990s revived the Heller myotomy, and the pendulum of achalasia treatment swung back in favor of surgery. The first mini-invasive Heller myotomy was performed in Dundee by Cuschieri via a laparoscopic approach. Two years later, Pellegrini reported performing the same operation through a thoracoscopic approach, and Ancona subsequently added an anterior fundoplication to the laparoscopic myotomy. Since then, the operation has gained in popularity and is now considered the gold standard treatment for esophageal achalasia.

DIAGNOSIS AND SURGICAL TECHNIQUE

Diagnostic work-up

Diagnostic work-up comprises esophageal high resolution manometry (HRM), barium swallow, and endoscopy. HRM provides detailed information on esophageal motility: using catheters incorporating 36 or more pressure sensors spaced 1 cm apart, it allows in-detail pressure recording from the pharynx to the stomach, and is currently considered the gold standard investigation to diagnose achalasia. The use of HRM has led to the subclassification of achalasia into three clinically relevant types based on the pattern of contractility in the esophageal body: type I (classical achalasia; no evidence of pressurization), type II (achalasia with compression or compartmentalization in the distal esophagus >30 mmHg), and type III (two or more spastic contractions). To quantify lower esophageal sphincter relaxation, a new manometric parameter was introduced: integrated relaxation pressure (IRP). This parameter calculates the mean post-swallow lower esophageal sphincter pressure over a 4-second period during which the lower esophageal sphincter pressure is at its lowest. The upper limit of normal for IRP is 10 mmHg for type I achalasia, 15 mmHg for type II achalasia, and 17 mmHg for type III achalasia, which differentiates the impaired relaxation in achalasia from non-achalasic individuals and from diffuse esophageal spasm patients.

The classical radiographic features of achalasia seen on contrast swallow investigations are esophageal dilatation and minimal lower esophageal sphincter opening, with a bird's-beak appearance of the cardia, sometimes with an air–fluid level in the gullet and no intragastric air bubble. In more advanced achalasia, severe dilatation with stasis of food and a sigmoid-like appearance can be noted. A "timed" barium swallow test has been proposed and is widely utilized in evaluating patients before and after treatment. A fixed amount of barium (200 mL) is ingested in 2 minutes, and pictures are taken after fixed intervals (at time 0, then after 1 minute, 2 minutes, and 5 minutes) to measure the height of the barium column.

Endoscopy is most commonly the primary investigation to be performed in a patient with dysphagia. Findings may appear normal in patients with achalasia, especially in the early stages, when the gullet is only mildly dilated. In more advanced cases, esophagitis ("stasis" esophagitis) may be identified and should not be confused with reflux esophagitis. Esophageal candidiasis, resistant to the usual treatments, can also be found, and is usually related to the functional obstruction. Malignant tumors can produce an achalasia-like syndrome called "pseudoachalasia" by infiltrating the gastro-esophageal junction and mimicking the clinical and manometric presentation of achalasia; they account for about 5% of cases of misdiagnosis. In general, patients with pseudoachalasia are older and have a shorter history of dysphagia and weight loss. Endoscopy, with a careful examination of the cardiac and fundic region, is therefore mandatory as part of the diagnosis work-up to avoid this potential catastrophic pitfall and, if the clinical suspicion is strong, computerized tomography and endoscopic ultrasound should be considered. These latter tests should be considered particularly in elderly patients with symptoms of recent onset.

Finally, all the tests routinely performed as part of preoperative assessment before surgery under general anesthesia (blood tests, chest X-rays, electrocardiogram) are required. Additional tests may be requested by the anesthesiologist for particular patients, based upon specific issues raised by the patients' physiological status and/or medical comorbidities.

Patient preparation and positioning

Patients should be kept on a liquid diet for 24 hours before the operation, and a dilated gullet should be mechanically washed and emptied via a naso-esophageal tube the night before the procedure. The required standard laparoscopic instrumentation is composed of two 12 mm trocars and three 5 mm trocars; a 30-degree laparoscope; a device for lifting the left liver lobe; atraumatic forceps, a cautery hook, scissors, and a needle holder for suturing. Small bipolar cautery forceps may be useful to control bleeding from the edges of the myotomy. The endoscope may be useful during the performance of the myotomy to facilitate the procedure and check for any mucosal perforation. We prefer to position endoscopically a guide wire in the stomach before starting the operation and to place a 3 cm Rigiflex balloon (Boston Scientific, Marlborough, Massachusetts, United States) across the cardia during the myotomy.

The operation is performed under general anesthesia and oro-tracheal intubation. The patient is placed supine on a steep reverse Trendelenburg position with legs abducted and the surgeon standing in between. The right arm is tucked against the patient's side and the left arm remains on an arm board. Prophylactic anti-thrombosis measures (low molecular weight heparin and stockings) are recommended.

Pneumoperitoneum is created using open technique, and the first 12 mm trocar for the laparoscope is positioned in the midline, halfway between the umbilicus and the xyphoid. A 5 mm trocar is inserted as laterally as possible on the patient's

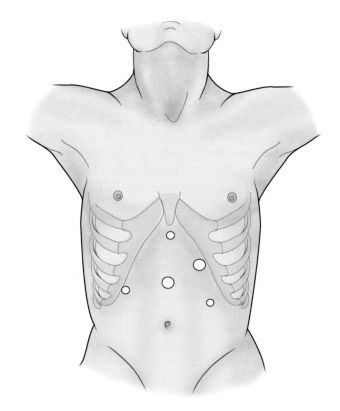

41.1 Position of the trocars for approaching the hiatus region.

right side, immediately below the costal margin, to lift the left lobe of the liver. A 5 mm trocar inserted immediately below the xyphoid is used for the operator's left hand, while a 12 mm trocar inserted laterally below the left costal margin provides access for the surgeon's right hand. Finally, a 5 mm trocar is positioned on the left mid-clavicular line to pull down the gastric fundus (see **Figure 41.1**).

Exposure of the anterior wall of the esophagus

An assistant on the surgeon's left-hand side lifts the left liver lobe using an atraumatic retractor, thus exposing the cardia region. An assistant on the surgeon's right-hand side grasps the gastric fundus with atraumatic forceps, maintaining a caudal traction on the esophagogastric junction. The operation begins with a minimal dissection of the anterior part of the esophagus. The fat tissue covering the esophagogastric junction is removed, paying attention to the small vessels coming from the gastric wall, which should be coagulated with the bipolar forceps; they usually mark the inferior limit of the myotomy. The left vagus nerve, which becomes anterior at this level by crossing the anterior esophageal wall from left to right, is clearly identified and must not be damaged.

Myotomy

The myotomy is started with the cautery hook 1–2 cm above the esophagogastric junction (see **Figure 41.2**). The cautery power is reduced to 15 W to avoid transmitting its coagulating

effect to the underlying mucosa. The longitudinal muscle fibers are hooked, lifted, and coagulated until the circular ones are exposed; then the latter are hooked, lifted, and divided using the same technique until the submucosal layer bulges slightly between the two margins of the myotomy. The margin of the myotomy is delicately lifted with forceps and scissors are used to bluntly dissect the muscle layer from the submucosal layer. The 30 mm Rigiflex balloon previously inserted at cardia level is gently inflated and deflated with 30–50 mL of air with a syringe while the myotomy is performed. This action exposes and stretches the circular fibers, which are cut or torn apart and allows the edges of the myotomy to be easily separated and peeled away from the submucosal plane. Minor bleeding from the edges of the myotomy can be carefully cauterized or simply controlled by inflating the balloon. On the gastric side, the myotomy is performed with a hook and the clasp and sling fibers are torn apart and coagulated. The myotomy that results should be 6–8 cm in length, extending 2 cm on the gastric side. The distal part of the myotomy is slightly directed toward the left, where the bundle of clasp and sling fibers is narrower (see **Figure 41.3**). Care must be taken during the myotomy to avoid injuring the anterior vagus nerve and prevent any esophageal perforation or spiraling of the myotomy.

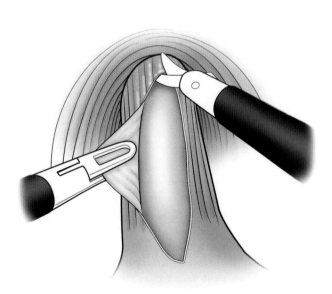

41.2 Once the submucosal plane is reached, the myotomy is easily extended using a scissor with no or minimal cautery.

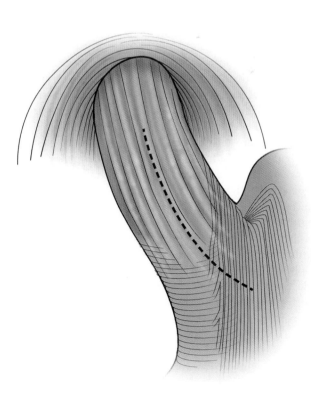

41.3 On the gastric side, the direction of the myotomy is shifted toward the left, where the bundle of clasp muscle fibers is narrow.

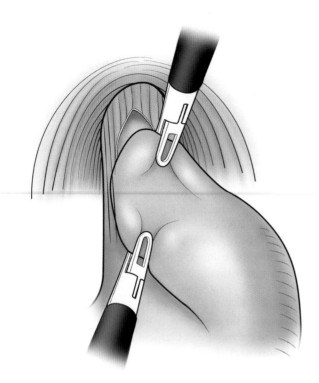

41.4 The operation is completed with a partial (180-degree) fundoplication. In general, there is no need to mobilize the gastric fundus by division of the short gastric vessels.

Antireflux fundoplication

Although some authors state that they perform only the myotomy, a fundoplication is frequently added to prevent postoperative gastro-esophageal reflux disease, which may be a severe complication in patients with a poor esophageal clearing ability due to the absence of peristalsis. Given this lack of any propulsive peristaltic activity of the esophageal body, a partial fundoplication is usually preferred (see **Figure 41.4**). The anterior 180-degree hemifundoplication (Dor) has the advantage of protecting the exposed esophageal mucosa and can be performed without completely mobilizing the esophagus, thus preserving the natural antireflux mechanisms. There is no need to mobilize the gastric fundus by dividing the short gastric vessels when a Dor hemifundoplication is performed. Three stitches are inserted on each side, the proximal one to include the stomach, the edge of the myotomy, and the diaphragm (for further detail, refer to Chapter 38, "Laparoscopic antireflux surgery").

Postoperative care

An esophagogram with a water-soluble contrast (Gastrografin) is obtained on the first postoperative day to rule out any mucosal perforation. A liquid diet is started and the patient is discharged 1–2 days after the operation. A soft diet is recommended for 8–10 days, after which a normal diet is introduced.

Patients usually return to the outpatient clinic a month later for a barium swallow to evaluate esophageal emptying. Endoscopy and function tests are performed after 6 months to rule out any postoperative gastro-esophageal reflux disease.

Complications

Laparoscopic Heller myotomy combined with partial fundoplication is a remarkably safe operation with a reported mortality of 0.1% (three deaths among 3086 patients). The most common complication is perforation of the esophageal or gastric mucosa during the myotomy. This can be caused directly by erroneous handling of the hook or scissors, or indirectly by excessive coagulation to the mucosa. Direct lesions are usually detected during the operation and can be sutured with 4-0 interrupted reabsorbable stitches. If a mucosal lesion is detected with a water-soluble swallow after the operation, a conservative treatment of gastric suction, nil by mouth, total parenteral nutrition, and antibiotics is usually sufficient. The overall complication rate is 6.3% (range 0%–35%), but clinical consequences are reported in only 0.7% (range 0%–3%) of cases.

DECOMPENSATED ACHALASIA

In cases of decompensated achalasia and sigmoid megaesophagus, the success of laparoscopic Heller myotomy is lower than in less advanced cases. In these patients, however, the alternative is an esophagectomy, so before embarking on such an invasive and aggressive approach, it is still worth performing a simpler laparoscopic Heller myotomy. The surgical technique is slightly modified and the distal esophagus is posteriorly dissected, encircled, and straightened. The myotomy and fundoplication are then performed as previously described.

OUTCOME

Clinical success rates of laparoscopic Heller myotomy are very high—on average, 89% (ranging from 76% to 100%) at a median follow-up of 35 months (range 8–38 months). It should be emphasized though that success rates drop (depending on the definition used) to 65%–85% at 5 years' follow-up, probably as a result of progression of the disease.

Positive prognostic factors for laparoscopic Heller myotomy are young age (<40 years) and a straight esophagus; that is, one with no tortuosities at its distal end (as in sigmoid esophagus). As for PD, the manometric pattern at diagnosis also affects clinical success rates following Heller myotomy; that is, patients with achalasia type II have the best outcome. Type III patients have the worse outcome; these patients, however, respond better to Heller myotomy than to PD, probably because the former entails a more extensive and more proximal disruption of the esophageal muscle than the latter.

FURTHER READING

Ancona E, Peracchia A, Zaninotto G, Rossi M, Bonavina L, Segalin A. Heller laparoscopic cardiomyotomy with antireflux anterior fundoplication (Dor) in the treatment of esophageal achalasia. *Surg Endosc.* 1993; 7(5): 459–61.

Andreollo NA, Lopes LR, Malafaia O. Heller's myotomy: a hundred years of success! *Arq Bras Cir Dig.* 2014; 27(1): 1–2.

Boeckstaens GE, Zaninotto G, Richter JE. Achalasia. *Lancet.* 2014; 383(9911): 83–93.

Campos GM, Vittinghoff E, Rabl C, Gadenstätter M, Lin F et al. Endoscopic and surgical treatments for achalasia: a systematic review and meta-analysis. *Ann Surg.* 2009; 249(1): 45–57.

Dor J, Humbert P, Paoli JM, Miorclerc M, Aubert J. [Treatment of reflux by the so-called modified Heller-Nissen technique.] *Presse Med.* 1967; 75(50): 2563–5. French.

Pellegrini C, Wetter LA, Patti M, Leichter R, Mussan G, Mori T et al. Thoracoscopic esophagomyotomy: initial experience with a new approach for the treatment of achalasia. *Ann Surg.* 1992; 216(3): 291–6; discussion 6–9.

Pandolfino JE, Kwiatek MA, Nealis T, Bulsiewicz W, Post J, Kahrilas PJ. Achalasia: a new clinically relevant classification by high-resolution manometry. *Gastroenterology.* 2008; 135(5): 1526–33.

Rohof WO, Salvador R, Annese V, Bruley des Varannes S, Chaussade S, Costantini M et al. Outcomes of treatment for achalasia depend on manometric subtype. *Gastroenterology.* 2012; 144(4): 718–25.

Shimi C, Nathason LK, Cuschieri A. Laparoscopic cardiomyotomy for achalasia. *J R Coll Surg Edinb.* 1991; 36(3): 152–4.

Tracey JP, Traube M. Difficulties in the diagnosis of pseudoachalasia. *Am J Gastroenterol.* 1994; 89(11): 2014–18.

Vaezi MF, Baker ME, Achkar E, Richter JE. Timed barium oesophagram: better predictor of long term success after pneumatic dilation in achalasia than symptom assessment. *Gut.* 2002; 50(6): 765–70.

Wang YR, Dempsey DT, Friedenberg FK, Richter JE. Trends of Heller myotomy hospitalizations for achalasia in the United States, 1993–2005: effect of surgery volume on perioperative outcomes. *Am J Gastroenterol.* 2008; 103(10): 2454–64.

Zaaijer JH. Cardiospasm in the aged. *Ann Surg.* 1923; 77(5): 615–17.

42

Per oral endoscopic myotomy (POEM) for achalasia

AMBER L. SHADA AND LEE L. SWANSTRÖM

HISTORY

Recent interest in natural orifice transluminal endoscopic surgery led to explorations of novel ways of exiting the gastrointestinal (GI) tract to perform extraluminal operations. One of these was submucosal endoscopy with a mucosal safety flap, which involved creating a submucosal tunnel before exiting the organ to minimize the chance of closure failure. Pasricha recognized the possibility this offered for endoscopic access to the circular muscles of the lower esophageal sphincter (LES), and used this approach to perform the first endoscopic myotomy in pigs in 2007. Subsequently, Inoue performed the first human per oral endoscopic myotomy (POEM) for achalasia in 2008. Since that time, POEM has been increasingly adopted as a technique to treat achalasia, and has expanded to the treatment of other esophageal motility disorders as well.

PRINCIPLES AND JUSTIFICATION

POEM is an effective treatment for all types of achalasia and has been reported for patients from age 3 to late 90s. It has been shown to be safe and effective for end-stage or "sigmoid" esophagus as well as reoperative cases. Aside from achalasia, POEM has been used for diffuse esophageal spasm (DES), hypertensive LES, spastic achalasia, and nutcracker esophagus.

The primary alternative approaches to the treatment of achalasia are either laparoscopic Heller myotomy or endoscopic balloon dilation. Injection of the LES with botulinum toxin (Botox) is regarded as a temporizing treatment due to its transient effectiveness. The advantages of POEM relate to its minimal access approach, resulting in less pain and shorter recovery. Additionally, the lack of dissection of the gastroesophageal junction (GEJ) to access the LES may minimize the chance of postprocedure gastroesophageal reflux and avoid external adhesions that might compromise subsequent surgical treatments. A further important benefit of POEM is the ability to extend the myotomy proximally in cases of esophageal body spastic motility disorders.

POEM requires general anesthesia and is therefore contraindicated in patients with severe pulmonary disease, cirrhosis, portal hypertension, and coagulopathy. Additionally, prior esophageal or mediastinal radiation, or recent mucosal ablation or endoscopic mucosal resection is a contraindication. While previous Heller myotomy is not a contraindication, previous esophageal resection would probably be.

While not an absolute contraindication, we typically do not perform POEM for achalasia patients who have an associated significant hiatal hernia, as there is a high rate of reflux afterward. Also, it is probably not resource efficient to perform POEM on someone needing a concomitant laparoscopic procedure, unless they have an indication for an extended thoracic myotomy.

PREOPERATIVE ASSESSMENT

Achalasia patients should always have a comprehensive symptom assessment covering typical presenting symptoms including dysphagia, chest pain, regurgitation of undigested foods, weight loss, and previous interventions—all of which have been shown to affect outcomes of any treatments. The Eckardt score, a useful standardized symptom tool, can score patients to stratify disease severity and predict treatment success (see **Table 42.1**). Upper endoscopy with biopsies is essential to exclude pseudoachalasia related to infiltrative cancers. Upper GI barium esophagogram—preferably a timed barium swallow—serves as a roadmap for the operation, excludes significant findings like diverticula and serves as a baseline study for long-term patient follow-up. Although "heartburn" is a frequent complaint of achalasia patients,

Table 42.1 Eckardt scoring system

Score	Symptom			
	Weight loss (kg)	Dysphagia	Retrosternal pain	Regurgitation
0	None	None	None	None
1	<5	Occasional	Occasional	Occasional
2	5–10	Daily	Daily	Daily
3	>10	Each meal	Each meal	Each meal

gastroesophageal reflux is physiologically extremely unlikely and thus 24-hour pH acid studies are not usually indicated.

Esophageal manometry is the single most important test, as it definitively establishes the diagnosis of achalasia. Introduced a decade ago, high resolution manometry (HRM) has increasingly become the gold-standard test, allowing classification of achalasia into three types that correspond as well to the degree of success following intervention: achalasia with minimal esophageal pressurization (Type 1, classic), achalasia with esophageal pressurization (Type 2), and achalasia with spasm (Type 3). Achalasia by definition is evidenced by complete loss of primary esophageal body motility and defective relaxation of the LES. Newer diagnostic modalities such as impedance planimetry have not been in use long enough to establish normal values and therefore are currently more intraoperative and research tools.

PATIENT PREPARATION

Preoperative informed consent should cover the following potential issues: possible anesthesia complications, esophageal perforation (salvageable with endoscopic approaches in the majority of cases), incomplete myotomy leading to continued dysphagia, inability to relieve symptoms (particularly if pain is a primary symptom), and postoperative gastroesophageal reflux.

Patients are prepared for surgery with 3 days of nystatin swish and swallow (given the high incidence of esophageal candidiasis in achalasia), and placed on a clear liquid diet 24 hours prior to surgery.

OPERATION

Anesthesia

General endotracheal anesthesia is always used, to better control carbon dioxide (CO_2) absorption and to compensate for elevation of the diaphragm from extravasated CO_2. Anesthesiologists should be reminded of the high risk for aspiration in achalasia patients and take appropriate induction precautions.

Positioning

1. The patient is positioned supine on the operating table with the left arm tucked at the patient's side. The operating room table should be moved away from the anesthesia machine to allow the surgeon and assistant adequate room at the head of the table (see **Figure 42.1**). The surgeon will operate facing toward the patient's feet, so the viewing monitor should be located at the foot of the bed, with the endoscope stack behind the surgeon. If using a scope cart with no secondary monitor, the endoscopic cart and monitor should be located across

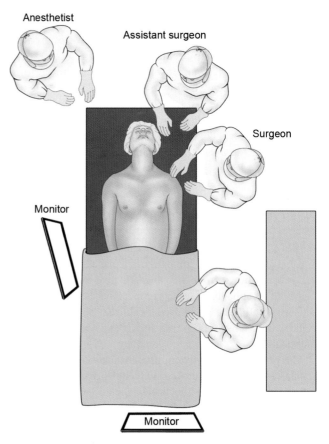

42.1 Patient and surgeon positioning for POEM.

the table at the patient's midbody. Pneumatic leg compression devices and forced-air patient warming should be used. Ready access to the chest and abdomen during the procedure is needed, most commonly for decompression of pneumoperitoneum or capnothorax.

Equipment

2. **Table 42.2** lists the endoscopic equipment required for POEM. A high-definition upper endoscope is critical. A standard overtube is usually placed, as it makes cleaning the esophagus easier, facilitates multiple scope withdrawal and reinsertions, and stabilizes the shaft of the endoscope to minimize bowing. Endoscopic bowing can tear the entry mucosotomy, making it more difficult to close (see **Figure 42.2**). The one exception to overtube use is when a long myotomy is performed, as it would require most of the overtube to be outside the mouth. Low-flow CO_2 insufflation is mandatory. Standard air insufflation leads to severe cardiopulmonary disturbances and complications. POEM uses a dissection cap on the end of the scope to create space and provide traction/countertraction on tissues. Monopolar cautery is used and the most common tools are the triangle tip cautery knife (Olympus Corporation, Tokyo, Japan), the hook cautery knife (Olympus Corporation), or combination cautery/injection devices like the ERBEJet (Erbe, USA, Inc., Marietta, Georgia, United States), or the FlushKnife (Fujifilm Corporation, Tokyo, Japan). The specific cautery device used is based on surgeon preference. A cautery unit optimized for endoscopic tools is advisable and we will here recommend settings based on the Erbe-brand cautery.

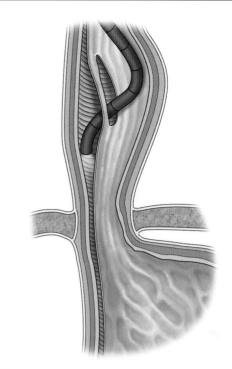

42.2 Without an overtube, endoscopic bowing can extend the mucosotomy, making closure more difficult.

Table 42.2   Endoscopic equipment used for POEM

Endoscopic equipment required for POEM	Essential, Yes/No
High-definition upper endoscope	Yes
Low-flow CO_2 insufflator	Yes
Endoscopic injection needle, 23 gauge	Yes
Combination injection needle, monopolar cautery (Apollo Medical†)	No
Biliary extraction balloon, 15 mm	No
Angled or straight dissecting cap (Olympus† or Cook§)	Yes
Standard overtube	No
Triangle tip cautery knife* Hook cautery knife* Needle knife cautery*	Yes
ERBEJet* (Erbe**) Flush Knife*	No
Endoscopic clips	Yes
Endoscopic suturing device (Overstitch, Apollo Medical)	No
Veress needle	Yes

Notes: *Surgeon preference dictates cautery device used. †Apollo Endosurgery, Inc., San Diego, California, United States; ‡Olympus Corporation; §Cook Group Inc., Bloomington, Indiana, United States; **Erbe USA, Inc.

Diagnostic endoscopy

3. A diagnostic endoscopy is performed, including retroflexion to evaluate the GE junction. As mentioned, all insufflation should be with CO_2 due to inevitable insufflation of the bowel as well as subsequent extramural CO_2 insufflation. The overtube is placed and taped in place and the esophagus carefully cleaned of all residual food.

Measurement of landmarks

4. Careful measurements, based on the endoscope position relative to the teeth or cap of the overtube, should be recorded. Landmarks include the GE junction, the eventual distal end of the myotomy 2–3 cm onto the gastric wall, the proximal aspect of the high-pressure zone and the proposed start of the myotomy. The myotomy length is dependent on the Chicago classification and increasingly by results of intraoperative testing such as EndoFLIP (Crospon Limited, Galway, Ireland) imaging. Type 3 achalasia, DES, and other spastic conditions may require a longer myotomy, sometimes all the way to the upper esophageal sphincter. If EndoFLIP imaging is used to guide surgery, it is performed at this point and values recorded. The site of the mucosotomy is based on the proximal extent of the myotomy, planning for a 2–4 cm mucosal flap for added protection. A small volume (0.5 mL) of undiluted methylene blue is injected into the deep submucosa of the anterior lesser curvature, 2–3 cm distal to the GE junction in the stomach, to mark the final extent of the myotomy (see **Figure 42.3**).

Submucosal lift

5. A submucosal lift is performed using a mixture of dilute methylene blue, normal saline, and a small amount of epinephrine on the anterior esophagus between 2 and 3 o'clock, according to premapped measurements. Obtaining a "good lift" is critical to ensure that the initial incision is into the correct plane versus adjacent mediastinal structures (pulmonary artery or right atrium). Injecting too deeply into the esophagus risks lifting the muscle and creating a full-thickness mucosotomy. A good lift is confirmed by seeing a blue blush and a globular raise of the mucosa. If these signs are not seen, the incision should not be performed and, instead, repeat lift should be attempted in another quadrant or more proximally.

Creation of mucosotomy and submucosal tunnel

6. The cautery device is used to create a 1.0–1.5 cm longitudinal mucosotomy at the proximal aspect of the methylene blue submucosal injection (see **Figure 42.4**). An Endo Cut mode for the cautery is used. Dissection using spray coagulation (50 W, mode 2 on an ERBEJ generator) is performed to carry the dissection through

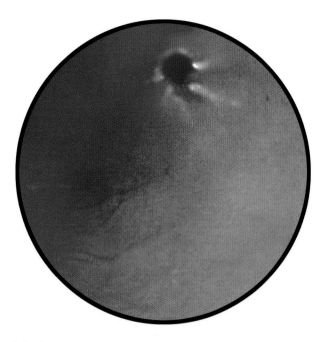

42.3   Retroflexed view of the gastric cardia demonstrating the tattoo made with undiluted methylene blue to mark the distal extent of dissection.

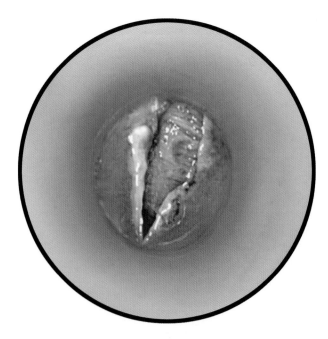

42.4   Mucosotomy creation in esophagus, with bluish hue of lift solution visible.

all layers of the submucosa until the circular muscle is visible. The endoscope with dissection cap is next introduced into the submucosal plane. We have found that the use of a 15 mm biliary extraction balloon can expedite insertion and minimize the size of the mucosotomy. The extraction balloon is inserted just inside the mucosotomy and the balloon inflated. The balloon is pulled back half-way into the dissecting cap while the scope is advanced. This effectively "shoehorns" the scope into the subcutaneous tunnel. The tunnel is created with a combination of blunt dissection and spray electrocautery, and is extended until it is 2–3 cm distal to the GE junction and well onto the gastric cardia (see **Figure 42.5**). Intermittent repeat injections of the methylene blue, normal saline, and epinephrine solution is necessary to assist safe dissection. The appropriate submucosal plane is identified by continuously visualizing the circular muscle fibers. This is an important technical point, as maintaining the submucosa with the mucosa helps to strengthen and protect it from full-thickness injury. It is critical that the tunnel extend well onto the gastric cardia, preferably along the lesser curvature of the stomach. The transition from the esophagus to the stomach is usually apparent due to the yellowish hue of the gastric mucosa, an increase in space, and the presence of larger vessels with more branching. The prominence of the LES fibers is another helpful landmark. The scope can also be intermittently removed from the submucosal tunnel to check progress of dissection, as marked by mucosal blanching, to ensure that the dissection is linear

and proceeds toward the target in the cardia. Finally, one should be able to identify the dark blue tattoo made at the beginning of the operation from the retroflexed approach.

Myotomy

7. The endoscope is next withdrawn to the premeasured level of the myotomy start and a selective circular myotomy of the LES is performed in an antegrade manner with the triangle tip or hook knife (40 W, mode 2 on ERBEJet) (see **Figure 42.6**). Initial proximal dissection is made using an Endo Cut mode for better visualization of tissue planes. Once the layer between the circular and longitudinal muscle is visualized, the circular muscle is progressively hooked and cauterized. Any substantial crossing vessels are coagulated using a coagulation grasper. Care is taken to ensure hemostasis for optimal visualization of the muscular fibers.

Examination of completed myotomy

8. After completing the myotomy, the endoscope is removed from the submucosal tunnel and passed through the esophageal lumen and GE junction to assess the tightness of the LES, ensure mucosal integrity, and inspect for adequate myotomy extension onto the stomach with retroflexion. The scope should now be able to easily pass through the LES.

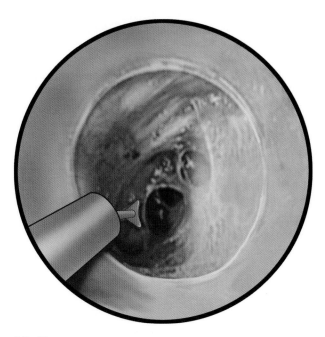

42.5 Creation of submucosal tunnel. Muscular layer is visible on the screen on the left, and submucosal layer on the right.

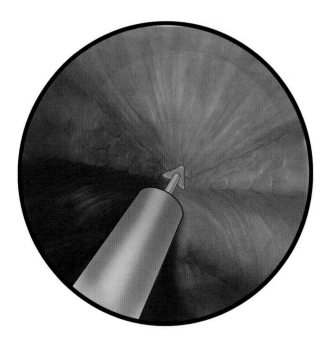

42.6 Myotomy of the circular muscle layer using the triangle tip cautery, with preservation of longitudinal layer.

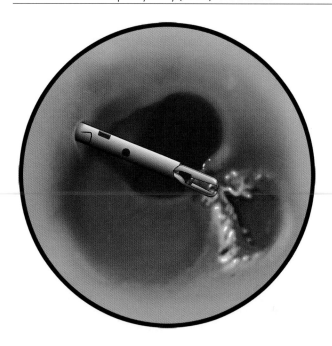

42.7   Closure of mucosotomy with endoscopic clips.

Closure of mucosotomy

9. Finally, the esophageal mucosotomy is closed with endoscopic clips (see **Figure 42.7**). These are sloughed postprocedure, usually within 2 to 6 weeks. Alternatively, the mucosotomy can be closed by endoscopic suturing, a technique that can be useful in cases of mucosotomy extension or edematous or thickened mucosa.

POSTOPERATIVE CARE

All patients undergo a water-soluble esophagogram on postoperative day 1, and are typically discharged after 23 hours' observation. They go home on a pureed diet for 1 week to avoid disrupting the clips. We routinely obtain a 24-hour pH impedance test, endoscopy, and timed barium swallow at 6 months after surgery.

OUTCOME

Eight years of clinical experience with POEM has shown it to be both safe and effective. With over 6000 cases performed worldwide, the procedure can no longer be considered experimental and now is one of the preferred options for treatment of achalasia at most major esophageal motility centers.

Early reports documented extremely effective dysphagia relief with a very low morbidity rate. One criticism of POEM is its relatively high incidence of postprocedure gastroesophageal reflux. The earliest clinical reports claimed very low reflux rates; however, objective testing has documented reflux rates up to 45%. As the procedure has been iterated over the years, particularly by modifying the myotomy length based on HRM or intraoperative EndoFLIP, the reflux rate has decreased. Several studies have shown that the current rate is around 32% and is, in fact, no different from late objective outcomes after laparoscopic Heller and partial fundoplication.

CONCLUSION

POEM represents a true minimally invasive advance in the treatment of achalasia. Its success in treating classic achalasia has spun-off into a new way of approaching a wide spectrum of benign esophageal and gastric motility disorders.

FURTHER READING

Bhayani NH et al. A comparative study on comprehensive, objective outcomes of laparoscopic Heller myotomy with per-oral endoscopic myotomy (POEM) for achalasia. *Ann Surg.* 2014 Jun; 259(6): 1098–103.

Carlson DA and Pandolfino JE. High resolution manometry and esophageal pressure topography: filling the gaps of conventional manometry. *Gastroenterol Clin North Am.* 2013 Mar; 42(1): 1–15.

Eckardt AJ and Eckardt VF. Treatment and surveillance strategies in achalasia: an update. *Nat Rev Gastroenterol Hepatol.* 2011 Jun;(8): 311–19.

Inoue H et al. Peroral endoscopic myotomy (POEM) for esophageal achalasia. *Endoscopy.* 2010 Apr; 42(4): 265–71.

Pandolfino JE et al. Achalasia: a new clinically relevant classification by high-resolution manometry. *Gastroenterol.* 2008 Nov; 135(5): 1526–33.

Pasricha PJ et al. Submucosal endoscopic esophageal myotomy: a novel experimental approach for the treatment of achalasia. *Endoscopy.* 2007 Sep; 39(9): 761–4.

Rieder E et al. Intraoperative assessment of esophagogastric junction distensibility during per oral endoscopic myotomy (POEM) for esophageal motility disorders. *Surg Endosc.* 2013 Feb; 27(2): 400–5.

Stavropoulos SN et al. The International Per Oral Endoscopic Myotomy Survey (IPOEMS): a snapshot of the global POEM experience. *Surg Endosc.* 2013 Sep; 27(9): 3322–38.

Sumiyama K et al. Submucosal endoscopy with mucosal flap safety valve. *Gastrointest Endosc.* 2007 Apr; 65(4): 688–94.

43

Left thoracic approach to esophageal diverticula

ANDRÉ DURANCEAU

PRINCIPLES AND JUSTIFICATION

Pulsion diverticula of the distal esophagus are considered to be complications of abnormal intraesophageal pressures. The work of Cross and colleagues supported the concept that spasm of the inferior sphincter accompanied by increased contraction pressures in the esophageal body is responsible for both the symptoms and the appearance of the diverticulum. Allen and Claggett, and Benacci et al. have reported significantly fewer leaks with secondary sepsis when a myotomy is combined with diverticulectomy than when a diverticulectomy alone is performed. When surgical treatment is indicated for a distal esophageal diverticulum, the diverticulum should be excised if it is large enough and the underlying motor abnormality corrected. After myotomy, a significant weakening of the gastroesophageal junction results, and an antireflux repair is added to the myotomy to prevent reflux damage to the esophageal mucosa. A partial fundoplication is preferred, as a more complete wrap causes functional obstruction to an esophagus made powerless by the myotomy.

While the traditional approach will be discussed in this chapter, newer approaches have been developed in the era of minimally invasive surgery. These are described in detail in the chapters that follow: Chapter 44, "Thoracoscopic management of esophageal diverticula," and Chapter 45, "Laparoscopic management of epiphrenic diverticula."

Indications

Significant symptoms related to swallowing and to the presence of the diverticulum constitute the main indication for surgical treatment. Asymptomatic diverticula do not require operative treatment.

PREOPERATIVE ASSESSMENT AND PREPARATION

Assessment

Radiological assessment is important to identify the size and location of the diverticulum. Videoscopic radiography usually allows visualization of the accompanying motor dysfunction. Although optional, radionuclide transit studies using liquid and solid markers quantify esophageal retention.

Esophageal motility studies are essential to characterize the motor disorder accompanying the diverticulum and to determine the extent of dysfunction.

Endoscopy and 24-hour pH monitoring are important to rule out reflux disease and mucosal damage or other mucosal abnormality.

Patient preparation

The patient is put on a liquid diet for 24 hours before the operation. If there is any possibility of significant esophageal retention, lavage of the esophageal cavity is performed with the patient awake on the morning of the operation.

A cephalosporin and antibiotics active against anaerobes (such as metronidazole [Flagyl], 500 mg, or clindamycin, 600 mg) are administered before induction of anesthesia. Subcutaneous heparin sodium, 5000 U, is administered routinely 2 hours before the operation and every 12 hours thereafter until the patient is fully ambulatory and ready to leave the hospital.

OPERATION

1. The esophagus is approached through a left thoracic incision. The pleura is opened at the superior border of the eighth rib, and a small posterior segment of the rib is removed. Anesthesia via a double-lumen endotracheal tube allows exclusion and retraction of the left lung during the operation. (See **Figure 43.1**.)

2. The mediastinum is opened 1 cm anterior to the aorta, from the aortic arch to the diaphragm. At the distal extent, the pleura is incised as an inverted T to provide free access to the hiatus. The inferior pulmonary ligament is divided up to the inferior pulmonary vein.

   The esophagus is mobilized proximally and at the level of the hiatus, below the diverticulum. Penrose drains are passed around it to facilitate traction and dissection. (See **Figure 43.2**.)

3. The esophageal body is freed completely from its fascial and vascular attachments up to the inferior border of the aortic arch.

   Progressive dissection of the diverticulum is then undertaken, with care taken to ensure that the right pleura is protected.

   If the hiatus is small and without a hernia, free access to the peritoneal cavity is obtained through a peripheral diaphragmatic incision 2–3 cm from its insertion at the chest wall. This allows complete and easy dissection of the fundus, gastrosplenic vessels, and hiatal structures. The phrenoesophageal ligament and the peritoneum are opened, and the whole gastroesophageal junction is delivered into the chest through the hiatus. The gastroesophageal fat pad is removed. (See **Figure 43.3**.)

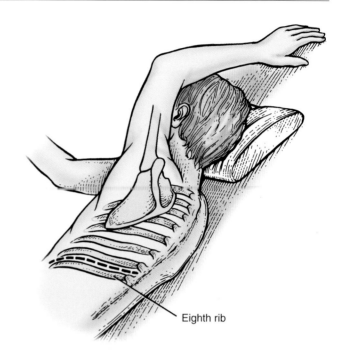

Eighth rib

43.1

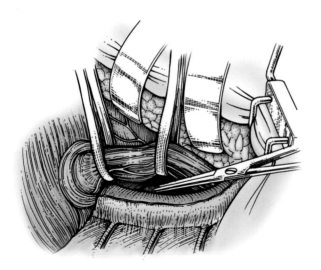

43.2

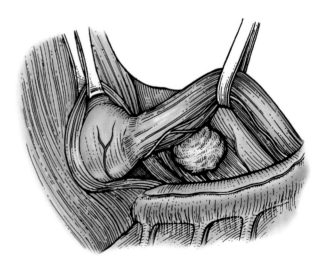

43.3

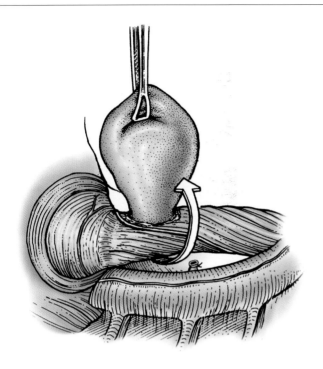

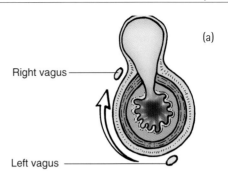

(a)

Right vagus

Left vagus

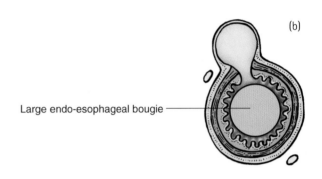

(b)

Large endo-esophageal bougie

43.4

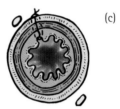

(c)

43.5a–c

4. When the esophagus and proximal stomach have been fully mobilized, the diverticulum and the distal esophagus are rotated toward the left chest. Usually, a layer of fibromuscular tissue invests the diverticulum. The mucosa of the diverticulum is freed progressively toward its neck, and the muscular defect surrounding the neck is thus clearly identified.

   If the diverticulum is not directed toward the right chest, it may have to be included in the planned myotomy and then suspended rather than removed. (See **Figure 43.4**.)

5. On completion of the dissection, a large mercury bougie (No. 50) is placed into the esophagus and stomach. This stent serves to distend the esophageal lumen and prevent undue narrowing at the point of excision of the diverticulum.

   With the bougie safely in place, resection of the diverticulum is now undertaken, using one of two methods. (See **Figure 43.5a through c**.)

6. The first technique is a manual one for resection of the diverticulum. Traction sutures are placed on the proximal and distal borders of the neck, and the diverticulum is resected by opening a straight line of mucosa. (See **Figure 43.6**.)

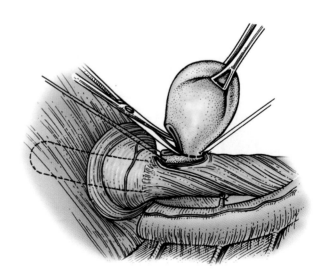

43.6

7. The esophagotomy is closed longitudinally, as for any esophageal anastomosis, with an interrupted single layer of inverting sutures. Both ends are closed with internal knots. The last three or four sutures are tied externally. (See **Figure 43.7**.)

8. The second technique is to use a 5–6 cm stapler to close the neck of the diverticulum. This is again accomplished with a large bougie protecting the esophageal lumen. A small cuff of mucosa is left distal to the stapling line, and a second row of sutures reapproximates the muscle over the staple line, anchoring it to the cut rim of the mucosa. (See **Figure 43.8**.)

9. When the rotation traction is eased, the site of the diverticulectomy resumes its normal position facing the right chest. A long myotomy is performed on the left posterolateral esophagus. The mercury bougie remains in place and serves as support for the mucosa. The use of magnifying spectacles helps in identifying the esophageal structures and encourages stringent hemostasis. A No. 15 scalpel blade is used, and the longitudinal muscle is opened along the whole length of the planned myotomy. The myotomy is then completed through the circular muscle layer, with care taken to avoid perforating the mucosa. The lower esophageal sphincter area may be recognized, as the muscle is usually thinner here. (See **Figure 43.9**.)

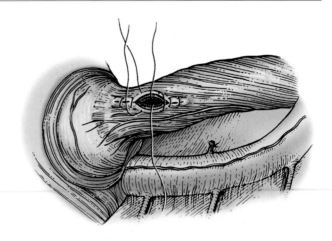

43.7

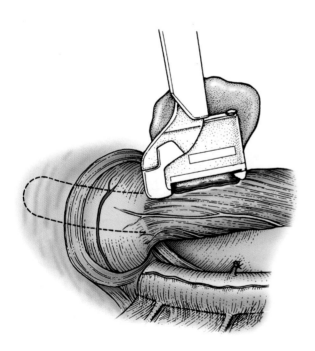

43.8

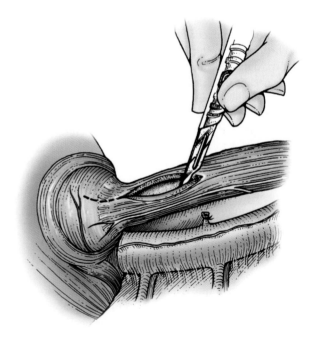

43.9

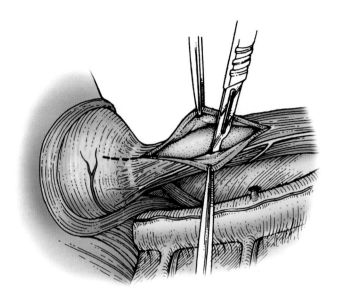

43.10

10. The myotomy is extended for 1 cm onto the gastric wall muscle, and the gastric submucosa can then be seen as a richly vascularized layer (see **Figure 43.10**).

11. Lateral dissection of the muscle from the mucosa is carried out with scissors. The assistant pulls the muscle outward while the surgeon holds the mucosa against the bougie with a dissector swab. This exposes a cellular tissue plane between the layers that affords easy dissection. Approximately 50% of the esophageal circumference is freed from the muscle. Once the myotomy is completed, hemostasis is obtained and the mucosa of the myotomized zone is checked to make sure that it has not been breached. The transverse sections show the points of dissection between layers, the placement of sutures to evert the dissected muscle, and the position of the sutures in relation to the right and left vagi.

   The bougie is removed, a nasogastric tube is placed in the esophageal cavity, and 50–100 mL of air is introduced into the esophagus while it is kept under saline. Any leak will be shown by bubbles of escaping air. (See **Figure 43.11**.)

12. A two-thirds fundic wrap of the Belsey type is next carried out. Two 2-0 silk sutures anchor the fundoplication on each side of the myotomized zone and at two levels. The two layers of the muscle are transfixed from outside to inside to evert the muscle while anchoring the seromuscular layer of the fundus to the esophageal wall. This is accomplished to prevent any closure of the myotomy at the gastroesophageal junction.

   The first two sutures are completed at the level of the former insertion of the phrenoesophageal ligament. The two sutures of the second layer are placed in a similar fashion, 2–3 cm more proximal, from the esophagus to the fundus and then through the diaphragm to tie both sutures on the thoracic side of the hiatus. (See **Figure 43.12**.)

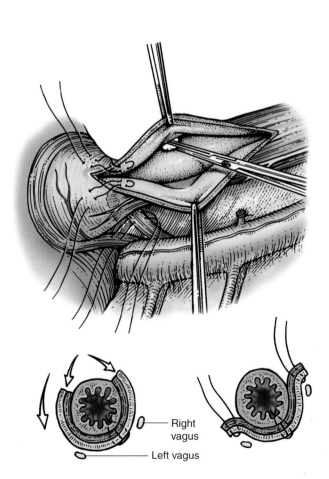

Right vagus

Left vagus

43.11

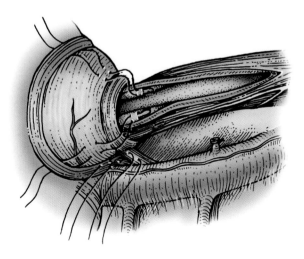

43.12

13. With this partial fundoplication, the distal 4–5 cm of the myotomized esophagus are reduced without any tension under the diaphragm, which affords good antireflux protection while allowing proper food transit at the gastroesophageal junction (see **Figure 43.13**).

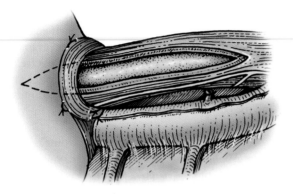

43.13

POSTOPERATIVE CARE

The nasogastric tube is left in place until normal bowel activity has resumed. Once gastric drainage is discontinued, an esophagogram is obtained using water-soluble contrast medium. If the mucosal configuration is considered adequate, liquid barium is added to complete the immediate postoperative evaluation.

The chest tube is removed when normal pulmonary reexpansion is obtained with less than 100 mL of drainage over a 24-hour period.

A liquid diet is resumed once the myotomy and diverticulectomy sites have been shown to be intact. The patient progresses to a semiliquid diet for the following 10 days. Normal alimentation is then resumed.

Complete functional reassessment is obtained 2 years after the operation and at regular intervals thereafter. Documentation of emptying capacity and reflux damage over time in these patients is particularly important.

FURTHER READING

Allen TH, Claggett OT. Changing concepts in the surgical treatment of pulsion diverticula of the lower esophagus. *Journal of Thoracic and Cardiovascular Surgery.* 1965; 50: 455–62.

Benacci JC, Deschamps C, Trastek V, Allen MS, Daly RC, Pairolero PC. Epiphrenic diverticulum: results of surgical treatment. *Annals of Thoracic Surgery.* 1993; 55: 1109–13.

Cross FS. Esophageal diverticula related neuromuscular problems. *Annals of Otology, Rhinology and Laryngology.* 1968; 77: 914–26.

Cross FS, Johnson GF, Gerein AN. Esophageal diverticula: associated neuromuscular changes in the esophagus. *Archives of Surgery.* 1961; 83: 525–33.

44

Thoracoscopic management of esophageal diverticula

THOMAS J. WATSON AND CHRISTIAN G. PEYRE

INTRODUCTION

Esophageal diverticula are uncommon and typically cause dysphagia, regurgitation, recurrent aspiration, or chest pain. Most clinically relevant esophageal diverticula are of the "pulsion" variety and result from an underlying esophageal motility disorder, most commonly achalasia. They occur over the mid to distal esophagus in an "epiphrenic" location. These are "false" diverticula, as they do not contain all layers of the esophageal wall, but rather only the mucosa and submucosa protruding through the circular and longitudinal muscles. "Traction" diverticula are the result of externally placed tension on the esophagus, typically due to mediastinal lymphadenopathy from infectious etiologies such as tuberculosis or histoplasmosis. These are "true" diverticula consisting of all esophageal layers, though are rarely of clinical consequence. For the purposes of this discussion, only pulsion diverticula are considered.

Traditional surgical treatment of esophageal diverticula has been the so-called triple-treat operation, consisting of diverticulectomy, esophageal myotomy, and partial fundoplication performed by an open left thoracotomy (refer to Chapter 43, "Left thoracic approach to esophageal diverticula"). The goals of surgery are to resect the diverticulum and to address the underlying motility disorder by performing a myotomy that extends from the proximal extent of the diverticulum across the lower esophageal sphincter. A partial fundoplication is added to prevent gastroesophageal reflux due to a lower esophageal sphincter rendered incompetent by myotomy. In the era of minimally invasive surgery, esophageal diverticula have been managed via laparoscopy and/or thoracoscopy. Given the epiphrenic location of most esophageal diverticula, laparoscopy is generally the minimally invasive procedure of choice (see Chapter 45, "Laparoscopic management of epiphrenic diverticula"). A myotomy of the lower esophageal sphincter and distal esophagus can be performed by this approach, a partial fundoplication added as an antireflux measure, and the diverticulum resected if it is situated sufficiently low within the mediastinum. Right- or left-sided thoracoscopy may be used as an adjunct to laparoscopy if the diverticulum cannot be reached through the hiatus. Only rarely should a thoracoscopic approach to diverticulectomy be performed as an independent procedure. Thoracoscopy hinders the performance of a myotomy that extends distally onto the stomach a sufficient length, increasing the risk of postoperative leak from the diverticulectomy site as well as the potential for persistent or recurrent symptoms. In addition, a fundoplication is not readily performed via a thoracoscopic approach.

As most epiphrenic diverticula are situated toward the right, right thoracoscopy typically allows optimal visualization. A limitation of the right-sided approach, however, is difficulty with exposure of the esophagogastric junction, hindering an adequate distal myotomy. A left-sided approach may facilitate the myotomy, but may provide inadequate visualization of many diverticula. In our experience, most epiphrenic diverticula are addressed first by laparoscopy, with a myotomy of the lower esophageal sphincter, a partial fundoplication, and a diverticulectomy, if feasible. Only if the diverticulum cannot be resected by this approach, and the patient continues to experience significant dysphagia or regurgitation, is subsequent thoracoscopy pursued.

OPERATIVE APPROACH

The operative principles are similar whether right or left thoracoscopy is being considered. The laterality of the diverticulum, as based upon preoperative barium esophagography, generally determines the side to be utilized. In most cases, a myotomy of the lower esophageal sphincter and partial fundoplication will have already been performed. Of course, the myotomy may need to be extended more proximally because of inadequate laparoscopic visualization of the thoracic esophagus.

Induction of anesthesia and positioning

The patient should be considered high risk for aspiration during induction of general anesthesia and intubation due to the presence of the diverticulum, the underlying esophageal motility disorder, and possible reflux that may have resulted from a prior myotomy. Rapid sequence induction with cricoid pressure and the patient in a semisitting position is generally utilized at our institution. The patient is then intubated with a double lumen endotracheal tube. Proper tube placement is confirmed bronchoscopically, and then the patient is rotated into the appropriate lateral decubitus position. Single lung ventilation is established to the contralateral lung, generally facilitating adequate thoracoscopic visualization of the esophagus and diverticulum. If exposure is inadequate, insufflation with carbon dioxide gas at a low pressure (5–8 mmHg) is feasible, though rarely necessary in our experience.

Trocar placement

The operation can usually be accomplished through three ports (see **Figure 44.1**). We prefer orienting the trocars so that the surgeon is standing toward the patient's back and working in a posterior to anterior orientation rather than an inferior to superior one. With this orientation in mind, an attempt is made to triangulate the placement of the trocars within the confines of the hemithorax. Due to the scapula, the most superior trocar is generally a bit more posterior than what ideal triangulation would require. We utilize a 5 mm, 30-degree thoracoscope placed through a 5 mm trocar positioned at approximately the 8th intercostal space at the posterior axillary line. This trocar may be placed somewhat more superiorly for diverticula of the mid esophagus. The surgeon's right- and left-hand operating ports are positioned at the mid to anterior axillary line (or slightly more posterior if the scapula tip is in the way), attempting to triangulate and being cognizant of the location of the ipsilateral hemidiaphragm. The deflated lung can generally be retracted with an instrument through the most superior port. Alternatively, the patient may be rotated more prone to aid in lung displacement away from the operative field. In addition, a stitch can be placed through the central tendon of the diaphragm and brought out through a small stab incision low on the lateral chest wall to retract the diaphragm inferiorly if necessary.

Exposure of the esophagus and diverticulum

The esophagus should be readily apparent. The mediastinal pleura overlying it is scored and the diverticulum identified. The false diverticulum is sharply and bluntly mobilized away from its surrounding soft tissue attachments until the neck is visualized as it emanates between the muscle layers of the esophageal wall (see **Figure 44.2**). Significant peridiverticular inflammation may be present, making dissection a challenge. The neck should be circumferentially mobilized until the esophageal muscle is seen in its entirety around it. If there is any concern for inadvertent esophageal or diverticular perforation, intraoperative flexible esophagoscopy should be performed, insufflating the lumen while submerging the esophagus under water within the chest and assessing thoracoscopically for air bubbles.

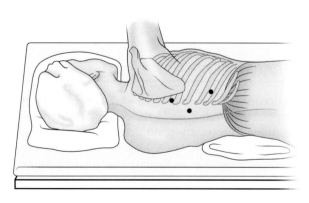

44.1

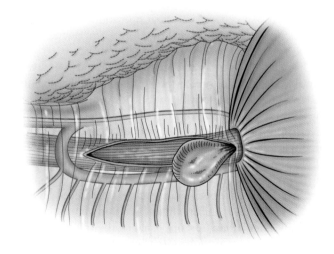

44.2

An adequate length of esophagus should be dissected to allow exposure of the diverticulum and a subsequent site for myotomy away from the diverticulectomy. At times, circumferential esophageal dissection will be necessary. If rotation of the esophagus is needed to facilitate exposure of the diverticulum, a Penrose drain may be placed circumferentially around the esophagus and brought out through a trocar incision (see **Figure 44.3**).

Diverticulectomy

A complete diverticular resection and closure is imperative without compromising the esophageal lumen. We routinely place a 48-51 Fr esophageal bougie to ensure an adequate luminal diameter; the diverticulectomy is performed with the bougie in place. The most inferior trocar generally can be utilized for passage of an Endo GIA stapler of an appropriate length, usually 45–60 mm, in an orientation parallel to the esophagus (see **Figure 44.4**). A single fire of the stapler is preferable to multiple fires. If that trocar site is not suitable, another trocar site or an additional incision may be necessary. The stapler is placed flush against the bougie in an inferior to superior orientation. After stapler firing, the bougie is then withdrawn and the staple line assessed for intactness. If there is any doubt, the endoscope may be inserted and insufflation performed. The staple line is then oversewn with longitudinal esophageal muscle using interrupted, permanent, monofilament or braided 3-0 suture of the surgeon's choosing (see **Figure 44.5**).

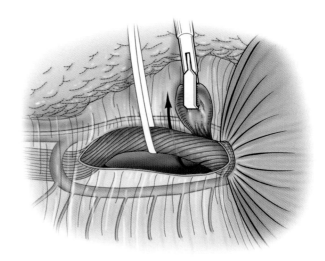

44.3

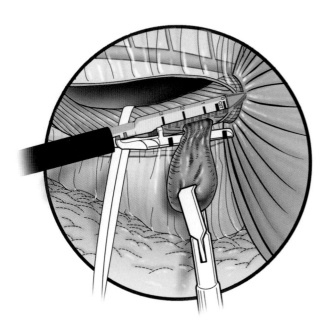

44.4

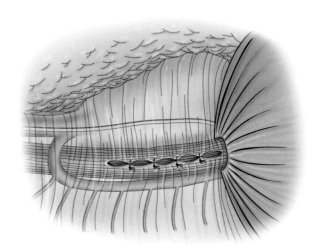

44.5

Myotomy

If an esophageal myotomy was not performed previously, or was inadequately extended proximally to reach the superior-most extent of the diverticular neck, it can be performed subsequent to completion of the diverticulectomy. The myotomy should be placed on the contralateral side of the esophagus, ideally 180 degrees from the diverticulectomy (see **Figure 44.6**). It is not imperative that the myotomy be placed along the same line as a previous one performed via the abdomen. It is critical, however, that the entire length of distal esophagus be myotomized along some portion. The myotomy can be performed with or without a bougie in place; we prefer the former.

We utilize endo scissors without cautery, reserving the use of cautery at low energy for specific bleeding sites. A blunt "peanut"-type dissector also may be beneficial. The myotomy should extend over one-third to one-half of the esophageal circumference, taking care not to extend it to the diverticulectomy site for fear of uncovering the region oversewn with esophageal muscle. We routinely extend the myotomy 2.5–3.0 cm beyond the esophagogastric junction, which mandates a partial fundoplication (performed via laparoscopy) to help prevent postoperative gastroesophageal reflux. Only in rare circumstances would we choose a more limited myotomy (1 cm across the esophagogastric junction) without addition of a fundoplication, though such a procedure could be completed entirely via thoracoscopy.

If a mucosal perforation occurs, it is repaired with interrupted fine monofilament suture. The adequacy of repair can be checked with intraoperative endoscopy and air insufflation. We do not routinely close the esophageal muscle over the myotomy site, though consideration may be given to doing so if a perforation is repaired.

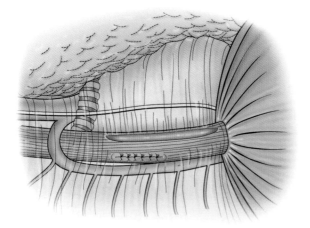

44.6

Closure

A pleural drainage catheter is routinely advanced via one of the trocar incisions, positioned near the diverticulectomy without abutting it, and left in place until an oral diet is resumed.

POSTOPERATIVE CARE

The vast majority of patients are extubated prior to leaving the operating room. The chest drain is placed to suction or water-seal drainage. A contrast esophagogram is obtained on postoperative day 1, and a clear liquid diet started at that time if no leakage is noted. The chest tube can be removed the next day and the patient discharged home if analgesia is adequate on an oral regimen. A liquid diet is continued for 1 week, and then a soft diet is allowed.

DISCUSSION

Esophageal diverticula are uncommonly encountered even in large esophageal surgery practices. Gaining adequate experience in their management, therefore, is a challenge even for the busy practitioner. An open left transthoracic approach, typically consisting of a diverticulectomy, distal esophageal myotomy, and partial fundoplication, has been the standard of care for decades. The results have been reliable, with excellent palliation of symptoms, infrequent recurrences, and low esophageal leak rates.

The desire to avoid the consequences of a thoracotomy, in particular the potential for significant and prolonged pain, has led to the introduction of minimally invasive alternatives to the management of esophageal diverticula, including both laparoscopic and thoracoscopic approaches. The results of such procedures, even in experienced hands, have demonstrated much higher leak rates compared with open operations, probably representing the technical difficulty associated with minimally invasive surgery. Surgeons must individualize the decision for surgical intervention and the operative approach, taking into consideration their own comfort and experience as well as the health and performance status of the patient. We still prefer a thoracotomy for younger, healthier individuals, and choose minimally invasive alternatives for more fragile or elderly patients. Perhaps with greater experience and refinement in techniques, minimally invasive treatment of esophageal diverticula will become the standard of care in the vast majority of cases.

FURTHER READING

Kilic A, Schuchert MJ, Awais O, Luketich JD, Landreneau RJ. Surgical management of epiphrenic diverticula in the minimally invasive era. *JSLS.* 2009; 13: 160–4.

Soares R, Herbella FA, Prachand VN, Ferguson MK, Patti MG. Epiphrenic diverticulum of the esophagus: from pathophysiology to treatment. *J Gastrointest Surg.* 2010; 12: 2009–15.

45

Laparoscopic management of epiphrenic diverticula

FERNANDO MIER AND JOHN G. HUNTER

Esophageal epiphrenic diverticula are pulsion diverticula located in the distal 10 cm of the esophagus. They represent the protrusion of the mucosa and submucosa through the muscular layers of the esophageal wall. (See **Figure 45.1**.)

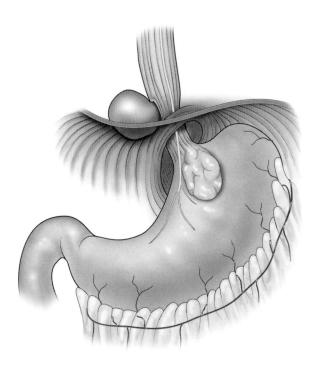

45.1 Anatomic overview of an epiphrenic diverticulum. (Reprinted with permission from the *Atlas of Minimally Invasive Surgical Operations*, JG Hunter and DH Spight, eds., McGraw-Hill [in press], Ontario, Canada.)

They are quite rare findings but the true incidence is unknown, as only 15%–20% are symptomatic, with the majority of cases diagnosed incidentally during a radiographic or endoscopic examination performed for other reasons. The pathophysiology of this rare disease is still uncertain. Many authors believe that the diverticulum is not a primary problem; rather, it is secondary to an underlying esophageal motility disorder that results in increased intraluminal pressure against a distal functional or mechanical obstruction leading to herniation of the esophageal mucosa. This is a critical concept because it mandates the need for a myotomy at the time of surgical resection. The most common treatment of symptomatic epiphrenic diverticula is myotomy, surgical resection, and the antireflux procedure. The approach has evolved from a thoracotomy (see Chapter 43, "Left thoracic approach to esophageal diverticula") to a laparoscopic transhiatal approach (as discussed in this chapter), or video-assisted thoracic surgery (refer to Chapter 44, "Thoracoscopic management of esophageal diverticula").

CLINICAL PRESENTATION

A large number of patients with epiphrenic diverticula are asymptomatic and the diverticulum is found incidentally as part of a work-up for other reasons. These patients do not require treatment. In the symptomatic patient, the most common presenting complaints are dysphagia and regurgitation of undigested food, but halitosis, chest pain, and unintentional weight loss are also common. Respiratory complaints such as chronic nocturnal cough and laryngitis are due to episodes of aspiration, and may be the only presenting symptoms in some patients. Generally, symptoms correlate with the degree of esophageal dysmotility and not with the size of the diverticulum. Complications such as bleeding perforation or malignant transformation are rarely seen.

WORK-UP AND TREATMENT

Barium swallow, endoscopy, and esophageal manometry

All patients with esophageal epiphrenic diverticula should be evaluated with the same diagnostic imaging and physiologic studies as any patient with any other gastroesophageal pathology. The barium esophagogram should be the first test performed, as it is essential for operative planning and helps the endoscopist identify the diverticulum. This diagnostic test defines the size of the diverticulum, size of its neck, location, and distance from the gastroesophageal junction. In 70% of the patients, the diverticulum is on the right side and 15% of patients may have two or more diverticula. Upper endoscopy should also be performed in all patients with dysphagia and epiphrenic diverticula, mainly to rule out any neoplastic process. Furthermore, the use of endoscopy can also be used to identify the side of the opening of the diverticulum, size of its neck, and distance to the gastroesophageal junction. Finally, either stationary or ambulatory esophageal manometry should be performed to determine the underlying motility disorder. Several studies have shown that the prevalence of primary esophageal motility disorders in patients with esophageal epiphrenic diverticula ranges from 85% to 100%, with achalasia being the most common.

Operative technique

PREOPERATIVE CONSIDERATIONS AND PATIENT POSITION

The patient is positioned on the operative table, pneumatic compression stockings are used for deep vein thrombosis prophylaxis, and preoperative antibiotics are used prior to skin incision. A rapid sequence induction is always performed to prevent aspiration of undigested food. Endoscopy to remove all food from the diverticulum is performed the day before surgery or on the operating table after the induction of anesthesia. A Foley catheter is placed and the patient's lower extremities are abducted and taped to the operating table. Once the abdomen is prepped and draped, the patient is positioned in steep reverse Trendelenburg.

PORT PLACEMENT

Our typical laparoscopic approach uses five ports placed in the same places we use for any surgery in the gastroesophageal junction or the hiatus (see **Figure 45.2**).

GASTROESOPHAGEAL JUNCTION DISSECTION, ESOPHAGEAL MOBILIZATION AND MEDIASTINAL DISSECTION, AND DIVERTICULECTOMY

The operation starts with opening the lesser omentum through the pars flaccida. Then the phrenoesophageal ligament is divided anteriorly from the apex of the right crus to the apex of the left crus, and the anterior vagus is identified and preserved. A window is then created posteriorly to the

esophagus with identification of the posterior vagus. This will expose the rest of the diaphragmatic crura. At this point, a Penrose drain can be passed around the esophagus to enable retraction. We then proceed to the posterior mediastinal dissection. Most of the dissection can be done bluntly or with a Harmonic scalpel. The diverticulum is identified in the posterior mediastinum. If difficulty is encountered in identifying the diverticulum, intraoperative endoscopy is indicated at this point. Once identified, the diverticulum is bluntly dissected free of the surrounding tissues. Care must be taken not to injure the pleura, especially in cases where inflammatory tissue is encountered. If the pleura is breached, a chest tube may be required at the end of the case. The diverticulum should be dissected entirely from the mediastinal connective tissue until the neck is clearly isolated. A 56 Fr bougie is placed into the esophagus, to prevent narrowing, and the diverticulum is divided with a laparoscopic stapler. We usually use a laparoscopic stapler with a 2.5 mm vascular load but a thickened or inflamed diverticulum may require the use of longer staples. The staple line should be oriented longitudinally. The bougie is removed. (See **Figure 45.3**.)

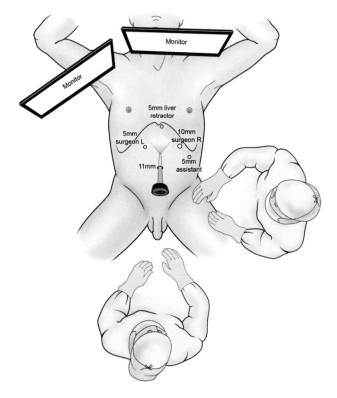

45.2 Port placement. Our typical laparoscopic approach uses five ports placed in the same places we use for any surgery in the gastroesophageal junction or the hiatus. (Reprinted with permission from the *Atlas of Minimally Invasive Surgical Operations*, JG Hunter and DH Spight, eds., McGraw-Hill [in press], Ontario, Canada.)

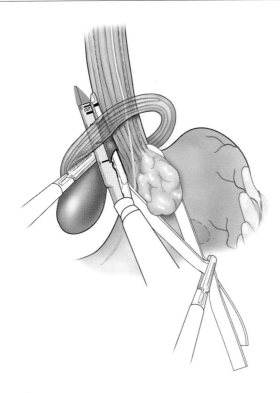

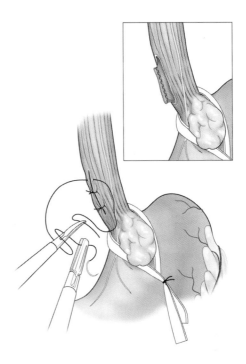

45.3 Diverticulectomy. The diverticulum should be dissected entirely from the mediastinal connective tissue until the neck is clearly isolated. This should be done with endoscopic guidance. A 56 Fr bougie is placed into the esophagus, to prevent narrowing, and the diverticulum is divided with a laparoscopic stapler. (Reprinted with permission from the *Atlas of Minimally Invasive Surgical Operations*, JG Hunter and DH Spight, eds., McGraw-Hill [in press], Ontario, Canada.)

45.4 Closure of diverticulectomy. Closure of the diverticulectomy staple line can be done with interrupted 2-0 silk sutures without tension. (Reprinted with permission from the *Atlas of Minimally Invasive Surgical Operations*, JG Hunter and DH Spight, eds., McGraw-Hill [in press], Ontario, Canada.)

MYOTOMY, OVERSEWING THE STAPLE LINE, AND FUNDOPLICATION

A contralateral myotomy should be performed from the most cranial portion of the staple line and continued caudally to 2–3 cm past the gastroesophageal junction. The myotomy can be performed with blunt dissection plus the use of myotomy scissors or cautery. Once this is performed, it usually allows the surgeon to pull longitudinal muscle together over the diverticulectomy staple line with interrupted 2-0 silk sutures without tension. (See **Figures 45.4 and 45.5**.)

Closure of the diaphragmatic hiatus can be done in the standard fashion with two to three pledgeted braided sutures if a hiatal hernia is present.

Finally, we proceed with the fundoplication to prevent gastroesophageal reflux. A partial fundoplication is preferred. After division of the short gastric vessels, the stomach fundus is used to form a Toupet (posterior) or Dor (anterior) fundoplication (for more detail, see Chapter 38, "Laparoscopic antireflux surgery"). Some surgeons suggest that a Toupet allows the myotomy edges to retract and prevent scarring and recurrence and also allows buttressing of the diverticulectomy staple line. A soft suction drain can be left in the

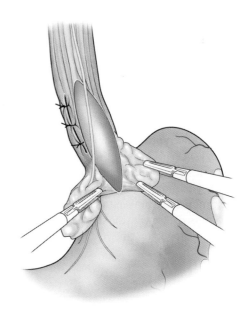

45.5 Myotomy. A contralateral myotomy should be performed from the most cranial portion of the staple line and continued caudally to 2–3 cm past the gastroesophageal junction. (Reprinted with permission from the *Atlas of Minimally Invasive Surgical Operations*, JG Hunter and DH Spight, eds., McGraw-Hill [in press], Ontario, Canada.)

Table 45.1 Laparoscopic repair of esophageal epiphrenic diverticula

Study	Number of patients	Leaks (%)	Mortality (%)	Symptom resolution (%)	Follow-up (months)
Fumagalli et al., 2012	30	3%	0%	90%	52
Zaninotto et al., 2012	24	16%	0%	76%	96
Fernando et al., 2005	10	10%	0%	72%	60
Del Genio et al., 2004	13	23%	1%	100%	58
Tedesco et al., 2005	7	14%	0%	100%	6
Melman et al., 2009	13	7%	0%	85%	13
Soares et al., 2011	19	10%	10%	92%	45
Klaus et al., 2003	11	9%	0%	100%	26

hiatus close to the staple line but there is no evidence to support the necessity of the drain. The ports are removed under direct vision and the fascia and port sites are closed in the standard fashion.

POSTOPERATIVE CARE

The patients are usually admitted to the surgical ward overnight and water-soluble contrast esophagography is performed on postoperative day 1 to evaluate for leaks. If no leak is identified, the diet is cautiously advanced to a soft pureed diet. The patient is usually discharged home on postoperative day 1 or 2, and their diet is usually advanced to a regular diet within the next 2–3 weeks. If a mediastinal or hiatal drain was left in place, this is usually removed prior to discharge.

RESULTS

Laparoscopic transhiatal surgery for esophageal epiphrenic diverticula has been proven feasible and safe in experienced hands. Several series have shown low complication and mortality rates with high symptom resolution rates (see Table 45.1). The most common complication, a staple line leak, can be minimized by using a staple load compatible with tissue thickness, oversewing the staple line, and adhering to a conservative postoperative diet.

SUMMARY

Esophageal epiphrenic diverticula are pulsion diverticula that result as part of a primary esophageal dysmotility disorder. Treatment is indicated for symptomatic diverticula only. Currently, laparoscopic management is safe and effective.

FURTHER READING

Del Genio A, Rossetti G, Maffetton V et al. Laparoscopic approach in the treatment of epiphrenic diverticula: long-term results. *Surg Endosc.* 2004; 18: 741–5.

Fernando HC, Luketich JD, Samphire J et al. Minimally invasive operation for esophageal diverticula. *Ann Thorac Surg.* 2005; 80: 2076–80.

Fisichella PM, Pittman M, Kuo PC. Laparoscopic treatment of epiphrenic diverticula: preoperative evaluation and surgical technique; how I do it. *J Gastrointest Surg.* 2011; 15: 1866–71.

Fumagalli UR, Ceolin M, Porta M, Rosati R. Laparoscopic repair of epiphrenic diverticulum. *Semin Thoracic Cardiovasc Surg.* 2012; 24: 213–17.

Klaus A, Hinder RA, Swain J, Achem SR. Management of epiphrenic diverticula. *J Gastrointest Surg.* 2003; 7: 906–11.

Melman L, Quinlan J, Robertson B et al. Esophageal manometric characteristics and outcomes for laparoscopic esophageal diverticulectomy, myotomy, and partial fundoplication for epiphrenic diverticula. *Surg Endosc.* 2009; 23: 1337–41.

Rosati R, Fumagalli U, Elmore U et al. Long-term results of minimally invasive surgery for symptomatic epiphrenic diverticulum. *Am J Surg.* 2011; 201: 132–5.

Soares R, Herbella FA, Prachand VN, Ferguson MK, Patti MG. Epiphrenic diverticulum of the esophagus: from pathophysiology to treatment. *J Gastrointest Surg.* 2010; 14: 2009–15.

Soares RV, Montenovo M, Pellegrini CA, Oelschlager BK. Laparoscopy as initial approach for epiphrenic diverticula. *Surg Endosc.* 2011; 25: 3740–6.

Tedesco P, Fisichella PM, Way LW, Patti MG. Cause and treatment of epiphrenic diverticula. *Am J Surg.* 2005; 190: 891–4.

Varghese TK, Marshall B, Chang AC et al. Surgical treatment of epiphrenic diverticula: a 30-year experience. *Ann Thorac Surg.* 2007; 84: 1801–9.

Zaninotto G, Parise P, Salvador R et al. Laparoscopic repair of epiphrenic diverticulum. *Semin Thoracic Surg.* 2012; 24: 218–22.

Index

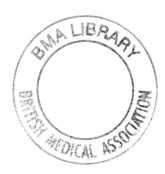